Cardiac Anesthesia
Second Edition

Volume 1

Cardiac Anesthesia
Second Edition

Volume 1

Edited by

Joel A. Kaplan, M.D.

Professor and Chairman
Department of Anesthesiology
Mount Sinai School of Medicine
New York, New York

Grune & Stratton, Inc.

Harcourt Brace Jovanovich, Publishers

Orlando   New York   San Diego   London
San Francisco   Tokyo   Sydney   Toronto

Library of Congress Cataloging-in-Publication Data
Cardiac anesthesia.

    Includes bibliographies and index.
    1. Anesthesia in cardiology. 2. Heart—Surgery.
I. Kaplan, Joel A. [DNLM: 1. Anesthesia. 2. Heart—
drug effects. 3. Heart Surgery. WO 245 C267]
RD598.C34   1987   617′.967412   87-147
ISBN 0-8089-1848-6

Grune & Stratton, Inc.
Orlando, FL 32887

Distributed in the United Kingdom by
Grune & Stratton, Ltd.
24/28 Oval Road, London NW 1

Library of Congress Catalog Number 87-147
International Standard Book Number 0-8089-1848-6
Printed in the United States of America

87 88 89 90 10 9 8 7 6 5 4 3 2 1

Contents

VOLUME 2

Preface

The second edition of *Cardiac Anesthesia* was written for the purpose of further improving anesthetic management of the patient with cardiac disease undergoing cardiac or noncardiac surgery. Since publication of the first edition of *Cardiac Anesthesia* in 1979, and *Cardiac Anesthesia, Volume 2: Cardiovascular Pharmacology* in 1983, the field of cardiac anesthesia has continued to grow at a very rapid pace. In order to maintain its place as the standard reference textbook in the subspecialty, this edition has been completely revised, expanded, and updated while combining all the subjects from the first two volumes.

The content of the book ranges from preoperative management of the cardiac patient, through selection of the anesthetic, monitoring, and cardiovascular support needed, to postoperative care of the patient in the intensive care unit. The book is organized into six parts, consisting of 32 chapters and hundreds of illustrations. The six major areas covered are (1) anesthetic pharmacology, with an emphasis on pharmacodynamics and pharmacokinetics; (2) monitoring, with details on new techniques such as transesophageal echocardiography; (3) preoperative management, with emphasis on proper drug therapy; (4) anesthetic management, ranging from congenital heart disease to heart transplantation; (5) circulatory support via mechanical and pharmacologic means; and (6) postoperative care and complications. The emphasis throughout is on using the most advanced monitoring techniques to determine the proper therapeutic interventions.

The material in this book was written by the acknowledged experts in each specific area of cardiac anesthesia. It is the most authoritative and up-to-date collection of material in the field. Each chapter aims to provide the scientific foundation in the area as well as the clinical basis for practice. All of the chapters have been coordinated in an effort to avoid unnecessary duplication and conflicting opinions. Whenever possible, material has been integrated from the fields of anesthesiology, cardiology, cardiac surgery, critical care medicine, and pharmacology to present a complete clinical picture. Thus, this book should continue to serve as the definitive text in the field for anesthesia residents, cardiac anesthesia fellows and attendings, cardiologists, cardiac surgeons, intensivists, and others interested in the management of the patient for cardiac surgery.

The first edition of *Cardiac Anesthesia* began with forewords written by a cardiologist, cardiac surgeon, and general anesthesiologist. They said that the field was responsible for reducing mortality and improving care provided by all anesthesiologists to cardiac patients, and Dr. J. Willis Hurst said that he viewed us with awe due to our multi-faceted skills. It is not necessary to have these types of introductions eight years later, because they were all correct and it is now well-known what we do! The development of the specialty of cardiac anesthesiology has been one of the major forces behind the surgeon's ability to tackle bigger challenges with better results. This fact is now widely recognized by our colleagues in both medicine and surgery.

I gratefully acknowledge the contributions made by the authors of the chapters. They are the dedicated experts who have made the field of cardiac anesthesia come of age. This book would not be possible without their hard work.

My sincere appreciation also goes to my personal secretary, Rosalind Brathwaite, and my administrative secretary Teresa Villafana, whose long hours at the word processor made this text a reality. In addition, thanks are in order for the secretaries of the contributing authors who sent us the original manuscripts from their institutions.

And, as always, my wife, Norma, found the many hours necessary to edit this book while making us comfortable and secure in resuming our role as "yankees."

Joel A. Kaplan, M.D.

Contributors

Jeffrey Askanazi, M.D., Assistant Professor, Department of Anesthesiology, College of Physicians and Surgeons, Columbia University, New York, New York

John L. Atlee, M.D., Professor, Department of Anesthesiology, University of Wisconsin Medical Center, Madison, Wisconsin

Paul G. Barash, M.D., Professor and Chairman, Department of Anesthesiology, Yale University Medical Center, New Haven, Connecticut

James G. Bovill, M.D., F.F.A.R.C.S.I., Professor, Department of Anaesthesia, University of Leiden, Leiden, Netherlands

Eva E. Buttner, M.D., Associate Professor, Department of Anesthesiology, University of Alabama at Birmingham, Birmingham, Alabama

Thomas J. Conahan, III, M.D., Associate Professor, Department of Anesthesiology, University of Pennsylvania Hospital, Philadelphia, Pennsylvania

Richard F. Davis, M.D., Associate Professor, Department of Anesthesiology, University of Florida College of Medicine, Gainesville, Florida

F.G. Estafanous, M.D., Chairman, Department of Cardiothoracic Anesthesiology, Cleveland Clinic, Cleveland, Ohio

Barry I. Feinberg, M.D., Chairman, Department of Anesthesiology, DePaul Health Center, Bridgeton, Missouri

Paolo Flezzani, M.D., Assistant Professor, Department of Anesthesiology, Duke University Medical Center, Durham, North Carolina

Robert E. Fowles, M.D., Adjunct Associate Professor, Department of Cardiology, University of Utah College of Medicine, Salt Lake Clinic, Salt Lake City, Utah

D. David Glass, M.D., Professor of Surgery (Anesthesiology) and Medicine, Chairman, Department of Anesthesiology, Dartmouth-Hitchcock Medical Center, Hanover, New Hampshire

Martin E. Goldman, M.D., Assistant Professor and Director of Echocardiography, Division of Cardiology, Department of Medicine, Mount Sinai School of Medicine, New York, New York

Randall B. Griepp, M.D., Professor and Chief, Division of Cardiothoracic Surgery, Department of Surgery, Mount Sinai School of Medicine, New York, New York

Linda B. Hertzberg, M.D., Assistant Professor of Surgery (Anesthesiology), Department of Anesthesiology, Dartmouth-Hitchcock Medical Center, Hanover, New Hampshire

Paul R. Hickey, M.D., Associate Professor, Department of Anaesthesia, Harvard Medical School, Senior Associate in Anesthesiology, Children's Hospital, Boston, Massachusetts

Zaharia Hillel, M.D., Ph.D., Assistant Professor, Division of Cardiothoracic Anesthesiology, Department of Anesthesiology, Mount Sinai School of Medicine, New York, New York

Roberta Hines, M.D., Assistant Professor, Department of Anesthesiology, Yale University School of Medicine, New Haven, Connecticut

Frederick O. Holley, M.D., Assistant Professor, Department of Anesthesiology, Stanford University School of Medicine, Stanford, California, Staff Anesthesiologist, Anesthesiology Service, Palo Alto Veterans Administration Medical Center, Palo Alto, California

Stanford Huber, M.D., Fellow, Cardiovascular Anesthesia, Department of Anesthesiology, University of Alabama at Birmingham, Birmingham, Alabama

John M. Jackson, M.D., Assistant Professor, Department of Anesthesiology, New York University School of Medicine, New York, New York

Stuart Jamieson, M.B., F.R.C.S., Professor and Head, Thoracic and Cardiovascular Surgery, Director of the Minnesota Heart and Lung Institute, University of Minnesota Medical Center, Minneapolis, Minnesota

Joel A. Kaplan, M.D., Professor and Chairman, Department of Anesthesiology, Mount Sinai School of Medicine, New York, New York

Robert A. Kates, M.D., Cardiac Anesthesiologist, Saint Francis Hospital, Roslyn, New York

Igor Kissin, M.D., Professor, Department of Anesthesiology, University of Alabama at Birmingham, Birmingham, Alabama

Steven N. Konstadt, M.D., Assistant Professor, Division of Cardiothoracic Anesthesiology, Department of Anesthesiology, Mount Sinai School of Medicine, New York, New York

Carol L. Lake, M.D., Associate Professor, Department of Anesthesiology, University of Virginia, Charlottesville, Virginia

Dwight C. Legler, M.D., (deceased), Assistant Professor and Consultant, Department of Anesthesiology, Mayo Clinic, Rochester, Minnesota

William A. Lell, M.D., Professor and Vice Chairman, Department of Anesthesiology, Director, Cardiovascular Anesthesia, University of Alabama at Birmingham, Birmingham, Alabama

Warren J. Levy, M.D., Assistant Professor, Department of Anesthesiology, University of Pennsylvania Hospital, Philadelphia, Pennsylvania

Robert S. Litwak, M.D., Professor, Division of Cardiothoracic Surgery, Department of Surgery, Mount Sinai School of Medicine, New York, New York

Edward Lowenstein, M.D., Professor, Department of Anaesthesia, Harvard Medical School, Anesthetist, Cardiac Anesthesia Group, Department of Anesthesiology, Massachusetts General Hospital, Boston, Massachusetts

Dennis T. Mangano, M.D., Ph.D., Professor-in-Residence and Vice Chairman, Department of Anesthesiology, University of California, San Francisco, California

Edward D. Miller, Jr., M.D., E.M. Papper Professor and Chairman, Department of Anesthesiology, Columbia University and Presbyterian Hospital, New York, New York

Michael Nugent, M.D., Assistant Professor, Department of Anesthesiology, Mayo Clinic, Rochester, Minnesota

J.P. O'Connor, M.D., Chief Resident in Anesthesiology, Royal Victoria Hospital, Montreal, Quebec

Ronald G. Pearl, M.D., Ph.D., Assistant Professor of Medicine and Anesthesiology, Associate Director of Intensive Care, Stanford University Medical Center, Stanford, California

Allen K. Ream, M.D., Associate Professor, Department of Anesthesiology, Director, Institute of Engineering Design in Medicine, Stanford University School of Medicine, Stanford, California

Sebastian Reiz, M.D., Ph.D., Professor of Anaesthesia, Umea University, Chairman, Department of Anaesthesiology, Regionsjukhuset, Umea, Sweden

J.G. Reves, M.D., Professor, Director and Chief, Cardiothoracic Anesthesia, Department of Anesthesiology, Duke University Medical Center, Durham, North Carolina

Sandra L. Roberts M.D., Assistant Professor, Department of Anesthesiology, University of Iowa College of Medicine, Iowa City, Iowa

John N. Roseberg, M.D., Fellow in Cardiovascular Anesthesiology, Department of Anesthesiology, Mayo Clinic, Rochester, Minnesota

Stanley H. Rosenbaum, M.D., Associate Professor of Clinical Anesthesiology and Medicine, College of Physicians and Surgeons, Columbia University, New York, New York

Myer H. Rosenthal, M.D., Professor of Anesthesiology, Medicine and Surgery, Director of Intensive Care, Stanford University Hospital, Stanford, California

John J. Savarese, M.D., Associate Professor, Department of Anesthesiology, Massachusetts General Hospital, Boston, Massachusetts

Ralph P.F. Scott, B.Sc., M.B.Ch.B., F.F.A.R.C.S., Department of Anaesthesia, Harvard Medical School, Massachusetts General Hospital, Boston, Massachusetts

Peter S. Sebel, Ph.D., F.F.A.R.C.S.I., Senior Lecturer and Honorary Consultant, The London Hospital Medical College, Whitechapel, London, England

Timothy Shine, M.D., Fellow in Cardiovascular Anesthesiology, Department of Anesthesiology, Mayo Clinic, Rochester, Minnesota

George Silvay, M.D., Ph.D., Professor, Division of Cardiothoracic Anesthesiology, Department of Anesthesiology, Mount Sinai School of Medicine, New York, New York

Stephen J. Thomas, M.D., Associate Professor, Department of Anesthesiology, Director, Cardiac Anesthesia, New York University School of Medicine, New York, New York

Daniel M. Thys, M.D., Associate Professor and Director of Cardiothoracic Anesthesiology, Department of Anesthesiology, Mount Sinai School of Medicine, New York, New York

John H. Tinker, M.D., Professor and Head, Department of Anesthesiology, University of Iowa College of Medicine, Iowa City, Iowa

Barbara Van de Wiele, M.D., Resident, Department of Anesthesiology, UCLA Medical Center, University of California, Los Angeles, California

David L. Wessel, M.D., Instructor in Anaesthesia (Paediatrics), Department of Anaesthesia, Harvard Medical School, Assistant in Anesthesiology and Cardiology, Children's Hospital, Boston, Massachusetts

J.E. Wynands, M.D., Professor, Department of Anesthesiology, Royal Victoria Hospital, Montreal, Quebec

PART I

Anesthetic Pharmacology

Edward Lowenstein, M.D.
Sebastian Reiz, M.D.

1

Effects of Inhalation Anesthetics on Systemic Hemodynamics and the Coronary Circulation

The circulatory effects of currently available inhalation anesthetics are dramatically different from those used a generation ago when diethyl ether and cyclopropane "supported" the circulation by liberating catecholamines. Only after more than a century of use was it recognized that both these drugs shared the counteracting properties of myocardial depression and sympathetic activation. Brewster et al studied normal dogs and dogs with a partial or complete sympathectomy produced by subarachnoid block, subarachnoid block plus adrenalectomy, or adrenalectomy alone.[1] They measured blood levels of diethyl ether, epinephrine, and norepinephrine, and, in some experiments, infused catecholamines. In the intact animals, increasing levels of ether were associated with catecholamine liberation and circulatory stimulation (Fig. 1-1). Blood levels of ether usually considered to be associated with circulatory collapse were well tolerated, since ventilation was provided and the consequences of respiratory arrest avoided. In contrast, animals with a total sympathectomy rapidly died of circulatory failure with high ventricular filling pressures and declining ventricular stroke work. While the intact animals had progressively greater blood levels of catecholamines as ether concentration increased, those with a sympathectomy failed to release catecholamines. Infusion of norepi-

nephrine in the latter animals reversed the circulatory consequences, however. Animals with a partial sympathectomy were intermediate between intact animals and those totally blocked. It thus was recognized that diethyl ether was a myocardial depressant, and the previously popular notion that circulatory collapse was due to loss of peripheral vascular resistance was countered.

Price et al studied the hemodynamic and sympathetic nervous system responses to cyclopropane, ether, thiopental, and halothane.[2] They demonstrated a lower incidence of hypotension with cyclopropane than with ether, though both drugs were associated with elevated norepinephrine levels. In contrast, neither thiopental nor halothane was associated with catecholamine liberation. On this basis, these authors concluded, "Cyclopropane is the anesthetic agent of choice in the presence of hemorrhagic and traumatic shock." However, the availability of new drugs raised questions about this approach. In 1974, Theye et al demonstrated that survival time in dogs subjected to progressive hemorrhage was greater during halothane or isoflurane anesthesia than cyclopropane.[3] Knowledge of this type has markedly changed the practice of anesthesia, particularly in patients with impaired circulatory reserve. Since halothane, enflurane, and isoflurane are ineffective liberators of

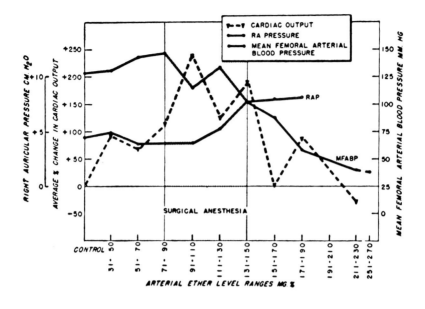

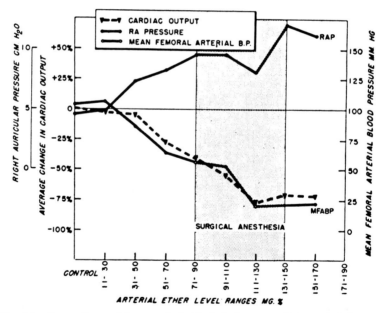

Fig. 1-1. Dogs with complete sympathetic blockade (lower panel) demonstrated severe myocardial depression with ether anesthesia, while intact dogs (upper panel) tolerated the same levels. Partial sympathetic blockade yielded intermediate results. (Reproduced from Brewster WR, Jr, Isaacs JP, Waino-Andersen T: Depressant effect of ether on myocardium of the dog and its modification by reflex release of epinephrine and norepinephrine. Am J Physiol 175:399–414, 1953, with permission.)

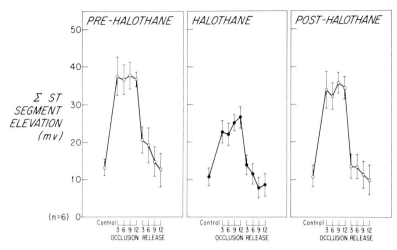

Fig. 1-2. Ischemia, as judged by the sum of the ST-segment elevations of multiple epicardial electrograms, was decreased during the addition of halothane anesthesia to dogs with obstruction of a coronary artery. Limited coronary blood flow in a non-failing heart is one setting in which myocardial depression associated with inhalation anesthesia may be beneficial. (Reproduced from Bland JHL, Lowenstein E: Halothane-induced decrease in experimental myocardial ischemia in the non-failing canine heart. Anesthesiology 45:287–293, 1976, with permission.)

catecholamines, their myocardial depressant properties must be compensated for by mechanisms other than endogenous catecholamine release. In addition, it has been recognized that a certain amount of myocardial depression is often well tolerated, and, in some circumstances, is even desirable[4] (Fig. 1-2).

MEASURES OF MYOCARDIAL PERFORMANCE

Myocardial muscle performance is most easily measured in isolated muscle strips bathed in nutrient solutions. Classical papillary muscle preparations are beloved by physiologists, who can confidently measure and change preload and afterload, and speak without reservation about contractility.[5] Under these conditions, preload refers to the force used to stretch the muscle prior to contraction, and afterload to the weight the muscle must lift in order to begin shortening.

Measurement of contractility is elusive in the intact heart. One major reason for this has been that evaluation of cardiac muscle physiology is based on measuring isolated muscle fiber length. Because of (1) the difficulty of measuring fiber length in the intact heart, (2) the existence of a relationship among pressure, length, and volume, and (3) the ease of measuring pressure in comparison to length, estima-

tion of ventricular performance has been based primarily on pressure measurements. For instance, the first time derivative of isometric left ventricular pressure development (LV dP/dt), which can be derived from a pressure recording, had great appeal and achieved wide popularity.[6] Unfortunately, a number of factors such as heart rate, "preload" (left ventricular end-diastolic volume), and "afterload" change the value obtained despite lack of any reason to believe that contractile state has changed. Modifications, such as the dP/dt/IP, which compared dP/dt at a given isometric pressure (typically 40 mm Hg), were developed but also proved to have limitations.

A second method for assessing contractility uses a combination of filling pressure and external work, based on the so-called Starling or Frank–Starling curve[7] (Fig. 1-3). This has achieved wide clinical popularity, as first dye dilution and then thermal dilution techniques for measuring flow (ie, cardiac output), and pulmonary artery balloon-tipped catheters for estimating left ventricular filling pressures became readily available. During the past decade and a half, patients with circulatory disturbances or impairment could have their cardiac performance estimated at a single point on the Starling curve to define a relationship to normality, and have their response to therapy gauged by repeatedly charting the same variables. Shifts to the left or right on these

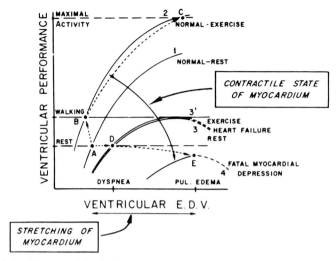

Fig. 1-3. Diagram of the classic Frank–Starling relationship. The development of balloon-guided pulmonary artery catheters with thermistors to measure cardiac output by thermal dilution, and an occlusive balloon to permit estimation of pulmonary capillary wedge pressure, led to guidance of therapy using this relationship. In the clinical setting, stroke work or stroke volume is plotted on the *y* axis and left ventricular filling pressure on the *x* axis. One major shortcoming of this approach is the lack of a linear relationship between ventricular end-diastolic volume and pressure. (Reproduced from Braunwald E, Ross J, Jr, Sonnenblick EH: Mechanisms of contraction of the normal and failing heart. Little, Brown & Co, Boston, 1968, with permission.)

ventricular function curves have been used to denote positive and negative changes of contractility, respectively. There are numerous limitations in this assessment, since it reflects pumping function rather than contractile state and is load dependent.

Aortic blood flow acceleration is another index of myocardial contractility and is thought to be relatively insensitive to changes in hemodynamic parameters.[8] Unfortunately, a flow recording is required to derive this variable. In the past, derived systolic time intervals have been shown to correlate with aortic acceleration, and, recently, Doppler techniques have been used to obtain aortic flow.

At present, the method for assessing myocardial contractility most widely considered load independent is the end-systolic pressure-volume relationship (ESPVR) developed by Suga and Sagawa[9,10] (Fig. 1-4). These measurements were originally obtained from an isolated heart, in which pressure generation took place without ejection (ie, isometrically), or with ejection of a saline-filled balloon through the mitral valve annulus. The aortic valve in this preparation was sutured closed, and coronary perfusion controlled by regulating either flow or pressure in the aortic root. This preparation has also proved useful

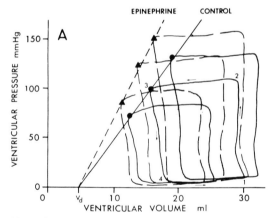

Fig. 1-4. Effect of increased contractile state upon pressure-volume loops, end-systolic pressure-volume lines, and the volume axis intercept (Vd). The left uppermost corners of the loops are connected to construct the pressure-volume lines. Note that the slope is rotated towards being more upright (ie, to the left) during epinephrine infusion, but Vd does not change. The triangles and broken lines represent the data during epinephrine; the circles and solid lines the data during the control state. (Reproduced from Suga H, Sagawa K, Shoukas AA: Load independence of instantaneous pressure-volume ratio of the canine left ventricle and effects of epinephrine and heart rate on the ratio. Circ Res 32:314–322, 1973, with permission.)

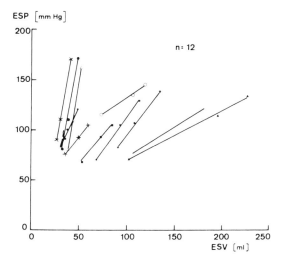

ESP [mm Hg]

n = 12

ESV [ml]

Fig. 1-5. ESPVR in 11 patients with coronary artery disease and one with a congestive cardiomyopathy. Each patient had been pretreated with propranolol and atropine. Measurements were then taken during methoxamine infusion and after sublingual isosorbide dinitrate. Note that the three points of each patient form a straight line. The slopes of the lines vary greatly, indicating differing inotropic states. ESP = end-systolic pressure; ESV = end-systolic volume. (Reproduced from Mehmel HC, Stockins B, Ruffmann K, et al: The linearity of the end-systolic pressure-volume relationship in man and its sensitivity for assessment of left ventricular function. Circulation 63:1216–1222, 1981, with permission.)

for deriving determinants of myocardial oxygen consumption.[10]

Four techniques have been used to estimate ventricular volumes and derive ESPV relationships in intact experimental animals and man. They are sonomicrometry, contrast ventriculography, echocardiography, and scintigraphy. Sonomicrometry and echocardiography are limited by their ability to measure only a finite number of dimensions; geometric assumptions thus are required to derive volumes. In the absence of ischemia or other causes of wall motion abnormalities, however, many of these assumptions appear valid. Rankin et al have developed a chronically instrumented dog model in which longitudinal and cross-sectional dimensions of the left ventricular cavity and thickness of the ventricular wall are measured by sonomicrometry and volume is derived.[11] Ventricular volume is rapidly decreased by transient caval occlusion, which is thought to avoid neurohumoral responses, and a family of pressure volume loops is obtained.

A number of studies using the ESPVR to gauge

contractility have been performed in man. Pressure or volume has been changed by pharmacologic interventions not thought to affect the contractile state, such as an infusion of methoxamine, sodium nitroprusside, or volume. Grossman et al have shown that ESPVR is steeper in man with normal ventricles than with poorly contractile ventricles.[12] Marsh et al have "afterloaded" patients with methoxamine infusions and shown that both end-systolic and peak systolic pressures are linearly related to end-systolic dimension measurements, and that postextrasystolic beats are shifted to the left, indicating an increase in inotropy or contractile state.[13] Mehmel et al studied patients who had been pretreated with beta-adrenergic blockade and atropine to minimize autonomic reflex responses to isosorbide dinitrate and methoxamine, thus generating three ESPVR points in each patient. The relationship with highly linear[14] (Fig. 1-5).

These studies indicate that in man, as in experimental preparations, ESPVR appears to provide a relatively load independent measure of the contractile state. As stressed by Sagawa, however, the load dependence or independence of the ESPVR of ejecting ventricles still needs to be validated in closed-chest preparations before acceptance is complete.[15]

EFFECT OF INHALATION ANESTHETICS ON MYOCARDIAL FUNCTION AND HEMODYNAMICS

Knowledge in three distinct areas is essential for rational use of these drugs: intrinsic properties of the drug including effects on normal myocardium, effects upon abnormal myocardium, and effects during clinical circumstances (ie, varying levels of stimulation, combined with other adjuvant drugs).

Studies in Animals

INTRINSIC PROPERTIES

In normal papillary muscle from a variety of mammalian species, dose-related decreases of indices of contraction, such as mean maximal velocity of contraction (Vmax) and developed force (Fm), have been observed with the inhalation anesthetics.[16] Vatner and Smith studied chronically instrumented normal intact dogs while awake breathing room air, awake breathing oxygen, and during 1 or 2% halothane.[17] These dogs were instrumented with left ventricular dimension crystals, and transducers for circumflex coronary artery, renal, mesenteric, and iliac artery flows, left ventricular and arterial pressures, and heart rate. Heart rate increased markedly with anesthesia, but declined with time (Fig. 1-6). Left ventricular and mean arterial pressures decreased initially and returned toward normal with time. Both changes were dose dependent. The LV dP/dt was also decreased in a dose dependent fashion, but did not change with duration of anesthesia. The most surprising aspect of the study was the change in ventricular dimensions. Left ventricular end-diastolic pressure and end-diastolic dimension (EDD) decreased significantly with 1% halothane, though the decrease lessened with time. With 2% halothane, end-diastolic dimension was unchanged from control until 90 minutes after induction when it was increased. End-systolic dimension (ESD) was decreased early during 1% halothane, but was not different from awake values 90 minutes later, and increased significantly during 2% halothane at all times. Ventricular dimension shortening (EDD-ESD), a reflection of stroke volume, was decreased during all phases of halothane anesthesia, regardless

of the end-diastolic pressure or volume relative to the awake state. This is evidence of dose dependent and time-related myocardial depression. The observed decreases in end-diastolic pressure (EDP) and EDD are unexpected, and are probably due to the increased heart rate. They tend to obscure the myocardial depression at low concentrations early in the course of anesthesia.

In contrast to Vatner's animals, heart rate during halothane anesthesia in unpremedicated human beings remains unchanged[18] or decreases.[19] Left ventricular filling pressure increases significantly only with high concentrations, and systemic vascular resistance (SVR) has consistently been reported as being unchanged in intact animals.

The myocardial depression associated with halothane, enflurane, and nitrous oxide was recently evaluated in both chronically instrumented intact, unpremedicated dogs and patients following cardiopulmonary bypass using the end-systolic pressure-volume relationship.[20] Contractility was assessed by the slope of this relationship (E_{es}) during different concentrations of anesthesia. Enflurane and halo-

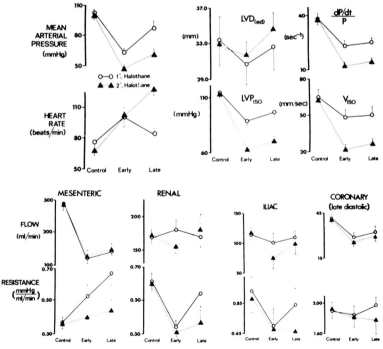

Fig. 1-6. Hemodynamic values in dogs before and during 1 and 2% halothane anesthesia. Control dogs were breathing oxygen. Early values were during peak halothane hypotension and late values were 90 minutes later. $LVD_{(ed)}$ = left ventricular end-diastolic diameter; $LVP_{(ISO)}$ = left ventricular pressure at isolength point; $V_{(ISO)}$ = left ventricular velocity at isolength point. (Reproduced from Vatner SF, Smith NT: Effects of halothane on left ventricular function and distribution of regional blood flow in dogs and primates. Circ Res 34:155–167, 1974, with permission.)

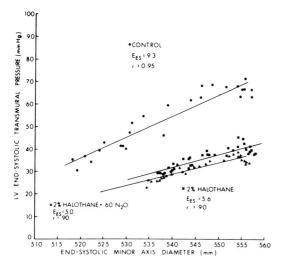

Fig. 1-7. Left ventricular end-systolic pressure-diameter relationship in one dog. Measurements were made awake and during 2% halothane with and without 60% nitrous oxide. Volume of the heart was decreased by transient caval occlusion. Note that halothane is associated with decreased contractility, and that the addition of nitrous oxide does not further change the inotropic state. E_{es} = slope of the curve. (Reproduced from Van Trigt P, Christian CC, Fagraeus L, et al: Myocardial depression by anesthetic agents [halothane, enflurane and nitrous oxide]: Quantitation based on end-systolic pressure-dimension relations. Am J Cardiol 53:243–247, 1984, with permission.)

thane depressed the hearts of dogs in a dose-related manner. Nitrous oxide, 60% added to the volatile anesthetic, did not further depress the slope (Fig. 1-7). In seven patients anesthetized with fentanyl, 0.5% halothane significantly decreased shortening velocity, magnitude of shortening, E_{es}, and cardiac output, while 60% nitrous oxide had no effect on these measurements. This confirmed the similarity of these responses in dogs and man. An index comparing similar levels of inhaled anesthetic-induced depression to the level of the minimum alveolar concentration (MAC) was derived in these studies and termed ID_{20}. This was defined as the dose of the anesthetic necessary to depress the inotropic state by 20 percent. For halothane and enflurane, the ID_{20} each averaged 0.7 MAC.[20]

STUDIES IN ABNORMAL MYOCARDIUM

Isolated papillary muscles from cats with heart failure have been studied to assess differences between abnormal and normal animals. In abnormal hearts, all indices of contractility are more sensitive to a given concentration of a volatile anesthetic than muscles from normal animals.[21] The control level of the force-velocity curve obtained in papillary muscles from cats with heart failure is similar to that from normal animals when exposed to anesthesia (Fig. 1-8). This phenomenon may contribute to the

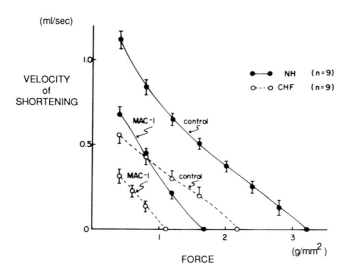

Fig. 1-8. Mean force velocity curves obtained from papillary muscles from normal cat hearts and muscles from hearts with congestive heart failure before and during administration of enflurane at 1 MAC in the perfusate. Note that the control level of CHF muscles is similar to that of normal muscles perfused with enflurane. NH = normal heart. (Reproduced from Kenmotsu O, Hashimoto Y, Shimosato S: The effects of fluroxene and enflurane on contractile performance of isolated papillary muscles from failing hearts. Anesthesiology 40:252–260, 1974, with permission.)

apparently narrower range of anesthetic concentrations tolerated by patients with congestive heart failure. The role of factors other than those acting directly on heart muscle, however, may be prominent.

Prys-Roberts et al studied the response to halothane and nitrous oxide after thiopental (10 mg/kg) in dogs 7–10 days after a myocardial infarction induced by ligation of three left ventricular branches of the left anterior descending coronary artery.[22] They noted no changes in heart rate, blood pressure, SVR, or LV dP/dt; decreases in stroke volume, cardiac output and aortic blood flow acceleration; and increases in LVEDP after 90 minutes of anesthesia. These data are similar to the findings of Vatner and Smith[17] and Roberts et al[23] with halothane in normal animals. They emphasized the greater sensitivity of aortic blood flow acceleration over LV dP/dt to assess contractile state changes, and indicated that, in their model of myocardial infarction, this inhalation anesthetic remained well tolerated. Subsequent studies have shown that when a region of ischemia is less than 25 percent of the LV myocardium, global hemodynamics are unchanged in response to halothane, despite severe local dysfunction.[24]

Studies in Man

INTRINSIC PROPERTIES

Young healthy volunteers have been extensively studied during enflurane, halothane, and isoflurane anesthesia.[25-27] Circulatory effects were different among these anesthetics in similarly conducted studies, with some of these differences being dramatic. At 1 MAC, isoflurane and enflurane did not increase right atrial pressure, whereas halothane did. Both isoflurane and enflurane were associated with an increased heart rate, while halothane was not; stroke volume was reduced about 20 percent by isoflurane and halothane, while the decrease was twice as great with enflurane. Cardiac output thus was maintained with isoflurane, but decreased about 20 percent by halothane and enflurane. Arterial pressure was decreased 20–30 percent by 1 MAC of halothane and isoflurane, and somewhat more by enflurane. Lastly, SVR was decreased to a progressively greater extent by 1 MAC of halothane, enflurane, and isoflurane, respectively.

These studies in young volunteers provide a powerful data base for comparison with other studies and clinical experience. In the Isoflurane New Drug Application, heart rate and blood pressure in 930 patients anesthetized with halothane were compared to those variables in 920 patients during isoflurane administration.[28] The similarities, rather than the differences between the values achieved, were impressive (Table 1-1). The lowest mean heart rate and blood pressure achieved were identical; isoflurane was associated with a maximal heart rate 4 beats per minute higher than halothane (102.2 vs 98.5) and a maximal blood pressure 8 mm Hg higher (150.2 vs 142.2).

A collaborative study was performed in 6798 patients in 165 institutions before the introduction of isoflurane into clinical practice.[29] Pulse rate during

Table 1-1

Hemodynamic Comparison of Isoflurane and Halothane

	Heart rate		Systolic pressure	
	Isoflurane	*Halothane*	*Isoflurane*	*Halothane*
	beats per minute		*mm Hg*	
Admission	79.0	80.3*	125.4	122.7*
Preinduction	83.1	83.4	139.9	134.3*
Operative (high value)	102.2	98.5*	150.2	142.4*
Operative (low value)	75.6	74.7	103.8	103.1
Last OR value	88.5	87.9	131.1	127.9*
First recovery value	89.3	89.0	138.1	133.7*

Source. Data are from the Isoflurane New Drug Application, 579–580.

Heart rate and blood pressure measurements were made in 920 patients before, during, and after anesthesia with isoflurane (average delivered MAC equalled 1.13) and in 930 patients anesthetized with halothane (average delivered MAC 1.46—a value significantly higher than that for isoflurane).

*Significant differences between isoflurane and halothane values.

induction and maintenance increased an average of
6.2 and 2.6 percent, respectively. Blood pressure
declined 2.4 percent during induction, and 11.7 percent during maintenance. Both values are far smaller
than the 20 percent elevation of heart rate and 35
percent decline in blood pressure reported in volunteer studies. In the collaborative study, most patients
received thiopental, half received a preoperative narcotic, and 58 percent received an anticholinergic
drug, whereas in the volunteer studies these drugs
were not used. Roizen et al previously noted that
changes in blood pressure and heart rate following
induction of anesthesia with halothane, morphine,
enflurane, or spinal block were similar to those
reported in the collaborative isoflurane study.[30]

The influences of age, premedication, and adjuvant drugs are striking when studying cardiovascular
responses to anesthesia. Isoflurane was associated
with greater declines in blood pressure in the elderly
and greater increases in heart rate in the young. However, no significant change in heart rate was observed
in patients with "cardiac disease."[29] The differences
in response between young volunteers and patients
have been documented in previous clinical studies.
For instance, in older patients, heart rate was not
increased during isoflurane in a number of studies,
either in the presence of surgery or before surgery
commenced.[31–33] Cahalan et al have demonstrated
that morphine premedication inhibits the increase in
heart rate normally observed with induction of
enflurane or isoflurane anesthesia and surgery[34] (Fig.
1-9). These data emphasize the importance of studying drugs under clinical circumstances and in actual
patients with illnesses.

Provocative studies by Smith and Corbascio[35]
and Winter et al[36] demonstrated that nitrous oxide is
also not without effects upon the circulation. They
showed that nitrous oxide stimulates the sympathetic
nervous system to release norepinephrine, and at 1.5
MAC, achieved under hyperbaric conditions, the circulation of human volunteers was hyperdynamic,
with clinical evidence of massive activation of the
sympathetic nervous system.[36] The addition of
nitrous oxide to halothane, enflurane, or isoflurane is
associated with an increase in systemic vascular
resistance.[35,37,38] In healthy human subjects, nitrous
oxide is associated with minimal myocardial depression, as judged by the IJ wave of the ballistocardiogram.[39] As a general summarizing principle, addition
of nitrous oxide to volatile anesthetics, while keeping
the depth of anesthesia constant, results in increased
SVR and higher blood pressure compared to breathing oxygen with or without nitrogen. Addition of

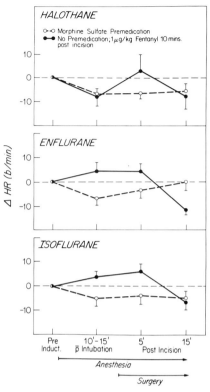

Fig. 1-9. Effect of narcotics upon heart rate during inhalation anesthesia. Morphine sulfate (0.15 mg/kg) premedication plus enflurane/nitrous oxide or isoflurane/nitrous oxide
resulted in a lower heart rate before and during surgery than
did the same inhalation anesthetic without morphine premedication. In the unpremedicated patients, fentanyl (1.0
μg/kg IV) was associated with a mean decrease in heart rate
of 13 bpm regardless of the anesthetic employed. Note that
heart rate during halothane/nitrous oxide did not rise until
the beginning of surgery in patients who had not received
morphine premedication. (Reproduced from Cahalan MK,
Lurz FW, Beaupre PN, et al: Narcotics alter the heart rate
and blood pressure response to inhalational anesthetics.
Anesthesiology 59:A26, 1983, with permission.)

nitrous oxide to a narcotic anesthetic results in circulatory depression, which is probably unrelated to a
direct myocardial action.[40]

Mechanism of the Effect of Volatile Anesthetics Upon Myocardial Contractility

There are several basic questions that have not
been resolved about the action of anesthetics upon
myocardial contractility including (1) the mecha-

nism(s) by which depression is induced, and (2) whether the mechanism is the same for all inhalation anesthetics. Brown and Crout documented that various inhalation anesthetics depress myocardial contractile force in a dose-related manner that correlates with the oil/gas partition coefficient.[41] Price showed that cat papillary muscle depression produced by 0.5% halothane was reversed by increasing the calcium ion concentration of the perfusing medium, and that the maximum force developed in the presence of calcium and halothane was identical to control.[42] The results suggest that restriction of calcium flow to the contractile proteins and/or inhibition of the reaction between calcium and the contractile proteins, rather than a metabolic effect, is responsible for the depression of contractility. Other investigators have also shown that anesthetics affect calcium within the myocardium in various ways. Because calcium is instrumental in so many of the steps involved in muscle contraction, it is not surprising that a calcium effect might be important in one or more of them. At present, however, the specific mechanism by which anesthetics achieve myocardial (or skeletal muscle) contractile depression has not been defined.

On the basis that the contractile depression associated with five inhalation anesthetics studied was qualitatively similar, Brown and Crout speculated that the mechanism of action of myocardial depression was identical at the molecular level.[41] Merin and Basch further supported this proposal by showing similarities between the contractile function and metabolism of all the anesthetics they studied.[43] However, Lynch has recently challenged this concept on the basis of differential depression of isolated guinea pig papillary muscle preparations by isoflurane, halothane, and enflurane.[44] A multitude of stimulation rates were used, while tension, intracellular action potential of the elicited twitch, and the time differentials of tension (dT/dt) and membrane potential (V) were recorded in the study. It was demonstrated that equivalent contractile depression by halothane was accompanied by greater depression of slow action potentials (Fig. 1-10). Furthermore, with normal action potentials, isoflurane depressed peak tension less at higher frequencies, and dT/dt_{max} less at all frequencies than halothane. While halothane in the presence of slow action potentials caused similar contractile depression at all frequencies, isoflurane and enflurane caused depression of the late-peaking twitch observed with less than 0.5 Hz stimulation, and isoflurane caused less depression than halothane or enflurane of early peaking tension and the dT/dt_{max} at frequencies greater than 1 Hz. These observations

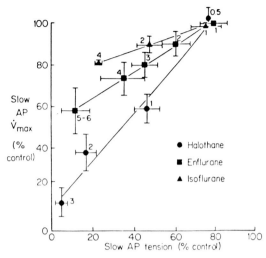

Fig. 1-10. Effect of three volatile anesthetics upon the relation of depression of slow action (calcium dependent) potential maximum rate of depolarization (V_{max}) to the simultaneously measured depression in peak tension of guinea pig papillary muscles at 0.30 Hz. The numbers beside the points represent the anesthetic concentration (in percent) bubbled through the perfusion medium. See text for details. (Figure courtesy of C. Lynch.)

strongly suggest that there are differences in the mechanism of myocardial contractile depression among anesthetics, and will undoubtedly constitute a major stimulus to further investigations searching for specific mechanisms.

Effects of Volatile Anesthetics Upon the Systemic Vasculature

Halothane, enflurane, and isoflurane induce relaxation of smooth muscles in blood vessels. For instance, Vatner and Smith infused halothane intra-arterially into a variety of vascular beds that had different responses to halothane inhalation in intact animals.[17] Intra-arterial halothane was associated with increased flow in all beds studied without change in perfusion pressure. Vasodilation was unaffected by blockade of the alpha-adrenergic, beta-adrenergic, cholinergic, or histaminergic systems. In addition, Price noted depression by halothane of rabbit aorta strips,[45] and Sprague et al studied the effects of halothane and isoflurane upon phenylephrine-induced isometric contraction of the rat aorta.[46] Both anesthetic drugs inhibited this response in a dose dependent manner. It is interesting that the potency

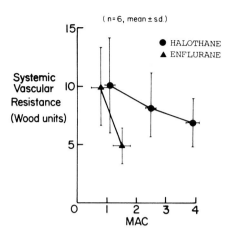

Fig. 1-11. Effect of volatile inhalation anesthetics upon systemic vascular resistance during cardiopulmonary bypass in man. Note that the systemic vascular resistance was similar when 1 MAC of halothane or enflurane was administered. However, a small increase in enflurane concentration was more effective than a large increase in halothane in reducing resistance. (Reproduced from Doherty F, Wilkinson PL, Robinson S: Enflurane reduces systemic pressure during cardiopulmonary bypass more effectively than halothane. Anesthesiology 55:A40, 1981, with permission.)

of halothane was greater than isoflurane (halothane 1 and 2% caused the same degree of relaxation as 4 and 6% isoflurane). The effect did not appear to be mediated by beta-adrenergic activity since propranolol did not block it. However, the cyclic adenosine monophosphate (AMP)/adenosine triphosphate (ATP) ratio increased in a dose dependent fashion with 6 and 8% isoflurane and 2 and 5% halothane, while phosphodiesterase activity was unchanged. Therefore, the authors attributed the aortic relaxation to increased cyclic AMP formation.

A "pure" way to compare the response of the systemic vasculature of humans to volatile anesthetics is to administer them during cardiopulmonary bypass. Doherty et al found similar SVR values during 1 MAC halothane and enflurane anesthesia (Fig. 1-11).[47] However, 2 MAC halothane reduced SVR by only about one-third as compared with 2 MAC enflurane.

The effect of anesthetics upon specific vascular beds is variable. For instance, regional blood flows and resistances showed striking disparities during halothane anesthesia in the studies of Vatner and Smith.[17] Coronary blood flow, estimated by measuring late diastolic blood flow, changed in accordance with oxygen demand. Changes in coronary vascular resistance never achieved statistical significance during early or late 1 or 2% halothane. Halothane's tendency to dilate the coronary bed thus was offset by a reduction in myocardial oxygen metabolic demand, which tended to constrict the coronary bed. Mesenteric flow was decreased at both 1 and 2% halothane. During the former, vascular resistance was increased, but during 2% halothane resistance was unchanged. The mesenteric bed was the only one that responded with vasoconstriction, and then only with 1% halothane. The renal vascular bed demonstrated the greatest reduction of vascular resistance of any organ studied. Renal flow remained unchanged at 1 and 2% halothane, and resistance declined by about 50 percent. With 1% halothane, resistance increased with time toward the control level, whereas it remained decreased at 2%. In the iliac artery, 1% halothane was associated with maintained flow, whereas flow declined with 2% halothane. Resistance during 1% halothane decreased by about 25 percent, and rose toward control with time. Iliac vascular resistance decreased with 2% halothane, and then remained at that level despite continued anesthetic administration. In summary, vascular dilation was apparent in the renal and iliac beds, constriction occurred in the mesenteric bed, and little change of tone occurred in the coronary bed in the intact animals studied by this group.[17]

Studies of Inhalation Anesthetics During Surgery

A number of recent investigations have examined the inhalation anesthetics during surgical stimulation. The questions addressed were (1) whether inhalation anesthetics were effective in preventing or reversing the adverse hemodynamic consequences of surgery, and (2) whether some inhalation anesthetics are preferable to others for this purpose.

Roizen et al documented the hemodynamic *stress* responses to halothane/N_2O, enflurane/N_2O, spinal anesthesia, and morphine/N_2O during anesthetic induction and surgical incision.[30] They found that approximately 1.5 MAC enflurane/N_2O or halothane/N_2O was necessary to inhibit the plasma norepinephrine response to surgical incision in 50 percent of patients; and over 2.0 MAC was required to provide inhibition in 95 percent of patients. Changes in heart rate and blood pressure did not correlate with changes in plasma norepinephrine. Increasing the concentration of halothane had a small effect on reducing the blood pressure and heart rate response to incision; however, this was not evident with enflurane/N_2O. These represent rather disappointing findings, which emphasize the well-recognized fact that whereas 1 MAC may be sufficient to prevent movement, this concentration of anesthetic does not predictably prevent other responses. The remaining endocrine and hemodynamic responses may result in adverse effects upon the heart, particularly if it is diseased. Furthermore, Roizen et al showed that although the modern inhalation anesthetics may not by themselves liberate catecholamines, consequences of catecholamine release cannot be ignored.

In other studies, Hess et al[48] and Roizen et al[49] investigated the efficacy of deepening inhalation anesthesia upon relief of stimulation-induced hypertension and elevation of the pulmonary capillary wedge pressure (PCWP). Hess et al compared isoflurane to halothane in acutely hypertensive patients anesthetized with flunitrazepam, fentanyl, nitrous-oxide, and pancuronium[48] (Fig. 1-12). Isoflurane appeared to achieve reduction of blood pressure primarily by vasodilation. Systemic vascular resistance and PCWP decreased markedly, car-

diac index increased, and heart rate and stroke volume were unchanged. In contrast, halothane seemed to act primarily by myocardial depression, since PCWP and SVR remained elevated, stroke volume and cardiac output decreased, and heart rate remained stable.

Roizen et al increased the inhaled concentration of volatile anesthetic agent when the PCWP became acutely elevated during a thiopental-nitrous oxide-pancuronium, enflurane, or halothane anesthetic.[49] Both anesthetics reduced the elevated blood pressure, PCWP, SVR, and plasma norepinephrine in the face of an unchanged heart rate and cardiac output (Fig. 1-13). The effects of enflurane and halothane were indistinguishable. Both appeared to act primarily by vasodilation under these circumstances, in dramatic contrast to the findings of Hess et al regarding halothane.

The interpretation of different results from such similar studies performed by two teams of reputable investigators is difficult. In fact, the literature is replete with such contradictions.[50] Why did the PCWP remain elevated despite halothane "treatment" in one study, whereas it normalized in the other? Why did vasodilation predominate when

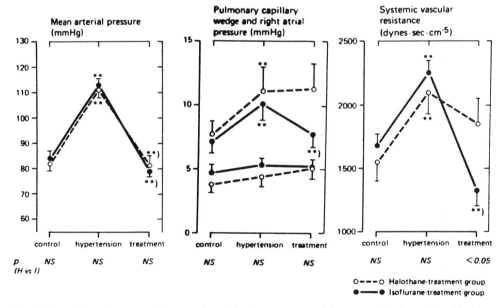

Fig. 1-12. Effect of treatment of hypertension, defined as a mean arterial pressure of 100 mm Hg, with either isoflurane (1.5–2.0 vol%) or halothane (1.0–1.5 vol%). While both anesthetics appeared to lower arterial pressure effectively, only isoflurane was associated with a decreased pulmonary capillary wedge pressure and systemic vascular resistance, and maintained stroke volume index. (Reproduced from Hess W, Arnold B, Schulte-Sasse U, Tarnow J: Comparison of isoflurane and halothane when used to control intraoperative hypertension in patients undergoing coronary artery bypass surgery. Anesth Analg 62:15–20, 1983, with permission.)

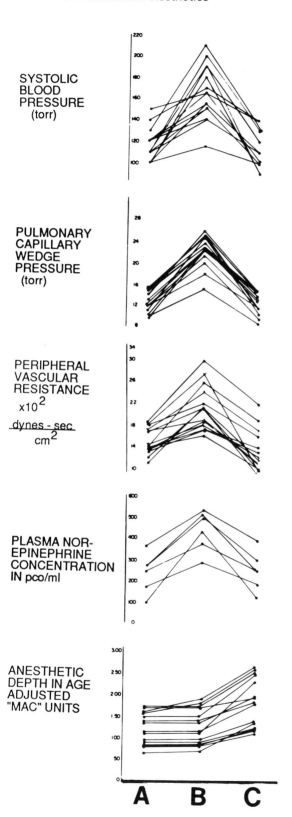

SYSTOLIC
BLOOD
PRESSURE
(torr)

PULMONARY
CAPILLARY
WEDGE
PRESSURE
(torr)

PERIPHERAL
VASCULAR
RESISTANCE
$x10^2$

$\dfrac{dynes - sec}{cm^2}$

PLASMA NOR-
EPINEPHRINE
CONCENTRATION
IN pco/ml

ANESTHETIC
DEPTH IN AGE
ADJUSTED
"MAC" UNITS

A   B   C

Roizen et al administered halothane whereas myocardial depression was most prominent when Hess et al used the same drug? The clinician is led to the conclusion that the circulatory similarities may outweigh the vaunted differences of the inhalation anesthetics on the circulation, and that, in most circumstances, factors other than myocardial contractility, heart rate, and vascular resistance may be most important when choosing among them.

PHYSIOLOGY OF THE NORMAL CORONARY CIRCULATION

Normal coronary artery tone and blood flow are governed primarily by local metabolic demand. Coronary blood flow will normally increase or decrease to provide close matching of flow to oxygen demand. When the factors governing demand are held constant, pressure autoregulation is prominent; within a wide range of coronary driving pressure, flow stays virtually constant. Above and below this pressure range, flow is linearly proportional to pressure[51] (Fig. 1-14). In normal coronary arteries, inflow pressure for the left ventricle has been considered the (mean) aortic diastolic pressure, and outflow pressure the coronary sinus or left ventricular end-diastolic pressure. The difference between the inflow and outflow pressure is usually defined as the coronary perfusion pressure (see Chapter 15).

Coronary blood flow has been measured by isotopically tagged microspheres, modifications of the Kety–Schmidt inert gas technique, flowmeters (Doppler, electromagnetic) placed on epicardial coronary arteries, and a retrograde thermodilution technique in the coronary sinus or great cardiac vein.[52] The first method requires sacrifice of the experimental subject and a limited number of measurements, but is excellent for estimating regional and transmural distribution of blood flow. The second requires steady-state conditions, and may be unreliable when there is inhomogeneity of perfusion. The third produces instanta-

Fig. 1-13. Effect of treatment of elevated pulmonary capillary wedge pressure with increased concentration of halothane or enflurane. Both anesthetics effectively lowered pulmonary capillary wedge pressure and systemic (peripheral) vascular resistance. Note the contrast of these results with those in Figure 1-12. A = values prior to surgical manipulation; B = values during surgical manipulation; C = values after treatment with myocardial depressant anesthetic (surgical manipulation continued). (Reproduced from Roizen MF, Hamilton WK, Sohn YJ: Treatment of stress-induced increases in pulmonary capillary wedge pressure using volatile anesthetics. Anesthesiology 54:446–450, 1981, with permission.)

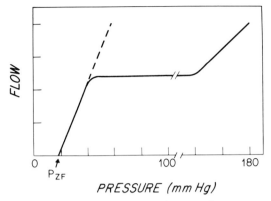

Fig. 1-14. Pressure-flow diagram demonstrating coronary arterial autoregulation. The dashed line illustrates the slope of maximum dilation.

neous flow measurements throughout the cardiac cycle, but is rarely applicable in man. The last technique is most often used in man, and can detect transient changes. It provides relative flow measurements, but is also sensitive to changes in catheter position and right atrial pressure. No ideal simple technique for clinical measurement thus exists.

Bellamy showed that the pressure at which flow stopped (P_{ZF} or $P_{F=0}$) in an epicardial coronary artery

was higher than left ventricular end-diastolic pressure[53] (Fig. 1-15). He interpreted these data to indicate that tissue pressure exceeded left ventricular cavity pressure, and that tissue pressure (rather than ventricular pressure) was the outflow pressure for coronary blood flow. It was also shown that the P_{ZF} could be changed. For example, Verrier et al showed that P_{ZF} in dogs receiving halothane was far lower than when the same dogs received nitrous oxide, and they interpreted this to mean that halothane produced a greater coronary vascular reserve than nitrous oxide.[54] This entire line of research ignores the capacitance of the coronary arteries. When blood is ejected into the aorta and the coronary arteries in systole, the elastic blood vessels expand, storing potential energy in the walls. During diastole, this energy provides additional impetus to drive blood forward through the small coronary vessels. Measurements of flow in intramyocardial coronary arteries indicate that downstream flow continues despite cessation in proximal epicardial vessels.[55] Therefore, the controversy surrounding the concept of P_{ZF} continues unabated, as exemplified by two recent articles, each championing an opposing view (Fig. 1-16).[56,57] In fact, new studies have negated the implications and interpretation of a great deal of

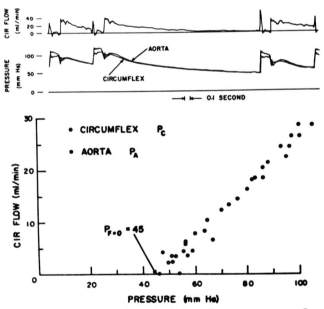

Fig. 1-15. Analogue recording of proximal circumflex coronary artery flow, aortic pressure and circumflex coronary artery pressure (top panel), and the flow/pressure relationship plotted from the long diastole in this dog (bottom panel). Note that the point of zero flow (denoted at $P_{F=0}$) is 45 mm Hg, far above the left ventricular end diastolic pressure. See text for details. (Reproduced from Bellamy RF: Diastolic coronary pressure-flow relation in the dog. Circ Res 43:92–101, 1978, with permission.)

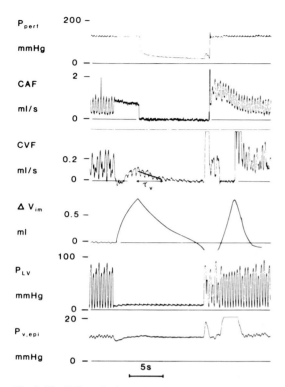

Fig. 1-16. Effect of a long diastole upon epicardial coronary artery flow, great cardiac vein flow, left ventricular pressure. Coronary perfusion was provided by a cannula in the main coronary artery, and clamped during diastole. Venous flow ceases immediately after cessation of systole and then resumes and plateaus. It decays and ceases when perfusion is stopped. This is consistent with the discharge of an intramyocardial capacitance system. Left ventricular diastolic pressure remains low throughout diastole. P_{PERF} = coronary perfusion pressure. (Reproduced from Spaan JAE: Coronary diastolic pressure-flow relation and zero flow pressure explained on basis of intramyocardial compliance. Circ Res 56:293–309, 1985, with permission.)

recent literature on P_{ZF}, and the outflow pressure for the coronary arteries is probably closer to the higher of either left or right ventricular end-diastolic pressures.

The well-oxygenated myocardium extracts lactate from the blood; but as oxygenation becomes deficient, the myocardium produces lactate.[58] Therefore, lactate production in the coronary sinus is accepted as a sensitive indicator of global myocardial ischemia. When oxygen imbalance is regional rather than global, coronary sinus measurements may reflect this by a decrease in lactate extraction, rather than lactate production. This interpretation of decreased extraction when only global (ie, coronary sinus) measurements are available as suggestive of regional ischemia is controversial. Previously unpublished data of the authors indicates that a 50 percent decrease in coronary sinus lactate extraction has a high likelihood of being associated with ST-segment depression and adds credence to this viewpoint (Fig. 1-17). Obviously, regional measurements are desirable to document disparate myocardial nutrition, and this can now be accomplished clinically by catheterizing and sampling blood from the great cardiac vein (draining the left anterior descending coronary artery and the anterior LV wall).

Coronary artery blood flow to the left ventricular myocardium is primarily diastolic, since compression of blood vessels during systole impedes flow.[53] In contrast, epicardial coronary blood flow to the normal low-pressure right ventricular myocardium is highest in systole, and never ceases during diastole, since the perfusion pressure always exceeds the intramyocardial pressure.[59] However, right ventricular hypertension causes the right coronary artery to act as though it were supplying left ventricular myocardium; epicardial flow ceases during systole, and a P_{ZF} can be demonstrated.

PHYSIOLOGY OF THE ABNORMAL CORONARY CIRCULATION

Until recently it was believed that an increase in oxygen demand through a flow-limited coronary artery was usually responsible for myocardial ischemia.[60] The single greatest conceptual change in the understanding of abnormal coronary blood flow is that decreased coronary blood flow (ie, oxygen supply) is also an extremely common cause of myocardial ischemia.[61] This ischemia frequently occurs without angina pectoris. The anatomical basis for the decreased flow may be an atherosclerotic plaque that is not totally occlusive and only partially circumferential. The remaining portion of the vessel wall is reactive or even hyperactive. The mechanism for the hyperactivity has not yet been elucidated, but the permanently reduced lumen due to atherosclerosis, plus the hyperactive contractile segment, is a powerful setting for flow-limiting narrowing.

When narrowing of a coronary artery occurs, there is initially no compromise of flow or pressure. When flow becomes impaired, the microvasculature distal to the constriction becomes fully dilated, loses autoregulation, and becomes pressure dependent.[60] Until recently, it was thought that no further dilation was possible in the ischemic myocardium. However, recent experiments have challenged even this basic

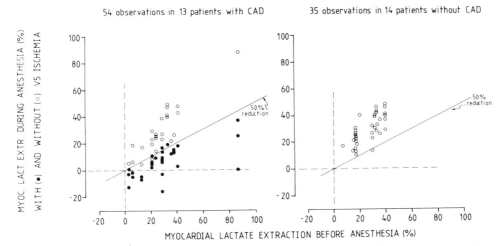

Fig. 1-17. Relationship of coronary sinus lactate extraction before anesthesia to lactate extraction during anesthesia in 13 patients with coronary artery disease (CAD) who demonstrated ischemia at least once during anesthesia, and in 14 patients without CAD. Presence of ischemia was defined as depression of 1.0 mm in the ST segment of ECG lead V_5. ECG depression occurred only in patients with CAD. In only one instance did lactate extraction decrease by more than 50 percent in normal patients. In contrast, ECG depression was evident in about half of the measurements in patients with CAD. Virtually all of these ECG changes were associated with reduction of greater than 50 percent in lactate extraction, though less than one-third were associated with lactate production. These data emphasize the insensitivity of lactate production as an index of ischemia when coronary sinus blood is sampled, and the desirability of regional blood sampling for estimation of ischemia in the heart with coronary artery disease. They suggest that large decreases of lactate extraction may be indicative of regional ischemia during anesthesia.

concept.[62] Unless the narrowing to all regions of the heart is uniform, it is likely that some areas will have a pressure-dependent blood supply at the same time that autoregulation will still be intact in other areas (Fig. 1-18).

The hydrodynamics of a constriction in a tube through which fluid is flowing are well defined. Flow across a constriction is proportional to the square root of the pressure difference across the stenosis.[60] At constant proximal pressure, flow is decreased only to a minor degree until a constriction is 80–90 percent complete. Then a precipitous decline of flow will occur with a small further decrement of cross-sectional area. In a critically narrowed tube, a small decrease in pressure gradient may similarly lead to a precipitous decline of flow. Other factors governing flow are the length of the constriction and the presence of sequential constrictions. For instance, in dogs in which a coronary artery was narrowed experimentally, Feldman et al demonstrated that a 60 percent stenosis, 15 mm in length, caused a compromise of flow similar to a 90 percent stenosis only 1 mm long.[63]

Coronary vessels in man are often completely occluded with remarkable preservation of myocardial function. Since heart muscle has virtually no capabil-

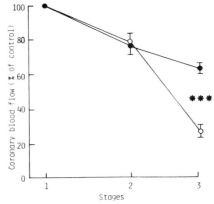

Fig. 1-18. Relationship of coronary blood flow to halothane concentration in dogs before and during narrowing of a coronary artery. Coronary blood flow decreases proportionately to myocardial oxygen demand prior to constricting the coronary artery. Following constriction, blood flow decreases proportionately until blood pressure declines sufficiently to compromise flow across the stenosis. When this point is reached, coronary blood flow declines further and regional dysfunction, indicative of myocardial oxygen imbalance, occurs. (Reproduced from Francis CM, Foex P, Lowenstein E, et al: The interaction between regional myocardial ischaemia and left ventricular performance under halothane anesthesia. Br J Anaesthesiol 34:965–979, 1982, with permission.)

ity to function anaerobically, this means that blood is nevertheless reaching the area beyond the occlusion. This blood supply may be antegrade from the original vessel or retrograde from another major coronary artery. In all cases, however, flow requires collateral vessels, which appear to be stimulated by oxygen deprivation.

In man with coronary artery disease, the situation is extremely complex, with stenoses varying in caliber, length, number, symmetry, and distensibility. Furthermore, coronary vasospasm is now recognized as a common and important factor in stable angina pectoris and preinfarction angina, rather than being limited to variant angina pectoris.[61] The combined effects of hydraulic physics and coronary artery physiology thus provide an infinite number of combinations of flow conditions, making it exceedingly difficult to accurately predict which combination of hemodynamic conditions will provide sufficient flow for adequate myocardial nutrition. This has provided the impetus for more sensitive and precise monitoring of the myocardial oxygen balance during anesthesia and the entire perioperative period. Four recently described examples of this complexity are the coronary steal syndrome, intramyocardial flow redistribution, the effect of distensibility upon stenotic resistance, and coronary vasospasm.

A *steal* is liable to occur in an area supplied by collateral vessels that are less responsive to vasodilator and vasoconstrictor stimuli than normal vessels, or in an area distal to a stenosis in which the vasculature is maximally dilated and the autoregulatory reserve is exhausted. Under these conditions, a coronary dilator may decrease flow through the collaterals or across the constriction, and flow may actually reverse from the area previously maximally dilated to the areas supplied by those vessels responsive to the vasodilator[64] (Fig. 1-19). It has been stated that both an occlusion of one vessel and a narrowing of another, as well as an intervention that dilates small intramural arteries (ie, nitroprusside as opposed to nitroglycerin) are required.[65] In addition, it has been postulated that an intervention that produces negative inotropy prevents the steal despite conductive coronary artery and small vessel dilation.[66] Neither of these postulates appears certain at present (see Chapter 15).

Intramyocardial blood flow redistribution during exercise was demonstrated by Gallagher et al in dogs with chronic stenosis of a single coronary artery.[67] Myocardial function and flow distribution were normal at rest, but during exercise, total flow to the stenotic segments remained unchanged rather than demonstrating the normal doubling. While subepi-

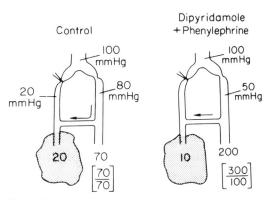

Fig. 1-19. Schematic diagram of the coronary circulation showing proposed mechanism for a vasodilator-induced coronary steal. The coronary artery divides into two branches, one completely occluded, and the other stenosed but providing collaterals to the first. In the control situation on the left, distal pressure is low in the occluded arterial bed and there is a small gradient in mean pressure across the stenosis. Flow in the ischemic region (dotted area) is 20 ml/min/100 g and is determined by the collateral driving pressure, or the difference between distal pressures in the bed supplying collaterals (80 mm Hg) and the ischemic bed (20 mm Hg). Flow in the distribution of the stenotic vessel is normal at 70 ml/min/100 g and is evenly distributed between subendocardium (lower value in bracket) and subepicardium (upper value). During dipyridamole administration, with blood pressure maintained constant by phenylephrine, flow increases in the nonischemic bed to 200 ml/min/100 g, but becomes maldistributed between subendocardium and subepicardium. In addition, pressure distal to the stenosis falls to 50 mm Hg, causing a reduction in collateral driving pressure. As a result, flow to the ischemic region decreases to 10 ml/min/100 g, interpreted as a coronary steal. (Reproduced from Becker LC: Conditions for vasodilator-induced coronary steal in experimental myocardial ischemia. Circulation 57:1103–1110, 1978, with permission.)

cardial flow doubled normally and midmyocardial flow was unchanged, flow to the subendocardium approached zero and myocardial function deteriorated (Fig. 1-20). Layers of the heart clearly vary in their net myocardial oxygen balance during these conditions.

Stenotic resistance remains constant in rigid stenoses, but varies in distensible stenoses. When distal pressure increases with a rigid stenosis, the pressure gradient across the stenosis is decreased, so flow decreases and calculated resistance increases; conversely, when distal pressure decreases, flow across the constriction increases.[68] With a distensible stenosis, increase in distal pressure may cause an increase in luminal stenosis area. The flow increases despite a decreased pressure gradient, because the

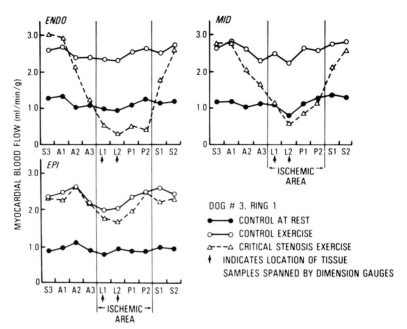

Fig. 1-20. Intramyocardial blood flow redistribution distal to a narrowed coronary artery is shown in one dog. Myocardial blood flow was measured in the absence of a stenosis at rest and during exercise, and in the presence of a stenosis during exercise. Flow to the subepicardial myocardium achieved normal levels during exercise, flow to the mid-myocardium was attenuated, and flow to the epicardium was virtually absent. (Reproduced from Gallagher KP, Osakada G, Matsuzaki M, et al: Myocardial blood flow and function with critical coronary stenosis in exercising dogs. Am J Physiol 12:H698–707, 1982, with permission.)

stenotic resistance is lowered. Conversely, when distal pressure falls, the stenosis lumen may narrow and flow decrease. This mechanism is effective primarily in the presence of an extremely tight stenosis, and only when it incorporates an elastic element.

Maseri's research group has been in the forefront of establishing the importance of coronary vasospasm in stable angina pectoris.[61] Unlike variant angina, which is associated with ST-segment elevation on the electrocardiogram (ECG) indicative of transmural ischemia, this type of coronary spasm may be associated with normalization or depression of the ST segment. Continuous monitoring has documented that ECG changes precede changes in heart rate or blood pressure, and scintigraphy has documented hypoperfusion (Fig. 1-21). Whereas oxygen demand-related angina pectoris is predictable and occurs in each individual at a characteristic workload or rate-pressure product, supply-related ischemia occurs unpredictably, often during sleep, or awake in the absence of effort. Most frequently, individuals have a combination of the two types of angina. It is likely that some, if not most, of the preoperative

ECG changes in premedicated patients with severe coronary artery disease reported by Slogoff and Keats were related to such vasospasm.[69] They observed an 18 percent incidence of new ST-segment depression greater than 0.1 mV by recording leads II and V_5 of the ECG every 2 minutes after arrival in the induction area. The importance of this type of ischemia during anesthesia needs to be studied further (see Chapter 15).

EFFECTS OF THE INHALATION ANESTHETICS UPON THE CORONARY CIRCULATION

Halothane

Animal studies using halothane anesthesia have demonstrated little effect upon coronary vascular tone or autoregulation.[54,70–72] Francis et al documented disproportionately decreased coronary blood flow associated with lowered blood pressure, resulting in dysfunction in regions of the myocardium supplied by a narrowed coronary artery, whereas regions

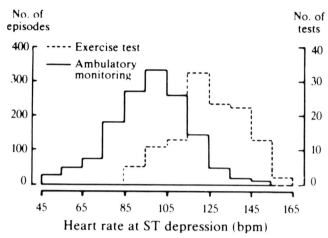

Fig. 1-21. Distribution of heart rates at onset of ST-segment depression during ambulatory monitoring and exercise testing in patients with stable angina pectoris. In 73 percent of episodes, heart rate was 20 beats per minute or more below that at ST depression during exercise. (Reproduced from Deanfield JE, Maseri A, Selwyn AP, et al: Myocardial ischaemia during daily life in patients with stable angina. Its relation to symptoms and heart rate changes. Lancet 2:753–758, 1983, with permission.)

supplied by a normal coronary artery had a decrease in coronary blood flow proportional to myocardial oxygen requirements.[73] The ischemia appeared to be a hydraulic phenomenon due to a decreased perfusion pressure rather than impairment of coronary autoregulation. Buffington has recently confirmed that regional function abnormalities are due to decreased perfusion pressure rather than a specific effect of halothane.[74]

One randomized clinical study compared the coronary hemodynamic effects of halothane (0.2–1 percent end-tidal) with those induced by morphine (2 mg/kg), both administered in conjunction with 50 percent nitrous oxide in oxygen, to patients scheduled to undergo coronary artery surgery.[75] Before surgical intervention, both techniques resulted in approximately a 20 percent reduction in myocardial oxygen consumption which was related to a decline in blood pressure. Coronary blood flow decreased less than 10 percent in both groups, and myocardial oxygen extraction decreased to a greater extent with halothane than with morphine. These results are in agreement with work reported by Sonntag et al in healthy subjects (halothane/air/oxygen),[76] Reiz et al (halothane/air/oxygen) in vascular surgical patients with a history of congestive heart failure,[77] and by Moffitt et al (halothane/oxygen, with and without 50% nitrous oxide) in patients with coronary artery disease and normal left ventricular function.[78] These four studies demonstrated an increase in coronary venous oxygen content during administration of halo-thane. One additional study in patients with coronary artery disease documented a comparable reduction of coronary blood flow and myocardial oxygen consumption, but with an unchanged coronary sinus PO_2.[79] In sum, the possible mild coronary vasodilating action of halothane appears to have little, if any, importance for development of myocardial oxygen supply/demand imbalance in man compared to the effects of an altered systemic circulation.

Enflurane

Enflurane is associated with coronary vasodilation in the acutely and chronically instrumented dog,[70,72] and administration of 1 MAC enflurane in oxygen-enriched air to unpremedicated patients with ischemic heart disease scheduled for vascular surgery resulted in coronary vasodilation.[80] Coronary blood flow decreased by 30 percent in association with a 47 percent reduction in coronary perfusion pressure, and myocardial oxygen extraction decreased from 68 to 57 percent. Moffitt et al investigated the effects of enflurane (0.5–3% inhaled concentration in oxygen) upon the coronary circulation of patients with coronary artery disease and normal left ventricular function.[81] With adequate premedication, beta-blockade, and fluid loading, enflurane decreased mean arterial pressure by 33 percent; myocardial oxygen consumption declined by 50 percent, in association with a 30 percent reduction in coronary blood flow, and an approximately 20 percent decrease in myocardial oxygen extraction. The combination of fentanyl (30 $\mu g/kg$) with enflurane and oxygen has also been shown to produce normal coronary metabolism.[82] Both the animal and available clinical data thus suggest that enflurane is associated with more coronary vasodilation than halothane; however, the myocardial oxygen balance is well maintained and myocardial ischemia does not occur.

The multiple thermistor technique allows for thermodilution measurements of regional coronary venous blood flow, making simultaneous estimation of the contribution of great cardiac venous blood flow (GCVF) to total coronary sinus blood flow (CSF) possible.[83] The former drains the left anterior descending coronary artery (LAD) territory; whereas coronary sinus blood flow represents virtually all left ventricular venous drainage. The normal GCVF/CSF ratio is 0.5–0.7.[84] Rydvall et al measured the GCVF/CSF ratio in four patients with coronary artery disease during enflurane/oxygen/enriched air and enflurane/nitrous oxide/oxygen anesthesia (constant MAC and constant inspired oxygen concentration).[80] They observed a decrease in GCVF/CSF with the former, but the ratio reverted to the awake control value with partial exchange of enflurane for nitrous oxide, despite further reduction of coronary perfusion pressure and myocardial oxygen demand (Table 1-2). The interpretation and clinical implications of this intriguing finding are not yet clear, but may relate to N_2O-induced myocardial ischemia.

Isoflurane

Much animal experimentation has demonstrated that isoflurane is a coronary vasodilator that interferes with autoregulation. Its potency appears considerably greater than halothane or enflurane, but less than adenosine (Fig. 1-22).[70,72,85-89]

In unpremedicated, vascular surgical patients with ischemic heart disease, Reiz et al demonstrated a coronary vasodilating action of 1 MAC isoflurane in oxygen-enriched air.[90] This anesthetic was associated with a 35 percent reduction in calculated coronary perfusion pressure, unchanged left ventricular filling pressure, and an increase in heart rate. Coronary blood flow remained constant despite a 36 percent reduction in myocardial oxygen consumption, and a decline in myocardial oxygen extraction from 68 to 48 percent. Similar results were obtained by Moffitt et al in premedicated, beta-blocked patients with coronary artery disease and normal left ventricular function receiving varying concentrations of isoflurane.[91]

Because adjuvant drugs might alter the pharmacologic effects of anesthetics upon the circulation, a double-blind comparison of two anesthetics with apparently different effects upon coronary vascular autoregulation (halothane and isoflurane) was recently conducted by the authors in patients with coronary artery disease. Many of the patients had a history of congestive heart failure and decreased left ventricular ejection fraction. They received their regular cardiac medications plus a morphine premedication one hour prior to study. Both anesthetics were administered in 60% nitrous oxide/40% oxygen after induction with fentanyl and thiopental. Muscle relaxation was provided by succinylcholine followed by pancuronium.

Strict intervention criteria were used to avoid major hemodynamic abnormalities which could themselves result in coronary hemodynamic changes. Hypotension was defined as a decline in the mean

Table 1-2
Regional Coronary Blood Flow During Enflurane–N_2O Anesthesia

Patient No.	Awake Ratio (GCVF/CSF)	Enflurane 30% oxygen in N_2 1 MAC Ratio (GCVF/CSF)	Enflurane 30% oxygen in N_2O 1 MAC Ratio (GCVF/CSF)
1	0.46 (54/117)	0.37 (29/73)	0.45 (27/60)
2	0.79 (132/167)	0.70 (112/161)	0.77 (102/132)
3	0.72 (103/144)	0.56 (93/167)	0.66 (92/139)
4	0.83 (181/217)	0.51 (98/192)	0.91 (212/232)

Regional left ventricular blood flow distribution before and during enflurane anesthesia without and with nitrous oxide at constant MAC. Despite further reduction in coronary perfusion pressure, part exchange of enflurane for nitrous oxide resulted in redistribution of blood flow.

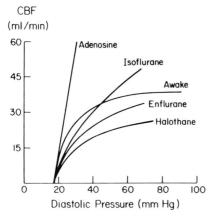

CBF
(ml/min)

Diastolic Pressure (mm Hg)

Fig. 1-22. Diastolic pressure—coronary blood flow relations in the awake and anesthetized dog. Halothane, enflurane, and isoflurane are effective vasodilators, though none impairs autoregulation comparably to adenosine. Isoflurane is more potent than either halothane or enflurane. (Reproduced from Sybert PE, Hickey RF, Hoar PF, et al: Effects of volatile anesthetics on the regulation of coronary blood flow. Anesthesiology 59:A24, 1983, with permission.)

arterial pressure of 30 percent, and phenylephrine was administered in 85 percent of patients before incision for this indication. Despite the rigid criterion for therapy, blood pressure and stroke volume were more effectively maintained at normal levels in isoflurane patients (Fig. 1-23, left panel). Halothane patients had significantly greater decreases in stroke volume index and mean arterial pressure at comparable changes in heart rate and PCWP, despite higher phenylephrine infusion rates.

In the halothane-anesthetized patients, coronary blood flow decreased in parallel to the perfusion pressure, and myocardial oxygen extraction moderately declined. In contrast, isoflurane-anesthetized patients did not experience a change in coronary blood flow, and had a pronounced fall in myocardial oxygen extraction (Fig. 1-23, right panel). These data, which are consistent with the studies summarized above, suggest that the multiple drugs used for treatment of underlying cardiac disease, premedication, induction of anesthesia, and maintenance of cardiovascular stability interfere little with the intrinsic actions of the inhaled anesthetics upon coronary vascular tone.

Coronary vasodilators, such as adenosine and dipyridamole, have been shown to produce ischemia by causing an adverse redistribution of myocardial blood flow, despite an unchanged coronary perfusion pressure. Other vasodilators, such as nitroglycerin,

sodium nitroprusside, and calcium channel blockers may also cause a redistribution of coronary blood flow when the coronary perfusion pressure is lowered.[65,92–95] Dipyridamole produces an inhomogeneous distribution of coronary blood flow when flow-limiting stenoses are present, and overperfusion of non-stenotic areas may coexist with underperfusion of poststenotic areas. This results in electrocardiographic ST-segment abnormalities in less than 5 percent, and angina in about 15 percent of patients with demonstrable lesions.[96–99] Vasodilation and relative hyperperfusion thus are associated with myocardial ischemia in a small proportion of patients with coronary artery disease.

It is likely that isoflurane, despite being a weaker coronary vasodilator than dipyridamole, sometimes produces a similar redistribution of coronary blood flow in patients with regions of myocardium supplied by collaterals distal to a stenosed coronary artery. Reiz et al observed ischemia in 5 of 10 patients during steady-state isoflurane anesthesia associated with a decreased perfusion pressure.[90] When blood pressure, heart rate, and filling pressure were adjusted to preanesthetic levels by pharmacologic intervention and atrial pacing, ischemia persisted in three of five patients (Fig. 1-24). Although calculated vascular resistance had returned towards control, myocardial oxygen extraction remained at a profoundly decreased level, suggesting persistent coronary vasodilation.

Moffitt et al demonstrated coronary sinus lactate production in 3 of 11 patients with coronary artery disease during an isoflurane/oxygen anesthetic that was sufficiently deep to reduce systolic blood pressure by 30 percent.[91] They previously observed no instances of lactate production during halothane/oxygen and enflurane/oxygen anesthesia given to the same end-point, and suggested that this supports the concept of an isoflurane-associated redistribution of coronary blood flow.[78,81]

Reiz and Ostman studied the effects of isoflurane/nitrous oxide/oxygen anesthesia upon the GCVF/CSF ratio and found a close correlation between the change in blood flow and oxygen consumption in the corresponding region of the myocardium (Fig. 1-25).[100] However, the regression line was shifted to the left of the line of identity. Of the 13 patients, 3 had an increase in great cardiac vein blood flow despite an unchanged or decreased oxygen consumption. These 3 patients were ischemic in the same region as detected by electrocardiography and/or lactate balance measurements. Despite a pronounced fall in blood pressure and impedance of

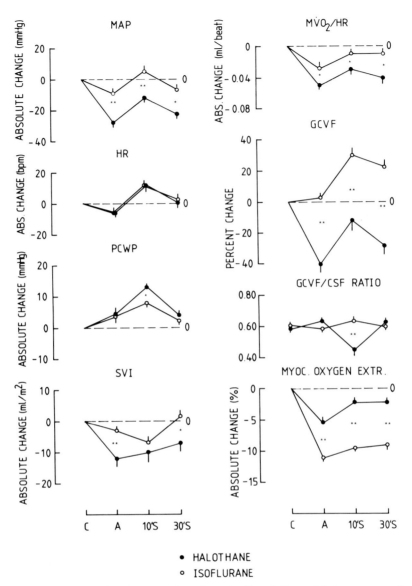

Fig. 1-23. Systemic and coronary hemodynamic effects before and during surgery and anesthesia with halothane or isoflurane administered in a blinded fashion in patients with ischemic heart disease undergoing aortoiliac reconstruction. Despite a higher infusion rate of phenylephrine, blood pressure was not as well maintained during halothane, and PCWP was higher. Nevertheless, oxygen extraction was lower with isoflurane, indicating markedly impaired coronary autoregulation. See text for details.

ejection, and an approximately 30 percent reduction in myocardial oxygen consumption in the area drained by the GCV, the GCVF/CSF ratio remained unaltered in only 2 of the 13 patients. Most ischemic patients had a reduction in this ratio. The GCVF/CSF ratio should remain unaltered unless one of the main coronary vessels is severely stenosed or redis-

tribution within the left ventricle is present. These data are again consistent with an isoflurane-associated impairment of coronary autoregulation with flow maldistribution.

Two other clinical studies of ischemia during isoflurane anesthesia derived data compatible with this theory, though interpreted to be in conflict.[48,101]

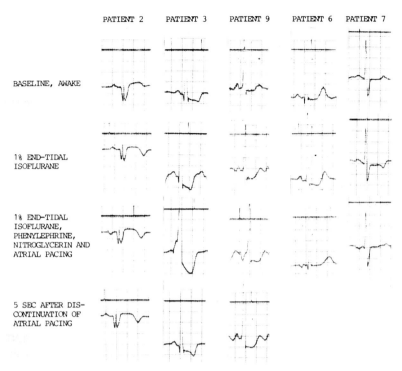

Fig. 1-24. ECG lead V_5 in five patients who developed ischemia during isoflurane anesthesia. Restoring blood pressure and left ventricular filling pressure to awake levels relieved ECG evidence of ischemia in only two patients. The data suggest that impaired coronary autoregulation could be responsible. (Reproduced from Reiz S, Balfors E, Sorensen MB, et al: Isoflurane—a powerful coronary vasodilator in patients with coronary artery disease. Anesthesiology 59:91–99, 1983, with permission.)

Hess et al studied the effects of adding isoflurane or halothane to patients in whom surgical stimulation during fentanyl/flunitrazepam anesthesia was causing hypertension.[48] Ischemia, as detected by a V_5 ECG lead, accompanied elevation of the blood pressure in 3 of 20 patients. Reduction of the blood pressure by either halothane (1 patient) or isoflurane (2 patients) was associated with reversal of the ECG changes, and both anesthetics reduced myocardial oxygen demand by reducing the left ventricular systolic pressure, SVR, and PCWP. The reduction in oxygen demand in the 2 isoflurane patients whose ischemia was relieved outweighed any adverse redistributive effect of the anesthetic, but does not permit conclusions regarding impairment of coronary autoregulation.

In the second study, Tarnow et al investigated the effects of atrial pacing on the ST segment of lead V_5 before and after induction of anesthesia with isoflurane/nitrous oxide/oxygen in patients with coronary artery disease.[101] When patients were paced to the same heart rate during anesthesia as awake, they had significantly less ST-segment depression, and the coronary perfusion pressure, left ventricular filling pressure, and rate pressure product (RPP) were lower. As in the previous study, myocardial oxygen demand was reduced. This may explain the lesser ST-segment depression, provided that the magnitude of ST-segment deviation is proportional to the metabolic severity of ischemia. The raw ECG data on 13 patients from this study have been plotted versus the RPP in Figure 1-26. Though RPP is a poor index of myocardial O_2 demand during anesthesia, it may adequately reflect myocardial oxygen demand during pacing or exercise-induced ischemia.[101-104] In 9 patients, decreases in RPP and ST-segment depression were closely correlated, and 4 of these patients had complete normalization of the ECG. In 3 of the remaining patients, the ST-segment abnormality was unchanged despite a comparable reduction in RPP. In the last patient, RPP was unchanged and the ST-segment depression increased from 0.015 to 0.020 mV. Thus, 4 of 13 patients did not have improvement of the index used to quantitate ischemia despite a

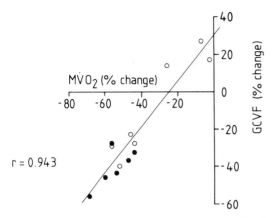

Fig. 1-25. Relationship between great cardiac vein blood flow (GCVF) and myocardial oxygen consumption in the corresponding area of the myocardium during isoflurane/ nitrous oxide anesthesia. The regression line is shifted to the left of the line of identity, suggesting interference with normal autoregulation. Note that three patients demonstrated ischemia despite elevated regional coronary blood flow and decreased regional oxygen consumption. Open symbols denote ischemic patients, closed symbols patients without ischemia. (Reproduced from Reiz S, Ostman M: Regional coronary hemodynamics during isoflurane-nitrous oxide anesthesia in patients with ischemic heart disease. Anesth Analg 64:570–576, 1985, with permission.)

reduction in the value used to quantitate myocardial oxygen demand. In these patients, it is not possible to exclude impairment of coronary autoregulation and flow redistribution as a contributing factor for ischemia.

Confirming evidence for the role of redistribution of coronary blood flow during isoflurane anesthesia has recently been obtained in animal models. Buffington et al performed experiments in dogs 4 weeks after gradual occlusion of the LAD, which permits collateralization of the LAD territory.[89] They demonstrated that 1% isoflurane shifted blood flow from collateral dependent to normal myocardium, despite constant heart rate, blood pressure, and total coronary blood flow. The maldistribution primarily affected the subendocardial zone (Fig. 1-27), and was associated with impairment of contraction in the area of the myocardium perfused by collaterals. Priebe has recently conducted crossover experiments in dogs with acutely narrowed LAD coronary arteries.* At the same perfusion pressure, heart rate, and left ventricular end-diastolic filling pressure, coronary blood flow to the region supplied by the stenosed artery was higher, and shortening was

*H Priebe, personal communication.

greater during halothane than during isoflurane anesthesia. In contrast, flow to the area supplied by the nonstenosed coronary artery was higher during isoflurane anesthesia, and contraction was normal during both anesthetics. Using quantitative angiography, Sill et al have demonstrated that distal coronary arterioles constitute the site of isoflurane-induced coronary vasodilation.[88]

There is compelling evidence that isoflurane, similar to other coronary vasodilators, can cause maldistribution of myocardial blood flow despite lowering myocardial oxygen demand. It appears prudent to maintain heart rate, blood pressure, and filling pres-

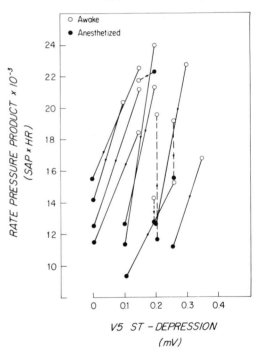

Fig. 1-26. Plot of rate-pressure product versus changes in ST segment of the ECG in patients with coronary artery disease while awake and during isoflurane anesthesia. Angina threshold was determined by atrial pacing while awake. The heart was paced to the same rate during isoflurane/nitrous oxide anesthesia. Of 13 patients, 3 had identical ECG changes despite achieving a lesser rate pressure product, and one had more severe depression. (Data replotted from Tarnow J, Markschies-Hornung A, Schulte-Sasse U: Isoflurane improves the tolerance to pacing-induced myocardial ischemia. Anesthesiology 64:147–157, 1986.)

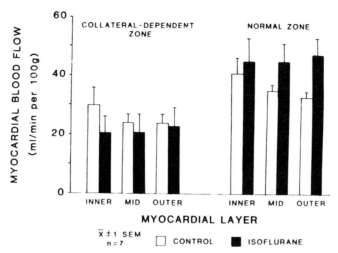

Fig. 1-27. Effect of isoflurane upon distribution of coronary blood flow in a canine model of chronic coronary occlusion. Isoflurane (1%) caused a redistribution of coronary blood flow away from collateral-dependent myocardium and away from the inner layers of the heart. (Reproduced from Buffington CW, Romson JL, Duttlinger NC: Does isoflurane cause coronary steal? Anesthesiology 63:A9, 1985, with permission.)

sure close to normal values if isoflurane is used in patients with coronary artery disease. Nevertheless, it is likely that instances of adverse redistribution of blood flow will still occur. The appropriate clinical response to recognition of this potentially adverse pharmacologic property is not immediately obvious and is certainly controversial. Some argue that isoflurane should not be administered to patients with coronary artery disease; while others remain unconvinced that adverse redistribution exists, or, if it exists, is unimportant compared to other beneficial properties of the drug.

Nitrous Oxide

Hemodynamic depression occurred when 50% nitrous oxide was added to enflurane or halothane anesthesia in patients undergoing myocardial revascularization.[105,106] Blood pressure, heart rate, cardiac index, SVR, and coronary sinus blood flow all decreased, but myocardial oxygen extraction increased. Mean lactate extraction diminished secondary to an increased coronary sinus lactate content without a change in arterial lactate levels. This suggests anaerobic glycolysis occurred distal to the coronary stenoses, but without ECG signs of ischemia.

Recently, Philbin et al studied dogs who had received high-dose fentanyl or sufentanil anesthesia, and observed postsystolic shortening in a region sup-

plied by a narrowed coronary artery when nitrous oxide was substituted for nitrogen (Fig. 1-28).[107] Coronary perfusion pressure, heart rate, and filling pressure were maintained constant, and regional coronary blood flow remained unchanged. These data are compatible with, but not diagnostic of, nitrous oxide-induced ischemia (see Chapter 3).

Effects of Interventions During Inhalational Anesthesia Upon the Coronary Circulation

Laryngoscopy, endotracheal intubation, and surgical stimulation appear to have profound effects on coronary autoregulation and the myocardial oxygen balance.

TRACHEAL INTUBATION

Moffitt et al reported the systemic and coronary effects of laryngoscopy and tracheal intubation in patients with coronary artery disease and good left ventricular function.[108] Anesthesia was provided with either thiopental/halothane or morphine/diazepam and pancuronium. Some patients received propranolol, 0.1 mg/kg IV, irrespective of pre-existing beta-adrenergic blockade. Systemic blood pressure declined 30 percent with induction and returned to control 1 minute postintubation. Heart rate increased significantly above control only in the halothane

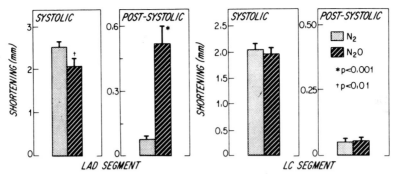

Fig. 1-28. Effect of nitrous oxide upon systolic and postsystolic shortening in regions supplied by a normal left circumflex or experimentally stenosed left anterior descending coronary artery. The data were acquired in seven dogs receiving a fentanyl infusion. The function of myocardium with a normal vascular supply was unchanged by nitrous oxide inhalation. Systolic shortening decreased and post-systolic shortening increased in the region supplied by the narrowed artery despite unchanged coronary artery blood flow, systemic hemodynamics or arterial oxygenation. The data are compatible with, but not diagnostic of, regional ischemia. (Reproduced from Philbin DM, Foex P, Drummond G, et al: Postsystolic shortening of canine left ventricle supplied by a stenotic coronary artery when nitrous oxide is added in the presence of narcotics. Anesthesiology 62:166–174, 1985, with permission.)

group. Coronary sinus blood flow increased significantly in the halothane group, but not in the morphine/diazepam group, and appeared to be related to the heart rate changes. Coronary sinus oxygenation decreased significantly (increased myocardial oxygen extraction) in both groups, suggesting that blood flow did not increase in proportion to the increased oxygen demand. However, none of the 29 patients was considered ischemic during intubation on the basis of the ECG or myocardial lactate balance studies.

In a large series of patients with coronary artery disease scheduled for vascular surgery, Reiz et al compared those who became ischemic as judged by the ECG, cardiokymography and/or myocardial lactate production ($n = 30$) with an age- and sex-matched control group of similar patients who did not ($n = 20$).[110] Patients received their usual cardiac medication approximately 1 hour before induction, along with a morphine premedication. Anesthesia was induced with low-dose fentanyl, thiopental, and enflurane, or isoflurane in oxygen to a mean systemic arterial pressure approximately 70 percent of their awake value. Muscle relaxation for intubation was provided by succinylcholine. Systemic and pulmonary arterial pressures, V_5 ECG, and coronary sinus blood flow were recorded continuously from immediately before insertion of the laryngoscope until well after the maximal hemodynamic changes had occurred (approximately 2 minutes). Patients

who became ischemic demonstrated an immediate decrease in coronary sinus blood flow in response to laryngoscopy (ie, within a few heart beats) (Fig. 1-29). In contrast, patients who did not become ischemic demonstrated no such change. Strikingly, mean arterial pressure, PCWP, and heart rate increased similarly in the two groups (Fig. 1-30). When the laryngoscope was removed, coronary sinus blood flow returned to control levels in the ischemic patients, though mean arterial pressure and PCWP, as well as heart rate, had progressively increased. This pattern persisted throughout the time of the maximal hemodynamic changes.

It is probable that neurogenically mediated vasoconstriction is responsible for the rapid initial decline of coronary blood flow. Interpretation of the subsequent changes in coronary sinus blood flow is more difficult, however, since an increase in flow in conjunction with the increase in myocardial oxygen demand is expected. Because Moffitt et al observed an increase in myocardial oxygen extraction, it is possible that all of these data are consistent with increased coronary vascular tone following intubation.[108]

Kleinman et al have recently demonstrated development of heterogeneous myocardial perfusion suggestive of myocardial ischemia in 45 percent of patients undergoing endotracheal intubation under either halothane or narcotic anesthesia. These observations were not accompanied by adverse hemody-

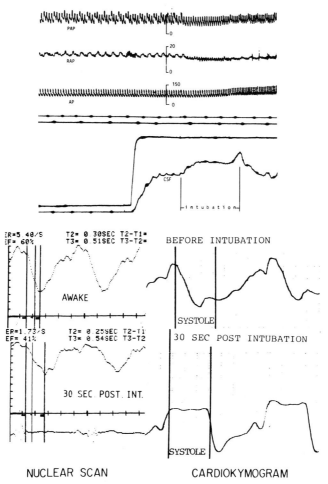

Fig. 1-29. Effects of laryngoscopy and intubation on hemodynamics and coronary blood flow (upper panel), scintigraphically-determined ejection fraction (lower left), and the cardiokymogram, which reflects anterior left ventricular wall motion (lower right) in one anesthetized patient with coronary artery disease. The upward shift of the mixed blood indicator resistance denotes a decrease in left ventricular coronary blood flow (CSF), which precedes changes in arterial pressure (AP), pulmonary artery pressure (PAP), or heart rate. Coronary blood flow returned to prelaryngoscopy levels when the laryngoscope was removed, despite the increased heart rate at this time. The associated ischemia is demonstrated by outward anterior wall motion and decreased ejection rate and ejection fraction. It is likely that the decreased coronary blood flow is due to vasospasm.

namic changes and are compatible with coronary vasospasm.[109]

SURGICAL STIMULATION

Only a few studies report coronary vascular responses to surgery, but the same lack of agreement noted previously exists in the hemodynamic response to surgery. In the study by Wilkinson et al,[75] sternotomy during high-dose morphine/nitrous oxide/oxy-gen anesthesia was associated with a greater increase in systemic blood pressure than during halothane/nitrous oxide/oxygen anesthesia, but there was a comparable increase in coronary blood flow. Myocardial oxygen extraction increased more in the halothane group, however. Myocardial oxygenation was inadequate, as judged by ECG changes or lactate production in 9 of 14 patients anesthetized with halothane, and 4 of 12 given morphine. In similar patients investigated by Hilfiker et al,[79] sternotomy

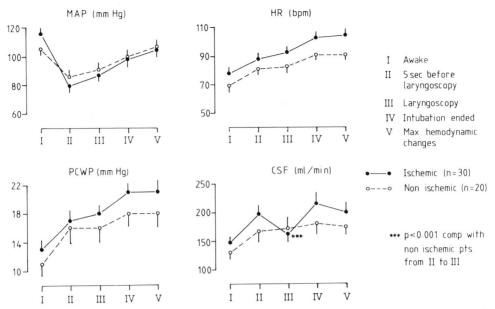

Fig. 1-30. Hemodynamics and coronary sinus blood flow before, during, and after laryngoscopy and tracheal intubation in 30 patients who became ischemic and 20 matched patients who did not. Note the similarity of changes in hemodynamics, but the immediate and transient decline of coronary sinus blood flow with laryngoscopy in the ischemic patients. The time course is suggestive of a neurogenic mechanism.

during halothane/nitrous oxide/oxygen anesthesia was not associated with either systemic or coronary hemodynamic changes, nor was ischemia recorded in any patient. Moffitt et al did not observe any systemic or coronary hemodynamic effects of sternotomy during enflurane/oxygen anesthesia.[81] Another group of patients with coronary artery disease subjected to aortoiliac reconstructive surgery during enflurane/nitrous oxide/oxygen anesthesia did not demonstrate any change in coronary blood flow or heart rate despite increases in systemic blood pressure, PCWP, and, hence, myocardial oxygen requirement.[110] Myocardial oxygenation was maintained, as judged by unchanged myocardial lactate extraction, by a pronounced increase in oxygen extraction to awake levels.

Larsen et al performed a randomized study comparing enflurane/nitrous oxide/oxygen with isoflurane/nitrous oxide/oxygen anesthesia.[111] The effects of anesthesia upon the systemic and coronary circulations were similar (Fig. 1-31). With sternotomy, however, important differences became apparent. As in the study of Reiz et al,[110] surgery during enflurane was associated with a return of coronary venous oxygen content to awake levels, and no instances of lactate production occurred. In contrast, coronary venous oxygen content remained elevated during isoflurane anesthesia, and myocardial lactate

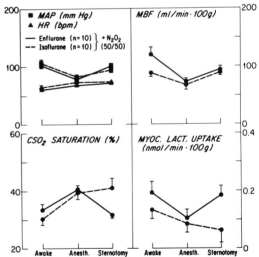

Fig. 1-31. Effect of anesthesia and sternotomy on hemodynamics and myocardial nutrition during enflurane/nitrous oxide or isoflurane/nitrous oxide anesthesia in patients with coronary artery disease. Heart rate and blood pressure responses were similar in the two groups of patients. Note that coronary sinus oxygenation remained elevated with sternotomy during isoflurane anesthesia despite decreasing lactate extraction. (Redrawn from data of Larsen R, Hilfiker O, Merkel G, et al: Myocardial oxygen balance during enflurane and isoflurane anesthesia for coronary artery surgery. Anesthesiology 61:A4, 1984, with permission.)

extraction continued to decline. Of 10 isoflurane patients, 1 produced lactate prior to sternotomy, and 3 thereafter.

Coronary hemodynamics during abdominal vascular surgery were also different between patients receiving halothane/ nitrous oxide /oxygen versus isoflurane/nitrous oxide/oxygen anesthesia in a blinded fashion (Fig. 1-23). Ten minutes after commencement of surgery, PCWP, heart rate, and mean arterial pressure were elevated relative to control in both groups. Mean arterial pressure was significantly lower and filling pressure higher in the halothane patients. Great cardiac vein blood flow increased similarly in both groups. Left ventricular oxygen extraction approached control during halothane, however, but remained profoundly decreased during isoflurane, indicating continued impairment of coronary autoregulation with the latter. In the halothane group, the GCVF/CSF ratio was decreased at this time, implying that flow through the LAD territory did not increase in proportion to total left ventricular blood flow. Flow-limiting stenoses in the LAD area, together with the lower driving pressure and higher filling pressure in the halothane patients, offer a possible explanation for this finding, and are compatible with animal experiments. Normalization of filling pressure by nitroglycerin after the 10-minute postincision measurement (needed in 80 percent of halothane patients) resulted in restoration of the GCVF/CSF ratio to normal.

Unfortunately, there are no studies of the impact of surgery on coronary hemodynamics and myocardial oxygenation in subjects with normal coronary vessels. Any conclusions derived thus may only be applicable to patients with ischemic heart disease, and, as noted above, such patients have abnormal coronary reactivity. Furthermore, because of the compromised vascular lumen, small changes in vascular tone (coronary spasm) may have profound flow-limiting effects (Fig. 1-32).

In summary, adjunctive drugs administered during anesthesia marginally affect the actions of the inhaled anesthetics upon the coronary circulation. In contrast, laryngoscopy, intubation, and surgical stimulation may partially or totally counteract the consequences of the inhalational anesthetics. This appears more effective during halothane or enflurane than isoflurane anesthesia. In the former, myocardial oxygen extraction increases and approaches normal, whereas in the latter, signs of persistent coronary vasodilation remain even when clear evidence of myocardial tissue oxygen deprivation exists. It thus appears that hyperperfusion and hypoperfusion may coexist with isoflurane.

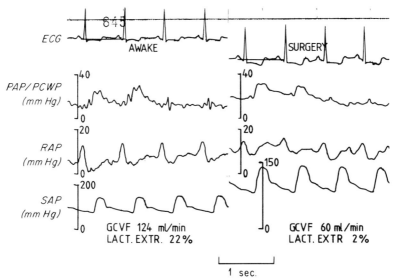

Fig. 1-32. The V_5 electrocardiogram, pulmonary artery, central venous and arterial pressures (top to bottom) before (left panel) and during fentanyl/isoflurane/nitrous oxide/oxygen anesthesia and surgery (right panel) in a vascular surgical patient with ischemic heart disease. ST-segment depression and reduction of myocardial lactate extraction developed despite comparable arterial blood pressure, pulmonary capillary wedge pressure, and heart rate. The marked decline in blood flow through the LAD area (GCVF) suggests coronary vasospasm as the mechanism.

REFERENCES

1. Brewster WR, Jr., Isaacs JP, Waino-Andersen T: Depressant effect of ether on myocardium of the dog and its modification by reflex release of epinephrine and norepinephrine. Am J Physiol 175:399–414, 1953

2. Price HL, Linde HW, Jones RE, et al: Sympathoadrenal response to general anesthesia in man and their relation to hemodynamics. Anesthesiology 20:563–575, 1959

3. Theye RA, Perry LB, Brizica SM: Influence of anesthetic agent on response to hemorrhagic hypotension. Anesthesiology 40:32–40, 1974

4. Bland JHL, Lowenstein E: Halothane-induced decrease in experimental myocardial ischemia in the non-failing canine heart. Anesthesiology 45:287–293, 1976

5. Sonnenblick EH: Implications of muscle mechanics in the heart. Fed Proc 21:975–990, 1962

6. Mahler F, Ross R, O'Rourke PA, et al: Effects of changes in preload, afterload and inotropic state on ejection and isovolumic phase measures of contractility in the conscious dog. Am J Cardiol 35:626–634, 1975

7. Cohn JD, Engler PE, Del Guercio LRM: The automated physiologic profile. Crit Care Med 3:51–58, 1975

8. Noble MIM, Trenchard D, Greg A: Left ventricular ejection in conscious dogs. The measurement and significance of maximum acceleration of blood from the left ventricle. Circ Res 19:139–144, 1966

9. Sagawa, K: End-systolic pressure-volume relationship in retrospect and prospect. Fed Proc 43:2399–2401, 1984

10. Suga H, Yamada O, Goto Y: Energetics of ventricular contraction as traced in the pressure-volume diagram. Fed Proc 43:2411–2413, 1984

11. Rankin JS, McHale PA, Arentzen CE, et al: The three-dimensional dynamic geometry of the left ventricle in the conscious dog. Circulation 56:304–313, 1976

12. Grossman, W, Braunwald E, Mann T, et al: Contractile state of the left ventricle in man as evaluated from end-systolic pressure-volume relations. Circulation 56:845–852, 1977

13. Marsh JD, Green LH, Wynne J, et al: Left ventricular end-systolic pressure-dimension and stress-length relations in normal human subjects. Am J Cardiol 44:1311–1317, 1979

14. Mehmel HC, Stockins B, Ruffmann K, et al: The linearity of the end-systolic pressure-volume relationship in man and its sensitivity for assessment of left ventricular function. Circulation 63:1216–1222, 1981

15. Sagawa K: The end-systolic pressure-volume relation of the ventricle: Definition, modifications and clinical use. Circulation 63:1223–1227, 1981

16. Kemmotsu O, Hashimoto Y, Shimosato S: Inotropic effects of isoflurane on mechanics of contraction in isolated cat papillary muscles from normal and failing hearts. Anesthesiology 39:470–477, 1973

17. Vatner SF, Smith NT: Effects of halothane on left ventricular function and distribution of regional blood flow in dogs and primates. Circ Res 34:155–167, 1974

18. Filner BE, Karliner JS: Alterations of normal left ventricular performance by general anesthesia. Anesthesiology 45:610–621, 1976

19. Lowenstein E, Clark JD, Villareal Y: Excess lactate production during halothane anesthesia in man. JAMA 190:110–113, 1964

20. Van Trigt P, Christian CC, Fagraeus L, et al: Myocardial depression by anesthetic agents (Halothane, enflurane and nitrous oxide): Quantitation based on end-systolic pressure-dimension relations. Am J Cardiol 53:243–247, 1984

21. Kemmotsu O, Hashimoto Y, Shimosato S: The effects of fluroxene and enflurane on contractile performance of isolated papillary muscles from failing hearts. Anesthesiology 40:252–260, 1974

22. Prys-Roberts C, Roberts JG, Foex P, et al: Interaction of anesthesia, beta-receptor blockade and blood loss in dogs with induced myocardial infarction. Anesthesiology 45:326–339, 1976

23. Roberts JG, Foex P, Clarke TNS, et al: Haemodynamic interactions of high-dose propranolol pretreatment and anaesthesia in the dog. I: Halothane dose-response studies. Br J Anaesthesiol 48:315–325, 1976

24. Lowenstein E, Foex P, Francis CM, et al: Regional ischemic ventricular dysfunction in myocardium supplied by a narrowed coronary artery with increasing halothane concentration in the dog. Anesthesiology 55:349–359, 1981

25. Calverley RK, Smith NT, Jones CW, et al: Cardiovascular effects of enflurane anesthesia during controlled ventilation in man. Anesth Analg 57:619–628, 1978

26. Eger EI, Smith NT, Stoelting RK, et al: Cardiovascular effects of halothane in man. Anesthesiology 32:396–409, 1970

27. Eger EI: Isoflurane: A review. Anesthesiology 55:559–576, 1981

28. Eger EI: Isoflurane: A compendium and reference. Published by Anaquest, a division of BOC Inc., Madison, WI, 1984

29. Clinical evaluation of isoflurane: Pulse and blood pressure. Can Anesth Soc J 29(Suppl):S15–S27, 1982

30. Roizen MF, Horrigan RW, Frazer BM: Anesthetic doses blocking adrenergic (Stress) and cardiovascular responses to incision—MAC BAR. Anesthesiology 54:390–398, 1981

31. Linde HW, Oh SO, Homi J, et al: Cardiovascular effects of isoflurane and halothane during controlled ventilation in older patients. Anesth Analg 54:701–794, 1975

32. Mallow JE, White RD, Cucchiara RF, et al: Hemodynamic effects of isoflurane and halothane in patients with coronary artery disease. Anesth Analg 55:135–138, 1976

33. Tarnow J, Bruckner JB, Eberlein HJ, et al: Haemodynamics and myocardial oxygen consumption during isoflurane (Forane) anesthesia in geriatric patients. Br J Anaesthesiol 48:669–675, 1976

34. Cahalan MK, Lurz FW, Beaupre PN, et al: Narcotics alter the heart rate and blood pressure response to inhalational anesthetics. Anesthesiology 59:A26, 1983

35. Smith NT, Corbascio AN: The cardiovascular effects of nitrous oxide during halothane anesthesia in the dog. Anesthesiology 27:560–566, 1966

36. Winter PM, Hornbein TF, Smith G: Hyperbaric nitrous oxide anesthesia in man. Determination of anesthetic potency (MAC) and cardiorespiratory effects. Abstracts of American Society of Anesthesiologists Annual Meeting, Boston, 103–104, October 1972

37. Dolan WM, Stevens WC, Eger EI II, et al: The cardiovascular and respiratory effects of isoflurane-nitrous oxide anesthesia. Can Anaesth Soc J 21:557–568, 1974

38. Smith NT, Calverley RK, Prys-Roberts C, et al: Impact of nitrous oxide on the circulation during enflurane anesthesia in man. Anesthesiology 48:345–349, 1978

39. Eisele JH, Smith NT: Cardiovascular effects of 40 percent nitrous oxide in man. Anesth Analg 51:956–963, 1972

40. Eger EI, II: Should we not use nitrous oxide? *In* Nitrous Oxide/N₂O, Elsevier/North Holland, New York and Amsterdam, 1985

41. Brown BR, Crout R: A comparative study of the effects of five general anesthetics on myocardial contractility: I: Isometric conditions. Anesthesiology 34:236–245, 1971

42. Price HL: Calcium reverses myocardial depression caused by halothane: Site of action. Anesthesiology 41:576–579, 1974

43. Merin RG, Basch S: Are the myocardial functional and metabolic effects of isoflurane really different from those of halothane and enflurane? Anesthesiology 55:398–408, 1981

44. Lynch C: Differential depression of myocardial contractility by halothane and isoflurane in vitro. Anesthesiology 64:620–631, 1986

45. Price ML, Price HL: Effect of general anesthetics on contractile response of rabbit aorta strips. Anesthesiology 23:16–20, 1962

46. Sprague DH, Yang JC, Ngai SH: Effects of isoflurane and halothane on contractility and the cyclic 3', 5'-adenosine monophosphate system in the rat aorta. Anesthesiology 40:162–167, 1974

47. Doherty F, Wilkinson PL, Robinson S: Enflurane reduces systemic pressure during cardiopulmonary bypass more effectively than halothane. Anesthesiology 55:A40, 1981

48. Hess W, Arnold B, Schulte-Sasse U, et al: Comparison of isoflurane and halothane when used to control intraoperative hypertension in patients undergoing coronary artery bypass surgery. Anesth Analg 62:15–20, 1983

49. Roizen MF, Hamilton WK, Sohn YJ: Treatment of stress-induced increases in pulmonary capillary wedge pressure using volatile anesthetics. Anesthesiology 55:446–450, 1981

50. Bailar JC, III: When research results are in conflict. N Engl J Med 313:1080–1081, 1985

51. Klocke FJ: Coronary blood flow in man. Prog Cardiovasc Dis 19:117–132, 1976

52. Ganz W, Tamura K, Marcus HS, et al: Measurement of coronary sinus blood flow by continuous thermodilution in man. Circulation 44:181–186, 1971

53. Bellamy RF: Diastolic coronary pressure-flow relation in the dog. Circ Res 43:92–101, 1978

54. Verrier ED, Edelist G, Macke C, et al: Greater coronary vascular reserve in dogs anesthetized with halothane. Anesthesiology 53:445–459, 1980

55. Chilian WM, Marcus ML: Phasic coronary blood flow velocity in intramural and epicardial coronary arteries. Circ Res 50:775–781, 1982

56. Klocke FJ, Mates RE, Canty JM, Jr., et al: Response to the article by Spaan on "Coronary diastolic pressure-flow relation and zero flow pressure explained on the basis of intramyocardial compliance." Circ Res 56:791–792, 1985

57. Spaan JAE: Controversies in cardiovascular research. Response to the article by Klocke et al on "Coronary pressure-flow relationships: Controversial issues and probable implications." Circ Res 56:789–790, 1985

58. Opie LH, Owen P, Thomas M, et al: Coronary sinus lactate measurements in assessment of myocardial ischemia. Am J Cardiol 32:295–305, 1973

59. Bellamy RS, Lowensohn HS: Effect of systole on coronary pressure-flow relations in the right ventricle of the dog. Am J Physiol 7:H481–H486, 1980

60. Lowenstein E, Hill RD, Rajagopalan B, et al: Winnie the Pooh revisited, or, the more recent adventures of piglet. Anesthesiology 56:81–83, 1982

61. Deanfield JE, Maseri A, Selwyn AP, et al: Myocardial ischaemia during daily life in patients with stable angina: Its relation to symptoms and heart rate changes. Lancet 2:753–758, 1983

62. Most AS, Williams DO, Gewirtz H: Elevated coronary vascular resistance in the presence of reduced resting blood flow distal to a severe coronary stenosis. Cardiovasc Res 19:599–605, 1985

63. Feldman RL, Nichols WW, Pepine CJ, et al: The

coronary hemodynamics of left main and branch coronary stenoses. J Thorac Cardiovasc Surg 77:377–388, 1979

64. Waltier DC, Gross GJ, Brooks HL: Coronary-steal induced increase in myocardial infarct size after pharmacologic coronary vasodilation. Am J Cardiol 46:83–89, 1980

65. Becker LC: Conditions for vasodilator-induced coronary steal in experimental myocardial ischemia. Circulation 57:1103–1110, 1978

66. Gewirtz H, Gross SL, Williams DO, et al: Contrasting effects of nifedipine and adenosine on regional myocardial flow distribution and metabolism distal to a severe coronary arterial stenosis. Observations in sedated, closed-chest domestic swine. Circulation 69:1048–1057, 1984

67. Gallagher KP, Osakada G, Matsuzaki M, et al: Myocardial blood flow and function with critical coronary stenosis in exercising dogs. Am J Physiol 12:H698–707, 1982

68. Schwartz JS: Effect of distal coronary pressure on rigid and compliant coronary stenoses. Am J Physiol 245:(Heart Circ Physiol 14) H1054–1060, 1983

69. Slogoff S, Keats AS: Does perioperative myocardial ischemia lead to postoperative myocardial infarction? Anesthesiology 62:107–114, 1985

70. Tarnow J, Eberlein HJ, Oser G, et al: Haemodynamik, Myokardkontraktilitat, Ventrikelvolumina, und Sauerstoffversorgung des Herzens unter verschiedenen Inhalationsanesthetika. Anaesthetist 26:220–226, 1977

71. Domenech RJ, Macho P, Valdes J, et al: Coronary vascular resistance during halothane anesthesia. Anesthesiology 46:236–240, 1977

72. Sybert PE, Hickey RF, Hoar PF, et al: Effects of volatile anesthetics on the regulation of coronary blood flow. Anesthesiology 59:A24, 1983

73. Francis CM, Foex P, Lowenstein E, et al: The interaction between regional myocardial ischaemia and left ventricular performance under halothane anesthesia. Br J Anaesthesiol 34:965–979, 1982

74. Buffington CW: Halothane, per se, does not cause ischemic myocardial dysfunction in the presence of coronary stenosis. Anesthesiology 63:A20, 1985

75. Wilkinson PL, Hamilton WK, Moyers JR, et al: Halothane and morphine-nitrous oxide anesthesia in patients undergoing coronary artery bypass operation—patterns of intraoperative ischemia. J Thorac Cardiovasc Surg 82:372–378, 1981

76. Sonntag H, Merin RG, Donath U, et al: Myocardial metabolism and oxygenation in man awake and during halothane anesthesia. Anesthesiology 51:204–210, 1979

77. Reiz S, Balfors E, Gustavsson B, et al: Effects of halothane on coronary hemodynamics and myocardial metabolism in patients with ischaemic heart disease and heart failure. Acta Anaesth Scand 26:133–138, 1982

78. Moffitt E, Sethna D, Gray R, et al: Nitrous oxide added to halothane reduces coronary flow and myocardial oxygen consumption in patients with coronary disease. Can Anaesth Soc J 30:5–9, 1983

79. Hilfiker O, Larsen R, Sonntag H: Myocardial blood flow and oxygen consumption during halothane-nitrous oxide anesthesia for coronary revascularization. Br J Anaesthesia 55:927–932, 1983

80. Rydvall A, Haggmark S, Nyhman H, et al: Effects of enflurane on coronary haemodynamics in patients with ischaemic heart disease. Acta Anaesthesiol Scand 28:690–695, 1984

81. Moffitt EA, Imrie DD, Scovil JE, et al: Myocardial metabolism and haemodynamic responses with enflurane anaesthesia for coronary artery surgery. Can Anaesth Soc J 31:604–610, 1984

82. Moffitt EA, McIntyre AJ, Barker RA, et al: Myocardial metabolism and hemodynamic responses with fentanyl-enflurane anesthesia for coronary artery surgery. Anesth Analg 65:46–52, 1986

83. Pepine CJ, Mehta J, Webster W, et al: In vivo validation of a dilution method to determine regional left ventricular blood flow in patients with coronary disease. Circulation 58:795–802, 1978

84. Roberts DL, Nakazawa HK, Klocke FJ: Origin of the great cardiac vein and coronary sinus drainage within the left ventricle. Am J Physiol 230(2):486–492, 1976

85. Lundeen G, Manohar M, Parks C: Systemic distribution of blood flow in swine while awake and during 1.0 and 1.5 MAC isoflurane anesthesia with or without 50% nitrous oxide. Anesth Analg 62:499–512, 1983

86. Gelman S, Fowler KC, Smith LR: Regional blood flow during isoflurane and halothane anesthesia. Anesth Analg 63:557–565, 1984

87. Vogel H, Gunther H, Harrison DK, et al: The influence of isoflurane and enflurane on tissue oxygenation and microcirculation of the dog myocardium. Anesthesiology 61:A5, 1984

88. Sill JC, Bove AA, Nugent M: Effects of isoflurane on proximal and distal coronary vasculature in intact dogs. Anesthesiology 63:A11, 1985

89. Buffington CW, Romson JL, Duttlinger NC: Does isoflurane cause coronary steal? Anesthesiology 63:A9, 1985

90. Reiz S, Balfors E, Sorensen MB, et al: Isoflurane—a powerful coronary vasodilator in patients with coronary artery disease. Anesthesiology 59:91–99, 1983

91. Moffitt EA, Barker RA, Glenn JJ, et al: Myocardial metabolism and hemodynamic responses with isoflurane anesthesia for coronary artery surgery. Anesth Analg 65:53–61, 1986

92. Harder DR, Belardinelli L, Sperelakis N: Differential effects of adenosine and nitroglycerine on the action potentials of large and small arteries. Circ Res 44:176–182, 1979

93. Becker LC: Effect of nitroglycerin and dipyridamole

on regional left ventricular blood flow during coronary artery occlusion. J Clin Invest 58:1287–1296, 1976

94. Henry PD, Shuchleib R, Borda LJ, et al: Effects of nifedipine on myocardial perfusion and ischemic injury in dogs. Circ Res 43:372–380, 1978

95. Chiariello M, Gold HK, Leinbach RC, et al: Deleterious effects of nitroprusside in myocardial injury during acute myocardial infarction. Circulation 54:766–773, 1976

96. Albro PC, Gould KL, Westcoot RJ, et al: Noninvasive assessment of coronary stenoses by myocardial imaging during pharmacologic coronary vasodilation. III. Clinical trial. Am J Cardiol 42:751–760, 1978

97. Leppo JA, O'Brien J, Rothendler JA, et al: Dipyridamole-thallium-201 scintigraphy in the prediction of future cardiac events after acute myocardial infarction. N Engl J Med 310:1014–1018, 1984

98. Leppo JA, Boucher CA, Okada RD, et al: Serial thallium-201 myocardial imaging after dipyridamole infusion: Diagnostic utility in detecting coronary stenoses and relationship to regional wall motion. Circulation 66:649–657, 1982

99. Boucher CA, Brewster DC, Darling RC: Determination of cardiac risk by dipyridamole-thallium imaging before peripheral vascular surgery. N Engl J Med 312:389–394, 1985

100. Reiz S, Ostman M: Regional coronary hemodynamics during isoflurane-nitrous oxide anesthesia in patients with ischemic heart disease. Anesth Analg 64:570–576, 1985

101. Tarnow J, Markschies-Hornung A, Schulte-Sasse U: Isoflurane improves the tolerance to pacing-induced myocardial ischemia. Anesthesiology 64:147–157, 1986

102. Reiz S, Haggmark S, Ostman M: Invasive analysis of noninvasive indicators of myocardial work and ischaemia during anesthesia soon after myocardial infarction. Acta Anaesth Scand 25:303–310, 1981

103. Moffitt EA, Sethna DH, Gray RJ, et al: Rate-pressure product correlates poorly with myocardial oxygen consumption during anesthesia in coronary patients. Can Anaesth Soc J 31:5–12, 1984

104. Gobel FL, Nordstrom LA, Nelson R, et al: The rate-pressure product as an index of myocardial oxygen consumption during exercise in patients with angina pectoris. Circulation 57:549–556, 1978

105. Moffitt EA, Scovill JE, Barker RA, et al: The effects of nitrous oxide on myocardial metabolism and hemodynamics during fentanyl and enflurane anesthesia in patients with coronary disease. Anesth Analg 63:1071–1075, 1984

106. Moffitt EA, Sethna DH, Gray RJ, et al: Nitrous oxide added to halothane reduces coronary flow and myocardial oxygen consumption in patients with coronary disease. Can Anaesth Soc J 30:5–9, 1983

107. Philbin DM, Foex P, Drummond G, et al: Postsystolic shortening of canine left ventricle supplied by a stenotic coronary artery when nitrous oxide is added in the presence of narcotics. Anesthesiology 62:166–174, 1985

108. Moffitt EA, Sethna DH, Bussell JA, et al: Effects of intubation on coronary blood flow and myocardial oxygenation. Can Anaesth Soc J 32:105–111, 1985

109. Kleinman F, Henkin RE, Glisson SN, et al: Qualitative evaluation of coronary flow during anesthetic induction using Thallium-201 perfusion scans. Anesthesiology 64:157–164, 1986

110. Reiz S, Rydvall A, Haggmark S: Coronary haemodynamic effects of surgery during enflurane-nitrous oxide anaesthesia in patients with ischaemic heart disease. Acta Anaesthesiol Scand 29:106–112, 1985

111. Larsen R, Hilfiker O, Merkel G, et al: Myocardial oxygen balance during enflurane and isoflurane anesthesia for coronary artery surgery. Anesthesiology 61:A4, 1984

Frederick O. Holley, M.D.

2

Pharmacokinetics in the Cardiac Patient

THE DOSE-RESPONSE RELATIONSHIP

It has long been recognized that the administration of anesthetic drugs is complicated by the presence of cardiac disease. As early as 1847, John Snow wrote in the London Medical Gazette:

"Any organic disease which impedes the flow of blood through the heart and lungs would seem to contraindicate the exhibition of ether by inhalation."[1]

As well as heralding a modern inclination toward intravenous agents in the compromised cardiac patient, Snow pointed out that this patient may have an altered anesthetic dose-response relationship. While Snow's experience was with the volatile anesthetic drugs, this observation certainly holds true for the intravenously administered agents as well.

The practical rationale for studying the dose-response relationship is one of predictive capacity and its impact on therapeutics. If a certain class of patients were all to deviate in one direction from normal in their response to a standard dose of a drug, the response might be brought back into line in a subsequent similar patient by altering the drug dose. For example, if elimination of an anesthetic drug should be found to be linearly related to cardiac output, future anesthetics could be tailored to the indi-

vidual patient on the basis of this physiologic measurement. Studies of pharmacology in disease states thus usually focus on correlating some aspect of the dose-response relationship with some measurement of abnormal physiology.

Under further scrutiny, the dose-response relationship can be separated into two components (Fig. 2-1). The first of these, pharmacokinetics, relates drug dose to its subsequent concentration in body fluids and tissues. It therefore encompasses such processes as drug absorption (for extravascular administration), distribution, and elimination. The second component, pharmacodynamics, relates drug concentration to response.

It should be conceptually clear that it is possible to study the pharmacokinetics of a drug while neglecting its pharmacodynamics. Drug doses are recorded, and concentrations, usually in blood, serum, or plasma, are measured. Abnormal pharmacokinetics are then related, qualitatively, to a previously observed or anticipated shift in the dose-response relationship. This reasoning process is correct only if the other part of the relationship, pharmacodynamics, remains constant. The inference of causality is not logically impeccable, only pragmatic. However, the vast majority of pharmacologic studies in disease states are of this nature. On the other hand,

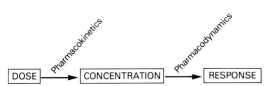

Fig. 2-1. The components of the dose-response relationship.

pharmacodynamics cannot be quantified while neglecting pharmacokinetics except in special cases of the in vitro preparation or at steady state when drug concentrations are unchanging and in equilibrium among all body tissues. Thus, pharmacodynamic studies require an integrative approach including simultaneous pharmacokinetic analysis. The requisite theory and conceptual model are complex and have only been described in detail in the last several years.[2] Pharmacodynamic data in disease states, particularly with respect to the cardiac patient, are thus understandably sparse. This chapter will focus on pharmacokinetics in the cardiac patient. Altered pharmacokinetics translate into an altered dose-response relationship with the premise, as noted above, that pharmacodynamics remain unchanged. Pharmacodynamic data will be presented whenever available. Before pharmacokinetic data on specific drugs can be appreciated, a summary of pharmacokinetic principles is essential. The reader who wishes more pharmacokinetic background than this summary can provide is referred to several recent textbooks for anesthesiologists on the subject.[3-5]

The purpose of this presentation is to aid in understanding such observations as are shown in Figures 2-2 and 2-3. Figure 2-2 depicts the effects of cardiopulmonary bypass (CPB) on fentanyl disposition.[6] Fentanyl, 500 μg, was injected intravenously at time zero. In contrast to the results in the control (nonbypass) patient in panel B, the initiation of CPB in panel A appears to cause a fall in plasma fentanyl levels; and the termination of CPB, a brief rise. The decline of fentanyl levels in the postoperative period appears slower in the CPB patient than in the control patient. This finding of slowed drug elimination is a common thread in the study of Walker et al,[7] who examined *d*-tubocurarine (dTc) disposition during surgery involving CPB (Fig. 2-3). However, in contrast to the findings with fentanyl, these authors observed that dTc concentrations increased on initiation of CPB; and, during bypass, actually remained higher than those observed in a group of normal subjects (shaded area). However, their drug administration regimen included an infusion rather than just the single bolus given in the fentanyl study. The extreme physiological changes of CPB can clearly produce striking pharmacokinetic alterations that may have widely differing effects on specific drugs, depending on their basic pharmacology. After a brief historical review, basic pharmacokinetic principles will be presented with the goal of understanding and explaining some of these effects.

The study of pharmacokinetics has its roots in the early part of this century in basic physiologic research; and, also, as noted above, in early investigations in anesthetic pharmacology. In 1924, continuing John Snow's interest, Haggard published a classic series of articles on the uptake, distribution, and elimination of diethyl ether.[8] To both Snow and Haggard, it was evident that any explanation of ether's effects had to take into account the factors influencing its uptake, distribution, and elimination (that is, its pharmacokinetics). Clearly, physiology (either normal or altered) was intimately involved.

Physiologically based pharmacokinetic models, or "perfusion" models, present the body as composed of a number of tissues each with known anatomical mass, perfusion, and drug solubility coefficient.[9] The rate and extent of drug distribution and the concentration of drug in any tissue at any time can be calculated from these parameters. Drug elimination from the body can be related to biochemically measured activity of hepatic enzymatic processes or renal transport mechanisms. An example of a physiologic pharmacokinetic model for thiopental is shown in Figure 2-4.

Characterization of the pharmacokinetic behavior of the volatile anesthetic agents using perfusion models has met with considerable success, particularly in the hands of Eger[10] and Mapleson.[11] In the 1960s, a number of investigators advanced physiologic pharmacokinetic models for thiopental[12-14] that were useful in understanding the relative roles of redistribution and metabolism in terminating thiopental's effects. The strengths of physiologic modeling lie in its ability to predict drug concentrations in any specified tissue at any time and in its ability to forecast the effect of any specific aberration in physiology (eg, altered organ blood flow or organ size) on drug disposition. The limitation of such an approach, however, is that a great deal of anatomic, physiologic, and physicochemical data (Fig. 2-4) is required in order to construct and to verify such a model. Tissue samples for determination of drug concentrations or the opportunity to measure individual organ blood flows are seldom available in humans.

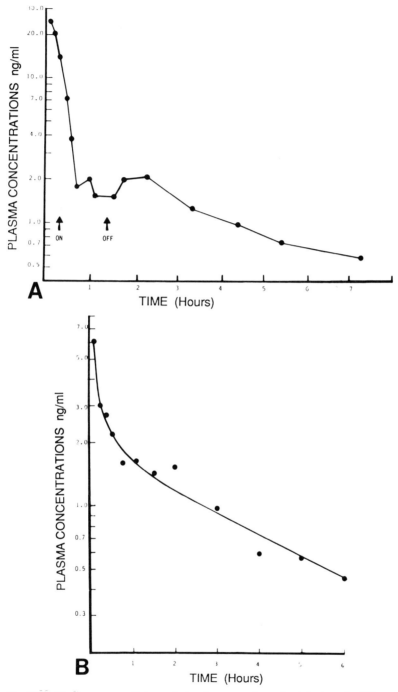

Fig. 2-2. The time course of plasma fentanyl concentrations after injection of a 500 μg IV bolus at time zero: (A) data from a cardiac surgery patient. Times of CPB are indicated by the arrows. (B) Data from a vascular surgery control patient. (From Koska AJ, Romagnoli A, Kramer WG: Effect of cardiopulmonary bypass on fentanyl distribution and elimination. Clin Pharmacol Ther 29:100–105, 1981, with permission.)

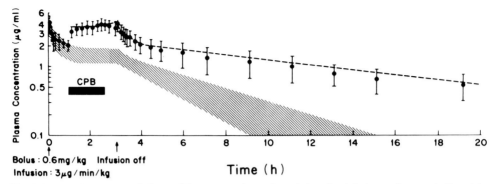

Fig. 2-3. The time course of plasma dTc concentrations after a bolus plus infusion regimen as indicated in patients undergoing cardiac surgery with CPB. Data is mean ± SD from 13 patients with a computer-predicted pharmacokinetic model (dashed line). The shaded area represents the range of concentrations in a group of normal subjects. (From Walker JS, Shanks CA, Brown KF: Altered d-tubocurarine disposition during cardiopulmonary bypass surgery. Clin Pharmacol Ther 35:686–694, 1984, with permission.)

Because of these practical limitations, investigators in pharmacology have turned, for the most part, to compartmental pharmacokinetic models such as that shown in Figure 2-5. In the two-compartment model depicted, drugs are administered into the central compartment (for intravascular administration) and also are considered to be eliminated from that compartment by organs of metabolism or excretion. Drugs may also distribute from the central to the peripheral compartment and back again, much as a drug might be taken up from the bloodstream by a

specified tissue in a perfusion model. The advantage of such a compartmental model is that differential equations can be written in the abstract to describe drug amounts and concentrations in each compartment. A whole series of such models and equations exists that describes systems of different volumes and different rates of distribution and elimination. These equations can then be compared with real blood level data (since intravascular doses are administered into the blood, it is assumed to be in the central compartment) to find the equation that fits the data best. That equation can then be used in a predictive fashion. The two-compartment model was first described by Teorell in 1937.[15] The mathematics are more fully explored below.

The beauty of such a model is in its conceptual simplicity, in its exact mathematical description, and in the fact that its parameters can be quantified using only blood-level data, which experimentally is most easily obtained. The price for this simplicity is that the exact anatomic and physiologic correspondences of the perfusion model are lost. The blood or plasma is the only tissue that can be stated unequivocally to be part of the central compartment. Other tissues of the vessel-rich group may or may not be part of the central compartment, and this may vary by drug, depending on the rapidity of blood/tissue equilibration. The peripheral compartment, in general, may be considered to be composed of less well-perfused tissues. However, it must be remembered that mathematically it is only an average of such tissues and, as such, may not correspond to any one specifically. Drug elimination is simply a mathematical description of the rate of fall of blood levels of drug once distribution is complete. The description does not

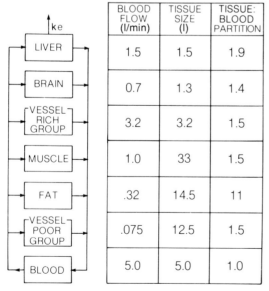

	BLOOD FLOW (l/min)	TISSUE SIZE (l)	TISSUE: BLOOD PARTITION
LIVER	1.5	1.5	1.9
BRAIN	0.7	1.3	1.4
VESSEL RICH GROUP	3.2	3.2	1.5
MUSCLE	1.0	33	1.5
FAT	.32	14.5	11
VESSEL POOR GROUP	.075	12.5	1.5
BLOOD	5.0	5.0	1.0

Fig. 2-4. A physiologic pharmacokinetic model of thiopental disposition constructed from the data of Saidman et al[13] by Stanski et al.[3]

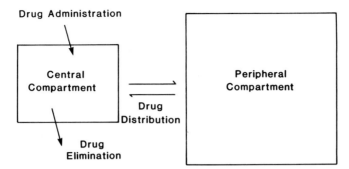

Fig. 2-5. A two-compartment pharmacokinetic model to describe drug disposition. Drug is administered into the central compartment (intravenously) and is assumed to be eliminated only from the central compartment.

imply any exact relationship to physiology. Clearly, a major reason for the interest in pharmacokinetics is to understand the effects of altered anatomy and physiology. It must be kept in mind, however, that for compartmental pharmacokinetic models the anatomic and physiologic correspondences are implied rather than implicit. This is the price that is paid for practical limitations in data collection and for the convenience of a mathematical solution.

BASIC PHARMACOKINETICS

The One-Compartment Model

Conceptually, it will be most straightforward to backtrack a little in the historical development of these ideas and to develop the basic pharmacokinetic concepts in terms of an even simpler model, the one-compartment model shown in Figure 2-6. Complexity will then be added by reintroducing the added

dimension of drug distribution as shown in Figure 2-5.

The one-compartment model is exactly analogous to the two-compartment model except that it lacks the peripheral compartment. Conceptually, the drug dose is placed into a volume of distribution (V_d) where it is assumed to be well mixed. (This assumption is a gross physiologic oversimplification and will be rectified in the discussion below of the multicompartment model.) The initial concentration of drug, C_o, in the volume of distribution is therefore:

$$C_o = \frac{\text{Dose}}{V_d} \qquad (2\text{-}1)$$

A sample (blood) is taken from V_d and the concentration of the drug in it is measured at time zero. If the concentration of drug is high, the drug is one with a small volume of distribution. If it is low, the volume of distribution is large. Thiopental and fentanyl are both drugs with relatively large volumes of distribution. In physicochemical and anatomic terms, this is true because these lipid soluble drugs distrib-

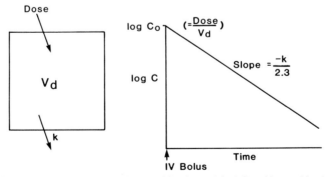

Fig. 2-6. A one-compartment pharmacokinetic model (left) with graphic depiction (right) of drug levels after an intravenous bolus.

ute extensively into body tissues, leaving only low concentrations in the blood. The volume of distribution may be larger than actual body size since it is only a conceptual volume.

Once the initial concentration, C_o, is defined, its rate of decline becomes of interest. Here, the compartmental pharmacokinetic model makes one assumption; that is, that the process of drug elimination from the body is first-order.*

In other words, the rate of change of the drug concentration, C, at any time, t, is proportional simply to that drug concentration, $C(t)$:

$$\frac{dC(t)}{dt} = k \cdot C(t) \qquad (2\text{-}2)$$

k is a proportionality constant or rate constant. First-order processes are extremely common in biology; and, empirically, almost all drugs behave in this fashion when administered in pharmacologic doses. Solving (integrating) Equation 2-2 for $C(t)$:

$$C(t) = C_o \cdot e^{-kt} \qquad (2\text{-}3)$$

This equation describes an exponential decline in drug concentration, $C(t)$, with time. At time zero, the concentration is C_o since e^{-kt} is equal to one. The exponential decline is, thus, a corollary to the first-order process.

Now for the sake of convenience in graphic display, the logarithm of Eq. 2-3 is obtained:

$$\log C(t) = \log C_o - \frac{kt}{2.3} \qquad (2\text{-}4)$$

where 2.3 is the logarithm of 10 to the base e. This equation describes a line with intercept log C_o and slope, $-k/2.3$, as shown in Figure 2-6. The concentration of drug, $C(t)$, in the volume V_d thus declines

---

*When related to the Michaelis-Menten equation[16] describing enzyme kinetics:

$$V = \frac{V_{max} \cdot C}{K_m + C}$$

This assumption implies that the drug concentration (C) must be well below K_m, the drug concentration that produces a reaction velocity (V), which is half the maximum (V_{max}). Notable exceptions are ethyl alcohol, salicylates, and thiopental when given in extremely high doses (cerebral resuscitation).

in a log-linear fashion with time. This semi-log display is a tremendous convenience, considering the frequency of first-order processes in biology.

Along with the concept of the first-order process goes the concept of half-life, the time for the original amount or concentration to be reduced by one-half. This occurs when:

$$e^{-kt} = \tfrac{1}{2} \text{ or } t = \frac{0.693}{k} \qquad (2\text{-}5)$$

where $0.693 = \ln(2)$. This half-life, or $t_{1/2}$, is an extremely important concept since it applies over any time interval because of the log-linear nature of the decline. After two half-lives, the original quantity is reduced by 75 percent; after three, by 87.5 percent, and so on. After four or five half-lives, the process is essentially complete.

The final important concept in describing the one-compartment model is that of clearance. Clearance may be thought of as analogous to creatinine clearance and is the volume that is totally cleared of drug per unit time. It can be calculated as:

$$\text{Clearance} = k \cdot V_d \qquad (2\text{-}6)$$

where k is the rate constant described above.

Clearance usually has the units of liters or milliliters per minute and may be adjusted for body weight (ml/kg/min). As the amount of drug in the volume, V_d, declines, the amount eliminated in any time interval will also decline (Eq. 2-2). However, the volume cleared per unit time (clearance) remains constant, resulting in the exponential decline of drug concentrations (Eq. 2-3) that is seen experimentally.

During ongoing, constant-rate drug administration, a condition of equilibrium known as steady state is eventually achieved. In this state, the concentration of drug in all body tissues is in equilibrium, and the amount of drug administered equals the amount eliminated. Since the amount of drug eliminated is simply the clearance multiplied by the plasma concentration, Cp_{ss}:

$$\text{Infusion rate} = \text{Clearance} \cdot Cp_{ss}$$

or

$$Cp_{ss} = \frac{\text{Infusion Rate}}{\text{Clearance}} \qquad (2\text{-}7)$$

This relationship is very useful in situations of chronic drug dosing or therapy by continuous infusion. If a disease process should affect drug clearance, the impact on the plasma concentration will be inversely proportionate. The possibility of calculating drug clearance by either of two methods is very useful.

Combining Equations 2-5 and 2-6:

$$\text{Clearance} = V_d \cdot \frac{0.693}{t_{1/2}}$$

$$\text{or} \qquad (2\text{-}8)$$

$$t_{1/2} = \frac{0.693\ V_d}{\text{Clearance}}$$

In other words, the half-life of the decline of drug concentrations, which will correlate in some manner with the rate of dissipation of drug effects, is related directly to the volume of distribution of the drug and inversely to its clearance. Drugs with large volumes of distribution will tend to have long half-lives. In contrast, drugs with high clearances will tend to have short half-lives. Clearance and volume are thus the fundamental pharmacokinetic parameters that contribute to what is clinically observed, the rate of decline of drug concentrations and effects.

Physiologic Correlates

VOLUME OF DISTRIBUTION

As Klotz wrote in 1976:

"Distribution is a physicochemical interaction between a drug and the body. Therefore, the pattern of this distribution is determined by the properties of these two partners."[17]

The properties of a drug that influence its ability to penetrate into body tissues are its pKa and degree of ionization at physiological pH, its molecular weight, and its polarity or lipid solubility. The non-depolarizing muscle relaxants are examples of a class of drugs of relatively high molecular weight (500–600) and polarity that do not penetrate well into tissues or red blood cells.[18] As a result, they have a relatively small volume of distribution, 0.3 to 0.6 l/kg, which closely approximates the size of the extracellular fluid space in which they are found. Smaller, less polar compounds, such as thiopental and fentanyl, have considerably larger distribution volumes, 2–3 l/kg and 3–4 l/kg, respectively.[3] Indices of lipid solubility such as the octanol/water partition coefficient are helpful in explaining pharmacokinetic differences between closely related compounds. For example, fentanyl has an octanol/water partition coefficient of 955, and the volume of distribution just indicated. Alfentanil, in contrast, has a much lower partition coefficient, 126, and a much smaller volume of distribution, less than 1 l/kg.[19] However, the chemically more distinct morphine has an octanol/water partition coefficient of 1.4 and a distribution volume of 4–6 l/kg.[19] Clearly, either octanol poorly represents human fat or morphine has a marked affinity for some other tissue component. The temptation to pursue this line of reasoning further is reduced by the limitations of physiologic/pharmacokinetic modeling.

Characteristics of the body, the other "partner" in the interaction, have marked influences on the volume of distribution as well. As noted in Equation 2-1, the volume of distribution is the ratio between the amount of drug in the body and its concentration in the blood or plasma. Conceptually, any conditions that alter the affinity of the blood or plasma for a drug will affect this ratio, if other factors remain unaltered. One such condition is the degree of drug/protein binding in plasma. As shown in Figure 2-7, it is only the free, unbound drug that is available to cross membranes and to penetrate tissues. Thermodynamic principles drive this free drug concentration into equilibrium between plasma and tissues. The total concentration in either area then depends on the capacity and affinity of binding by both plasma proteins and tissue components. In plasma, acidic drugs like thiopental bind largely to albumin.[20] When albumin levels decrease in liver disease, or binding affinity or capacity is reduced as in renal failure or in the presence of a competing drug, volume of distribution may increase in the absence of changes in tissue affinity. In contrast, basic drugs like fentanyl and its analogues, amide local anesthetics, and propranolol principally bind in plasma to alpha-1-acid glycoprotein (AAG). This compound, in contrast to albumin, is an acute phase reactant and tends to increase with chronic disease or after major surgery, trauma, or myocardial infarction.[21] If tissue affinities remain unaltered, the resulting increase in plasma drug binding will produce an apparent contraction of the volume of distribution.

Finally, changes in tissue-drug affinities or body composition can affect the volume of distribution by altering the amount of drug on the tissue side of Figure 2-7. Well-known differences in body composition are found at the extremes of age, with neonates having an increased proportion of body water and the elderly having a reduced muscle mass/fat ratio.[17] Obese patients may have increased volumes of distribution for certain drugs although here the drug's

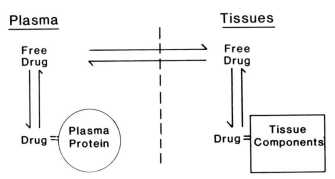

Fig. 2-7. The relationship between free, protein-bound, and tissue-bound drug. The free drug is in equilibrium between plasma and tissues. The relative amounts of total drug in plasma and tissues depend on the degree of plasma protein binding and tissue binding of drug.

physicochemical properties play an important role. For example, the water-soluble digoxin does not distribute into excess body weight, whereas the lipid-soluble diazepam disproportionately distributes there.[22] Lastly, extreme reductions in peripheral perfusion may contract a drug's apparent volume of distribution.[23]

CLEARANCE

Drug clearance, more so than volume, has obvious relations to physiology since processes that rid the body of drugs can be explicitly studied. This discussion will focus primarily on hepatic and renal processes, leaving the details on drugs eliminated in the blood (succinylcholine, atracurium) or by the lungs (volatile anesthetics) to other chapters.

Hepatic drug clearance has received a great deal of attention from both physiologists and biochemists in the past decade. A pivotal concept has been that of extraction ratio, E:

$$E = \frac{C_A - C_V}{C_A} \qquad (2\text{-}9)$$

where C_A is the concentration of drug in blood perfusing the liver (mixed hepatic arterial and portal venous), and C_V is the concentration in hepatic venous blood. The same concept can be applied to any organ that eliminates a drug. E is simply the fraction of drug removed from blood on a single pass through that organ. The hepatic clearance of a drug (Cl_H) can then be expressed in terms of E and hepatic blood flow Q_H:

$$Cl_H = E \cdot Q_H \qquad (2\text{-}10)$$

The product has the familiar units for clearance, volume per unit time.

It is evident that for drugs that are efficiently extracted by the liver, where E is close to one, hepatic drug clearance will approximate liver blood flow. The elimination half-life will thus depend on liver blood flow and volume of distribution and will be altered by physiologic processes that affect these terms. Etomidate and ketamine are examples from anesthetic practice of high hepatic extraction ratio compounds. Such compounds, in general, have poor systemic availability when administered orally, since they undergo first-pass hepatic extraction from portal venous blood before reaching the systemic circulation. Propranolol, when given orally, is also subject to such effects, explaining the large (compared to intravenous) and variable oral dose needed to achieve systemic effects.

When the hepatic extraction ratio is low, factors other than liver blood flow limit hepatic drug clearance (Fig. 2-8). These factors include the fraction of drug bound to plasma proteins (which is less available to the liver than the unbound fraction) and the ability of the liver to remove drug from the blood in the absence of blood flow or protein binding limitations.[24] This latter capability, termed intrinsic clearance, is related to hepatic enzymatic activity and may be increased by hepatic enzyme induction or possibly decreased by hepatocellular disease.[25] In general, for low extraction ratio drugs, increased intrinsic clearance or unbound fraction will raise hepatic drug clearance, if other factors remain unchanged. Thiopental and benzodiazepines (except midazolam) are examples of low extraction ratio compounds whose clearance is affected by these physiological variables.

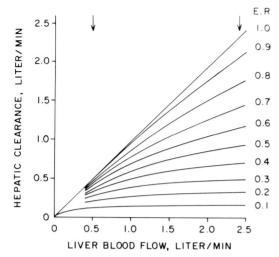

Fig. 2-8. The dependence of hepatic drug clearance on liver blood flow for compounds of different hepatic extraction ratio, E.R. When extraction ratio is high, clearance is said to be flow limited. At low extraction ratios, enzymatic capacity and protein binding are limiting instead. Arrows indicate the physiologic range of liver blood flow. (From Wilkinson GR, Shand DG: A physiological approach to hepatic drug clearance. Clin Pharmacol Ther 18:377–390, 1975, with permission.)

All of these factors result in the following principles of hepatic drug clearance, which are useful in understanding the interaction of physiology and pharmacology in the cardiac patient:

1. Drugs of high hepatic extraction ratio (clearance of 1–2 liters/min in the adult) are "flow-limited." Their hepatic clearance is sensitive to factors that affect hepatic blood flow (low output syndromes, congestive heart failure, CPB, general anesthesia, posture, etc.) It is relatively insensitive to factors that alter intrinsic clearance or protein binding.
2. Low extraction ratio drugs (clearance of 500 ml/min or less) are sensitive to factors that affect intrinsic clearance (enzyme induction, liver disease) or protein binding (many disease states). Clearance of these drugs is little affected by altered liver blood flow.
3. Drugs of intermediate extraction ratio are affected by all of the above factors, but to a less pronounced degree than compounds at extremes of the spectrum.

Renal clearance is of particular importance for polar, water-soluble drugs such as the nondepolarizing muscle relaxants, many antibiotics, and antiar-rhythmics. Lipid-soluble drugs, although filtered by the glomerulus, are passively reabsorbed and, in general, depend on hepatic elimination. Their polar metabolites, however, do accumulate in patients with renal insufficiency. Metabolites of meperidine and morphine have been held responsible for CNS side effects in patients with renal failure.[26,27]

Concepts of drug extraction developed in the discussion of hepatic drug clearance are useful in considering renal processes. A drug with high renal extraction must be one that undergoes active tubular secretion. The clearance of such a drug would be sensitive to changes in renal perfusion. Drugs that are simply filtered by the glomerulus are insensitive to changes in renal blood flow as long as glomerular filtration rate (GFR) is preserved by autoregulation.[28] When renal blood flow drops below the autoregulatory range or when renal disease compromises the GFR, however, renal clearance decreases for such drugs. The decreased clearance and prolonged elimination of gallamine, metocurine, and pancuronium in renal failure are well-known examples of this phenomenon. Finally, plasma protein binding influences renal drug clearance by, in effect, shielding the drug from renal excretion unless it is actively secreted. Changes in protein binding with disease can thus affect a drug's renal clearance.

Multicompartment Models

In order to be useful in a predictive and comparative way, a pharmacokinetic model must be able to describe experimental data in a reasonably accurate fashion. Fairly early in the development of pharmacokinetic concepts, it became obvious that thinking of the body as a single compartment was an indefensible oversimplification.[29] The principal observation that conflicted with the single compartment concept was the finding that after rapid intravascular drug administration, drug concentrations decline quickly at first (Fig. 2-9) before settling into a slower log linear elimination phase. This observation is supported by physiologic reasoning; it is obvious that drugs that have any degree of tissue disposition cannot mix and equilibrate instantaneously in the body. The period of rapid, early decline of drug concentrations represents drug distribution from blood into tissues or, in the terms of the two-compartment pharmacokinetic model (Fig. 2-5), from the central to the peripheral compartment. If blood samples are taken at appropriate times, almost all drugs follow this type of behavior.

A number of modifications to the previous dis-

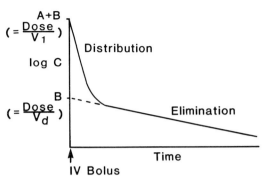

Fig. 2-9. The time course of plasma drug concentrations, C, after bolus administration into the central compartment of a two-compartment model (Fig. 2-5). Drug distribution and elimination phases are indicated. The *y*-intercepts B and (A + B) relate to volumes of distribution. Note the logarithmic scale of concentration.

cussion follow from the addition of the peripheral body compartment. These involve issues of the time course and volumes of drug distribution. The basic definition of drug clearance and its physiologic correlates remain unaltered. However, the calculation of drug clearance is somewhat more complicated and is further explored elsewhere.[3-5,30] Once drug distribution is complete, the familiar log-linear process of drug elimination can be discerned. In the multicompartment model, the elimination half-life remains directly related (although not strictly proportional) to volume of distribution and inversely related to clearance.

The new process in the multi-compartment model is that of drug distribution. Empirically, it has been determined that, like drug elimination, drug distribution is a first-order process. It can thus be described by an exponential term, and the overall behavior of drug concentrations becomes the sum of two exponential terms:

$$C(t) = Ae^{-\alpha\tau} + Be^{-\beta\tau} \qquad (2\text{-}11)$$

where α is related to the distribution rate constant, and β to the elimination rate constant (k in the one-compartment model). Distribution, like elimination, thus has a half-life. Distribution half-lives of commonly used anesthetic drugs when described by a two-compartment model are on the order of 5–20 minutes.[3] For anesthetic drugs like thiopental and fentanyl, distribution is often far more important than elimination in the termination of effects, giving clinical relevance to this parameter. In a recent study by

Burch and Stanski,[31] the relative importance of metabolism and distribution were assessed for the recovery from thiopental anesthesia. In the first 15 minutes after a bolus induction dose, blood levels dropped by over ten-fold to levels consistent with only mild sedation. Of this marked decline in drug levels, 82 percent was due to thiopental distribution and only 18 percent to metabolism.

Volume of distribution as the proportionality constant between the plasma concentration and the total amount of drug in the body is clearly not constant during drug distribution. It increases as drug distributes out of the blood into tissues and the plasma concentration falls. The initial volume of distribution (V_1 or volume of the central compartment) is that calculated after initial mixing in the blood, but before any peripheral distribution has occurred. It is obtained by extrapolating the concentration-time profile in Figure 2-9 back to zero (to the initial concentration A + B, see Eq. 2-1). The smaller the V_1, the higher is the initial drug concentration in blood and the greater is the potential for pronounced initial drug effects in rapidly equilibrating tissues. The apparent volume of drug distribution (after peripheral distribution is complete) is obtained by extrapolating the log-linear elimination phase back to time zero (to the concentration B in Fig. 2-9). This volume is an approximation of the steady-state volume of distribution (Vd_{ss}), the sum of the central and peripheral compartment volumes, which exists when all compartments are in equilibrium. The ratio of Vd_{ss} to V_1 is an index of the relative importance of drug distribution in causing blood levels to fall. This ranges from 20-fold or more for thiopental[32] and fentanyl,[33] to only 4- or 5-fold for most nondepolarizing muscle relaxants.[18]

In many recent investigations of pharmacokinetics, drugs have been said to exhibit three-compartment behavior, meaning that the plasma concentration-time profile can be characterized with three exponential phases, and the compartmental model supplemented by a second peripheral compartment. This type of model has two distribution half-lives rather than one; otherwise, it is conceptually identical to the simpler two-compartment model. Whether a drug exhibits two- or three-compartment behavior depends more on the timing and site of blood sampling and the assay precision than on the drug or the patient. Two- and three-compartment analyses of the same data will, however, produce systematically different pharmacokinetic results. Comparisons should, therefore, be made within a uniform modeling scheme.

PHARMACODYNAMICS

The drug concentration-time profile shown in Figure 2-9, based on the compartmental model (Fig. 2-5) and understood in terms of its pharmacokinetic parameters (clearance, volumes of distribution, half-lives) with their physiologic correlates, is the foundation for a discussion of intravenous anesthetic pharmacology in the cardiac patient. At this point, however, a note of caution regarding pharmacokinetics should be reiterated. The concentration-time profile in Figure 2-9 does not explain the time course of drug effects; it only deals with concentrations. For example, a finite (and sometimes considerable) period of time is required between intravenous drug injection and peak drug effects; yet, peak concentration is achieved immediately. To explain this observation, it is necessary to postulate that the site of drug effect is not in the blood or central compartment, but is some distance removed. A pharmacokinetic model containing a distinct effect site has been developed that incorporates this concept.[2] The final stepping stone in the dose-response relationship is pharmacodynamics, the relationship between drug concentration (at the effect site) and drug effect. Several different possible forms for this relationship are shown in Figure 2-10. In the simplest case (panel A), drug effect is proportional to concentration. This simple model, however, fails to explain the maximum effect that is observed with many drugs. If the model is made more complex (panels B and C), a maximum effect is predicted. The sigmoid relationship (panel C) also predicts a negligible drug effect at low concentrations, which agrees with clinical observations on many anesthetic drugs; perhaps most notably, the nondepolarizing muscle relaxants. In addition to pharmacokinetics, then, both the relationship between drug concentrations and effects (pharmacodynamics) and the time lag entailed in that relationship (the pharmacokinetic/dynamic interface) are crucial to an understanding of anesthetic pharmacology. The state of knowledge in this area is summarized in a recent review.[34] However, few studies in this area have specifically focused on the cardiac patient.

In considering the concentration-response relationship, it must also be specified whether the concentrations in question are total plasma concentrations (free and protein-bound drug) or free-drug concentrations. There is considerable experimental evidence and an excellent theoretic rationale for the principle that the free-drug concentration is the one available to diffuse into tissues and to exert a

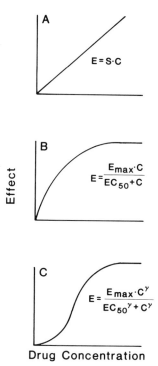

Fig. 2-10. Three alternative pharmacodynamic models for the relationship between drug concentration C, and drug effect, E. (A) A linear model. S is the slope of the relationship. (B) A hyperbolic model. E_{max} is the maximal effect and EC_{50} is the concentration that produces half of that effect. (C) A sigmoid model. E_{max} and EC_{50} are analogous to the hyperbolic model, and γ is a sigmoidicity term. The appropriate model is chosen by statistical criteria and inspection of the data.

pharmacological effect.[35,36] Nonetheless, total drug concentrations are usually the ones monitored in clinical practice. As pointed out above, disease and altered physiology often change drug-protein binding, altering not only pharmacokinetics, but also the relationship between free and total drug concentration. With the customary clinical monitoring tools, pharmacodynamics may thus appear to change with disease. For example, 3 days after cardiac surgery, lidocaine free fraction in plasma decreases from 30 to 16 percent, coincident with a rise in alpha-1-acid glycoprotein levels.[37] As well as altering lidocaine pharmacokinetics, this increase in binding may render a normally effective total lidocaine concentration subtherapeutic and a normally toxic, total concentration safe. Altered drug-protein binding must be considered whenever the concentration-response relationship appears changed by disease.

PHARMACOKINETIC METHODOLOGY IN THE CARDIAC PATIENT

The interpretation of pharmacokinetic data in the cardiac patient is also colored by a number of significant methodologic issues. First is the assumption that the pharmacokinetic parameters being estimated are constant during the period of study. Although it is recognized that there are significant minute-to-minute fluctuations in physiologic and pharmacokinetic parameters, pharmacokinetic analysis produces time-averaged values over the period of study.[38] If substantial physiologic perturbations (eg, CPB) occur during the study period, their effect on pharmacokinetics will be averaged out over the entire study interval. That interval is often long (many hours) since, for statistical accuracy, the study period should be at least twice the duration of the longest half-life estimated. The effect of CPB on drug clearance, for example, thus may be difficult to estimate for many intravenous anesthetics that have elimination half-lives of several hours. The application of invasive physiological techniques is a route around this limitation of static modeling of pharmacokinetics in flux.[38]

Secondly, the issue of the site of blood sampling and of drug administration becomes a real one in the cardiac patient since a number of options are available. Pharmacokinetic analysis has traditionally employed venous blood sampling. In recent years, however, some analyses of arterial blood samples have been performed. Theoretically, arterial sampling may be preferable since arterial concentrations reflect those delivered to extracting organs and sites of drug effect better than does the venous efflux from tissues.[39] Arterial sampling may produce systematically different values than venous sampling,[32,40] depending on the timing of blood sampling and the hepatic extraction ratio of the drug in question. In addition to arterial and venous sites, blood may be removed from different parts of the pump oxygenator during the period of its use. These concentrations, theoretically, should be identical to both mixed venous and arterial levels during CPB. Drug extraction by the CPB apparatus, however, as has been shown to occur with fentanyl in certain types of membrane oxygenators,[41,42] and with nitroglycerin in a bubble oxygenator,[43] will considerably complicate the pharmacokinetic analysis. Drugs may also be administered via the CPB apparatus. Although this point has received little emphasis, the exact site of drug administration has considerable effect on the mixing volume, which will determine the initial systemic drug concentration. In the setting of CPB, pulmonary drug distribution no longer buffers the systemic circulation.[44] This consideration may have particular relevance for antiarrhythmic drug therapy during CPB.

Thirdly, there is the issue of heparin effect on drug-protein binding and, hence, on pharmacokinetics. This issue is unavoidable in procedures involving CPB and affects the comparison of pharmacokinetics in the cardiac patient with those in the patient without heart disease. It is well accepted that heparin causes a release and activation of the enzyme lipoprotein lipase, which, in turn, hydrolyzes plasma triglycerides into nonesterified fatty acids.[45-47] These compounds have been shown to competitively inhibit the binding of many drugs to plasma proteins that may potentially alter drug kinetics.[48-53] After heparin administration, even in subtherapeutic doses, there is a severalfold rise in nonesterified fatty acid concentrations.[53,54] However, it has now become clear through several studies that this increase is largely a test-tube artifact,[54-56] with, presumably, an efficient clearance mechanism for these compounds in the intact organism. When lipoprotein lipase activation is prevented, the effect of heparin on drug-protein binding is largely abolished.[54,56] However, lipoprotein lipase inactivators may have their own effects on protein binding. These issues render difficult the interpretation of protein binding measurements in the heparinized patient.

DRUG DISPOSITION IN THE CARDIAC PATIENT

From one perspective, pharmacokinetic parameters are simply tools for comparing different classes of patients in an attempt to predict or to explain why they may differ in their pharmacologic response to a drug dose. These tools have been developed conceptually in the preceding sections with this goal in mind. Using the pharmacokinetic approach and vocabulary, the various aspects of cardiac pathophysiology will be explored for their effects on drug disposition.

Congestive Heart Failure

The pathophysiology of congestive heart failure is covered more fully in Chapter 14. However, some aspects of the pathophysiology that may impinge on drug disposition are summarized in Table 2-1. Briefly, pump failure ultimately leads to a reduced cardiac output, with blood pressure maintained by a

Table 2-1
Potential Effects of Congestive Heart Failure
on Drug Disposition

Pathophysiology	Pharmacokinetic Sequelae
↓ Cardiac output	↓ Hepatic and renal clearance
↓ Vital organ perfusion	↓ Distribution volume
↓↓ Peripheral perfusion	↓ GI and IM absorption
↑ Sympathetic activity	Slower onset of drug effects
Visceral congestion	

sympathetically mediated increase in peripheral vascular resistance. The sacrifice of peripheral perfusion may reduce the peripheral tissue distribution of some drugs and can markedly slow the absorption of drugs administered orally or intramuscularly.[57] Reduced hepatic and renal perfusion, which may follow in later stages of the syndrome, will adversely affect the clearance of high-extraction ratio drugs. In addition, the redistribution of renal blood flow from outer cortex to medulla that occurs in congestive heart failure may further reduce renal drug clearance.[58,59] Hepatic congestion or hypoperfusion may reduce the clearance of low-extraction ratio drugs by impairment of microsomal drug oxidation or actual hepatocellular damage.[57,60] Finally, for drugs that depend on tissue perfusion to exert their effects, onset may be delayed by impaired cardiac performance. Reduced volume of distribution or clearance can both lead to higher than anticipated drug levels. Slow onset of drug effects can lead to further unneeded drug administration. All of these phenomena predispose the patient with congestive heart failure to toxic drug reactions if conventional dosage guidelines are followed. However, overgeneralization is to be avoided. The variability of these effects from drug to drug is illustrated by the following examples.

LIDOCAINE

Lidocaine is a favorite drug of pharmacokineticists. Its disposition has been characterized in many disease states, and it will be used again as an example in subsequent sections of this chapter. Lidocaine is used frequently in the patient with heart failure for dysrhythmia management. It was noted in the late 1960s that such patients have an increased incidence of toxicity from standard doses of lidocaine.[61,62] The investigations that elucidated the mechanism of this effect were important historically in establishing the utility of pharmacokinetic predictions and in pointing out the need for therapeutic drug level monitoring.

In 1971, Stenson et al demonstrated a pharmacokinetic explanation for this increased toxicity.[63] In a study of 17 patients undergoing cardiac catheterization, they demonstrated an inverse relationship between cardiac index and arterial lidocaine concentration after a bolus plus infusion regimen (Fig. 2-11). Hepatic blood flow was estimated by indocyanine green clearance and correlated well with

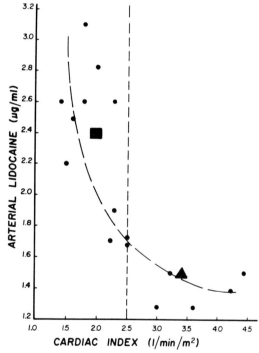

Fig. 2-11. Arterial lidocaine concentrations related to cardiac index after a bolus plus infusion regimen in 17 patients undergoing cardiac catheterization. Average values for groups with low and normal cardiac indices are indicated by the large square and triangle. (From Stenson RE, Constantino RT, Harrison DC: Interrelationships of hepatic blood flow, cardiac output, and blood levels of lidocaine in man. Circulation 43:205–211, 1971, with permission.)

cardiac index. Lidocaine, as a moderate-to-high extraction ratio drug, is the type of compound whose clearance is directly related to liver blood flow. The reduced clearance explains the higher levels (see Eq. 2-7).

In a subsequent study, Thomson et al formally determined the pharmacokinetics of lidocaine in patients with heart failure.[64] In comparison with normal subjects, the 11 patients in their study with heart failure had a smaller V_1 (21 vs 37 liters), a smaller Vd_{ss} (62 vs 93 liters), and a lower clearance (6.3 vs 10.0 ml/kg/min). Because both clearance and Vd_{ss} were reduced in the heart failure group, the elimination half-life was unchanged. Lidocaine levels were significantly higher in patients with heart failure, however, correlating both with the pharmacokinetic calculations and with the earlier study.[63] On the basis of their findings, the authors recommended reduced lidocaine doses for dysrhythmia management in patients with congestive heart failure.

When congestive heart failure is due to myocardial infarction, there are further alterations in lidocaine pharmacology. Lidocaine levels often rise by as much as 60–100 percent during the period when steady state should have been achieved.[65] Based on interpretation of total drug levels, this finding was used as the basis for a further reduction in lidocaine doses in patients with myocardial infarction. With further investigation, however, it appears that free lidocaine concentrations do not increase.[66] The phenomenon of increased lidocaine levels (and decreased clearance) after myocardial infarction is attributed to increases in the stress-reactant plasma protein, AAG, with increased lidocaine binding.[66] Although the rationale for reducing lidocaine doses in heart failure remains, the impetus for doing so after uncomplicated myocardial infarction is less powerful.

PROCAINAMIDE

Like lidocaine, procainamide tends to produce higher blood levels than normal when given in standard doses to patients with congestive heart failure. Fifty to sixty percent of a dose of procainamide is excreted by the kidneys in unchanged form, with the remainder metabolized. One of its metabolites, *N*-acetyl procainamide, has antiarrhythmic activity, is excreted by the kidneys, and accumulates when renal function is impaired.[57] To the extent that renal function is diminished in congestive heart failure, a reduction in procainamide clearance and that of its polar metabolites would be expected. This prediction

was experimentally confirmed in 1971 by Koch-Weser and Klein,[68] who showed that steady state procainamide concentrations were directly related to blood urea nitrogen (BUN). In addition, the volume of distribution of procainamide was 1.5 liters/kg in patients with cardiac failure, as compared to 2.0 liters/kg in patients with normal circulatory function.[68] Both of these pharmacokinetic changes predispose the patient with heart failure to higher drug levels and a greater likelihood of toxic response after either acute or chronic dosing.

QUINIDINE

Like lidocaine and procainamide, pharmacokinetics of quinidine are altered by congestive heart failure. After intravenous administration in patients with congestive heart failure, quinidine clearance (largely hepatic) was reduced to 3.2 ml/kg/min from 4.7 ml/kg/min in cardiac patients without heart failure.[69] Volume of distribution was also smaller in the patients with heart failure, 1.8 vs 3.0 liters/kg. Like the other antiarrhythmics, quinidine thus will tend to produce higher levels in cardiac failure after either acute or chronic intravenous administration. Interestingly enough, after chronic oral administration, quinidine levels are apparently not affected by heart failure.[70] This finding, in conjunction with the intravenous study, would suggest that quinidine absorption (bioavailability) is reduced in cardiac failure.

THEOPHYLLINE

Theophylline is occasionally used in the patient with an acute exacerbation of congestive heart failure to reduce the degree of bronchospasm associated with pulmonary fluid accumulation. The patient with heart failure is already prone to dysrhythmias and is at particular risk for serious complications from theophylline toxicity. As a low-clearance drug (1–2 ml/kg/min), theophylline is not susceptible to effects of cardiac pathophysiology on hepatic blood flow. Nonetheless, a number of reports have documented that theophylline clearance is reduced and elimination half-life is prolonged in patients with cardiac failure.[71,72] Volume of distribution is apparently unchanged. These data suggest that a desired therapeutic theophylline level can be achieved with a normal loading dose, but it should be maintained with a 50 percent reduced maintenance dose.[71,72] These reports also document that cardiac failure can have a direct effect on hepatic metabolism in addition to hemodynamic effects on hepatic drug clearance.

DIGOXIN

The need for a reduction of digoxin dosage in congestive heart failure is a well-known example of the interaction of pathophysiology and pharmacology. As a drug with extensive tissue distribution that undergoes renal excretion, digoxin is susceptible to the renal effects of congestive heart failure. In fact, digoxin clearance correlates better with urea clearance than with creatinine clearance,[73] suggesting that, like urea, digoxin is reabsorbed by the renal tubule in states of severe prerenal azotemia and low urine flow.

Drug Disposition and Beta-Adrenergic Blockade

Beta-adrenergic blockade is a mainstay of the management of ischemic heart disease (Chapter 13). Beta-blocker therapy has well-recognized hemodynamic effects including a reduction of total cardiac output, which may significantly decrease liver blood flow.[74] The implications of this observation for the clearance of high hepatic extraction ratio drugs are apparent. Unfortunately, cardiac patients are not usually available for controlled pharmacokinetic studies both with and without concurrent beta-blockade, either because of ethical concerns for withholding

therapy or because other conditions change as well (eg, surgery is performed). Therefore, most studies of the effects of beta-blockade on drug disposition have been performed in healthy volunteers or in animal models, and the results must be extrapolated to the cardiac patient with some degree of caution.

The interaction of beta-blockade with lidocaine disposition is the most extensively studied. In 1973, Branch et al examined the propranolol/lidocaine interaction in anesthetized dogs.[75] They found that propranolol administration decreased lidocaine clearance by 25 percent and similarly prolonged its elimination half-life. Hemodynamic changes were also measured in these animals; cardiac output and liver blood flow were both significantly diminished by propranolol, while hepatic lidocaine extraction ratio was unchanged. The same interaction was later documented in young, healthy volunteers by Ochs et al.[76] They found that propranolol, 80 mg every 8 hours, reduced lidocaine clearance from 18 to 11 ml/kg/min with a prolongation of the elimination half-life from 65 to 101 minutes in bolus-dose studies. There was no change in lidocaine volume of distribution. The same authors also infused lidocaine to assess the effect of propranolol therapy on steady-state levels. Figure 2-12 shows lidocaine concentrations in the same subject with and without propranolol therapy.

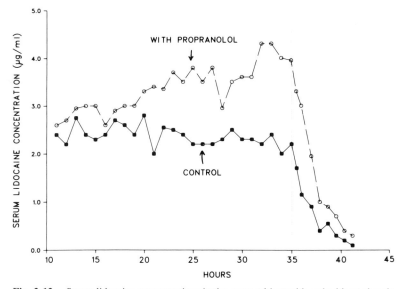

Fig. 2-12. Serum lidocaine concentrations in the same subject with and without chronic propranolol therapy (80 mg orally every 8 hours). On both occasions, the subject received a 100-mg lidocaine loading dose followed by an infusion of 2 mg per minute, which was terminated at 35 hours. Propranolol reduces lidocaine clearance. (From Ochs HR, Carstens G, Greenblatt DJ: Reduction in lidocaine clearance during continuous infusion and by coadministration of propranolol. N Engl J Med 303:373–377, 1980, with permission.)

The demonstrated reduction in lidocaine clearance by propranolol correlates with higher steady state lidocaine levels (see Eq. 2-7). Another high hepatic-extraction ratio compound that has been studied, indocyanine green, has also shown a reduction in clearance by propranolol.[77]

If the effect of propranolol on hepatic drug clearance is purely a hemodynamic one, it should also be demonstrable with therapeutic doses of other beta-blockers. Conrad et al compared the effects of metoprolol and propranolol in approximately equipotent doses on lidocaine pharmacokinetics.[78] They found that propranolol produced a 47 percent reduction in lidocaine clearance, whereas metoprolol produced only a 31 percent reduction. In another study with equivalent metoprolol doses, investigators were unable to demonstrate any significant effect on lidocaine disposition.[79] This disparity between the effects of different beta-antagonists and the disproportionate effect of propranolol on lidocaine clearance in relation to liver blood flow observations has led to suspicion of another effect of propranolol on hepatic drug metabolism.[74,75]

In order to demonstrate a nonhemodynamic effect on drug disposition, a drug whose clearance is not blood-flow dependent must be studied. Such compounds are drugs with low hepatic extraction ratios. Antipyrine, a commonly used marker compound, has its clearance reduced 30–40 percent by propranolol treatment.[80,81] Of more therapeutic relevance, diazepam clearance is decreased by 17 percent,[82] and theophylline clearance by approximately one-third.[83] The clearance of alprazolam and lorazepam, however, are unaffected.[82] On the basis of this evidence, it has been suggested that propranolol may have an additional effect on oxidative drug metabolism that is independent of beta-adrenoreceptor blockade.[84]

Drug Disposition in Aging

The cardiac surgery population includes increasing numbers of elderly patients as analyses begin to show relative benefit.[85] There is no question that the elderly exhibit an increased incidence of adverse drug reactions,[86] and many clinicians believe that the elderly are more sensitive to a variety of drugs.[87] Pharmacokinetic studies in this area are legion. Common themes include higher drug levels and prolonged elimination in the elderly. Pharmacokinetic explanations include changes in volumes of distribution (with altered body composition) and reduced drug clearances (with reduced vital organ perfusion or

age-related impairment of the microsomal mixed-function oxidase system).[87] Recent work of particular importance to anesthesiologists shows that the elderly are more sensitive to thiopental and etomidate because of a smaller initial distribution volume (V_1).[32,88] On the other hand, the elderly are more sensitive to the narcotics fentanyl and alfentanil on a pharmacodynamic basis, while drug disposition is unaltered.[89] The reader is referred to recent reviews for further details on this important subject.[34,87]

Drug Disposition in Renal Disease

Hypertensive nephropathy and renovascular disease are common in the cardiovascular surgery population. Principles of renal drug clearance and the effects of renal failure on plasma protein binding were discussed in previous sections. In brief, the types of drugs whose clearance is most affected by renal impairment are polar, water-soluble compounds that normally are filtered by the glomerulus and excreted. In particular, some of the nondepolarizing muscle relaxants and many antibiotics have a reduced renal clearance and prolonged elimination in renal insufficiency.[18] Nomograms have been developed relating drug dosage to serum creatinine or creatinine clearance. Further details can be found in recent comprehensive reviews.[59,90]

DRUG DISPOSITION DURING CARDIAC SURGERY

All of the preceding interactions of pathophysiology and pharmacokinetics impinge on the preoperative medical therapy of the cardiac surgery patient. Medical problems seldom disappear in the operating room, although they may be eclipsed by more acute issues. The above-mentioned effects of congestive heart failure, beta-blockade, advanced age, and renal disease upon drug disposition thus must be considered in planning therapy with intravenous anesthetic drugs. For the cardiac patient undergoing noncardiac surgery, these pre-existing abnormalities may be the primary influence on drug disposition. But for the patient undergoing cardiac surgery, there is one additional factor, CPB, which looms large in importance as a factor affecting pharmacokinetics.

Considered as a state of circulatory pathophysiology, CPB produces changes probably more profound than those of any other. The relatively extreme nature of the perturbations led one early writer to describe CPB as a controlled form of shock.[91] Although perfusion techniques have certainly improved in the interim, the magnitude of the hemo-dynamic effects probably exceed those of congestive heart failure. Both the critical nature of the therapy involved and the potential for discovering significant pharmacokinetic alterations have spawned numerous studies in the last decade on drug disposition in the cardiac surgical patient. Before considering these studies in detail, the individual aspects of the physi-ology of CPB that may affect drug disposition will be considered. These alterations and their poten-tial impact on pharmacokinetics are summarized in Table 2-2.

Hypotension and Altered Regional Blood Flow

Initiation of CPB is usually accompanied by a drop in mean arterial pressure and systemic vascular resistance due to hemodilution. In many centers, selection of a pump flow lower than a normal cardiac output may also contribute to the observed hypoten-sion. The combination of hypotension, hypothermia, and nonpulsatile blood flow has a significant impact on the distribution of circulation, with a marked reduction in peripheral flow and relative preservation of the central circulation.[92,93]

There is little information on the effects of hypo-tension on drug disposition in man. However, there is data from a primate model that has considerable relevance to CPB. Benowitz et al produced a 30 per-cent reduction in blood pressure and a 35 percent reduction in cardiac output in rhesus monkeys by phlebotomy, and measured the effects on both regional blood flow and lidocaine disposition.[94] Lidocaine clearance in the hypotensive animals was reduced by 46 percent. Since total hepatic blood flow measured by microsphere injection was unchanged, this decrease was attributed to hepatocellular impair-ment or to intrahepatic shunting. In addition, lido-caine steady-state volume of distribution was 19 percent lower in the hypotensive animals, and blood flow to skeletal muscle, kidney, skin, bone, and adi-pose tissue was markedly diminished. As a result of these pharmacokinetic differences, steady-state lido-caine concentrations were 60 percent increased by hypotension, and elimination half-life was 40 percent prolonged. The same authors used a perfusion model for lidocaine disposition to predict concentrations in hypotensive man after a bolus dose (Fig. 2-13A).[95] When lidocaine concentrations are actually measured in a patient undergoing CPB (Fig. 2-13B), the profile is remarkably similar.

Table 2-2
Effects of Cardiopulmonary Bypass on Drug Disposition

Pathophysiology	Pharmacokinetic Sequelae
Hypotension	↓ Hepatic and renal clearance
Altered regional blood flow	↓ Distribution volume
Hypothermia	
Hemodilution	↓ Protein binding ↑ Distribution volume
↓ Pulmonary blood flow	↓ Pulmonary drug distribution ↑ Systemic drug levels
Vasoactive drug therapy	Altered drug clearance and distribution
↑ Postoperative protein binding	↓ Distribution volume ↓ Hepatic drug clearance (low extraction ratio) Altered drug level interpretation

Hypothermia

Hypothermia also appears to affect liver function in animals. In one study, when the hepatic tempera-ture of cats was lowered by only $1°-2°C$, the rate of hepatic extraction of both ethanol and glycerol was reduced by approximately 40 percent.[96] For these compounds that exhibit zero order hepatic extrac-tion, the effect of hypothermia on liver blood flow is irrelevant. The observed effect thus represents either a temperature dependence of hepatic enzymatic activity or a marked intrahepatic redistribution of blood flow with the development of significant intra-hepatic shunting. In any event, the effect of hypo-thermia upon metabolic drug clearance is demonstrated and may well be more profound with greater temperature changes.

Hypothermia affects renal function as well, with an impact on renal drug clearance. Glomerular filtra-tion rate is decreased by 65 percent in the dog at $25°C$.[97] In a study of dTc pharmacokinetics in the hypothermic cat, Ham et al documented a 60 percent decrease in drug clearance, and a concomitant reduc-tion in the amount of dTc excreted in the urine.[98]

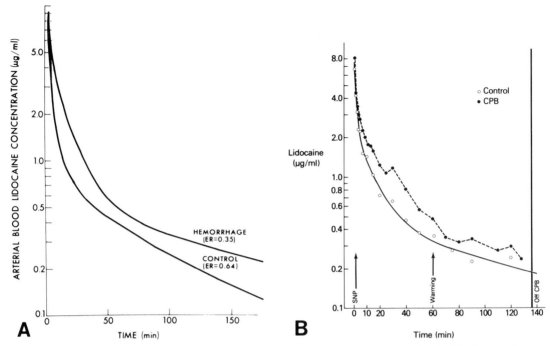

Fig. 2-13. (A) Predicted lidocaine concentrations in a 100-kg man after a 100-mg IV bolus, both in the control state and following hemorrhage. Data on hemorrhage including hypotension, altered regional blood flow, and reduced hepatic extraction (E.R.) of lidocaine were obtained in a primate model. (From Benowitz N, Forsyth RP, Melmon KL: Lidocaine disposition kinetics in monkey and man. II. Effects of hemorrhage and sympathomimetic drug administration. Clin Pharmacol Ther 16:99–109, 1974, with permission.) (B) Lidocaine concentrations in a cardiac surgical patient after a 100 mg intravenous bolus. The same subject was studied before surgery (control) and during CPB. The times of initiation of vasodilators (SNP), warming, and CPB termination are indicated. (Holley FO, unpublished data.)

Hemodilution

Hemodilution, in addition to its effect on vascular resistance and blood pressure, has a pronounced effect on drug binding to plasma proteins. Typically, a target hematocrit in the mid-20s is achieved in adults with a crystalloid pump prime.[99] The unintended consequence of this dilution of red cells is a proportionate 40–50 percent dilution of plasma proteins. When free and protein-bound drug and plasma proteins are all diluted equally, equilibrium considerations dictate that drug/plasma protein binding will diminish, and free drug fraction will increase accordingly. Figure 2-14 demonstrates this phenomenon for lidocaine with the dilutions performed in vitro.

Other consequences of acute hemodilution for drug disposition include the following:

1. Since plasma drug concentration is reduced without any change in the amount of drug in the body, the apparent volume of distribution increases acutely (Eq. 2-1).

2. After acute hemodilution, drug redistribution from tissues may occur in order to bring free drug concentrations in plasma and tissues back into equilibrium. The magnitude of this flux of drug depends on the relative amounts in tissues and plasma and on the degree of protein binding change.

3. As noted above, focus on total drug concentration can be misleading if the free fraction changes significantly, and the degree of drug effect is to be predicted.

4. For drugs whose plasma/red cell partitioning is not equal, blood and plasma clearance will no longer bear the same relationship to each other after hemodilution and must be distinguished.

5. The largely artifactual effect of heparin on drug protein binding is discussed above.

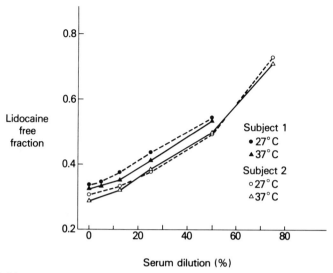

Fig. 2-14. In vitro demonstration of the effects of hemodilution on lidocaine protein binding. Serum from two subjects was studied at the indicated temperatures. Serum dilution represents the fraction of lactated Ringer's solution in the final sample. (Ponganis KV, Holley FO, Stanski DR, unpublished data.)

Reduction in Pulmonary Blood Flow

Although the exact amount depends on techniques of atrial cannulation and venting,[100] the reduction in pulmonary blood flow during CPB is often nearly total. This alteration in the circulation may significantly affect the disposition of basic drugs such as lidocaine, propranolol, and fentanyl, which are thought to distribute significantly into the lungs.[101] The metabolism of biogenic amines may be impaired by what is essentially an abolition, albeit temporary, of the pulmonary circulation, contributing perhaps to the elevation in plasma catecholamines, which has now been documented to occur during CPB.[102] In addition, during CPB, the lungs may serve as a reservoir for drugs that cannot be rapidly eliminated or distributed. Upon weaning from CPB, washout of a significant mass of drug into the systemic circulation might conceivably account for a rise in plasma drug concentrations.

Postoperative Drug Therapy

The hemodynamic effects of drugs given after CPB and in the postoperative period may alter drug disposition. An example from a primate model demonstrates this fact very clearly for the interactions of isoproterenol and norepinephrine with lidocaine

(Fig. 2-15).[94] These data suggest that isoproterenol increased lidocaine's volume of distribution and clearance, whereas norepinephrine decreased them. The interpretation of this data, however, becomes more complicated in the clinical setting where vasoactive drugs are generally employed in an attempt to correct pathophysiology rather than to create it.

Postoperative Changes in Protein Binding

Postoperative drug binding to plasma proteins may be mildly affected by the small decrease in serum albumin that is often seen after major surgery. However, of greater importance is the rise in the concentration of AAG that occurs after major surgery as well as after trauma and myocardial infarction.[21] AAG concentration has been shown to double several days after cardiac surgery (Fig. 2-16), correlating with changes in lidocaine kinetics.[37] Other drugs that may be affected are those that bind to AAG: amide local anesthetics, antiarrhythmics, fentanyl and its derivatives, and propranolol. In addition, the change in free fraction affects the pharmacodynamic interpretation of measured total drug levels as discussed above.

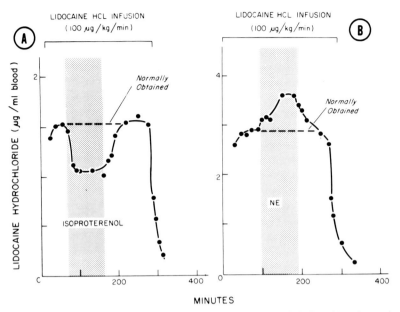

Fig. 2-15. Data from primates on the effects of isoproterenol infusion (A) and norepinephrine (NE) infusion (B) on serum lidocaine levels during a constant-rate lidocaine infusion. Isoproterenol appears to increase lidocaine clearance and volume of distribution, while norepinephrine has the opposite effect. (From Benowitz N, Forsyth RP, Melmon KL: Lidocaine disposition kinetics in monkey and man. II. Effects of hemorrhage and sympathomimetic drug administration. Clin Pharmacol Ther 16:99–109, 1974, with permission.)

Effects of Cardiopulmonary Bypass on the Disposition of Specific Drugs

Because of the methodologic limitations discussed above, and because some of the effects operate in opposite directions upon a given parameter (eg, volume of distribution), studies of individual drugs have demonstrated the influence of CPB on pharmacokinetics with varied degrees of success. A brief review of data on specific drugs does, however, permit some general principles to emerge.

LIDOCAINE

Lidocaine is an ideal probe to investigate the effects of CPB on drug disposition. Its pharmacokinetics in a variety of disease states (including relevant cardiovascular conditions) have already been characterized. Therapeutic concentrations are well defined and are monitored clinically, and, unlike some other drugs (cephalosporin antibiotics, for example), excessive concentrations are also to be avoided. Finally, unlike anesthetic drugs, it can be administered repeatedly with safety in the perioperative period for investigational purposes.

Lidocaine pharmacokinetics have been com-

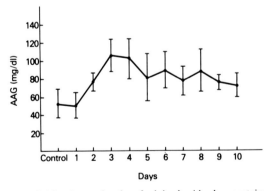

Fig. 2-16. Serum levels of alpha-*l*-acid glycoprotein (AAG) in 10 patients who underwent cardiac surgery between the control measurement and day 1 (mean ± SD). Concentrations of this plasma protein, which binds basic drugs, had increased significantly by 3 days after surgery and then returned slowly toward normal. (From Holley FO, Ponganis KV, Stanski DR: Effects of cardiac surgery with cardiopulmonary bypass on lidocaine disposition. Clin Pharmacol Ther 36:617–626, 1984, with permission.)

pared before and after CPB by Holley at al in a study that used each patient as his own control. No differences could be demonstrated in lidocaine pharmacokinetics after a bolus injection of 100 mg when compared preoperatively, 15 minutes after termination of CPB, or one day postoperatively.[37] A reduction in lidocaine clearance immediately after CPB would not have been surprising, considering the hemodynamic and temperature differences that persist at this time. The clearance of indocyanine green, a high hepatic-extraction ratio compound, is decreased by 30 percent after CPB.[6] However, the authors attributed the lack of observed effect to the withdrawal of propranolol therapy that occurred concurrently. These coronary artery bypass graft (CABG) patients were beta-blocked with propranolol during the control study, but therapy was discontinued postoperatively. The increase in lidocaine clearance that would be expected with propranolol withdrawal may have counteracted the anticipated effects of CPB. The fact that immediately after CPB no volume of distribution change could be demonstrated may mean that opposing effects of peripheral vasoconstriction and reduced plasma protein binding offset each other.

Of interest, however, is that in the same study, no significant changes in lidocaine pharmacokinetics could be demonstrated somewhat later, 3 days after surgery.[37] The importance of this finding is that it runs opposite to the clinical suspicion. These patients appear more normal physiologically 3 days after surgery than they do 15 minutes after CPB. The changes demonstrated were a 42 percent decrease in lidocaine clearance and a 40 percent decrease in steady-state volume of distribution, coincident with a 46 percent decrease in lidocaine free fraction because of increased AAG levels (Fig. 2-16). The reductions in clearance and volume of distribution would both tend to produce higher lidocaine levels in these patients recovering from CABG surgery; however, toxicity may be mitigated by the decreased lidocaine free fraction at this time. Assessment of antiarrhythmic efficacy, in relation to the usual therapeutic and toxic levels, must be made cautiously in this period since the relationship between free and total levels is not normal. In the final portion of the study, 1 week after surgery, all of these pharmacokinetic and protein binding alterations had begun to resolve. In the patient who suffers postoperative complications, however, the situation may be different.

Lidocaine disposition has been studied during CPB as well, since antiarrhythmic therapy is sometimes crucial during this period. Methodologic limitations are severe during CPB, however, since the period of interest is shorter than lidocaine's elimination half-life. These considerations precluded accurate calculation of lidocaine pharmacokinetics in one recent study.[103] However, those authors found that their data suggested an increased volume of distribution that they attributed to hemodilution and decreased protein binding. On that basis, they recommended a larger than normal loading dose, 2.5 mg/kg. To date, lidocaine protein binding has not been measured during CPB because of the heparin artifact.[54,55]

NARCOTIC ANALGESICS

Because of its long half-life and the nature of its effects, investigators studying fentanyl during cardiac surgery have not had the liberty of making repeated pharmacokinetic measurements in the same patient. To those proposing high-dose fentanyl in the late 1970s as an alternative to morphine for cardiac anesthesia,[104] the time-course of fentanyl levels during and after CPB and their relationship to adequacy of anesthesia were obviously of extreme interest. The earliest studies thus did not attempt formal pharmacokinetic analysis, but focused simply on the time course of fentanyl concentrations during CPB. As shown in Figure 2-2, fentanyl levels drop abruptly on initiation of CPB, 30–50 percent in most studies.[6,105,106] Although exact data have not been reported, this drop may be attributed to decreased protein binding secondary to hemodilution. Fentanyl is normally 80–85 percent protein bound.[107] Until the reason for the abrupt decline was understood, it was sometimes given as a rationale for administering a supplemental fentanyl dose after initiation of CPB. However, the rationale is much less cogent if the free fentanyl concentration, which changes much less, is considered. Fentanyl levels in the CNS do not change with hemodilution, except to the extent that re-equilibration of free concentrations occur. It can be predicted that the flux of drug will be small since most of the fentanyl in the body at this time is found in tissues.[108]

The acute fall in fentanyl concentrations without a change in the amount of drug in the body implies an acute increase in fentanyl's volume of distribution (Eq. 2-1). The subsequent lack of decline in fentanyl levels during CPB, documented by many,[6,105,106,109] suggests a markedly reduced fentanyl clearance, perhaps because of hypothermia and reduced non-pulsatile liver blood flow. When fentanyl administration is continued during CPB at a rate that produces stable levels before CPB, concentrations tend to rise,[110,111] suggesting either reduced hepatic clearance, impaired peripheral drug distribution, or both. Some investigators have actually noted a rise in fentanyl levels with termination of CPB.[6,109] Bentley et al have shown that this is due to washout of fentanyl from the lungs with resumption of ventilation and reperfusion of the pulmonary circulation.[109] A significant fall in fentanyl levels, if observed during CPB, may point to extracorporeal drug extraction by adsorption onto certain types of membrane oxygenators.[40,42] The usual stability of fentanyl levels during CPB, however, would suggest that further empiric fentanyl administration is not necessary during this period unless specifically suggested by signs of light anesthesia.

After CPB, fentanyl's elimination half-life is prolonged, 5.2 hours in one study compared with 3.3 hours in a vascular surgery control group[6] (Fig. 2-2). This prolongation, measured as 11–12 hours by Hug et al in a more recent study, is attributed to both an increased volume of distribution and a decreased clearance.[112] The slow decline of fentanyl levels in the postoperative period is of concern with respect to spontaneous ventilation and the timely extubation of these patients. The success of ventilatory weaning and extubation on the morning after surgery is dose related,[113] with CPB patients taking longer than vascular surgery patients to resume spontaneous ventilation after equivalent fentanyl doses[114] (see Chapter 3).

Alfentanil, like fentanyl, is eliminated more slowly after CPB ($t_{1/2}\beta$, 195 minutes vs 72 minutes before CPB).[115] The difference here was attributed solely to an increased volume of distribution. In a preliminary report,[116] which correlated this information with data on protein binding, the volume of distribution increase was explained by a tripling of alfentanil free fraction after CPB. Although total alfentanil levels declined markedly at the start of CPB, the free concentration was practically unchanged.[116]

For phenoperidine, a narcotic analgesic used widely in Europe, the pattern is remarkably similar to that for fentanyl. In one study, the initiation of CPB produced a 19–86 percent fall in plasma level, but the effect was only transient.[117] Continued drug administration at an infusion rate that produced stable levels before CPB caused concentrations to rise, eventually to a level above the pre-CPB baseline, again suggesting impaired drug clearance and/or peripheral distribution during CPB. The phenoperidine elimination phase was not studied.

NONDEPOLARIZING MUSCLE RELAXANTS

It is natural that the effects of CPB on the disposition of the nondepolarizing relaxants should be investigated since these drugs represent an essential part of the anesthetic management of the cardiac surgical patient. These studies are also interesting as probes of the mechanisms of CPB's effects since the muscle relaxants (with their small volumes of distribution and low clearances) differ pharmacokinetically from lidocaine and fentanyl. The concern for avoiding excessive drug levels, however, which is great for lidocaine and fentanyl, is mitigated for the muscle relaxants both by the development of drugs with minimal cardiovascular side effects and by the current preference for high-dose narcotic anesthesia and postoperative ventilatory support.

The pharmacokinetic effects of CPB on the muscle relaxants are summarized in Table 2-3.[118-120] Figure 2-3 depicts the dTc plasma level profile when given by bolus plus maintenance infusion as compared to predicted values in a group of normal subjects.[7] The higher-than-predicted levels are a common theme in the studies of dTc, gallamine,[118] and alcuronium.[119] These increases appear to represent the effects of decreased drug clearance and a contraction of the initial distribution volume. The shrinkage of this volume would not normally produce an increase in drug levels except that muscle relaxant administration is ongoing in these bolus plus infusion studies. The effect of CPB on the steady-state volume of distribution is not apparent perhaps because plasma protein binding is only moderate (less than 50 percent) for these drugs. The situation may be different in the pediatric population, where the volume of the pump prime is relatively large in relation to muscle relaxant volumes of distribution (see Chapter 5).

A number of other studies have examined the maintenance requirements of pancuronium,[121-123] vecuronium,[122] and atracurium[124] in order to maintain a standard reduction in twitch height during hypothermic CPB. This requirement is uniformly reduced, probably representing pharmacokinetic effects like those in Table 2-3. However, the factor of pharmacodynamic sensitivity has an impact upon dose requirement as well. In one study of pancuronium during CPB,[121] the sensitivity appeared greater than normal, which would also tend to reduce dose requirement. Such a trend has also been noted in the past for dTc in patients undergoing neurosurgical procedures under hypothermia.[125] The clinical relevance of these studies of muscle relaxant disposition

Table 2-3

Effects of CPB on Some Nondepolarizing Relaxants

Drug	Administration	Elimination Half-Life after CPB	Clearance	Volume of Distribution	Initial Volume of Distribution	Levels During CPB	Maintenance Requirement
d-Tubocurarine[7]	Bolus + Infusion	↑ 268%	↓ 78%	Unchanged	↓	↑↑	↓ (predicted)
Gallamine[118]	1 or 2 boluses	↓ 27%	Unchanged	↓ 15%	↓	↑	Minimal change (predicted)
Alcuronium[119]	Bolus + Infusion	↑ 167%	↓ 40%	Unchanged	↓	↑	↓ (predicted)
Metocurine[120]	Bolus + Infusion	Unchanged	Unchanged	Unchanged	Unchanged	↓	Unchanged

is in the recovery period, which may be prolonged because of the effects of CPB.

HYPNOTICS

Midazolam, lorazepam, etomidate, and thiopental have been investigated in the setting of CPB. After bolus doses, both lorazepam and midazolam demonstrated abrupt declines in levels with initiation of bypass, followed by rises in levels during the warming period.[126-128] Although pharmacokinetic calculations were not performed nor protein binding measured, similar pharmacokinetic mechanisms were probably operative as in the case of fentanyl. After bypass, the elimination half-life of midazolam was prolonged (281 vs 120 minutes) compared with earlier studies in young, healthy subjects.[126] Etomidate levels, when delivered by infusion, show a decrease with initiation of bypass, an increase with hypothermia, followed by a decrease during warming.[129] These changes are compatible with physiologically-induced alterations in peripheral drug distribution and clearance. However, drug levels in this study remained within the range that the authors felt was compatible with adequate anesthesia. In a recent study, where thiopental was administered during CPB,[130] drug distribution appeared normal, but metabolic clearance was significantly impaired, perhaps by hypothermia. Since drug metabolism is important for recovery from thiopental only after very high doses, these authors recommended normal dosing during CPB. Morgan et al[131] have recently investigated thiopental plasma protein binding during CPB. They found that the unbound fraction nearly doubled (from 16.6–29.3 percent) with hemodilution upon initiating bypass. Thus, although total drug lev-

els fell by 50 percent as CPB began, free drug levels (and presumably drug effects) were much more constant (see Chapter 4).

PROPRANOLOL

As a mainstay of antianginal treatment, propranolol therapy is a factor in the care of a large percentage of cardiac surgery patients and is generally continued up until the time of surgery.[132] It also is often reinstituted in low doses after surgery for prophylaxis against supraventricular tachyarrhythmias.[133] In addition to its effects on the disposition of other drugs, propranolol disposition is itself influenced by CPB. Any perturbations are of considerable significance for the continuation or initiation of propranolol therapy after CPB, when both the hyperdynamic state and excessive myocardial depression are to be avoided.

Plachetka et al studied patients who received either chronic oral or chronic oral plus acute intravenous propranolol prior to CPB.[134] Propranolol levels in both groups dropped by approximately 50 percent on initiation of CPB and then remained constant for the duration of bypass. Although protein binding was not measured, the abrupt decline in propranolol levels almost certainly represents hemodilution with an increase in propranolol free fraction. Normally, propranolol is highly bound, 90–95 percent.[130] Wood et al found a doubling of propranolol free fraction during CPB, but did not correct for the heparin artifact.[135] Thus, the profile of free propranolol concentrations, the concentrations producing drug effects, is not known during CPB, but may not be as greatly perturbed as is the total concentration.

At the end of CPB, Plachetka et al found that

propranolol concentrations actually rose and remained elevated without declining significantly for 4 hours.[134] Subsequently, they did decline but with a half-life almost twice normal (5.5 hours vs 3.2 hours). In a study of hypothermic dogs not placed on bypass, McAllister et al found that propranolol clearance was only half normal.[136] Plachetka's data would suggest a similar alteration in man.[134] The rise of drug levels at the end of CPB may represent drug washout with pulmonary reperfusion as found with fentanyl.

The implications of this work for propranolol therapy after CPB are clouded by the lack of information on free propranolol levels and the neglect in all the studies of measurements of propranolol's effects. It is probably safe to say that propranolol should be administered cautiously after CPB because drug levels may be rising from pulmonary washout, distribution and elimination may be impaired, and pharmacodynamic sensitivity may be altered.

DIGOXIN

Digoxin therapy in the preoperative cardiac surgery patient is less common today than in the early days of cardiac surgery when valve replacement was more frequent. However, it is more often used in the early postoperative period for prophylaxis of supraventricular dysrhythmias.[133,137] Digoxin toxicity is often difficult to identify in the early postoperative period and is potentiated by CPB-induced hypokalemia and hypomagnesemia.

Several investigators[138-140] have compared digoxin levels before and after CPB in patients receiving chronic therapy and found no difference. This is not surprising since digoxin has a 40-hour elimination half-life and is minimally protein bound with extensive tissue distribution. However, after CPB digoxin clearance is reduced, coincident with a reduced creatinine clearance.[138,140] These data would suggest that not only is perioperative supplementation unnecessary for the patient on chronic digoxin therapy, but also that maintenance doses should be reduced in the early postoperative period until renal function normalizes.

CEPHALOSPORINS

Perioperative prophylaxis with cephalosporins is common in cardiac surgery, with the purpose of preventing such disastrous complications as prosthetic valve endocarditis and sternal wound infection. Interest in the effects of CPB on the pharmacokinetics of

the cephalosporins was fueled by the need to know if levels adequate for prophylaxis were being achieved. Miller et al have shown that the pharmacokinetics of cephalothin[141] and cefaxolin[142] are indistinguishable on preoperative and first postoperative days. However, the clearance of both drugs is reduced intraoperatively by 50–70 percent with prolonged elimination resulting. Cefamandole is also eliminated more slowly after cardiac surgery.[143] Cefazolin, which is normally 80 percent protein bound, shows a not unanticipated drop in concentration at the beginning of CPB and an increase in its volume of distribution.[142] Cephalosporin dosing after cardiac surgery, therefore, need not be any more frequent than after other types of surgery in order to maintain prophylactic levels.

Patterns of Drug Disposition During CPB

The following patterns emerge from this discussion of data on specific drugs and from consideration of the interaction of altered physiology and pharmacokinetics.

1. The concentrations of most drugs drop with initiation of CPB. However, the magnitude of this decline may overestimate the decrease in free drug concentration, which is often relatively well maintained because of an increase in free drug fraction. In addition, pharmacodynamic relationships may be altered by hypothermia, but little is known about this effect.

2. The administration of drugs during CPB may produce higher than expected levels because of either reduced peripheral drug distribution, impaired drug clearance, or the abolition of the normal first-pass pulmonary drug distribution.

3. Elimination of many drugs is markedly prolonged after CPB, either because of impaired hepatic or renal drug clearance or because of increases in drug distribution volumes, secondary to hemodilution. Recovery from drug effects may likewise be prolonged.

4. The free fraction of drugs with significant plasma protein binding is abnormal during and after CPB, being increased early by hemodilution and decreased several days after surgery by the production of stress-reactant binding proteins. This phenomenon affects the interpretation of measured total drug levels in relation to recommended therapeutic concentrations.

RATIONAL, PHARMACOKINETICALLY GUIDED DRUG THERAPY IN THE CARDIAC PATIENT

The administration of intravenous anesthetics or therapeutic agents of any sort is certainly complicated by the presence of cardiac disease. Surgery and CPB simply add to the complexity. Not only are drug disposition and response different in the cardiac patient, they are almost certainly more variable than in the normal population. Some cardiac patients will have very little of the disease-induced physiologic/pharmacokinetic interaction in question, while others have the maximum compatible with life. Pharmacokinetic parameters in the cardiac patient thus may range from the normal to the extreme. The current extent of knowledge of pharmacokinetics in the cardiac patient has been reviewed in order to give the reader some predictive capabilities to apply to his or her own practice. To the (variable) extent that drug disposition can be correlated with clinically measurable aspects of anatomy or physiology, those measurements are helpful in designing drug administration regimens to achieve desired drug concentrations and, ideally, effects.

At the risk of oversimplification, it is evident that many processes at work in the cardiac patient (congestive heart failure, beta-blockade, old age, renal disease, CPB) all tend to lower drug clearance. Data on specific drugs and conditions can be used to reduce the maintenance dose of the drug, according to Equation 2-7. The risk of not doing so is an undesirably high drug level and an adverse drug reaction. Equation 2-1 can be used, likewise, to adjust the loading dose of a drug according to available information on its volume of distribution and the impact of disease or surgery on that volume.

As pharmacokineticists who are interested in optimizing drug levels point out,[144,145] a very small amount of data from the individual patient is worth as much as a tremendous amount of mean population data in disease states in predicting that patient's response. If rapid measurement of drug levels can be made within the time frame of cardiac anesthesia and surgery, so much the better. But failing that, observation of clinical response to a drug dose, with the best possible estimate of the time course of drug disposition in that patient in mind, will aid in staying within that ideal zone, the therapeutic window.

REFERENCES

1. Snow J: On the inhalation of the vapour of ether. London Medical Gazette 39:539–542, 1847
2. Holford NHG, Sheiner LB: Understanding the dose-effect relationship. Clinical application of pharmacokinetic-pharmacodynamic models. Clin Pharmacokinet 6:429–453, 1981
3. Stanski DR, Watkins WD: Drug Disposition in Anesthesia. Orlando, FL, Grune & Stratton Inc, 1982
4. Prys-Roberts C, Hug CC, Jr (eds): Pharmacokinetics of Anaesthesia. Oxford, Blackwell Scientific Publications, 1984
5. Wood M, Wood AJJ (eds): Drugs and Anesthesia: Pharmacology for Anesthesiologists. Baltimore, Williams and Wilkins, 1982
6. Koska AJ, Romagnoli A, Kramer WG: Effect of cardiopulmonary bypass on fentanyl distribution and elimination. Clin Pharmacol Ther 29:100–105, 1981
7. Walker JS, Shanks CA, Brown KF: Altered d-tubocurarine disposition during cardiopulmonary bypass surgery. Clin Pharmacol Ther 35:686–694, 1984
8. Haggard HW: The absorption, distribution, and elimination of ethyl ether. J Biol Chem 59:737–802, 1924
9. Rowland M: Physiologic pharmacokinetic models: Relevance, experience, and future trends. Drug Metab Rev 15(1&2):55–74, 1984
10. Eger EI: Anesthetic Uptake and Action. Baltimore, Williams and Wilkins, 1974
11. Mapleson WW: The rate of uptake of halothane vapour in man. Br J Anaesth 34:11–18, 1962
12. Bischoff KB, Dedrick RL: Thiopental pharmacokinetics. J Pharm Sci 57:1346–1351, 1968
13. Saidman LJ, Eger EI: The effect of thiopental metabolism on duration of anesthesia. Anesthesiology 27:118–126, 1966
14. Price HL, Kornat PJ, Safer JN, et al: The uptake of thiopental by body tissues and its relation to the duration of narcosis. Clin Pharmacol Ther 1:16–22, 1960
15. Teorell T: Kinetics of distribution of substances administered to the body. Arch Int Pharmacodyn 57:205–240, 1937
16. Michaelis L, Menten ML: Die kinetik der invertinwirking. Biochem Z 49:333–369, 1913
17. Klotz U: Pathophysiological and disease-induced changes in drug distribution volume: Pharmacokinetic implications. Clin Pharmacokinet 1:204–218, 1976
18. Ramzan MI, Somogyi AA, Walker JS, et al: Clinical pharmacokinetics of the non-depolarizing muscle relaxants. Clin Pharmacokinet 6:25–60, 1981
19. Hug CC, Jr: Pharmacokinetics and dynamics of narcotic analgesics, In Prys-Roberts C, Hug CC Jr.

(eds): Pharmacokinetics of Anaesthesia. Oxford, Blackwell, 1984, pp 187–234

20. Koch-Weser J, Sellers EM: Binding of drugs to serum albumin. N Engl J Med 294:311–316, 526–531, 1976

21. Piafsky KM: Disease-induced changes in the plasma binding of basic drugs. Clin Pharmacokinet 5:246–262, 1980

22. Abernethy DR, Greenblatt DJ: Pharmacokinetics of drugs in obesity. Clin Pharmacokinet 7:108–124, 1982

23. Wilkinson GR: Pharmacokinetics of drug disposition: Hemodynamic considerations. Annu Rev Pharmacol 15:11–25, 1975

24. Wilkinson GR, Shand DG: A physiological approach to hepatic drug clearance. Clin Pharmacol Ther 18:377–390, 1975

25. Williams RL, Mamelok RD: Hepatic disease and drug pharmacokinetics. Clin Pharmacokinet 5:528–547, 1980

26. Szeto HH, Inturrisi CE, Houde R, et al: Accumulation of nor-meperidine in patients with renal failure or cancer. Ann Intern Med 86:738–741, 1977

27. Don HF, Dieppa RA, Taylor P: Narcotic analgesics in anuric patients. Anesthesiology 42:745–747, 1975

28. Tucker GT: Measurement of the renal clearance of drugs. Br J Clin Pharmacol 12:761–770, 1981

29. Riegelman S, Loo JKC, Rowland M: Shortcomings in pharmacokinetic analysis by conceiving the body to exhibit properties of a single compartment. J Pharm Sci 57:117–123, 1968

30. Gibaldi M, Perrier D: Pharmacokinetics. New York, Marcel Dekker, Inc, 1982, pp 45–111

31. Burch PG, Stanski DR: The role of metabolism and protein binding in thiopental anesthesia. Anesthesiology 58:146–152, 1983

32. Homer TD, Stanski DR: The effect of increasing age on thiopental disposition and anesthetic requirement. Anesthesiology 62:714–724, 1985

33. Mather LE: Clinical pharmacokinetics of fentanyl and its newer derivatives. Clin Pharmacokinet 8:422–446, 1983

34. Swerdlow BN, Holley FO: Pharmacokinetic and pharmacodynamic relationships for intravenous anesthetic drugs. Clin Pharmacokinet 12: In press, 1987

35. Rowland M: Plasma protein binding and therapeutic drug monitoring. Ther Drug Monit 2:29–37, 1980

36. Levy RH, Moreland TA: Rationale for monitoring free drug levels. Clin Pharmacokinet 9 (Suppl 1): 1–9, 1984

37. Holley FO, Ponganis KV, Stanski DR: Effects of cardiac surgery with cardiopulmonary bypass on lidocaine disposition. Clin Pharmacol Ther 35:617–626, 1984

38. Ruciman WB, Ilsley AH, Mather LE, et al: A sheep preparation for studying interactions between blood flow and drug disposition. I. Physiological profile. Br J Anaesth 56:1015–1028, 1984

39. Stanski DR, Hudson RJ, Homer TD, et al: Pharmacodynamic modeling of thiopental anesthesia. J Pharm Biopharm 12:223–240, 1984

40. Lam G, Chiou WL: Arterial and venous blood sampling in pharmacokinetic studies: Propranolol in rabbits and dogs. Res Commun Chem Pathol Pharmacol 33:33–48, 1981

41. Koren G, Crean P, Klein J, et al: Sequestration of fentanyl by the cardiopulmonary bypass. Eur J Clin Pharmacol 27:51–56, 1984

42. Rosen DA, Rosen KR, Davidson B, et al: Absorption of fentanyl by the membrane oxygenator. Anesthesiology 63:A281, 1985

43. Dasta JF, Jacobi J, Wu LS, et al: Loss of nitroglycerin to cardiopulmonary bypass apparatus. Crit Care Med 11:50–52, 1983

44. Rebuck AS, Brande AC: Assessment of drug disposition in the lung. Drugs 28:544–553, 1984

45. Fielding PE, Shore VG, Fielding CJ: Lipoprotein lipase. Properties of the enzyme isolated from post heparin plasma. Biochem 13:4318–4323, 1974

46. Krauss RM, Levy RI, Fredrickson DS: Selective measurement of two lipase activities in postheparin plasma from normal subjects and patients with hyperlipoproteinemia. J Clin Invest 54:1107–1124, 1974

47. LaRosa JC, Levy RI, Windmueller HG, et al: Comparison of the triglyceride lipase of liver, adipose tissue, and postheparin plasma. J Lipid Res 13:356–363, 1972

48. Desmond PV, Roberts RK, Wood AJJ, et al: Effect of heparin administration on plasma binding of benzodiazepines. Br J Clin Pharmacol 9:171–175, 1980

49. Kessler KM, Leech RC, Spann JF: Blood collection techniques, heparin and quinidine protein binding. Clin Pharmacol Ther 25:204–210, 1979

50. Routledge PA, Bjornsson TD, Kitchell BB, et al: Heparin administration increases plasma warfarin binding in man. Br J Clin Pharmacol 8:281–282, 1979

51. Storstein L, Janssen H: Studies on digitalis. VI. The effect of heparin on serum protein binding of digitoxin and digoxin. Clin Pharmacol Ther 20:15–23, 1976

52. Van der Vijgh WJF, Oe PL: Pharmacokinetic aspects of digoxin in patients with terminal renal failure. III. Effect of heparin. Int J Clin Pharmacol Biopharm 15:560–562, 1977

53. Wood M, Shand DG, Wood AJJ: Altered drug binding due to the use of indwelling heparinized cannulas (heparin lock) for sampling. Clin Pharmacol Ther 25:103–108, 1979

54. Brown JE, Kitchel BB, Bjornsson TD, et al: The artifactual nature of heparin-induced drug protein binding alterations. Clin Pharmacol Ther 30:636–643, 1981

55. Giacomini KM, Swezey SE, Giacomini JC, et al: Administration of heparin causes *in vitro* release of nonesterified fatty acids in human plasma. Life Sci 27:771–780, 1980

56. Giacomini KM, Giacomini JC, Blaschke TF: Absence of effect of heparin on the binding of prazosin and phenytoin to plasma proteins. Biochem Pharmacol 29:3337–3340, 1980

57. Benowitz NL, Meister W: Pharmacokinetics in patients with cardiac failure. Clin Pharmacokinet 1:389–405, 1976

58. Kilcoyne MM, Schmidt DH, Cannon PJ: Intrarenal blood flow in congestive heart failure. Circulation 47:786–797, 1973

59. Duchin KL, Schrier RW: Interrelationship between renal haemodynamics, drug kinetics, and drug action. Clin Pharmacokinet 3:58–71, 1978

60. Dunn GD, Hayes P, Breen KJ, et al: The liver in congestive heart failure: A review. Am J Med Sci 265:174–189, 1973

61. Seldon R, Sasahara AA: Central nervous system toxicity induced by lidocaine. JAMA 202:908–909, 1967

62. Anderson ST, Pitt A: Lignocaine in the management of ventricular arrhythmias. Med J Aust 1:208–211, 1969

63. Stenson RE, Constantino RT, Harrison DC: Interrelationships of hepatic blood flow, cardiac output, and blood levels of lidocaine in man. Circulation 43:205–211, 1971

64. Thomson PD, Melmon KL, Richardson JA, et al: Lidocaine pharmacokinetics in advanced heart failure, liver disease, and renal failure in humans. Ann Intern Med 78:499–508, 1973

65. Prescott LF, Adjepon-Yamoah KK, Talbott RG: Impaired lignocaine metabolism in patients with myocardial infarction and cardiac failure. Br Med J 1:939–941, 1976

66. Routledge PA, Shand DG, Barchowsky A, et al: Relationship between alpha-1-acid glycoprotein and lidocaine disposition in myocardial infarction. Clin Pharmacol Ther 30:154–157, 1981

67. Gibson TP, Matusik EJ, Briggs WA: N-acetyl procainamide levels in patients with end-stage renal failure. Clin Pharmacol Ther 19:206–212, 1976

68. Koch-Weser J, Klein SW: Procainamide dosage schedules, plasma concentrations, and clinical effects. JAMA 215:1454–1460, 1971

69. Ueda CT, Dzindzio BS: Quinidine kinetics in congestive heart failure. Clin Pharmacol Ther 23:158–164, 1978

70. Kessler KM, Lowenthal DT, Warner H, et al: Quinidine elimination in patients with congestive heart failure or poor renal function. N Engl J Med 290:706–709, 1974

71. Powell JR, Vozeh S, Hopewell P, et al: Theophylline disposition in acutely ill hospitalized patients. The effect of smoking, heart failure, severe airways obstruction and pneumonia. Am Rev Respir Dis 118:229–238, 1978

72. Piafsky KM, Sitar DS, Rangno RE, et al: Theophylline kinetics in acute pulmonary edema. Clin Pharmacol Ther 21:310–316, 1977

73. Halkin H, Sheiner LB, Peck CC, et al: Determinants of the renal clearance of digoxin. Clin Pharmacol Ther 17:385–394, 1975

74. Nies AS, Evans GH, Shand DG: The hemodynamic effects of beta-adrenergic blockade on the flow-dependent hepatic clearance of propranolol. J Pharm Exp Ther 184:716–720, 1973

75. Branch RA, Shand DG, Wilkinson GR, et al: The reduction of lidocaine clearance by dl-propranolol: An example of hemodynamic drug interaction. J Pharm Exp Ther 184:515–519, 1973

76. Ochs HR, Carstens G, Greenblatt DJ: Reduction in lidocaine clearance during continuous infusion and by coadministration of propranolol. N Engl J Med 303:373–377, 1980

77. Shepherd AN, Hayes PC, Jocyna M, et al: The influence of captopril, the nitrates and propranolol on apparent liver blood flow. Br J Clin Pharmacol 19:393–397, 1985

78. Conrad KA, Byers JM, Finley PR, et al: Lidocaine elimination: Effects of metoprolol and of propranolol. Clin Pharmacol Ther 33:133–138, 1983

79. Jordö L, Johnsson G, Lundborg P, et al: Pharmacokinetics of lidocaine in healthy individuals pretreated with multiple doses of metoprolol. Int J Clin Pharmacol 22:312–315, 1984

80. Greenblatt DJ, Franke K, Huffmann DH: Impairment of antipyrine clearance in humans by propranolol. Circulation 57:1161–1164, 1978

81. Bax NDS, Lennard MS, Tucker GT: Inhibition of antipyrine metabolism by beta-adrenoreceptor antagonists. Br J Clin Pharmacol 12:779–784, 1981

82. Ochs HR, Greenblatt DJ, Verburg-Ochs B: Propranolol interactions with diazepam, lorazepam, and alprazolam. Clin Pharmacol Ther 36:451–455, 1984

83. Conrad KA, Nyman DW: Effects of metoprolol and propranolol on theophylline elimination. Clin Pharmacol Ther 28:463–467, 1980

84. Wood AJJ, Feely J.: Pharmacokinetic drug interactions with propranolol. Clin Pharmacokinet 8:253–262, 1983

85. Gersh BJ, Kronmal RA, Schaff HV, et al: Comparison of coronary artery bypass surgery and medical therapy in patients 65 years of age or older. N Engl J Med 313:217–223, 1985

86. Krupka L, Verner A: Hazards of drug use among the elderly. Gerontologist 19:90–95, 1979

87. Schmucker DL: Aging and drug disposition. An update. Pharmacol Rev 37:133–148, 1985

88. Arden JR, Holley FO, Stanski DR: Increased sensitivity to etomidate in the elderly: Initial distribution

versus altered brain response. Anesthesiology 65:19–27, 1986

89. Scott JC, Stanski DR: Decreased fentanyl/alfentanil dose requirements with increasing age. A pharmacodynamic basis. Anesthesiology 63:A374, 1985

90. Gibson TP: Influence of renal disease on pharmacokinetics, In Evans WE, Schentag JJ, Jusko WJ (eds): Applied Pharmacokinetics. San Francisco, Applied Therapeutics, Inc, 1980, pp 32–56

91. Lillehei RC, Longerbeam JK, Bloch JH, et al: The nature of irreversible shock: Experimental and clinical observations. Ann Surg 160:682–710, 1964

92. Mavroudis C: To pulse or not to pulse. Ann Thorac Surg 25:259–271, 1978

93. Stanley TH: Arterial pressure and deltoid muscle gas tensions during cardiopulmonary bypass in man. Can Anaesth Soc J 25:286–290, 1978

94. Benowitz N, Forsyth RP, Melmon KL, et al: Lidocaine disposition kinetics in monkey and man. II. Effects of hemorrhage and sympathomimetic drug administration. Clin Pharmacol Ther 16:99–109, 1974

95. Benowitz N, Forsyth RP, Melmon KL, et al: Lidocaine disposition kinetics in monkey and man. I. Prediction by a perfusion model. Clin Pharmacol Ther 16:87–98, 1974

96. Larsen JA: The effect of cooling on liver function in cats. Acta Phys Scand 81:197–207, 1971

97. Boylan JW, Hong SK: Regulation of renal function in hypothermia. Am J Physiol 211:1371–1378, 1966

98. Ham J, Miller RD, Benet LZ, et al: Pharmacokinetics and pharmacodynamics of d-tubocurarine during hypothermia in the cat. Anesthesiology 49:324–329, 1978

99. Nadjmabadi MH, Rastan H, Saidi MT, et al: Haemodynamic effects of acute intraoperative haemodilution in open heart surgery. Anaesthetist 27:364–369, 1978

100. Utley JR, Stephens DB: Venting during cardiopulmonary bypass. *In* Utley JR (ed): Pathophysiology and Techniques of Cardiopulmonary Bypass. Baltimore, Williams and Wilkins, 1983, pp 115–127

101. Roth RA, Wiersma DA: Role of the lung in total body clearance of circulating drugs. Clin Pharmacokinet 4:355–367, 1979

102. Merlone S, Gaba D, Dauffenbach R, et al: High time resolution catecholamine sampling during cardiopulmonary bypass. Anesthesiology 63:A37, 1985

103. Morrell DF, Harrison GG: Lignocaine kinetics during cardiopulmonary bypass. Br J Anaesth 55:1173–1177, 1983

104. Stanley TH, Webster LR: Anesthetic requirements and cardiovascular effects of fentanyl-oxygen and fentanyl-diazepam-oxygen anesthesia in man. Anesth Analg 57:411–426, 1978

105. Lunn KJ, Stanley TH, Eisele J, et al: High dose fentanyl anesthesia for coronary artery surgery. Plasma fentanyl concentrations and influence of nitrous oxide on cardiovascular responses. Anesth Analg 58:390–395, 1979

106. Bovill JG, Sevbel PS: Pharmacokinetics of high dose fentanyl. Br J Anaesth 52:795–801, 1980

107. Meuldermans WEG, Hurkmans RMA, Heykants JJP: Plasma protein binding and distribution of fentanyl, sufentanil, alfentanil and lofentanil in blood. Arch Int Pharmacodyn Ther 257:4–19, 1982

108. Hug CC, Murphy MR: Tissue redistribution of fentanyl and termination of its effects in rats. Anesthesiology 55:369–375, 1981

109. Bentley JB, Conahan TJ, Cork RC: Fentanyl sequestration in lungs during cardiopulmonary bypass. Clin Pharmacol Ther 34:703–706, 1983

110. Sprigge JS, Wynands JE, Whalley DG, et al: Fentanyl infusion anesthesia for aortocoronary bypass surgery: Plasma levels and hemodynamic response. Anesth Analg 61:972–978, 1982

111. Wynands JE, Townsend GE, Wong P, et al: Blood pressure response and plasma fentanyl concentrations during high- and very high-dose fentanyl anesthesia for coronary artery surgery. Anesth Analg 62:661–665, 1983

112. Hug CC, Moldenhauer CC: Pharmacokinetics and dynamics of fentanyl infusion in cardiac surgical patients. Anesthesiology 57:A45, 1982

113. Holley FO: Prolonged respiratory depression in cardiac surgery patients: The contribution of fentanyl. Anesthesiology 61:A80, 1984

114. Koska AJ, Romagnoli A, Kramer WG: Pharmacodynamics of fentanyl citrate in patients undergoing aortocoronary bypass. Bull Tex Heart Inst 8:405–412, 1981

115. Hug CC, DeLange S, Burm AGL: Alfentanil pharmacokinetics in patients before and after cardiopulmonary bypass. Anesth Analg 62:266, 1983

116. Hug CC, Burm AGL, DeLange S, et al: Alfentanil pharmacokinetics and protein binding before and after cardiopulmonary bypass (CPB). Society of Cardiovascular Anesthesiologists, Annual Meeting Program:76–77, 1983

117. Fischler M, Levron JC, Trang H, et al: Pharmacokinetics of phenoperidine in patients undergoing cardiopulmonary bypass. Br J Anaesth 57:877–882, 1985

118. Shanks CA, Ramzan IM, Walker JS, et al: Gallamine disposition in open-heart surgery involving cardiopulmonary bypass. Clin Pharmacol Ther 33:742–799, 1983

119. Walker JS, Brown KF, Shanks CA: Alcuronium kinetics in patients undergoing cardiopulmonary bypass surgery. Br J Clin Pharmacol 15:237–244, 1983

120. Shanks CA, Avram MJ, Kinzer J, et al: Pharmacokinetics and pharmacodynamics of metocurine in cardiac surgery patients. Anesth Analg 65:S138, 1986

121. d'Hollander AA, Duvaldestin P, Henzel D, et al:

Variations in pancuronium requirement, plasma concentration, and urinary excretion induced by cardiopulmonary bypass with hypothermia. Anesthesiology 58:505–509, 1983

122. Buzello W, Schluermann D, Schlinder M, et al: Hypothermic cardiopulmonary bypass and neuromuscular blockade by pancuronium and vecuronium. Anesthesiology 62:201–204, 1985

123. Futter ME, Whalley DG, Wynands JE, et al: Pancuronium requirements during hypothermic cardiopulmonary bypass in man. Anaesth Int Care 11:216–219, 1983

124. Flynn PJ, Hughes R, Walton B: Use of atracurium in cardiac surgery involving cardiopulmonary bypass with induced hypothermia. Br. J Anaesth 56:967–972, 1984

125. Ham J, Stanski DR, Newfield P, et al: Pharmacokinetics and dynamics of d-tubocurarine during hypothermia in humans. Anesthesiology 55:631–635, 1981

126. Kanto J, Himberg JJ, Heikkila A, et al: Midazolam kinetics before, during, and after cardiopulmonary bypass surgery. Int J Clin Pharm Res 5:123–126, 1985

127. Aaltonen L, Kanto J, Arola M, et al: Effect of age and cardiopulmonary bypass on the pharmacokinetics of lorazepam. Acta Pharmacol Toxicol 51:126, 1982

128. Boscoe MJ, Dawling S, Thompson MA, et al: Lorazepam in open-heart surgery—plasma concentrations before, during, and after bypass following different dose regimens. Anaesth Int Care 12:9–13, 1984

129. Oduro A, Tomlinson AA, Voice A, et al: The use of etomidate infusions during anaesthesia for cardiopulmonary bypass. Anaesth 38 (Suppl):66–69, 1983

130. Nancherla AR, Narang PK, Kin YD, et al: Sodium thiopental kinetics during cardiopulmonary bypass. Anesth Analg 65:S111, 1986

131. Morgan DJ, Crankshaw DP, Prideaux PR, et al: Thiopentone levels during cardiopulmonary bypass. Anaesth 41:4–10, 1986

132. Kaplan JA, Dunbar RW, Bland JW, et al: Propranolol and cardiac surgery: A problem for the anesthesiologist? Anesth Analg 54:571–578, 1975

133. Roffman JA, Fieldman A: Digoxin and propranolol in the prophylaxis of supraventricular tachydysrhythmias after coronary bypass surgery. Ann Thorac Surg 31:496–501, 1981

134. Plachetka JR, Salomon NW, Copeland JG: Plasma propranolol before, during, and after cardiopulmonary bypass. Clin Pharmacol Ther 30:745–751, 1981

135. Wood M, Shand DG, Wood AJJ: Propranolol binding in plasma during cardiopulmonary bypass. Anesthesiology 51:512–516, 1979

136. McAllister RG, Bourne DM, Tan TG, et al: Effects of hypothermia on propranolol kinetics. Clin Pharmacol Ther 25:1–7, 1979

137. Csicsko JF, Schatzlein MH, King RD: Immediate postoperative digitalization in the prophylaxis of supraventricular arrhythmias following coronary artery bypass. J Thorac Cardiovasc Surg 81:419–422, 1981

138. Coltart DJ, Chamberlain DA, Howard MR, et al: Effect of cardiopulmonary bypass on plasma digoxin concentrations. Br Heart J 33:334–338, 1971

139. Morrison J, Killip T: Serum digitalis and arrhythmia in patients undergoing cardiopulmonary bypass. Circ 47:341–352, 1973

140. Krasula RW, Hastreiter AR, Levitsky S, et al: Serum, atrial, and urinary digoxin levels during cardiopulmonary bypass in children. Circulation 49:1047–1052, 1974

141. Miller KW, Chan KKH, McCoy HG, et al: Cephalothin kinetics before, during, and after cardiopulmonary bypass surgery. Clin Pharmacol Ther 26:54–62, 1979

142. Miller KW, McCoy HG, Chan KKH, et al: Effect of cardiopulmonary bypass on cefazolin disposition. Clin Pharmacol Ther 27:550–556, 1980

143. Polk RE, Archer GL, Lower R: Cefamandole kinetics during cardiopulmonary bypass. Clin Pharmacol Ther 23:473–480, 1980

144. Sheiner LB, Beal SL, Rosenberg B, et al: Forecasting individual pharmacokinetics. Clin Pharmacol Ther 26:294–305, 1979

145. Vozeh S, Berger M, Wenk M, et al: Rapid prediction of individual dosage requirement for lidocaine. Clin Pharmacokinet 9:354–363, 1984

Peter S. Sebel, Ph.D., F.F.A.R.C.S.I.
James G. Bovill, M.D., F.F.A.R.C.S.I.

3

Opioid Analgesics in Cardiac Anesthesia

Opioid analgesics are used extensively in current anesthetic practice, both as a component of a *balanced* anesthetic technique, and in cardiac anesthesia in a high-dose opioid anesthetic technique. The rationale for a high-dose technique is that opioids appear to produce less myocardial depression than conventional intravenous and inhalational agents. Furthermore, it appears that opioids, in large doses, may suppress the hormonal and metabolic responses to surgery, producing *stress-free* anesthesia. In this chapter, current information about opioid receptors and the body's own opioids, endorphins, and enkephalins will be reviewed. The use of opioid analgesics as sole anesthetics will be considered, and an attempt will be made to develop a rationale for the use of these agents in cardiac anesthesia based on their general pharmacology and pharmacokinetic properties.

There is some confusion about terminology in this field, with the terms "narcotic," "opiate," and "opioid" being used more or less interchangeably throughout the literature. The term "narcotic" is derived from the Greek word for stupor and was used to mean any drug that produced sleep. For this reason it was used to describe morphine and morphine-like drugs. It also applies to other drugs that may produce sleep, such as barbiturates. The term "opiate"

applies to drugs derived from the opium poppy: morphine, codeine, and the other semi-synthetic morphine derivatives such as diacetylmorphine (heroin). Goodman and Gilman define the term "opioid" as a generic designation for all exogenous substances that bind specifically to any of the several subspecies of opioid receptors and produce some agonist action. Substances such as naloxone that bind to opioid receptors with little or no agonist action are termed "opioid antagonists."[1]

OPIOID RECEPTORS

The existence of specific opioid receptors was suggested by the observation that all morphine-like drugs were not only structurally similar, but also exhibited stereospecificity, with only the levorotatory(−)isomer being active. The dextrorotatory, mirror image of the naturally occurring (−)-morphine, (+)-morphine, is devoid of analgesic activity.[2] The (+)-isomer of lofentanil, a fentanyl analogue, is a short-acting partial antagonist; whereas the (−) isomer is a pure, potent, and extremely long-acting opioid agonist.[3] That the opioid receptor system might be heterogenous rather than homogenous was suggested by studies on the *N*-allyl derivative of mor-

Table 3-1

Classification of Opioid Receptors

Receptor	Effect	Agonist	Antagonist
Mu	Supraspinal analgesia Ventilatory depression Euphoria Dependence Miosis	Beta-endorphin Morphine	Naloxone Pentazocine Nalbuphine
Delta	Modulates mu-receptor activity Supraspinal analgesia Ventilatory depression	Leu-enkephalin Beta-endorphin	Naloxone Met-enkephalin
Kappa	Spinal analgesia Ventilatory depression Sedation Miosis	Dynorphin Morphine Nalbuphine	Naloxone
Sigma	Dysphoria Vasomotor stimulation Hallucinations Mydriasis	? Pentazocine ? Phenylcyclidine	Naloxone

phine, nalorphine. Nalorphine, originally introduced as a morphine antagonist, was shown to have analgesic properties.[4] The antagonist effects of nalorphine were originally explained on the basis of a homogenous receptor system. It was thought that nalorphine was a partial agonist with low intrinsic activity.[5] The further observation that large doses of nalorphine were less effective than small doses in antagonizing the effects of morphine was, however, inconsistent with a single-receptor hypothesis. Martin first proposed that nalorphine acted as a competitive antagonist at the morphine receptor, and was an agonist at a second receptor site where its own analgesic actions were mediated.[6] This was described as receptor dualism. Following a series of pharmacologic experiments in dogs with spinal section, this hypothesis was expanded to a three-receptor system (Table 3-1). The morphine receptor (mu) was associated with analgesia, tolerance, and dependence. The kappa-receptor, the typical agonist being ketocyclazozine, produced analgesia, sedation, and some dependence. Dysphoric effects were mediated by the sigma receptor, the typical agonist being *n*-allylnormetazocine (SKF-10 047). Nalorphine was described as a mu-receptor antagonist and a kappa- and sigma-receptor agonist.[7,8] Subsequently, a delta-receptor, with a high affinity for leucine-enkephalin was described.[9] An epsilon-receptor, identified in rat vas deferens, is thought to be specific for beta-endorphin.[10] It is believed that the delta- and mu-receptors coexist within the same physical complex, and that endogenous mu-receptor activation by beta-endorphin is regulated by the enkephalins. Binding of enkephalins at the delta-receptor can either promote or inhibit mu-receptor activity, depending on whether Leu- or Met-enkephalin predominates.[11,12] Leu-enkephalin potentiates opioid-induced analgesia; whereas Met-enkephalin antagonizes it (Fig. 3-1). The mu-receptor is now known to consist of two subtypes, a high-affinity mu_1-receptor and a low-affinity mu_2-receptor.[13] Analgesia is associated with the mu_1-, but not the mu_2-receptor. Respiratory depression, an unwanted side effect of opioid drugs, is not mediated by mu_1-receptors, but is probably a property of mu_2- or delta-receptors.[14,15]

In 1973, the existence of stereospecific opioid receptors in rat brain was demonstrated by three independent groups of researchers by isolated tissue and biochemical studies using tritiated opioid.[16-18] Autoradiographic techniques allowed specific microscopic localization of the sites associated with the opioid receptor.[19] Within the spinal cord, receptors are located in a dense band in the substantia gelatinosa. In the brain stem, opioid receptors are found within the periacqueductal gray matter and the solitary nuclei that receive input from the vagus and glossopharyngeal nerves. Opioid receptors are also found in the area postrema, which contains the chemoreceptor trigger zone. This is the site where opioids induce nausea and vomiting. In the brain the

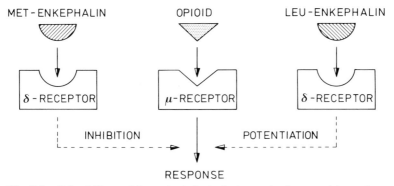

Fig. 3-1. Role of Met- and Leu-enkephalin in the interaction between delta- and mu-receptors.

highest receptor concentration is in the amygdala. This area is associated with emotional rather than analgesic behavior.

If specific receptors exist in the brain and spinal cord, sensitive to the effects of morphine-like drugs, then it is likely that endogenous substances exist within the body that are active at these receptors. This reasoning led to the isolation of two pentapeptides with opioid activity in pig brain, methionine enkephalin and leucine enkephalin, by Hughes et al in 1975.[20] These pentapeptides are specific neurotransmitters, involved in the integration of information relating to pain and emotional behavior. The amino-acid sequence of methionine enkephalin is the same as residues 61–65 of beta-lipotrophin, a pituitary peptide containing 91 amino acids.[21] Various fragments of beta-lipotrophin were found to have opioid activity, and the most potent of these, residue 61–91, was designated beta-endorphin. The biologic function of opioid peptides within the pituitary remains unclear, but they are probably involved in regulating pituitary function and hormone secretion.[19]

It is likely that understanding of the opioid receptor system and endogenous opioid systems will become more complete with time. What is already apparent is that the existence of the various subspecies of receptors helps in understanding the pharmacology of the opioid agonists, antagonists, and mixed agonist/antagonists.

USE OF OPIOID ANALGESICS

History

Opium, the juice of the unripe seedhead of the poppy, Papaver somniferum, has been known as a narcotic from the time of the Sumarians, 5000 years

ago. Raw opium contains 25 active alkaloids, including morphine, codeine, and papaveretum. Opioid administration only became possible on a scientific basis, however, with the isolation by Serturner in 1806 of an active principle, which he called "morpheum," after Morpheus, the Greek god of dreams. Reliable parenteral administration was made possible by the invention of the syringe by Pravaz in 1853, and the hollow needle by Wood in 1855. In 1869, Claude Bernard was probably the first to investigate the use of morphine for premedication; and it was being used by subcutaneous injection during minor surgery by 1872.[22] In 1900, Schneiderlein introduced an anesthetic technique involving the intramuscular administration of morphine in divided doses, up to 70 mg, and scopolamine. Using this technique, patients were oblivious to pain and only 70 percent required restraint during surgery! This anesthetic technique was, in a way, a forerunner of today's high-dose opioid techniques; but at the turn of the century, the patients were required to breathe for themselves and this method of anesthesia caused several deaths and was soon abandoned.

The use of morphine-like drugs virtually disappeared from anesthetic practice for the next four decades, and it was not until the 1940s that they again assumed an important role along with the use of curare and the rapid-acting barbiturates. Curare allowed muscle relaxation without the need for deep levels of anesthesia; and the barbiturates, although producing unconsciousness, did not provide analgesia. An important development was the introduction of meperidine supplementation of nitrous oxide anesthesia.[23,24] Meperidine, the first synthetic opioid, was produced by Eisleb and Schaumann in 1939. Since then many synthetic and semisynthetic opioid compounds have been produced. The phenylpiperidine derivatives, including fentanyl, have largely replaced meperidine for intraoperative use. The introduction of nalorphine (N-allyl-morphine) into clinical practice in 1951 gave anesthesiologists the opportunity to selectively reverse opioid-induced respiratory depression for the first time.[25]

Use of Opioids in Balanced Anesthesia

The anesthetic state consists of four essential components: amnesia, analgesia, muscle relaxation, and abolition of autonomic reflexes to surgery.[26,27] Modern general anesthesia uses a combination of different drugs to achieve this state, a technique commonly referred to as *"balanced anesthesia."* This term was introduced by Lundy in 1926 to describe a combination of premedication, regional analgesia, and general anesthesia with one or more agents so that unconsciousness and pain relief were obtained via a balance of agents and techniques.

The inclusion of an opioid as the specific analgesic component of balanced anesthesia offers several advantages. When an opioid is given either as part of the premedication or as a small bolus along with the intravenous induction drug, induction of anesthesia is smoother, less induction agent is required, and the cardiovascular responses to laryngoscopy and intubation of the trachea are reduced or abolished.[28] The course of anesthesia also tends to be associated with fewer hemodynamic fluctuations, and there is a decreased need for inhalation anesthetics. The use of opioids is particularly advantageous in operations that involve sudden painful manipulations, eg, traction on visceral organs during intra-abdominal surgery. Anticipation of these events and prior supplementation with a small dose of an opioid (eg, 50–100 μg fentanyl) will often be sufficient to prevent increases of arterial blood pressure and heart rate associated with these manipulations.

The sympathoadrenal responses to laryngoscopy and intubation of the trachea, resulting in hypertension, tachycardia, and dysrhythmias, are well known.[29,30] They are particularly dangerous in patients suffering from hypertension or coronary artery disease. Many different approaches have been tried to attenuate these hemodynamic responses, including topical analgesia,[31] prior administration of beta-adrenergic blocking drugs,[32] and the use of vasodilators such as nitroprusside[33] and hydralazine.[34] Topical analgesia is not always effective, and vasodilators, while effective in controlling hypertension, may accentuate tachycardia. The ability of low doses of fentanyl (5–8 μg/kg) given intravenously at

the time of induction, to significantly reduce or abolish these hemodynamic responses, has been well documented.[35]

The cardiovascular changes during laryngoscopy and intubation are a reflex response to stimulation in an area richly innervated by the 9th and 10th cranial nerves. In the rat, high concentrations of opioid receptors are found in the nuclei of these nerves and in the closely associated solitary nuclei.[36] The efficacy of low doses of opioids to suppress these responses may be due, therefore, to a specific blockade at the level of these nuclei of afferent nerve impulses arising in the pharynx and larynx.

Use of Opioids in Cardiac Anesthesia

A technique of anesthesia for cardiac surgery, involving high doses of morphine, was developed in the late 1960s and early 1970s. It was based on the observation by Lowenstein et al that patients requiring mechanical ventilation for respiratory failure tolerated large doses of morphine for sedation without discernible circulatory effects.[37] This observation led them to administer equivalent doses of morphine as the anesthetic for patients undergoing cardiac surgery for acquired valvular disease. The publication of their results in 1969 stimulated considerable interest and research, and, today, high-dose opioid anesthesia is extensively used, alone or in combination with other drugs, in cardiac anesthesia. It soon became apparent, however, that whereas morphine in the doses described by Lowenstein et al (0.5–3 mg/kg) was adequate for critically ill patients who often had end-stage valvular heart disease, in other, less critically ill patients, it did have serious disadvantages. Many problems were reported, including sporadic episodes of incomplete amnesia, occasional histamine-related reactions (cutaneous flushing, hypotension, bronchospasm), hypertension and tachycardia during periods of maximum surgical stimulation, and increased intra- and postoperative blood and fluid requirements.[38] Attempts to overcome these problems by increasing the dose of morphine were only partially successful, least so in patients undergoing coronary artery surgery. The latter patients, who usually did not have a history of chronic heart failure and were often relatively young and fit, sometimes were extremely resistant to morphine anesthesia. Stanley et al[39] reported requirements of 8–11 mg/kg in their patients. Dosages of this nature introduced further problems. Excessive volumes of blood and fluids were needed to maintain adequate cardiac filling pressures, and patients were described as "plum-colored" with generalized edema on return to the intensive care unit. Prolonged respiratory depression was another unacceptable side effect following such large doses of morphine.

A variety of supplements were used in an effort to reduce the incidence of awareness, control hypertension, and reduce the total dose of morphine required, thereby attenuating the extent of postoperative respiratory depression. The most commonly used supplements were nitrous oxide and diazepam. Although by themselves these drugs cause minimal hemodynamic changes, when combined with high-dose morphine they result in significant circulatory depression, with decreases in cardiac output and arterial blood pressure.[40-42] The addition of low-to-moderate concentrations of halothane after large doses of morphine also produced marked cardiovascular depression in patients with coronary artery disease.[43]

Because of the above problems associated with the use of morphine, several other opioids were investigated in an attempt to find a suitable alternative. Both meperidine and alphaprodine, a methyl-substituted derivative of the reversed ester of meperidine, were studied but caused significant hypotension, tachycardia, and marked myocardial depression when given in anesthetic doses.[44,45] Hydromorphone, a hydrogenated-ketone derivative of morphine, that is 7–10 times as potent and 8–10 times as lipid soluble as morphine, has also been investigated.[46] Like morphine, hydromorphone did not reliably induce anesthesia in patients undergoing coronary artery surgery, and supplementation with nitrous oxide and halothane was necessary for unconsciousness and complete suppression of sympathetic responses during surgery.

Fentanyl, and its two newer derivatives, sufentanil and alfentanil, have proved to be the most reliable and effective of the opioids for producing anesthesia. The use of fentanyl as a total anesthetic was first reported by Stanley and Webster in 1978.[47] They induced anesthesia in patients undergoing mitral valve replacement with fentanyl, 50 μg/kg, and gave additional fentanyl as needed. The average total dose of fentanyl, 74 μg/kg, provided complete anesthesia with minimal hemodynamic disturbances. In a subsequent study involving patients undergoing coronary artery surgery, the same group also used a total dose of 75 μg/kg of fentanyl.[48] Since then, extensive investigations and reports on the use of fentanyl in cardiac surgery have appeared in the anesthetic literature. These have been reviewed recently.[49]

GENERAL ASPECTS OF OPIOID PHARMACOLOGY

Structure–Activity Relationships

The large number of naturally occurring, semi-synthetic and synthetic compounds with opioid activity have an apparently wide diversity of chemical structures. However, closer examination reveals many basic similarities among the various compounds. Two basic opioid structures exist, the rigid molecules of the morphine-like compounds, and more flexible molecules of the phenylpiperidine group, of which meperidine is the prototype.

Morphine consists of a skeleton of five rigidly interlocking rings bearing several peripheral functional groups. This rigid pentacyclic structure has a T-shape, with the piperidine ring forming part of the crossbar, and a hydroxylated aromatic ring lying in the vertical stem (Fig. 3-2). This rigid T-structure is common to all compounds of this class. Certain portions of the morphine molecule are important for pharmacologic activity, whereas others play no role in activity and can be removed without altering potency or receptor binding.[50]

The basic amino site in the piperidine ring is essential for opioid activity, and substitution at this site profoundly alters activity.[51] In all morphine-like compounds the nitrogen atom is at a constant distance, 4.55 Å, from the center of the aromatic ring.[52] Replacing the nitrogen methyl with short-chain alkyl groups results in potent opioid antagonists. The most effective substitutions have three carbon-chains, eg,

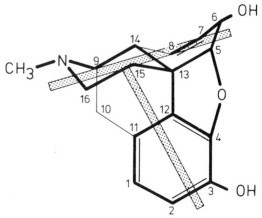

Fig. 3-2. Structure of morphine illustrating the T-shape of the molecule. The bonds C9-C10, C10-C11, and C8-C14 appear to be nonessential for opioid activity.

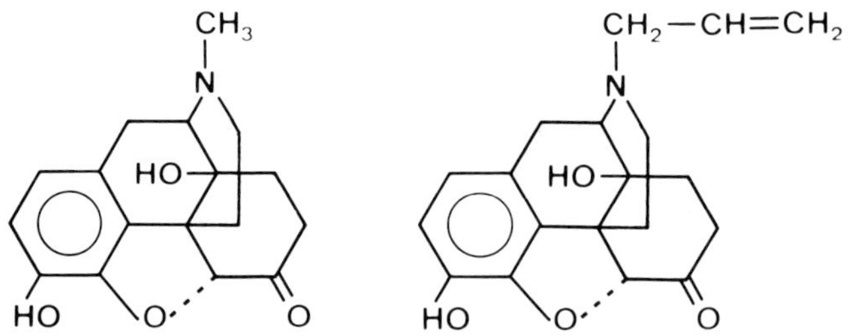

OXYMORPHONE   NALOXONE

Fig. 3-3. Structure of oxymorphone and naloxone. Hydroxylation at the C14 carbon atom is responsible for naloxone being a pure antagonist rather than a mixed agonist-antagonist.

allyl ($-CH_2 - CH = CH_2$) or cyclopropylmethyl ($-CH_2-\Delta$). Substitution of an antagonist subgroup alone results in compounds with mixed agonist-antagonist properties, eg, nalorphine. When this is combined with hydroxylation or bromination at the C-14 position, pure antagonists are formed.[53] Hydroxylation alone at the C-14 site confers antagonist activity (eg, oxymorphone vs naloxone, Fig. 3-3). Substitution of a phenylethyl group onto the nitrogen increases agonist activity. Fentanyl, which has a phenylethyl subgroup, is 600 times as potent as meperidine, which has a similar molecular structure but no phenylethyl subgroup.

Dismantling the morphine skeleton by removing the oxide bridge generates more potent tetracyclic compounds known as morphinans. Additional removal of the methylene bridge leaves a phenylpiperidine structure (a phenyl ring connected to a 6-membered ring containing 5 carbon atoms and 1 nitrogen atom), which is the vital part of the morphine molecule. This dismantling results in an unfolding of the molecule so that the aromatic ring reorients to an equational position on the piperidine ring, compared with an axial position in morphine. The distance between the aromatic ring and the piperidine nitrogen increases to 5.66 Å.[54] The phenylpiperidine opioids are an extremely important class of opioids, containing meperidine and fentanyl and its congeners.

Structural similarity can also be observed between opioid drugs and the endogenous opioid peptides. The enkephalins contain sequences of amino acids in which tyrosine and phenylalanine are separated by two glycine molecules and terminated by either leucine (Leu-enkephalin) or methionine (Met-enkephalin). Morphine is synthesized by the poppy plant from two molecules of tyrosine, and the skeletal backbone of tyrosine is evident in the morphine molecule.[55]

Examination of structure–activity relationships in opioids and opioid peptides has allowed a model of the opioid receptor to be developed. This receptor model consists of two active sites: an aromatic subsite (T-site) that preferentially binds hydroxylated rings (as in morphine and the tyrosine residue in enkephalin), separated 4.5 Å from an anionic site; and a second aromatic site (P-site), 5.5 Å from the anionic site, that preferentially binds nonhydroxylated aromatic rings (as in the phenylpiperidines and the phenylalanine residue in enkephalin). This P-site also binds the alkyl groups in antagonists and in doing so pulls the bound nitrogen away from the anionic site, thereby interrupting agonist activity. Potent agonists such as fentanyl can bind to both P- and T-sites; whereas less potent compounds can only bind to one site. Binding to the P-site seems to play a greater role at the delta-receptor than the mu-receptor.[56]

Respiratory Depression

All pure agonist opioids produce dose-related respiratory depression. The primary effect is a reduction in the sensitivity of the respiratory center to carbon dioxide so that, initially, respiratory rate is affected more than tidal volume, which may even increase. With increasing doses, respiratory rhythmicity and reflexes are also disturbed, resulting in the irregular, gasping breathing characteristic of opioid overdose. This has been described as "pharmacological decerebration" or "Ondine's curse." These responses are the result of drug action at centers in the medulla and pons. Several areas on the ventral surface of the medulla have been credited with being specific chemoreceptors that, by detecting central changes in [H^+], regulate respiration.[57] Application of opioids directly to the medulla selectively depresses tidal volume and CO_2 response; whereas the frequency of respiration is actually increased.[58] Application to the rostral surface of the pons induces a selective depression of frequency, without modifying tidal volume, progressing at higher doses to respiratory arrest. On a dose basis, pontine structures are considerably more sensitive to the depressant effects of opioids than those in the medulla. Therefore, the observed clinical effects are a combination of both medullary and pontine depression.

Maximum respiratory depression occurs within 5 to 10 minutes after intravenous injection with most opioids, but depression will last for much longer and may persist beyond the period of effective analgesia. Even with small doses of fentanyl (2–9 μg/kg), responses to CO_2 may be depressed for 2–4 hours[59,60]; whereas the analgesic effect will have subsided by 1–1 1/2 hours.[61] This shorter duration of analgesia relative to respiratory depression may be a reflection of the sensitivity of current methods to measure these variables. It may also, however, be a reflection of different affinities for the receptors responsible for analgesia (mu_1) and respiratory depression (mu_2 and/or delta).[62] Elderly patients are more sensitive to the respiratory depressant effects of opioids than younger patients, and the dosage used needs to be adjusted accordingly. It is also important to remember that other central nervous system depressants such as barbiturates, alcohol, and inhalational anesthetics will potentiate the respiratory effects of opioids.

Reversal of Respiratory Depression

Opioid–antagonist drugs will reverse both the respiratory depression and analgesia induced by an opioid agonist. Naloxone, a pure antagonist, is the drug most frequently used, but the mixed agonist-antagonists, eg, nalorphine, are equally effective and, in some situations, may be preferred, since they cause a less abrupt and complete reversal of analgesia due to their inherent analgesic effects.

Extreme caution must be exercised when naloxone is given to reverse respiratory depression after high doses of opioids have been given. There are several reports of intense pressor responses and tachycardia occurring when naloxone was used to reverse the effects of opioids in animals[63,64] and humans.[65] Attempts to reverse high-dose morphine anesthesia with naloxone, 0.4 mg IV, caused immediate hypertension and severe pulmonary edema.[66] Large doses of naloxone have been reported to cause death.[67] In animals, these hemodynamic changes have been associated with 60 percent increases in coronary blood flow and myocardial oxygen consumption.[64] Such changes obviously are potentially detrimental for patients with coronary artery disease. They have been attributed to release of catecholamines and sympathetic overactivity resulting from acute reversal of analgesia.[68] Naloxone administered to subjects who have not been given opioids has no influence on blood pressure or plasma catecholamines.[69] Another explanation for the pressure response after naloxone administration in patients given opioids may be alteration of baroreceptor reflexes so that an exaggerated hemodynamic response occurs to subsequent stimulation.[70] Naloxone may also have an analeptic action unrelated to opioid receptor antagonism.[71]

When using antagonists, respiratory depression may recur if the antagonist has a shorter action than the agonist. The elimination half-life of naloxone, 1–1 1/2 hours, is shorter than most opioids with the exception of alfentanil.[72] The duration of the effect of 0.4 mg/70 kg naloxone was estimated to be only 45 minutes.[73]

Opioids are known to inhibit the release of acetylcholine from neurons in the central nervous system;[74] while direct application of acetylcholine to the floor of the fourth ventricle has been shown to stimulate respiration.[75] Physostigmine, an anticholinesterase, increases the level of acetylcholine in the brain and can antagonize morphine-induced respiratory depression in animals, without antagonizing analgesic activity.[76] Studies in humans have clearly demonstrated that physostigmine, 13–33 μg/kg IV, can rapidly reverse the somnolent effect of morphine and restore ventilation to predrug values without altering analgesia.[77,78] The effect lasts approximately 35–45 minutes. The use of physostigmine may be accompanied by an increased incidence of nausea and vomiting.

Recently, the use of the mixed agonist-antagonist, nalbuphine, to reverse fentanyl-induced respiratory depression has been described.[79–83] Latasch et al gave a standardized dose of nalbuphine, 20 mg IV, at the end of surgery to patients anesthetized with nitrous oxide and 23 μg/kg fentanyl for elective general surgery.[81] Within 2 minutes of nalbuphine administration, all patients had progressed from apnea to spontaneous ventilation and became so alert that they would not tolerate the endotracheal tube. Analgesia was not reversed, and 80–98 percent of the patients had marked or complete pain relief for up to

3 hours. There were no significant changes in blood pressure or heart rate. No major side effects were observed. However, others have reported significant increases in blood pressure after satisfactory reversal of fentanyl-induced respiratory depression with nalbuphine, 0.1 mg/kg.[82,83] This was associated with a significant increase in epinephrine, but not norepinephrine or dopamine levels.[83]

Nalbuphine may prove to be a useful alternative to naloxone for reversal of opioid-induced respiratory depression. The persistence of analgesia may prevent many of the undesirable sympathetic side effects associated with the use of naloxone, especially after high doses of opioids. Since nalbuphine has a considerably longer plasma half-life (5 hours) than naloxone (1–1½ hours), the risk of recurrence of respiratory depression will be reduced.

Cardiovascular Effects

All opioids, with the exception of meperidine, produce bradycardia. Meperidine often produces tachycardia, possibly due to the similarities in structure between it and atropine. The mechanism of opioid-induced bradycardia is not completely understood although there is experimental evidence that it is caused by central vagal stimulation. It is totally blocked by bilateral vagotomy[84] or pharmacologic vagal blockade with atropine.[85] Morphine, in concentrations found clinically, has no effect on the sinoatrial node.[86]

Fentanyl-induced bradycardia is more marked in anesthetized than conscious subjects, although the severity is less when nitrous oxide is used.[87] This may be due to the sympathomimetic effect of nitrous oxide.[88] Interestingly, second and subsequent doses of fentanyl produce less bradycardia than the initial dose,[85] suggesting a possible tolerance mechanism.

Premedication with atropine can minimize, but may not totally eliminate opioid-induced bradycardia, especially in patients taking beta-adrenoreceptor–blocking drugs. The speed of injection appears to be important, particularly with the more potent drugs; slow administration minimizes bradycardia. Although severe bradycardia should obviously be avoided, moderate slowing of heart rate is not harmful, and, by reducing myocardial oxygen consumption, may be beneficial, especially in patients with coronary artery disease. The negative chronotropic action of fentanyl is an important factor in its protective effect on the heart during periods of ischemia.[89]

Isolated heart or heart muscle studies have dem-

onstrated consistent dose-related negative inotropic effects for morphine,[90-92] meperidine,[91] and fentanyl.[90,91] All of these experiments used concentrations of the drugs 100 to several thousand times those found clinically, however, even during high-dose opioid anesthesia. After a bolus dose of fentanyl, 75–100 μg/kg, peak plasma concentrations are seldom above 100 ng/ml, and fall rapidly to about 20 ng/ml within 5 minutes.[93,94] In the experiments described by Strauer, fentanyl had no significant effect on papillary muscle function with concentrations up to 1000 ng/ml, and only a 30 percent depression when the concentration was 5000 ng/ml.[91] Morphine depressed the contractility of the isolated heart only in concentrations equivalent to 285 μg/ml.[95] Peak concentrations only rarely exceed 1 μg/ml immediately after an intravenous dose of 2 mg/kg in man.[96,97]

In humans, 0.5–3 mg/kg morphine[37] or 50–100 μg/kg fentanyl[49] have no deleterious effects on myocardial function. Meperidine, however, even in low doses (2–2.5 mg/kg) causes significant decreases in arterial blood pressure and cardiac output, accompanied by tachycardia in intact animals[63,98] and in humans.[44] Anesthetic doses of meperidine (more than 10 mg/kg IV) cause marked decreases in cardiac output and, frequently, cardiac arrest in dogs.[63]

Peripheral Vascular Effects

Hypotension can occur after even small (10 mg) doses of morphine given intravenously, and is primarily related to decreases in systemic vascular resistance. Morphine reduces arteriolar resistance and increases venous capacitance.[99,100] The most important mechanism responsible for these changes is probably histamine release. Basic drugs like morphine can displace histamine from its binding sites in most cells and cause a significant elevation in plasma histamine, the changes correlating with vasodilatation and hypotension.[101] The amount of histamine released is reduced by slow administration (less than 10 mg/min). Pretreatment with either diphenylhydramine or cimetidine does not block these reactions, but they are significantly attenuated by combined H_1 and H_2 antagonist pretreatment.[102] Venodilatation lasts much longer than arteriolar dilation and causes a significant increase in intraoperative fluid requirement during high-dose morphine anesthesia.[100] Stanley et al found that patients receiving a mean dose of 9.3 mg/kg of morphine needed significantly more blood and crystalloid intra- and postoperatively to maintain filling pressures, blood pressure, and urinary output than a similar group given 2.7 mg/kg of morphine.[39] Postoperatively, the patients given the higher dose were described as edematous, plum-colored, and prone to hypotension, especially on change of position. These changes are not necessarily due to falls in vascular resistance alone, and there is evidence that there is loss of fluid and protein into the interstitial compartment. Up to 11 ml/kg of blood is pooled or lost from the circulating blood volume in dogs after 1 mg/kg of intravenous morphine.[103] Others have reported losses of plasma from the circulation to the interstitial spaces of 17–20 percent of total blood volume, which they attributed to histamine release.[104] Neither fentanyl nor sufentanil in high doses releases histamine, and they have minimal effect on vascular resistance.[105] Neither morphine nor fentanyl, in clinically equivalent concentrations, blocks alpha-adrenergic receptors in isolated vascular tissue studies.[106,107] Morphine may have a direct action on vascular smooth muscle, independent of histamine release.[108,109]

Gastrointestinal Tract

The gastrointestinal tract is the only system outside the central nervous system (CNS) with significant concentrations of opioid receptors. They are distributed throughout the gut, with highest concentrations in the upper small intestine and stomach antrum. Morphine and related drugs delay gastric emptying, and the passage of food through the duodenum may be delayed for up to 12 hours after morphine administration. Opioids also delay transit time through the ileum and colon by increasing resting tone and diminishing propulsive activity. This latter effect accounts for a major part of the constipating effect of morphine-like drugs, frequently used in the treatment of diarrhea. The use of opioids during anesthesia and postoperatively can contribute to postoperative ileus.

Opioids also affect the biliary system, increasing common bile duct pressure and decreasing bile production and flow, primarily as a result of spasm of the sphincter of Oddi, but also due to increased tone in the bile duct itself.[110] Meperidine, perhaps due to its atropine-like activity, is often thought to produce less biliary spasm than other opioids. The weight of evidence suggests that this is not true, however. In a study assessing changes in biliary mechanics intraoperatively, Radney et al found that meperidine, 1 mg/kg IV, caused a 61 percent increase in common bile duct pressure, compared to a 53 percent increase after morphine, 0.125 mg/kg.[110] Reversal of biliary

spasm with atropine is unreliable in humans,[111] but it is reversible with naloxone.[112] Opioids should be avoided in patients with biliary colic and in those undergoing radiographic investigations of the biliary system. Spasm of the sphincter of Oddi can be a cause of pain after opioid administration that, in the patient with coronary artery disease, may be difficult to distinguish from angina pectoris.

Emetic Effects

Nausea and vomiting are common and undesirable side effects of opioids, resulting from stimulation of the chemoreceptor trigger zone (CTZ). They are more common in ambulatory patients, due to vestibular stimulation of the CTZ, which is sensitized by opiates. Opioids depress the vomiting center, and with increasing plasma concentrations this effect overcomes the CTZ stimulant effect.[113,114] Emetic effects are less common after second and subsequent doses, and are rare after anesthetic doses.

Muscle Rigidity

All opioids in high doses produce muscle rigidity. It is a particular problem with the more lipophilic drugs like fentanyl. An 88 percent incidence was reported in patients anesthetized with fentanyl, 50 μg/kg, for cardiac surgery.[115] The phenomenon is characterized by increased muscle tone, progressing to severe stiffness, particularly in the abdominal and thoracic muscles although limb muscles are also affected. Rigidity of the thoracic muscles, so-called *wooden chest,* can cause severe difficulties with ventilation in nonparalyzed anesthetized patients.[116] Chest wall rigidity has also been reported during recovery from high-dose fentanyl anesthesia.[117] The severity of rigidity is increased by rapid injection[116] and by concomitant use of nitrous oxide.[118,119] Fentanyl-induced muscle rigidity is not due to a direct action on muscle fibers since it can be blocked by neuromuscular blocking drugs.[120] Opioids do not have significant effects on nerve conduction and cause only minimal depression of the monosynaptic spinal reflexes associated with muscle stretch receptors.[121] Muscle rigidity is probably a manifestation of the catatonic state, a basic pharmacologic property of all opioids, which may be related to enhancement of dopamine biosynthesis in the caudate nucleus[122,123] or an interaction at gamma-aminobutyric acid (GABA)-ergic neurons.[124]

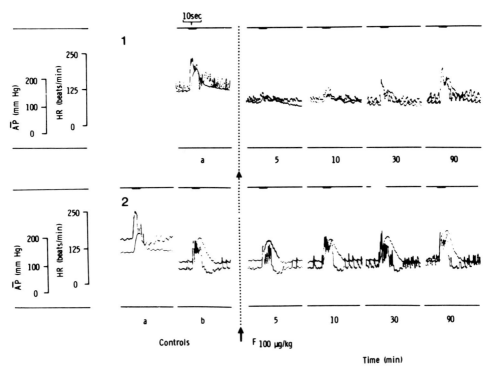

Fig. 3-4. Effect of a bolus intravenous injection of fentanyl, 100 μg/kg, on reflex-evoked changes in heart rate (HR) and mean arterial pressure (AP) produced by electrical stimulation of an exposed radial nerve in two dogs. In dog 1 (upper trace) fentanyl abolished the reflex responses at 5 min and reduced them at 10 and 30 min. Dog 2 (lower trace) was preconditioned with incremental doses of fentanyl—controls a and b are before and after conditioning, followed by a bolus of fentanyl, 100 μg/kg, that had no effect on reflex cardiovascular responses. Preconditioning had thus caused tolerance to fentanyl. (From Askitopoulou H, Whitwam JG, Al-Khudhairi, et al: Acute tolerance to fentanyl during anesthesia in dogs. Anesthesiology 63:255–261, 1985, with permission.)

Tolerance

The phenomenon of tolerance, ie, the decreased intensity and shortened duration of pharmacologic effect with repeated doses, is a characteristic feature of all opioid drugs.[1] Tolerance to a variety of effects including analgesia,[125,126] hypothermia,[127] and circulatory responses[128] has been demonstrated for morphine in animals. Short-term tolerance to the analgesic effects of fentanyl occurs in conscious rats within 2–5 days.[129] Acute tolerance to the effect of fentanyl on cardiovascular responses in dogs has been shown to occur within 3 hours.[130] Askitopoulou et al studied the effect of fentanyl on blood pressure and heart rate responses to electrical stimulation of the radial nerve in two groups of dogs.[130] One group received a single bolus of fentanyl, 100 μg/kg IV; while the second group received logarithmically increasing boluses from 1.5 μg/kg to 63 μg/kg at 20-minute intervals during 180 minutes (preconditioning). In group one, a bolus of 100 μg/kg of fentanyl depressed evoked changes in heart rate and blood pressure by 82 and 75 percent, respectively, in 5 minutes, and recovery occurred within 90 minutes. In group two, the 100-μg/kg bolus, given after preconditioning, had no significant effect on the evoked cardiovascular responses (Fig. 3-4).

In humans, tolerance to fentanyl has been reported to develop within hours after intravenous administration[131] and during prolonged infusion.[132] The clinical relevance of acute tolerance for patients is difficult to ascertain. It could be responsible for the occasional reports of awareness during fentanyl anesthesia.[133-135] The practice of administering large boluses of fentanyl at the start of anesthesia may predispose to tolerance developing and might explain the subsequent inability of even large subsequent boluses to suppress the cardiovascular responses during and after sternotomy.

DRUG	RESEARCH #	YEAR DISCOVERED	CHEMICAL STRUCTURE
Fentanyl	R 4263	1960	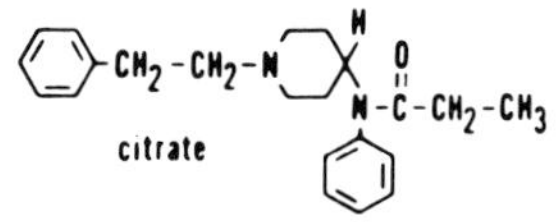
Carfentanil	R 33799	1974	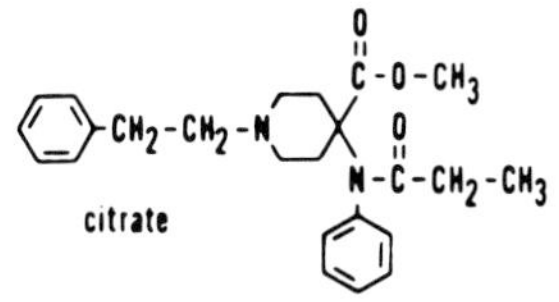
Sufentanil	R 33800	1974	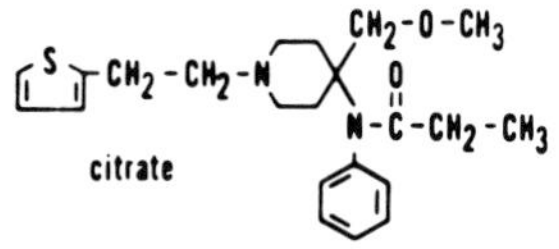
Lofentanil	R 34995	1975	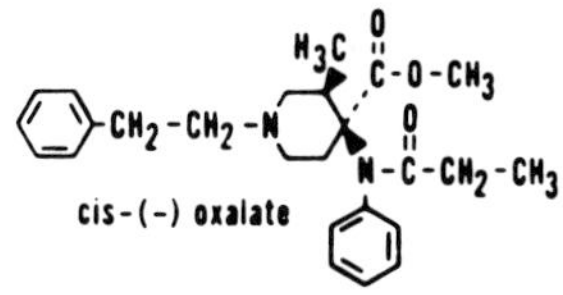
Alfentanil	R 39209	1976	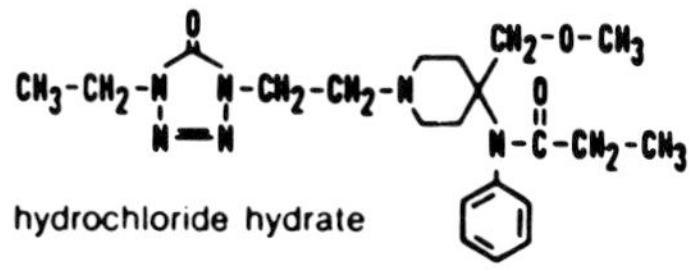

Fig. 3-5. Structure of fentanyl and its analogues.

FENTANYL AND ITS ANALOGUES

Fentanyl is used extensively in anesthesia, both as an analgesic supplement and as a sole anesthetic, and the emphasis in this chapter will be on it and its newer derivatives. Although a very useful drug, fentanyl does not represent the definitive opioid. Chemists have continued to search for compounds that are more potent and shorter acting. Various chemical adjustments of the anilopiperidine ring have resulted in the development of four fentanyl analogues of interest to anesthesiologists (Fig. 3-5). Of these, sufentanil and alfentanil are available in the United States and certain European countries, carfentanil is used as a calming agent in large-animal work, and the future of lofentanil is uncertain.

The comparative pharmacology of these opioids has been studied in rats (Table 3-2). The most notable feature is the exceptional potency of sufentanil, carfentanil, and lofentanil; between 8000 and 18,000 times as potent as meperidine.[136] They are also much less toxic than meperidine or morphine in spontane-ously breathing rats, the safety margin (LD_{50}/ED_{50}) being greater than 25,000 for sufentanil.

De Castro et al studied the effects of very large doses of eight opioids in dogs, in an attempt to define the acute toxicity of these agents.[137] The dogs received only the opioid being studied, with neuro-muscular blocking agents, and were mechanically ventilated with air/oxygen (Table 3-3). Only dogs who received meperidine died. Despite signs of sympathetic hyperactivity, those in the other groups survived. It should be noted that dogs are less sensitive to opioids than humans; the anesthetic dose of fentanyl in dogs is 2 mg/kg,[85] and in humans, 50–70 μg/kg.[138] De Castro et al proposed that the more potent an opioid, the more specific its site of action and the lower the incidence of side effects. The more potent opioids thus would be expected to be more effective in binding to opioid receptors. Indeed, after 5 μg/kg of lofentanil, the opioid receptors in the rat forebrain are fully occupied, and at 24 hours after administration 45 percent of the receptors were still occupied.[3,139] There is good correlation between the

Table 3-2

Therapeutic Index of Several Analgesics in Spontaneously Breathing Rats*

	ED_{50}	LD_{50}	Therapeutic index	Potency ratio
	mg/kg/IV	*mg/kg/IV*	*LD_{50}/ED_{50}*	
Sufentanil	0.00071	17.9	25,211	8500
Carfentanil	0.00034	3.4	10,000	17,800
Alfentanil	0.044	47.5	1,080	137
Fentanyl	0.011	3.1	277	550
Lofentanil	0.00059	0.066	112	10,200
Morphine	3.21	22.3	69.5	—
Pentazocine	9.1	48.0	30.8	—
Meperidine	6.0	29.0	4.8	1

Source: Data modified from Janssen PAJ: Potent, new analgesics, tailor-made for different purposes. Acta Anaesth Scand 26:262–268, 1982, and from Cookson RF: Carfentanil and lofentanil. Clinics in Anaesthesiology 1(1):156–158, 1983, with permission.

*The ED_{50} is defined as the dose that provides surgical anesthesia in 50 percent of rats. In this case, surgical anesthesia is defined as absence of tail withdrawal within 10 seconds of immersion in hot water. The LD_{50} is the dose at which 50 percent of the animals die. The therapeutic index is also referred to as the safety margin.

opioid-binding properties of an opioid and its analgesic potency. Lofentanil, in particular, binds very strongly to the receptors and this, rather than any pharmacokinetic or redistributive phenomena, accounts for its prolonged duration of action.

Tritiated sufentanil binds extensively with mu-opioid receptors.[140] The ratio for specific (receptor) versus nonspecific (nonreceptor) binding is 90 percent, compared with 75 percent for fentanyl and 60 percent for morphine. This, together with a high receptor affinity, makes sufentanil an ideal ligand for

opioid binding studies. Leysen et al studied the inhibition of stereospecific sufentanil binding by 37 opioid agonists and antagonists[140] (Fig. 3-6). They found competitive inhibition for all substances studied and the binding affinities correlated well with analgesic potency as measured by the rat tail withdrawal test. Lipophilicity and degree of ionization have little influence on binding affinity. The fact that binding affinity and analgesic potency correlate well supports the view that opioid analgesic action is mediated by the same receptor site, namely the mu-

Table 3-3

Acute Toxicity of Narcotics in Paralyzed and Mechanically Ventilated Dogs

	Potency ratio (relative to morphine)	Loading dose*	Severe hyperactivity†	Lethal dose	Safety margin between loading dose and severe side effects
		mg/kg IV	*mg/kg IV*	*mg/kg*	
Meperidine	1/3	7.5	15	20–32‡	2
Morphine	1	2.5	80	>200	32
Alfentanil	31	0.08	10	>20	125
Fentanyl	124	0.02	10	>10	500
Sufentanil	1240	0.002	2	>4	1,000

Source: Data modified from de Castro J, van de Water A, Wouters L, et al: comparative study of cardiovascular, neurological, and metabolic side-effects of eight narcotics in dogs. Acta Anaesthesiol Belg 30:5–99, 1979, with permission.

*The loading dose was the dose that permitted intubation and catheterization of the dog without significant changes in heart rate or blood pressure.

†The severe sympathomimetic hyperactivity was associated with endogenous catecholamine release and very large increases in heart rate, blood pressure, left ventricular end-diastolic pressure, and oxygen consumption.

‡Only dogs receiving meperidine died. Despite severe sympathetic hyperactivity, dogs in all other groups survived even after massive doses of opioids.

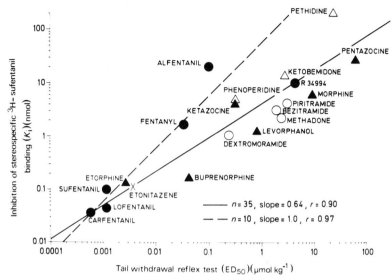

Fig. 3-6. Correlation between inhibition constants measured in vitro for stereospecific sufentanil binding in rat forebrain membranes; and analgesic ED_{50} values measured in the rat tail withdrawal test. Lines represent analysis of linear regression. (— for all compounds, n = 35, r = 0.9; – – – for fentanyl analogues, n = 10, r = 0.97). Not all compounds are plotted. (From Leysen JE, Gommeren W, Niemegeers CJE: [³H] Sufentanil, a superior ligand for μ-opiate receptors. Binding properties and regional distribution in rat brain and spinal cord. Eur J Pharmacol 87:209–225, 1983, with permission.)

receptor. Figure 3-6 shows a possible separate correlation of unity for the 4-anilopiperidine series (fentanyl derivatives). This may reflect their better access to central receptor sites.

The fact that lofentanil and sufentanil bind effectively to mu-receptors supports De Castro's thesis that the more potent opioids are more specific in their actions and have fewer side effects. This is further supported by the fact that neither fentanyl nor sufentanil cause histamine release, whereas morphine does.[101] The lack of the histamine release is responsible for the better cardiovascular stability obtained during anesthesia with fentanyl[141] or sufentanil[142] compared with morphine.

Fentanyl

Fentanyl is a phenylpiperidine of the 4-anilopiperidine series, structurally related to, but not derived from meperidine. It is commercially available as the citrate salt in an aqueous, preservative-free solution containing 50 μg of fentanyl base per ml. On a milligram basis, fentanyl is considerably more potent than either morphine or meperidine; estimates have ranged from 60 to 270 times as potent as morphine as an analgesic, depending on species. In humans fentanyl is 60 to 80 times as potent as morphine.

At the opioid receptor, however, this potency difference becomes less obvious and the intrinsic affinities of fentanyl and morphine differ only by a factor of two to three (Table 3-4).[140,143] The differences between the receptor affinities and clinical potency ratios arise from differing physicochemical and phar-

Table 3-4
Receptor Binding Characteristics of Opioids

	Binding affinity	Specific binding
	K_i, nM	%
Carfentanil	0.036	80
Lofentanil	0.044	70
Sufentanil	0.1	92
Fentanyl	1.6	75
Morphine	5.7	60
Alfentanil	19.0	—
Meperidine	193.0	—

Source: Based on data from Leysen JE, Gommeren W, Niemegeers CJE[140] and Gommeren W, Leysen JE.[139]

Binding affinity is measured by K_i, the equilibrium inhibition constant for [³H]sufentanil. The lower the value of K_i, the higher the affinity for the mu-receptor. Because of its extremely rapid dissociation from the receptor, the binding affinity of alfentanil may be underestimated. Specific binding is the percentage of drug bound to specific (receptor) sites as opposed to nonspecific (nonreceptor) sites.

Table 3-5
Pharmacokinetic Parameters

	Morphine	Meperidine	Fentanyl	Alfentanil	Sufentanil
pKa	7.9	8.5	8.4	6.5	8.0
% Unionized of pH 7.4	23.0	7.4	8.5	89.0	19.7
Lipid solubility (octanol-water partition coefficient)	6.0	525.0	816.0	129.0	1757.0
Protein binding (%)	63.0	82.0	84.0	92.0	93.0
Vd^{ss} (liters/kg)	3.4	4.4	4.0	0.7	1.7
Cl (ml/kg/min)	2.3	7.7	12.6	5.1	12.7
$T_{1/2} \beta$ (hr)	1.7	6.7	3.6	1.6	2.7

macokinetic properties of these drugs, especially the differences in lipid solubility.

PHARMACOKINETICS OF FENTANYL

Pharmacokinetics has been defined as what the body does to a drug; in contrast to pharmacodynamics, which is what a drug does to the body.[144] Obviously kinetics and dynamics are closely interrelated, and the better understanding of the pharmacokinetics of fentanyl that has resulted from the extensive research in this field has facilitated an improved understanding of its pharmacodynamics (see Chapter 2).

The absorption, distribution, and elimination of a drug are determined by many factors including lipid solubility, tissue and protein binding, and degree of ionization at physiologic pH. These properties of fentanyl and related opioids are summarized in Table 3-5. Fentanyl is a highly lipid-soluble drug, as measured by either the heptane/water[145] or octanol/water[146] partition coefficient. Lipid solubility is an important factor determining the rate of entry and exit to and from organs and tissues, especially the CNS, which has a high lipid content. Fentanyl is rapidly transferred across the blood-brain barrier, resulting in a rapid onset of action after intravenous injection.[147,148] After intravenous administration in rabbits, high concentrations of fentanyl are rapidly reached in well-perfused tissues such as the lungs, kidney, heart, and brain, with peak concentrations attained within 0.5 to 1 minute after injection.[149] Tissue uptake is slower in muscle, with maximum concentration reached at 5 minutes. In adipose tissue, due to its low perfusion and high capacity, the maximum concentration only occurs after about 30 minutes. Very similar results have been reported in the rat.[147]

Morphine has a much slower onset time since its very low lipid solubility limits its rate of entry into the CNS.[150] The relative potential for entering the

CNS is 156 times greater for fentanyl than for morphine.[146] Large quantities of fentanyl are taken up by adipose tissue acting as a reservoir that slowly releases fentanyl back into the circulation when plasma concentrations fall below that in fat. This slow re-entry serves to maintain the plasma concentration and is one factor in the relatively long plasma elimination half-life of fentanyl, 3.1–3.7 hours in volunteers.[145,151] In contrast, the elimination half-life of morphine is shorter, 1.7–2.9 hours.[97,152,153]

The properties that enable fentanyl to cross the blood-brain barrier also ensure rapid penetration across the placental barrier. Craft et al studied the kinetics of intravenous fentanyl in the chronic maternal fetal sheep preparation.[154] Fentanyl was detected in fetal blood within 1 minute of maternal administration, and peak concentrations occurred at 5 minutes. Thereafter, equilibrium was established between maternal and fetal blood, with maternal concentrations remaining on average 2 1/2 times those in the fetus. In patients undergoing cesarean section, given fentanyl, 1 µg/kg IV, within minutes of delivery, the highest concentration in cord blood occurred at 2 minutes after injection.[155] The maternal/fetal concentration ratios averaged 3.3, in close agreement with those found in the sheep model. These differences between maternal and fetal plasma concentration are higher than would have been expected from the high lipid solubility and rapid transplacental transfer. They are probably related to the high protein binding of fentanyl.

In vitro studies have shown that, at pH 7.4, fentanyl is 80–85 percent bound to plasma proteins, so that only 15–20 percent remains unbound and available for placental transfer.[146,151] The acute-phase protein, alpha$_1$-acid glycoprotein (alpha$_1$-AGP), accounts for about 60 percent of the protein binding of fentanyl.[146] The fetal concentration of alpha$_1$-AGP is, however, only about 40 percent that in maternal plasma, so that the unbound fraction of fentanyl in fetal plasma, and thus the pharmacodynamic effect, may be higher than would be predicted from the assayed concentration, which measures both bound and unbound fraction.[156]

Within the concentration ranges encountered clinically, protein binding of fentanyl is independent of drug concentration.[146,151] Although pH changes alter the degree of binding (binding decreases with acidosis and increases with alkalosis), the clinical relevance of this is uncertain and is probably of limited importance. Because of the large volume of distribution of fentanyl, any change in binding will have minimal effect on the concentration of the unbound (free) fraction since the latter will either be rapidly diluted by widespread distribution throughout the extravascular tissues or replaced from these tissues. Additionally, changes in pH will alter the physicochemical characteristics of fentanyl in such a way that the effect of any change in free fraction will be counterbalanced. Fentanyl is a basic drug (pKa 8.4), and an increase in pH will increase the ionized fraction and increase lipid solubility. These changes will enhance CNS penetration, and will at least partially compensate for the decrease in free-fraction concentration.

Fentanyl is rapidly and extensively metabolized by the liver to inactive metabolites. Only 4–7 percent of an administered dose is excreted unchanged in the urine.[157] In the rat, the main metabolic pathways involve N-dealkylation to norfentanyl and amide hydrolysis to desproprionylfentanyl.[158] Goromaru et al were unable to detect any desproprionylfentanyl in the urine of patients given fentanyl (0.4 mg) during general anesthesia.[157] In their patients 30–50 percent of the fentanyl was excreted as norfentanyl. In contrast, van Rooy et al were able to detect both metabolites in urine of patients undergoing cardiac surgery, given fentanyl 60 μg/kg.[159] The difference in the findings of these two studies probably reflects the differences in the doses used. An additional factor may be the use of halothane in Goromaru's study; whereas no inhalational anesthetic drug was given by van Rooy et al. Halothane is known to influence the pharmacokinetics of fentanyl, causing a 50 percent reduction in drug clearance.[160] Halothane can influence drug elimination by decreasing liver blood flow or by altering the ability of the liver to metabolize fentanyl. It is known that halothane can inhibit cytochrome P-450 metabolism of many compounds.

The disposition of fentanyl in plasma has been extensively studied in animals, healthy human volunteers, and patients undergoing surgery. After bolus intravenous injection, plasma fentanyl concentrations decrease rapidly due to distribution from the plasma to tissues. In the dog, after a 10- or 100-μg/kg intravenous dose of fentanyl, 98 percent of the dose is cleared from the plasma in 5 minutes, and by 30 minutes 99 percent of the drug is eliminated from the plasma.[160] In human volunteers, 98.6 percent of a 10-μg/kg intravenous dose is eliminated from plasma in 60 minutes.[151] This rapid distribution of fentanyl explains why, after moderate 10-μg/kg doses, fentanyl has a short duration of action. The mechanism is analogous to the rapid recovery from thiopental as a result of redistribution. However, attempts to increase the intensity of effect by giving a larger initial dose converts fentanyl from a short-acting to a long-acting drug, as illustrated in Figure 3-7. A 10-fold increment in dose produces an 8-fold increase in the time that plasma levels remain above the threshold for respiratory depression. With the larger dose, the distribution phase is completed before the fentanyl concentration declines to threshold levels. Thus, the duration of action now becomes dependent on the decrease in concentration during the much slower terminal elimination phase. Distribution to the tissues increases the likelihood of accumulation with regularly repeated doses of fentanyl. Since after the first dose the tissues already contain some fentanyl, they take up a lesser proportion of subsequent doses during the distribution phase. Therefore, plasma levels decline to a lesser degree during the distribution phase, and they remain above the threshold concentration for progressively longer periods after each dose due to their slow decline during the elimination phase (Fig. 3-8). To avoid accumulation of fentanyl, doses should be titrated according to the response and needs of the patient. Successive doses at regular intervals should be progressively reduced in amount, or the interval between doses of the same size should be progressively lengthened.

There is remarkable inconsistency in the reported pharmacokinetic parameters for fentanyl.[161] Estimates of terminal half-life range from 100 minutes[162] to 347 minutes,[163] volume of distribution (Vdss) from 55 liters[162] to 257 liters,[151] and total body clearance from 194 ml/min[163] to 1530 ml/min.[151] This great variability in fentanyl kinetics probably reflects differences in methodology, analytical techniques, and subjects studied. Some have studied groups of healthy young volunteers;[145,151,162] whereas others have investigated patients undergoing a variety of surgical procedures under general anesthesia.[163–165] Anesthesia and surgery are known to influence hepatic blood flow and drug metabolizing

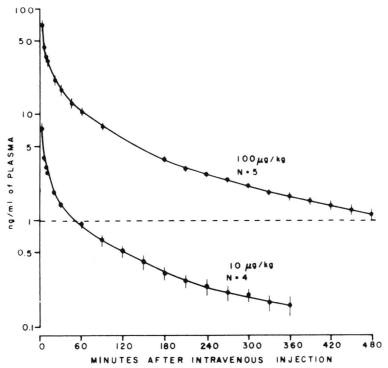

Fig. 3-7. Plasma concentration of unchanged fentanyl after doses of 10 μg/kg and 100 μg/kg. Each data point represents the mean ± SEM for the number of dogs indicated by N. The dashed horizontal line is the threshold for respiratory depression in the dog lightly anesthetized with enflurane. (From Murphy MR, Olson WA, Hug CC, Jr: Pharmaco-kinetics of ^{3}H-fentanyl in the dog anesthetized with enflurane. Anesthesiology 50:13–19, 1979, with permission.)

ability.[166,167] Hepatic clearance of fentanyl is flow dependent and is thus sensitive to reduction in liver perfusion. Halothane and enflurane inhibit fentanyl biotransformation in rat hepatic tissue homogenates,[168] and halothane has been shown to affect fentanyl disposition in humans.[168,169]

The nature of the surgery will also influence fentanyl disposition in surgical patients. Major surgery may be associated with blood loss and fluid shifts between intra- and extravascular spaces and changes in distribution volume. In addition, trauma, including surgical trauma, increases the concentration of alpha$_1$-AGP, a major determinant of fentanyl binding. This will further alter fentanyl distribution. Patients undergoing abdominal aortic surgery anesthetized with fentanyl, 100 μg/kg, had an elimination half-life of fentanyl of 8.7 hours, about double that of normal volunteers.[170] This was due to a lower clearance and a greater volume of distribution. Not surprisingly, fentanyl kinetics is significantly altered in

patients undergoing cardiac surgery with cardiopulmonary bypass. Koska et al found an elimination half-life of fentanyl of 5.2 hours in cardiac patients, compared with 3.3 hours in a control group undergoing vascular surgery without cardiopulmonary bypass.[171] In addition, indocyanine green (ICG) clearance studies were performed. ICG clearance, which is closely related to hepatic plasma flow, was reduced about 30 percent during and after bypass. Other studies during cardiac surgery have reported even longer elimination half-lives, 7.1 hours[93] and 11 hours.[172] Clearance was diminished (7.6 ml/kg/min) and volume of distribution (7.9 liters/kg) increased[172] (see Chapter 2).

A variety of assay methods have been used to measure plasma fentanyl concentrations. Earlier animal studies used ^{3}H-labeled fentanyl, and this was also used in one human volunteer study.[151] The majority of human studies have used a radioimmunoassay (RIA) that is sensitive and specific, allowing

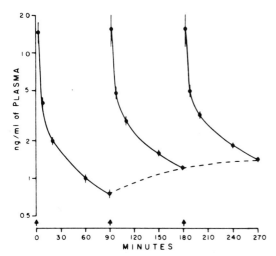

Fig. 3-8. Plasma fentanyl concentrations after three successive 10-µg/kg boluses of fentanyl administered intravenously at 90-min intervals. The dotted line connecting values at the end of successive intervals indicates accumulation of fentanyl with repeated doses. (From Murphy MR, Olson WA, Hug CC, Jr: Pharmacokinetics of ³H-fentanyl in the dog anesthetized with enflurane. Anesthesiology 50:13–19, 1979, with permission.)

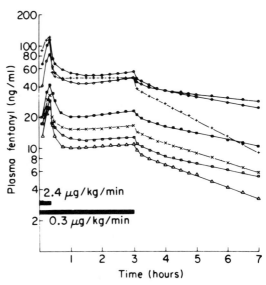

Fig. 3-9. Computer-predicted plasma fentanyl concentrations, based on published pharmacokinetic data from seven studies, during an infusion of fentanyl, 2.7 µg/kg/min, for 20 min, followed by 0.3 µg/kg/min for a further 160 min, when the infusion was stopped. (From Reilly CS, Wood AJJ, Wood M: Variability of fentanyl pharmacokinetics in man. Computer predicted plasma concentrations for three intravenous dosage regimens. Anaesthesia 40:837–843, 1985, with permission.)

measurement of concentrations as low as 0.1 ng/ml.[173] This assay is commercially available as a kit containing antiserum to fentanyl obtained from rabbits immunized with a fentanyl analogue coupled to bovine albumin.[174] The accuracy of these RIA kits has recently been questioned[175] since they give drug levels significantly higher than those obtained using a gas chromatographic technique.[176] This inaccuracy is related to the sequence in which the reagents are added to the patient sample. The suggested sequence when using the RIA kits is to add antiserum prior to the labelled fentanyl, in contrast to the classical method of performing RIA where the antiserum is added last to the patient sample-labeled drug mixture. Using spiked serum samples containing known concentrations of fentanyl from 0.5 to 40 ng/ml, the RIA kit significantly overpredicted the concentration by 29–76 percent. In contrast, when the assay was performed using the classical RIA technique, the results were accurate to ±7 percent.[175]

An accurate knowledge of kinetic parameters is needed when designing continuous infusion regimens to achieve a desired effect. Reilly et al compared predicted plasma fentanyl concentrations using computer simulation based on derived pharmacokinetic data obtained from seven previously published studies.[177] They found marked differences in predicted plasma concentrations. The peak predicted concentration after a bolus of 500 µg of fentanyl ranged from 8.4 to 114 ng/ml and took from 3 to 19 hours to decline to 0.5 ng/ml. Following a simulated two-stage infusion of fentanyl (2.7 µg/kg/min for 20 minutes, then 0.3 µg/kg/min), steady-state plasma concentrations ranged from 11 to 51 ng/ml (Fig. 3-9). Until the pharmacokinetics of fentanyl are more accurately defined, it remains illogical to use fixed infusion regimens based on published data in an attempt to achieve a predicted plasma concentration. Ideally, such a regimen should be based on data previously obtained from the same patient, but this is possible only in exceptional circumstances. At the present time, infusion rates should be individually adjusted to achieve the desired effect rather than relying on a fixed-rate regimen. The use of variable infusion rates of fentanyl produces greater hemodynamic stability and the need for adjuvant drug intervention is significantly lower compared to a fixed infusion rate during coronary artery surgery.[178]

FACTORS THAT POTENTIALLY INFLUENCE FENTANYL PHARMACOKINETICS

Dose. Increasing the dose of a drug to a level where saturation of metabolizing enzymes occurs can potentially alter the pharmacokinetics from first-order (linear) to zero-order (nonlinear). Despite the wide range of doses used clinically, from 1.5 μg/kg for analgesia and anesthetic supplements to 150 μg/kg or more for anesthesia, there is no evidence that the pharmacokinetics of fentanyl is dose dependent. The pharmacokinetics of fentanyl have been shown to be independent of dose in dogs over a 6.4–640-μg/kg dose range.[179]

Age. With increasing age, the elimination of many drugs is prolonged.[180] Bently et al compared fentanyl pharmacokinetics in two groups of adult patients, one group aged less than 50 years and the other aged over 60 years, undergoing elective intra-abdominal surgery.[164] Serum fentanyl concentrations were significantly higher in the older patients, despite equivalent (10 μg/kg) doses of fentanyl. The average terminal elimination half-life in the older patients was 15.8 hours, compared with 4.4 hours in the younger patients. This prolonged elimination in the older patients was due to decreased clearance: 4.0 $\pm$ 0.6 ml/kg/min versus 15.4 $\pm$ 1.6 ml/kg/min in the younger patients. The volumes of distribution were not significantly different between the groups. The most likely explanation for the decreased clearance in older patients is reduction in hepatic blood flow, which decreases with aging.[181] Hepatic clearance of fentanyl approximates hepatic blood flow and is thus flow dependent.[145] In addition, microsomal enzyme activity has been shown to be decreased in the elderly.[182] The decreased clearance and longer elimination half-life in elderly patients have important clinical implications. Less fentanyl will be required to reach a desired analgesic effect, and the pharmacologic effects, including respiratory depression, will be more prolonged than in younger patients. Based on the data of Bently et al,[164] the time to reach a threshold concentration for respiratory depression of 1 ng/ml after fentanyl, 10 μg/kg, would take 150 minutes in the younger patients and approximately 560 minutes in the elderly.[151] These differences will be even more pronounced with doses of 50–100 μg/kg often used in cardiac surgery.

Renal and liver disease. There is limited data concerning the influence of severe renal disease on fentanyl pharmacokinetics. It is likely that accumula-

tion of fentanyl metabolites will occur with impaired renal function, but this is unlikely to have clinical consequences since they are pharmacologically inactive. This is in contrast to meperidine and morphine. Normeperidine, the main metabolite of meperidine, is a CNS stimulant and its accumulation in the presence of renal failure can produce toxic effects, including convulsions.[183] Accumulation of morphine-3-glucuronide, the principal metabolite of morphine, has been implicated in the prolonged narcotic effect of morphine in patients with renal failure.[184] Fentanyl has been given to anephric patients without untoward side effects.[185] In these patients fentanyl clearance was higher than in surgical patients with normal renal function.

Since the liver is the principal organ for biotransformation of fentanyl, decreases in hepatic function due to liver disease would be expected to alter the pharmacokinetics of fentanyl. Fentanyl clearance may be modified by three factors that are altered in liver disease: (1) reduced hepatic blood flow, (2) diminished activity of metabolizing enzymes, and (3) changes in plasma proteins. The intrinsic hepatic clearance of fentanyl is several times that of normal hepatic blood flow.[145,151] Total intrinsic clearance gives an indication of the maximum ability of the liver to metabolically remove drug in the absence of flow limitations. For drugs such as fentanyl with high intrinsic clearance, hepatic elimination will be sensitive to changes in liver blood flow, but much less so to alterations in the drug metabolizing capacity of the liver. Plasma clearance of fentanyl is the same in patients with moderate cirrhosis as in patients with normal hepatic and renal function.[186] No studies are available of the influence of severe hepatic insufficiency on fentanyl pharmacokinetics, but it is to be expected that clearance would be prolonged. In anhepatic animals there is a marked prolongation of the elimination half-life of fentanyl.[149,187] Interestingly, in hepatectomized dogs, 8 percent of the administered dose of fentanyl was excreted in the urine as fentanyl metabolites, indicating possible extrahepatic sites of metabolism for fentanyl.[187]

Hepatic dysfunction is often associated with hypoproteinemia. Since fentanyl is 60 to 80 percent protein bound, there will be an increased amount of free fentanyl available. Because of the large volume of distribution of fentanyl, however, which is likely to be even greater in patients with liver disease due to edema and an increased circulating blood volume, the intensity of effect after a single dose is not likely to be increased beyond that in a normal subject. A single dose of moderate size also will have a relatively normal duration of action, since the termination of the effect depends primarily on the distribution of fentanyl from the plasma to peripheral tissues.[151] The reduced clearance of fentanyl in these patients means that large or repeated doses will more rapidly lead to accumulation and an unusually long duration of action.

Obesity. Because of its high lipophilicity, it might be expected that the distribution volume would be increased, and thus plasma elimination half-life prolonged, in the obese patient. Bently et al studied the pharmacokinetics of a 10-μg/kg intravenous bolus of fentanyl in three nonobese and five morbidly obese (body weight greater than two times ideal weight) patients.[188] There were no significant differences in the terminal elimination half-lives, the clearance, or the apparent volumes of distribution between the obese and the nonobese. However, since fat has an enormous capacity for holding lipophilic drugs such as fentanyl, obesity may alter the pharmacodynamic effect after very large doses, especially if these are given by repeated increments or by a continuous infusion.

Drug interactions. Few studies have investigated the effects of specific drugs on fentanyl pharmacokinetics. As mentioned above, anesthetic drugs, especially the volatile anesthetics, are likely to influence fentanyl disposition, primarily by reducing hepatic blood flow. Surgical patients anesthetized with halothane or enflurane have reduced fentanyl clearances compared to a control group receiving only intravenous anesthesia.[168] Studies in sheep have shown that meperidine disposition is significantly altered by general anesthesia but not by spinal anesthesia.[189] In the sheep, general anesthesia with halothane, 1.5 percent, caused a 71 percent decrease in hepatic blood flow from the awake control value.[190] Similar decreases in hepatic blood flow during 2 minimum alveolar concentration (MAC) halothane anesthesia have been reported in humans.[191,192] Hepatic arterial blood flow, of most importance for hepatic clearance of drugs, is more compromised than portal blood flow during halothane anesthesia.[190]

Cimetidine reduces hepatic metabolism and clearance of a variety of drugs by inhibiting oxidative drug metabolism by binding to cytochrome P-450. Borel et al studied five dogs pretreated with cimetidine, 10 mg/kg, IM the night before, and 5 mg/kg/, IM 90 minutes before receiving 100 μg/kg of fentanyl intravenously.[193] The dogs served as their own

controls in a double-crossover protocol with a minimum of 3 weeks between studies. Cimetidine significantly increased the elimination half-life of fentanyl from 155 minutes to 340 minutes. Cimetidine also prolongs fentanyl elimination half-life in humans.[194]

CONCENTRATION-EFFECT RELATIONSHIPS

Highly lipophilic drugs like fentanyl rapidly cross the blood-brain barrier, and thus a close relationship between plasma concentration and effect is to be expected. The relationship among plasma concentration, cerebrospinal fluid (CSF) concentration, and ventilatory depression has been examined in dogs[148] and in humans.[163] In dogs anesthetized with enflurane-oxygen, given fentanyl (10 μg/kg IV), maximum concentrations of fentanyl in cisternal CSF occurred between 2.5 and 10 minutes, and by 20 minutes after injection CSF concentration had equilibrated with that in plasma.[148] A linear relationship was found between the log-concentration of fentanyl in plasma or CSF and ventilatory depression as indicated by the rise in end-tidal CO_2. The apparent threshold for ventilatory depression was about 1 ng/ml. There is a good correlation between plasma fentanyl concentrations and the slope of the CO_2 response curve.[195] Cartwright et al studied the relationship between ventilatory depression and plasma fentanyl concentrations postoperatively in patients given either 10 or 25 μg/kg of fentanyl during anesthesia.[196] Plasma fentanyl concentrations associated with 50 percent depression of CO_2 responsiveness were in the range of 1.5 to 3.0 ng/ml. In patients who had been hyperventilated during anesthesia, however, lower values were found than in patients who were maintained normocapnic. In patients given a continuous infusion of fentanyl, a steady-state plasma concentration of 2.9 ng/ml was associated with a 45 percent depression of CO_2 responsiveness.[197] A plasma concentration of 4.6 ng/ml was associated with a 50 percent depression in young healthy volunteers who had not received anesthesia or other drugs.[198]

Delayed respiratory depression in the postoperative period several hours after recovery from anesthesia has been reported after small (50–500 μg) intravenous doses of fentanyl given during anesthesia.[199,200] This biphasic respiratory depression may be related to secondary peaks in plasma fentanyl concentrations during the elimination phase.[201] Stoeckel et al demonstrated enterohepatic recirculation of fentanyl, with sequestration in the stomach and subsequent reabsorption from the small intestine.[202] Peak concentrations in gastric juice occurred within about

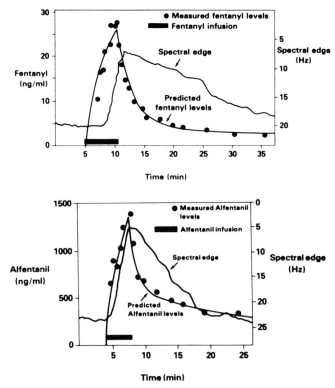

Fig. 3-10. Time course of spectral edge and plasma concentrations during and after infusions of fentanyl and alfentanil. Note the inverted spectral edge axis and how the spectral edge changes lag the concentration changes (From Scott JC, Ponganis KV, Stanski DR: EEG quantitation of narcotic effect. The comparative pharmacodynamics of fentanyl and alfentanil. Anesthesiology 62:234–241, 1985, with permission.)

15–30 minutes of intravenous fentanyl administration and were about 5–10 times higher than those in the plasma. Partitioning of fentanyl into gastric juice occurs as a result of the difference between gastric pH and the high pKa (8.43) of fentanyl. As much as 16 percent of an administered dose may accumulate in the stomach. Since the average volume of gastric juice is small (25–100 ml), however, the amount of fentanyl involved is likely to be of little consequence. Also, because the hepatic extraction of fentanyl is high, little of the fentanyl reabsorbed into the portal circulation would reach the systemic circulation. Indeed, direct administration of fentanyl by nasogastric tube results in almost indetectable plasma fentanyl concentrations.[203] A more likely explanation for the observed secondary peaks is release of fentanyl from body stores, especially muscle, as a result of increased patient activity in the postoperative period. Because of its large mass, muscle can store up to 55 percent of fentanyl present in the body.

The relationship between fentanyl and alfentanil serum concentrations, during and after slow infusions, and electroencephalogram (EEG) changes have recently been investigated in volunteers, using the spectral edge parameter as a measure of EEG changes.[204] The spectral edge is the frequency below which 95 percent of the total power in the EEG occurs. Spectral edge changes paralleled opioid concentrations but lagged behind them in time, with a well-defined hysteresis effect (Figs. 3-10 and 3-11). This hysteresis was more marked for fentanyl than for alfentanil, and could be related to changes in an *effect* compartment and differing pharmacokinetic properties of the two drugs.

Little is known about the relationship between fentanyl plasma concentration and analgesia, the principal pharmacologic effect of this and other opioids. This is probably because analgesia as an entity is extremely difficult to quantify in humans. Plasma concentrations of 1.7 ± 0.24 ng/ml provide

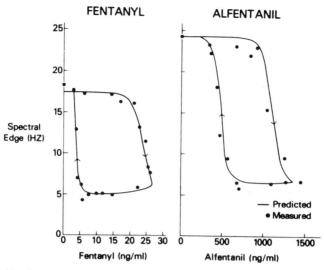

Fig. 3-11. Spectral edge versus serum concentrations of fentanyl and alfentanil, illustrating the hysteresis effect that is greater for fentanyl than for alfentanil. (From Scott JC, Ponganis KV, Stanski DR: EEG quantitation of narcotic effect. The comparative pharmacodynamics of fentanyl and alfentanil. Anesthesiology 62:234–241, 1985, with permission.)

good postoperative analgesia.[205] The range of fentanyl concentrations associated with different effects is summarized in Table 3-6.

FENTANYL IN CARDIAC ANESTHESIA

Since the first report, in 1978, by Stanley and Webster[47] of high-dose fentanyl anesthesia for patients undergoing mitral valve surgery, and the subsequent report from the same group in patients undergoing coronary artery surgery,[48] the advantages and disadvantages of fentanyl in cardiac anesthesia have been extensively documented. Stanley and his colleagues reported that fentanyl, in an average dose of 75 μg/kg, provided complete anesthesia with minimal cardiovascular depression for both groups of patients. Not all investigators, however, have been able to replicate these good results. Hicks et al studied 10 patients, with normal left ventricular function, during induction of anesthesia for coronary artery surgery.[206] Fentanyl was given at a rate of 100–200 μg/min and cardiovascular profiles were obtained after 15, 30, and 50 μg/kg. Metocurine was given for muscle relaxation and the study was completed before intubation of the trachea. Cardiac index and left ventricular stroke work index were decreased significantly after fentanyl, 15 and 30 μg/kg. These decreases could not be attributed to a decrease in metabolic oxygen demand and were taken as evidence of fentanyl-induced myocardial depression. Hicks' results, however, are at variance with those of several other investigators who found no evidence that induction of anesthesia with fentanyl, 28–50 μg/kg, caused myocardial depression.[141,207-210] Barash et al, using technetium-99m-labeled red cells and a left ventricular nuclear probe, demonstrated that fentanyl, 75 μg/kg, not only maintained hemodynamic parameters within the range of awake control values,

Table 3-6

Fentanyl Effects Related to Plasma Concentration

Fentanyl concentration in plasma	Effect
ng/ml	
>1	Slight analgesia and ventilatory depression
>3	Analgesia and 50% decrease in ventilatory response to carbon dioxide
8–10	50% decrease in MAC
>20	Unconsciousness and 65% decrease in MAC

Source: From Hug CC Jr: Pharmacokinetics and dynamics of narcotic analgesics. *In* Prys-Roberts C, Hug CC Jr (eds): Pharmacokinetics of Anaesthesia. Oxford, Blackwell, p 218, 1984, with permission.

Table 3-7
Hemodynamic and Left Ventricular Function Changes Following Induction of
Anesthesia with Fentanyl, 75 μg/kg

	Ejection fraction (%)	Heart rate (bpm)	Systolic blood pressure (mm Hg)	Pulmonary capillary wedge pressure (mm Hg)	Cardiac index (liters/min/m^2)
Pre-induction	51±5	55±3	139±6	14±2	3.1±0.3
Pre-intubation	51±5	55±4	136±6	18±2	3.1±0.2
Intubation	52±6	53±4	133±7	17±2	2.7±0.2
1 min	52±6	56±4	136±7	18±2	2.7±0.2
3 min	55±6	52±4	132±5	17±2	2.8±0.2
5 min	53±8	47±6	129±5	16±3	2.8±0.1
10 min	54±6	50±4	127±6	17±2	2.7±0.2

Source: From Barash PG, Tarabadkar S, Giles R, et al: Preservation of global left ventricular function during intubation in patients with ischemic heart disease. Anesthesiology 55: A6, 1981, with permission.

Data (mean±SEM) were obtained from 10 patients undergoing elective coronary artery surgery. Ejection fraction was measured by a radionuclear probe after injection of red blood cells labeled with technetium (Tc-99 m).

but also preserved left ventricular ejection fraction, an index of global ventricular function, in patients with ischemic heart disease (Table 3-7).[211] This was in marked contrast to the changes that occurred during diazepam, enflurane, and nitrous oxide anesthesia in a comparable group of patients.[212] In the latter group, there was a 31 percent increase in heart rate and a 37 percent increase in blood pressure after intubation. Although cardiac index did not change from control value, the ejection fraction decreased by 35 percent, and, in four patients, remained depressed.

Although induction of anesthesia with fentanyl generally causes minimal hemodynamic disturbances, this stability is not always maintained during surgery. During and after sternotomy, arterial hypertension, increases in systemic vascular resistance, and decreases in cardiac output frequently occur. Waller et al reported that 8 of 12 patients given fentanyl (50–89 μg/kg) before sternotomy required additional anesthetic drugs and a nitroglycerin infusion in order to control systolic hypertension during and after sternotomy.[207] Edde found that poststernotomy hypertension occurred in all 12 patients anesthetized with fentanyl (50 μg/kg).[208] Sebel et al reported that 45–50 percent of patients given fentanyl (60–70 μg/kg) at induction needed nitroprusside within 3 to 5 minutes after sternotomy to control hypertension.[141] The variability in the hemodynamic

responses to surgical stimulation, even with similar doses of fentanyl, is probably a reflection of differences in the patient populations (eg, degree of beta-blockade) studied by different authors. De Lange et al found that in patients undergoing coronary artery surgery anesthetized with fentanyl (122 μg/kg), 86 percent of those not taking beta-adrenoreceptor blocking drugs became hypertensive during sternal spread; whereas only 33 percent of those taking beta-blocking drugs became hypertensive.[209]

The degree of myocardial impairment will also influence the response. Critically ill patients, or patients with significant myocardial dysfunction, appear to require lower doses of fentanyl for complete anesthesia. This may reflect altered fentanyl kinetics in those patients. A decrease in hepatic blood flow consequent to decreased cardiac output and congestive heart failure will reduce the plasma clearance of fentanyl. Patients with poor left ventricular function thus may develop higher plasma and brain concentrations of fentanyl for a given loading dose or infusion rate than patients with good ventricular function. Additionally, patients with depressed myocardial function may lack the ability to respond to surgical stress by increasing cardiac output in the face of progressive increases in systemic vascular resistance. Wynands et al compared two groups of patients undergoing coronary artery surgery anesthetized with a loading dose of fentanyl (30 μg/kg), followed by an infusion of fentanyl at a rate of 0.3 μg/kg/min.[213] One group was comprised of 7 patients with poor left ventricular function (ejection fraction less than 0.3, left ventricular end-diastolic pressure [LVEDP] greater than 20 mm Hg, and at least one area of myocardial dyskinesia). The second group comprised 12 patients with good left ventricular function. Despite similar plasma fentanyl concentrations in both groups, all patients with good ventricular function, as compared with only 3 of the 7 patients with poor ventricular function, became hypertensive at some period before cardiopulmonary bypass.

The previous lifestyle also appears to influence hemodynamic responses during cardiac surgery. Patients in the Netherlands required considerably larger amounts of fentanyl (143 μg/kg) than a group of patients undergoing similar surgery in Salt Lake City, who only required 74 μg/kg fentanyl.[214] It was postulated that the Dutch patients, perhaps because of their exposure to caffeine, alcohol, and tobacco, were more tolerant to CNS depressants than the Mormon patients in Salt Lake City.

In an attempt to reduce the incidence of hypertension and other hemodynamic disturbances associated with sternotomy, the dose of fentanyl has been increased, although not always with success. Vasodilators were required in 42 to 45 percent of patients given fentanyl, 122–127 μg/kg.[209,215] Zurich et al gave fentanyl (150 μg/kg) over 5 minutes to 10 patients undergoing coronary artery surgery and found no significant changes from the awake control values in mean blood pressure or vascular resistance up to the start of bypass.[216] Cardiac output, however, decreased significantly after sternotomy. Although doses of the magnitude used by Zurich et al can provide cardiovascular stability during surgery, they are likely to be associated with prolonged respiratory depression and delayed recovery after surgery.

The technique of administering fentanyl by a single large bolus at induction of anesthesia is neither pharmacokinetically logical nor efficient. Although high plasma and brain concentrations are obtained almost immediately, these decline rapidly and may be below the minimum effective level at the time of maximum stimulation, ie, sternotomy and aortic dissection. Several authors have investigated infusion schemes designed to maintain stable plasma fentanyl concentrations. Sprigge et al studied three groups of patients given loading doses of fentanyl, 30, 40, or 50 μg/kg followed by infusions of 0.3, 0.4, or 0.5 μg/kg/min, respectively, until the time of rewarming on cardiopulmonary bypass or until a total dose of

100 μg/kg had been given.[94] Stable plasma concentrations were reached within 20 minutes, the mean concentrations being 10–12 ng/ml in group 1, 12–14 ng/ml in group 2, and 15–18 ng/ml in group 3. Although fewer patients in group 3 than in the other groups responded to surgical stimulation, 50 percent of patients with a plasma fentanyl concentration of 15 ng/ml had an increase in systolic blood pressure requiring treatment. Stable plasma fentanyl concentrations of 20 ± 1 ng/ml, produced by a loading infusion of 2.4 μg/kg/min for 20 minutes and a maintenance infusion of 0.3 μg/kg/min thereafter, were adequate to maintain heart rate and blood pressure within ± 20 percent of preanesthetic values.[217] Wynands et al found that no patients with a plasma fentanyl concentration above 18 ng/ml became hypertensive at sternotomy.[218] Significantly more patients, however, became hypertensive at aortic dissection (35 percent) than during sternotomy (16.3 percent), suggesting that either the intensity, or more likely the nature, of the stimulus is different during aortic dissection than during sternotomy. The incidence of hypertensive response to aortic dissection in patients with plasma levels above 20 ng/ml was 33 percent (2/6), and in those with a level less than 20 ng/ml, 62 percent (13/21). Although these differences were not statistically significant, the number of patients involved is relatively small and the evidence from this study and that of Moldenhauer and Hug[217] suggests that plasma fentanyl concentrations of about 20 ng/ml may provide optimal hemodynamic stability in the prebypass period. Plasma concentrations in excess of 20 ng/ml may result in patients needing prolonged periods of postoperative ventilatory support.[218] Indeed it is likely that beyond this plasma concentration little additional anesthetic benefit will accrue.

The ability of fentanyl to reduce the MAC of enflurane in dogs reaches a plateau of about 65 percent reduction at fentanyl plasma concentrations of 30 ng/ml (Fig. 3-12).[219] Assuming that reduction of enflurane MAC is a reflection of anesthetic depth, this suggests a ceiling to the effectiveness of fentanyl as an anesthetic. A similar concentration/effect relationship for a fentanyl-induced decrease in cardiac output in dogs has been demonstrated (Fig. 3-13).[220] Since dogs are less sensitive than humans to opioids, it is likely that the higher doses of fentanyl used in cardiac surgery, especially those achieving plasma fentanyl concentrations of 20 to 30 ng/ml, may already be producing a maximal effect.

During surgery, including cardiac surgery, the intensity of the surgical stimulus varies, and it

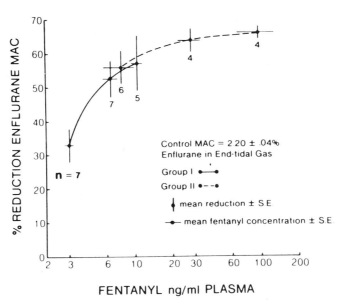

Fig. 3-12. Reduction of enflurane MAC as a function of plasma fentanyl concentration. (From Murphy MR, Hug CC, Jr: The anesthetic potency of fentanyl in terms of its reduction of enflurane MAC. Anesthesiology 57:485–488, 1982, with permission.)

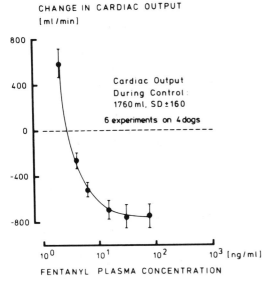

Fig. 3-13. Changes in cardiac output with increasing plasma concentrations of fentanyl in four unanesthetized, spontaneously breathing dogs with chronically implanted electromagnetic flow probes on the ascending aorta. The maximum decrease in cardiac output from preinjection control value occurred at a plasma fentanyl concentration of about 30 ng/ml. (From Arndt JO, Mikat M, Parasher C: Fentanyl's analgesic, respiratory, and cardiovascular actions in relation to dose and plasma concentration in unanesthetized dogs. Anesthesiology 61:355–361, 1984, with permission.)

would, therefore, seem logical to vary the concentration of the anesthetic drug to meet these differing demands. Although this is standard practice when using volatile anesthetic drugs, it has not been possible until recently with intravenous drugs such as fentanyl that have a relatively slow plasma clearance. The use of computer-assisted continuous infusion pumps have, however, made this feasible. Alvis et al compared two computer-assisted methods of fentanyl infusion with a manual fentanyl administration method in 30 patients undergoing coronary artery surgery.[178] After premedication with oral diazepam (10 mg), intramuscular scopolamine (0.4 mg), and morphine (0.1 mg/kg), anesthesia was induced with diazepam (0.3 mg/kg) and pancuronium (0.1 mg/kg). The lungs were ventilated with 50 percent nitrous oxide in oxygen. In the control (manual) group, fentanyl, 150–250 μg, was given prior to laryngoscopy and similar boluses were given to prevent anticipated hemodynamic responses to surgical stimulation. Fentanyl by continuous infusion was started prior to laryngoscopy in the two automated infusion groups. In group S (stable fentanyl level), the infusion rate was adjusted by computer to maintain a predicted constant plasma fentanyl concentration of 7.5 ng/ml. A similar initial plasma concentration was chosen in the third group V (variable fentanyl level). However, in this latter group the anesthesiologist

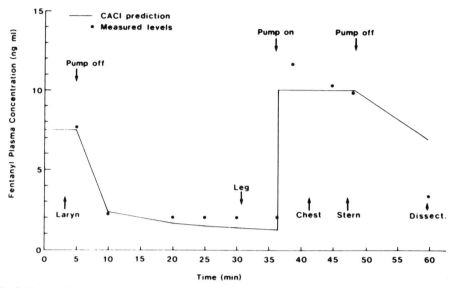

Fig. 3-14. Predicted and measured plasma fentanyl concentrations during a variable fentanyl level computer-assisted continuous infusion (CACI) for a single patient. The continuous infusion of fentanyl was adjusted to different levels according to different surgical stimulation or non-stimulation. Laryn = laryngoscopy; leg = leg incision; chest = chest incision; stern = sternotomy; dissect = mediastinal dissection. (From Alvis JM, Reves JG, Govier AV, et al: Computer-assisted continuous infusions of fentanyl during cardiac anesthesia. Comparison with a manual method. Anesthesiology 63:41–49, 1985, with permission.)

could instruct the computer to adjust the infusion rate to achieve different fentanyl levels according to the response of the patient (Fig. 3-14). The study was continued for 1 hour, up to mediastinal dissection. The stable fentanyl group of patients received significantly more fentanyl (27.1 ± 0.09 μg/kg) than either groups C (19.6 ± 0.85 μg/kg) or V (22.8 ± 1.41 μg/kg). Patients in group V had greater hemodynamic stability, required significantly fewer adjuvant drugs, and experienced fewer hypotensive or hypertensive episodes than the other groups. Although the plasma fentanyl concentrations reported by Alvis et al, because of the concomitant use of diazepam, are not directly comparable with those in which fentanyl alone was used, the message of this study is clear. The most efficient manner of fentanyl administration, both in terms of total drug needed and hemodynamic stability, is by continuous infusion with the infusion rate adjusted according to variations in patient requirements. Improvements in computer control of infusion pumps and a better understanding of dose-(or concentration) effect relationships should allow anesthesiologists to administer fentanyl and other opioids to their patients on a more rational basis in the future.

DRUG INTERACTIONS

To limit the total dose of fentanyl and yet maintain good hemodynamic stability during surgery and ensure unconsciousness and amnesia, fentanyl has been combined with other drugs. Diazepam is often used as a supplement to fentanyl anesthesia. As with morphine, however,[42] addition of diazepam in patients anesthetized with fentanyl can cause profound decreases in blood pressure, systemic vascular resistance, and cardiac output.[47,221] Neither fentanyl nor diazepam, when given alone, produces important hemodynamic depression. Tomichek et al found that when fentanyl (50 μg/kg) was given after doses of diazepam from 0.125 to 0.5 mg/kg, plasma concentrations of epinephrine and norepinephrine decreased significantly compared to a control group who received fentanyl alone.[221] Urinary levels of epinephrine and norepinephrine have been reported to decrease after anesthesia with diazepam and fentanyl.[222] Reduction in plasma catecholamine levels could explain the observed cardiovascular changes. However, in Tomichek's study, pulmonary capillary wedge pressure did not change, despite a decrease in cardiac output and systemic vascular resistance. This suggests the possibility that the diazepam–fentanyl

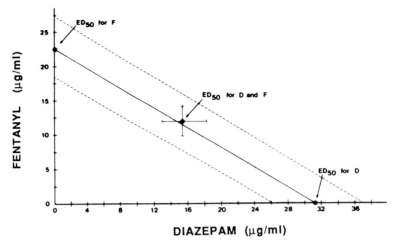

Fig. 3-15. Isobologram for the interaction of the negative inotropic effects of fentanyl and diazepam at ED_{50} level (50% decrease from control in dP/dt_{max}) in isolated perfused rat hearts. Isobols are lines connecting equipotent doses. The solid line connects ED_{50} points for fentanyl alone and diazepam alone. The dashed lines represent the 67% confidence limits. The combined drug value lies close to the isobol line, indicating that the combined effects are additive. Had the point been above and to the right of the isobol line, the interaction would have been infra-additive; below and to the left supra-additive. (From Reves JG, Kissin I, Fournier SE, et al: Additive negative inotropic effect of a combination of diazepam and fentanyl. Anesth Analg 63:97–100, 1984, with permission.)

combination causes some myocardial depression. In the isolated rat heart preparation, both fentanyl and diazepam have a negative inotropic effect; but the combination of the two drugs produces an additive, and not a supraadditive, negative inotropy (Fig. 3-15).[223] In this study, however, negative inotropic effects occurred at concentrations about 400 times in excess of those encountered in patients. Also, in humans the reflexes that counteract negative inotropic effects of drugs are preserved while these are absent in the isolated heart preparation. This would suggest, therefore, that the hemodynamic changes caused by diazepam and fentanyl in combination are unlikely to be the result of significant myocardial depression, but rather are due to a peripheral vascular effect of this drug combination.

Addition of nitrous oxide to the inspiratory gas in patients who have been given large doses of fentanyl produces hemodynamic changes similar to those described above with diazepam. Nitrous oxide alone causes minimal myocardial depression in normal volunteers[224] and in patients with coronary artery disease.[225] In the dog, the myocardial depressant effects of nitrous oxide and fentanyl are additive.[226]

In patients undergoing coronary artery surgery in whom anesthesia was induced with fentanyl (50 μg/kg) while breathing 100% oxygen, ventilation with 50% nitrous oxide in oxygen resulted in a significant decrease in cardiac index, an increase in systemic vascular resistance, and no change in mean arterial blood pressure in patients with poor left ventricular function. In a similar group of patients with good left ventricular function, the addition of nitrous oxide produced no significant hemodynamic changes. The detrimental effect of nitrous oxide in combination with both enflurane and fentanyl on ventricular function in patients with coronary artery disease has been demonstrated by others.[227] This has also been confirmed in dogs with coronary artery constriction anesthetized with fentanyl[228] or sufentanil.[229]

It has been suggested that the reduction in inspired oxygen concentration, when nitrous oxide/oxygen is substituted for 100% oxygen in the inspired gas, may be partially responsible for the above changes, although the evidence is conflicting. In one study, either 70% nitrous oxide or 70% nitrogen was randomly added 15 minutes after induction of anesthesia with fentanyl (100 μg/kg) and ventilation with 100% oxygen.[230] Both resulted in significant reductions in blood pressure, and statistical analysis revealed that 50 percent of the reduction caused by nitrous oxide could be attributed to the reduction in F_IO_2. Conversely, changing the inspired gas mixture from 100% oxygen to 60% helium after administration of fentanyl (75 μg/kg) produced no significant hemodynamic effects in cardiac surgical patients.[48] However, when the same patients were ventilated with 60% nitrous oxide, cardiac output decreased by 33 percent with significant increases in systemic vascular resistance and central venous pressure.

The influence of nitrous oxide on hemodynamic function may be related to the extent of myocardial dysfunction. In dogs anesthetized with 100 μg/kg fentanyl followed by an infusion of 1 μg/kg/min of fentanyl no evidence of regional myocardial dysfunction was seen in the absence of a critical coronary artery stenosis either with or without nitrous oxide.[228] Once a critical stenosis in the left anterior descending coronary artery was produced, however, the introduction of 66% nitrous oxide caused rapid and significant dysfunction, measured by systolic shortening, in only the area of the LAD distribution. This was not accompanied by any significant changes in coronary blood flow, coronary vascular resistance, heart rate, or arterial oxygen tension. The dysfunction was usually, but not always, reversible by elimination of nitrous oxide. This evidence raises doubts about the wisdom of using nitrous oxide in patients with significant coronary artery stenosis. In such patients, anesthetized with fentanyl, 50 μg/kg, cardiac depression produced by 66% nitrous oxide was most prominent in those with left ventricular hypokinesis and ejection fractions less than 55 percent.[231]

The choice of neuromuscular blocking drug for patients anesthetized with high doses of opioids may have important consequences. Pancuronium, because of its vagolytic action, has been recommended since it prevents or minimizes opioid-induced bradycardia.[232,233] Pancuronium, given 10 minutes after induction of anesthesia with 75 μg/kg of fentanyl, returned heart rate and cardiac index, which had decreased significantly after fentanyl, to awake control values.[234] In contrast, after administration of vecuronium, which has no vagolytic activity, heart rate and cardiac index decreased further. Of 10 patients receiving vecuronium 5 had a heart rate below 45 beats per minute; heart rates this low were not seen in patients given pancuronium.

The use of pancuronium during high-dose fentanyl anesthesia may, however, produce adverse effects. In patients undergoing coronary artery surgery anesthetized with fentanyl (100 μg/kg), those given pancuronium (0.1 mg/kg) had a significantly higher heart rate and rate-pressure product postinduction than patients given either 0.42 mg/kg metocurine or a combination of 0.108 mg/kg metocurine and 0.027 mg/kg pancuronium.[235] More significantly, myocardial ischemia, indicated by new ST-segment depression, occurred in 3 of 12 patients given pancuronium alone. This was associated with tachycardia and increases in systolic arterial pressure during induction. None of the patients given metocurine or the pancuronium/metocurine combination showed evidence of myocardial ischemia.

FENTANYL AND MYOCARDIAL METABOLISM

Although the effect of fentanyl on the myocardium has been extensively studied in animals, only limited information is available about the direct myocardial effects of high-dose fentanyl in humans. The recent availability of special catheters for insertion into the coronary sinus has made possible the direct measurement of coronary sinus blood flow (an approximation of total myocardial blood flow) and estimations of myocardial oxygen consumption and lactate extraction or production.[236] Lactate production by the myocardium is an indicator of myocardial ischemia. Sonntag et al reported lactate production, before the start of surgery, in 5 of 9 patients given fentanyl, 100 μg/kg.[215] However, they gave the fentanyl as a slow infusion over about 30 minutes. They also gave etomidate (0.3 mg/kg) after patients had received fentanyl, 10 μg/kg. It is possible that the prolonged induction could have caused patient stress and, thereby, myocardial ischemia. During sternotomy, myocardial blood flow and oxygen uptake increased significantly, and in 7 of the 9 patients lactate production was observed. Other studies, using different techniques of fentanyl administration, found lower incidences of lactate production.[237-239] Moffitt et al induced their patients with 75 μg/kg of fentanyl over 12 minutes and observed lactate production in only 1 of 10 patients at intubation.[237] No lactate production occurred at sternotomy. Of the 10 patients in the study of Skourtis et al, 1 also produced lactate at intubation.[238] Unfortunately, these authors failed to report the dose of fentanyl used in their study. Rapid induction of anesthesia with fentanyl, (100 μg/kg) given over 2–4 minutes, was not associated with lactate production in any of the 20 patients studied by Bovill et al.[239] Rapid induction resulted in a significant decrease in coronary sinus blood flow and myocardial oxygen consumption.

"Stress-free" Anesthesia

In recent years, considerable interest has been expressed in the possible modification of the metabolic and endocrine responses to surgical trauma by anesthesia. This so-called stress response consists of increases in plasma concentrations of glucose, cortisol, catecholamines, antidiuretic hormone, lactate, and other hormones and metabolites. These responses, part of the body's reaction to trauma, cause a catabolic state designed to stimulate and increase the healing process. This normal physiologic response is of obvious benefit to the body when the injury is minor, but the response to major surgery may be inappropriate. The profound and often prolonged reaction that results can have undesirable consequences. These include increased cardiac work due to hypertension and tachycardia, and vasoconstriction resulting in tissue hypoxia and acidosis. Hormonal responses may depress both inflammatory and immune mechanisms, while excessive protein catabolism may impair tissue repair. The increase in stress hormones is related to the severity of the operative trauma, being much greater during intra-abdominal surgery than body surface procedures. Increases in the plasma concentrations of stress hormones and metabolites occur during general anesthesia with inhalation and intravenous agents. These responses are significantly modified, however, by moderate-to-high doses of opioids.

Morphine, even in small doses, inhibits ACTH release and blocks at least part of the pituitary-adrenal response to surgical stimulation.[240] Morphine (1 mg/kg) suppresses surgically induced increases in plasma cortisol, but not human growth hormone during major abdominal surgery.[241] Although morphine is known to stimulate antidiuretic hormone (ADH) secretion in dogs and rats,[242] it does not do so in humans in the absence of surgical stimulation. Plasma ADH rises significantly during cardiac surgery, before cardiopulmonary bypass, in patients anesthetized with morphine (1 mg/kg) plus nitrous oxide; and further increases occur during bypass.[243]

Fentanyl (50 μg/kg) as a supplement to nitrous oxide/oxygen anesthesia abolishes the hyperglycemic response and reduces the cortisol and human growth hormone responses to abdominal surgery more than halothane/nitrous oxide/oxygen anesthesia.[244,245] However, suppression of the stress response is transient and does not compensate for the prolonged postoperative respiratory depression that may occur when doses of a magnitude great enough to effect stress responses are used.[245] High doses of fentanyl (50 μg/kg) are not effective in altering an established metabolic response during surgery.[246]

High doses of fentanyl, sufficient to produce anesthesia, prevent or significantly modify the endocrine changes and metabolic substrate mobilization during the prebypass period of cardiac surgery, although significant changes occur during and after bypass.[247-249] The continued administration of fentanyl, 0.5 μg/kg hourly for 12–18 hours after surgery, also fails to prevent postoperative endocrine and metabolic responses.[249] The mechanism whereby opioids can minimize the endocrine and metabolic stress responses is unknown. It may be related to the resulting analgesia or to a specific effect due to interaction with opioid receptors. The hypothalamus and pituitary, which possess high concentrations of opioid receptors, play major roles in mediation of endocrine and metabolic responses to trauma. The naturally occurring opioid peptides are involved in the modulation of pituitary function by varying dopamine turnover, and it is likely that the interaction of opioid drugs with receptors in that region thereby modify stress responses.[250]

It is of interest that prolactin is the only hormone that significantly increases during anesthesia with fentanyl or sufentanil.[247,251] There is experimental evidence that hyperprolactinemia may be an overt physiologic response to stimulation of the mu$_1$ subtype of opioid receptor.[252] Meptazinol, a selective mu$_1$ agonist,[253] causes greater elevation of prolactin in postoperative patients than morphine; and there is a significant correlation between plasma prolactin and meptazinol concentrations.[254]

FENTANYL "ANESTHESIA" AND RECALL

The absence of awareness of events during surgery is, by definition, an essential element of anesthesia. A high incidence of recall of intraoperative events was a feature of morphine anesthesia,[38] and, although this problem diminishes when fentanyl is used, sporadic incidences of recall have been reported in the anesthetic literature (Table 3-8).[94,133-135,216] Even with very high doses of fentanyl, total amnesia for the surgical procedure cannot be guaranteed. Of 10 patients given 150 μg/kg of fentanyl, 2 could recall sternotomy.[216] A common feature of the cases of recall reported has been the lack of benzodiazepine use either as premedication or intraoperatively. In one report, awareness occurred during the second, but not the first, of two fentanyl anesthetics that were 6 days apart.[135] The total doses of fentanyl were similar in both cases (75.8 and 72

Table 3-8

Recall or Awareness During High-dose Fentanyl/Oxygen Anesthesia

Investigators	Surgery	Premedication	Fentanyl dose ($\mu g/kg$)	Additional anesthetic agents	Comment
Mummaneni et al (1980)[135]	CABG	Morphine 0.1 mg/kg	75.8	Diazepam 10 mg	No recall
	Emergency CABG	Morphine 0.1 mg/kg	72	—	Same patient as above 6 days after first CABG. Recall before and after CPB.
Hildenberg (1981)[134]	MVR	Morphine 0.15 mg/kg Scopolamine 0.4 mg	90	—	Recall of sternotomy, yet no signs of light anesthesia (no increase in HR, BP, tears, sweating or movement).
Waller et al (1981)[207]	CABG	Diazepam 0.2 mg/kg Scopolamine 0.3 mg Fentanyl 0.5–1.0 $\mu g/kg$	50–90	— —	No recall but one patient opened eyes and moved at skin incision.
Zurich et al (1982)[216]	CABG	Morphine 0.15 mg/kg Scopolamine 0.4 mg	150	—	2/10 patients with recall of sternotomy, yet no signs of light anesthesia. Plasma fentanyl concentration at sternotomy = 33 ± 6 ng/ml.
Sprigge et al (1982)[94]	CABG	Diazepam 0.15 mg/kg Morphine 0.15 mg/kg Scopolamine 0.4 mg	60	—	1/10 patients recalled leg incision. BP increased more than 20%. Plasma fentanyl concentration = $10 - 12$ ng/ml.
Sonntag et al (1982)[215]	CABG	Diazepam 10 mg	100	Etomidate 0.3 mg/kg	No recall but 4/9 patients obeyed verbal commands or opened eyes during sternotomy.
Moldenhauer et al (1982)[217]	CABG	Lorazepam 0.03 mg/kg Morphine 0.1 mg/kg	107 (constant infusion)	—	No recall but 1/6 patients opened eyes on command after CPB. Plasma fentanyl concentration = 20 ± 1 ng/ml.
Mark et al (1983)[133]	CABG	Morphine 0.12 mg/kg	96	Diazepam 13 mg	Recall with hypertensive crisis after CPB. Patient was alcoholic.

CABG = coronary artery bypass graft; CPB = cardiopulmonary bypass; MVR = mitral valve replacement; HR = heart rate; BP = blood pressure.

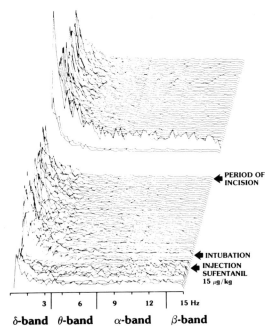

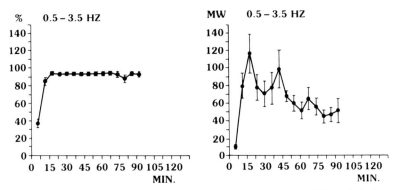

Fig. 3-16. Typical example of a compressed spectral array analysis of a single EEG derivative (T3 - Co) during anesthesia with sufentanil, 15 μg/kg. The shift in frequency to high-power delta activity with induction of anesthesia is illustrated. Similar changes occur with high-dose fentanyl anesthesia. The blank period after incision is because of electrocautery interference. (From Bovill JG, Sebel PS, Wauquier A, et al: Electroencephalographic effects of sufentanil anaesthesia in man. Br J Anaesth 54: 45–52, 1982, with permission.)

μg/kg), although diazepam was given during the first and not the second anesthetic. Awareness during surgery is not always associated with autonomic responses indicative of light anesthesia. For this reason, when using high-dose opioid anesthesia, especially when no hypnotic or amnesia supplements are used, muscle relaxants should be carefully titrated to avoid complete paralysis. This will allow signs of responsiveness to be recognized by patient movement and treated appropriately.

These occasional incidences of awareness have raised the question as to whether high doses of fentanyl, and other opioids, produce true anesthesia. The electroencephalographic changes produced by fentanyl and its analogues, sufentanil and alfentanil, are consistent with anesthesia.[138,255-257] General anesthesia with conventional agents is associated with a progressive slowing of the EEG as anesthesia deepens. With high doses of fentanyl and sufentanil there is marked slowing of the EEG, with significant reduction of frequencies above the delta (0.5–3.5 Hz) band, consistent with deep anesthesia (Fig. 3-16). Additionally, the decrease in absolute power in the delta band with time roughly parallels the decrease in opioid concentrations (Fig. 3-17). A preliminary report, based on aperiodic analysis during fentanyl anesthesia, suggests that this technique can reliably estimate depth of anesthesia.[258] There was a very good correlation between EEG stages and clinical levels of anesthesia (based primarily on cardiovascular responses).

Fig. 3-17. Mean ± SEM changes with time in relative EEG power (left) and absolute EEG power (right) in the delta (0.5–3.5 Hz) band after sufentanil, 15 μg/kg. Relative power is the power in the delta band expressed as a percentage of the total power in the EEG in the frequency range 0.5–40 Hz. (From Bovill JG, Sebel PS, Wanquier A, et al: Electroencephalographic effects of sufentanil anaesthesia in man. Br J Anaesth 54:45–52, 1982, with permission.)

CARFENTANIL

Carfentanil is formulated as the citrate and is a white crystalline powder soluble in water and common organic solvents. It is approximately twice as potent as sufentanil and has attracted particular interest for the immobilization of large wild animals, including elephants, rhinos, and buffalo.[259] Immobilization occurs rapidly and reliably in 5–15 minutes. Respiratory depression appears to be benign in large animal species, and mortality is very low. Carfentanil has also been used in nebulized form for inhalation anesthesia.[260] Dogs and monkeys have surgical analgesia within 10 minutes of exposure to carfentanil. Further evaluation of this method for inducing anesthesia in uncooperative subjects has been suggested.

LOFENTANIL

Lofentanil is obtained by substituting a methyl group in the piperidine ring of carfentanil. It has a similar potency to carfentanil but, in contrast to the other 4-anilino piperidines, is extremely long-acting. A single intravenous dose of 0.7 μg/kg in humans will cause respiratory depression for 48 hours.[261] The long duration of action can be attributed to prolonged fixation of the drug at receptor sites.[3] The extremely long-acting nature of the drug should render it suitable for epidural administration. Administered epidurally in the cat, it was found to produce naloxone-reversible analgesia with few side effects.[262] In humans (20 subjects), 5 μg of lofentanil administered epidurally produced analgesia for 72 hours.[263] However, prolonged respiratory depression is likely to complicate epidural lofentanil administration.[261] Lofentanil has also been used in very low doses (0.25–0.75 μg total dose) intravenously for relief of postoperative pain. Analgesia lasted approximately 4 hours, but was not very effective.[264] This may reflect the extremely small doses used.

It is not yet possible to determine if lofentanil and carfentanil will find a place in clinical practice. Experience in humans has so far been too limited. It is feasible that lofentanil will be used epidurally, perhaps for control of chronic pain.

ALFENTANIL

Two major disadvantages to the use of large doses of opioids as anesthetics for cardiac surgery are the occurrence of hypertension related to the period of sternotomy and, when adequate anesthetic doses are used, prolonged respiratory depression. Alfen-

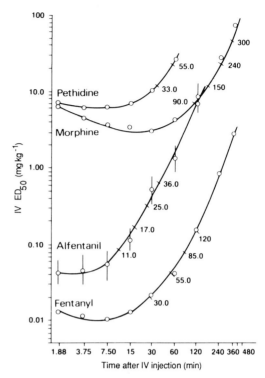

Fig. 3-18. ED$_{50}$ of pethidine, morphine, alfentanil and fentanyl measured at differing times following IV injection in the rat tail withdrawal test. Numbers next to curves indicate time (min) at which the ED$_{50}$ is 2, 4, 8, and 16 times the minimum ED$_{50}$. (From Niemegeers CJE, Janssen PAJ: Alfentanil a particularly short-acting intravenous narcotic analgesic. Drug Devel Res 1:83–88, 1981, with permission.)

tanil is of interest to the cardiac anesthesiologist because, although not as potent as fentanyl, it has a short elimination half-life. This property renders it suitable for administration by continuous intravenous infusion which can keep plasma alfentanil concentration high enough to suppress "break-through hypertension" and yet enable a reasonably fast recovery.

Among the initial evaluations of alfentanil was the rat-tail withdrawal test.[265] This is a quantifiable test for comparing duration of action and potency of opioids. The tail of the animal is immersed in water at 55°C. A control rat will withdraw its tail within 3 to 4 seconds, but withdrawal will be delayed or absent in an animal treated with an opioid. The onset of action of alfentanil is a rapid, measurable effect being discernible within 15 seconds, and peak effect occurs within 1 minute of intravenous injection, compared with meperidine, 4 minutes, fentanyl, 8 minutes, and morphine, 30 minutes (Fig. 3-18). The

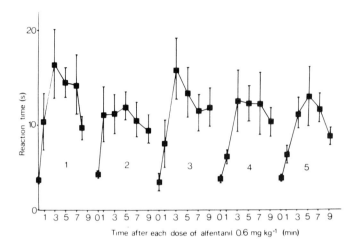

Fig. 3-19. Mean ± SEM hot-plate reaction times of 12 mice after repeat injections of alfentanil, 0.6 mg/kg. Each repeat injection was given when reaction times had returned to saline control values. (From Williams JG, Brown JH, Pleuvry BJ: Alfentanil: A study of its analgesic activity and interactions with morphine in the mouse. Br J Anaesth 54:81–85, 1982, with permission.)

duration of action of alfentanil is also short. At twice its lowest ED_{50}, analgesia lasts for 11 minutes (fentanyl, 30 minutes, meperidine, 35 minutes, morphine, 115 minutes). In rabbits, the duration of respiratory depression produced by 10 μg/kg of alfentanil was 5 minutes, whereas the effects of an equipotent dose of fentanyl lasted for 15 minutes.[265] The respiratory depressant effect of the drug was also found to be noncumulative following injections every 10 minutes.[266] Fentanyl, on the other hand, produced a stepwise decrease in respiratory rate. Repeat injections of alfentanil were similarly non-cumulative in duration of analgesic effect following five repeat doses in mice during the hotplate test (Fig. 3-19).[267] Alfentanil is about 30–70 times as potent as morphine (depending on species), and one-quarter as potent as fentanyl, with one-quarter the duration of action.[137,265]

In five volunteers, alfentanil (1.6–6.4 μg/kg) produced the typical subjective effects of an opioid, and a dose-related respiratory depression lasting for less than 30 minutes at all doses studied.[268]

Pharmacokinetics

The pharmacokinetics of a single bolus injection of alfentanil have been studied in volunteers[145] and in surgical patients.[269-271] Plasma concentrations have been assayed using either RIA[272] or gas chromatography.[273] Both two- and three-compartment models have been used to describe the kinetics of alfentanil

(Table 3-9). The elimination half-life of alfentanil, about 90 minutes, is substantially shorter than that of other opioids. The comparative pharmacokinetic properties of fentanyl and alfentanil have been reviewed by Stanski and Hug who consider alfentanil, when compared with fentanyl, to be a pharmacokinetically predictable analgesic.[274] The comparative pharmacokinetics of the two drugs are summarized in Table 3-9. It should be noted that, for a single small bolus injection of drug, the action of fentanyl or alfentanil is terminated by redistribution. The drug diffuses rapidly into the brain and is then redistributed to muscle and fat. After very large or repeated doses of drug, redistribution is less effective in reducing brain concentration, and the duration of action then becomes elimination dependent. The volume of distribution of alfentanil is approximately one-quarter that of fentanyl, and its clearance one-half that of fentanyl. Since the volume of distribution is so much smaller than that of fentanyl, more alfentanil is effectively available for clearance. Stanski and Hug suggest that the reduced volume of distribution of alfentanil is related to its lower lipid solubility, limiting its penetration into red blood cells, muscle, and fat.[274] They also suggest that the duration of effect of a large bolus injection of alfentanil, or an infusion discontinued from steady state, will be much shorter for alfentanil than fentanyl.

In a study of alfentanil kinetics following a large bolus injection of 200 μg/kg, one patient was found to have a prolonged elimination half-life (151 min-

Table 3-9

Comparative Pharmacokinetics of Fentanyl, Alfentanil, and Sufentanil in Humans

Investigators	Drug	Dose (μg/kg)	T1/2π (min)	T1/2α (min)	T1/2β (min)	Vd (liters/kg)	Cl (ml/kg/min)
McClain, Hug[151]	Fentanyl	6.4	1.7	13.4	219	4.0	12.7
Bower, Hull[145]	Fentanyl	2.4	—	—	185	4.7	22
Bower, Hull[145]	Alfentanil	2.4	—	—	96	0.4	3.4
Camu et al[270]	Alfentanil	120	3.5	16.8	94	1.0	7.9
Schuttler, Stoeckel[271]	Alfentanil	82	—	4.3	70	0.5	5.5
McDonnell et al[275]	Alfentanil	200	—	8.2	103	0.5	5.0
Bovill et al[269]	Alfentanil	50	1.3	9.4	94	1.0	7.6
Bovill et al[269]	Alfentanil	125	1.0	14.4	94	0.7	5.1
Bovill et al[321]	Sufentanil	5	0.6	17.7	164	2.9	12.7

utes) and a slow clearance (1.65 ml/kg/min).[275] This subject was also found to be a poor metabolizer of phenacetin, suggesting that alfentanil oxidation has the debrisoquine type of genetic polymorphism.[276] Up to 10 percent of some populations are known to be hypometabolizers of debrisoquine, and they also are poor metabolizers of phenacetin. It is possible, therefore, that a certain (as yet undetermined) proportion of the population will have an abnormal oxidative phenotype for alfentanil, which is metabolized by O-demethylation and N-dealkylation.[277] This phenotype, if it is found to be extensive, will have important implications for the use of alfentanil. A drug described as pharmacokinetically predictable may turn out to be very unpredictable.

Infusion Kinetics

The pharmacokinetics of an empirically derived dosage scheme of a single bolus of 80 μg/kg alfentanil, followed by a 1-hour infusion of 3 μg/kg/min, was studied in patients undergoing elective surgery.[278] The calculated pharmacokinetic parameters after discontinuation of infusion (T1/2β 87 min, Cl 3.33 ml/kg/min and Vd 0.44 1/kg), were similar to those found by Bovill et al after a single bolus.[269] During the infusion, plasma alfentanil concentrations remained above 300 ng/ml, the level suggested as being necessary to suppress hemodynamic responses during surgery.[269] In contrast, in patients undergoing major abdominal surgery, Reitz et al found a clearance of 2.6 ml/kg/min and an elimination half-life of 198 minutes.[279] There were, however, only two patients in their series. An infusion scheme as described by Fragen[278] (ie, a single bolus followed by a fixed-rate infusion), would only be expected to reach steady-state after four half-lives,[280] and,

indeed, plasma concentrations increased throughout the infusion (Fig. 3-20). Infusion schemes based on a bolus followed by an initial fast infusion and a slow maintenance infusion would be expected to reach steady-state plasma concentrations within 30 minutes.[280] Two such infusion regimens for alfentanil have been assessed during neurosurgery in an attempt to maintain a steady plasma concentration of 300 ng/ml.[281] The first regimen was based on a scheme proposed by Wagner and consisted of a bolus of 100 μg/kg, 10 μg/kg/min for 10 minutes and 2 μg/kg/min thereafter.[282] The second regimen, based on a scheme described by Rigg and Wong, consisted of a bolus of 32.5 μg/kg, 7.5 μg/kg/min for 10 minutes, and 1.6 μg/kg/min thereafter.[283] For each group of patients, steady-state plasma concentrations were reached as judged by mean concentrations. However, there was considerable intrapatient variation. Alterations in the volume of the central compartment, by hemorrhage, for example, are likely to disturb alfentanil kinetics. Wide patient-to-patient variation in plasma concentrations, and the possibility of abnormal metabolism, suggest that alfentanil infusion regimens should be designed to "dose to effect" rather than to computer predictions.

The pharmacokinetics of a bolus injection of alfentanil before and after cardiac surgery were studied[284] and used as a model to define an infusion regimen to keep a steady-state concentration of 1000 ng/ml.[285] The bolus data (based on a dose of 125 μg/kg) suggested similar kinetics in cardiac patients to those found by Bovill et al.[269] The bolus dose repeated after cardiopulmonary bypass showed a prolonged elimination half-life as a result of an increase in the volume of distribution (Vd) from 0.31 liters/kg before bypass to 0.87 liters/kg after bypass. Using the data obtained from this study and Wagner's

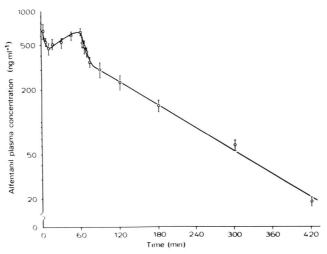

Fig. 3-20. Plasma concentrations of alfentanil after a 30-s bolus injection of 80 μg/kg and a 1-h continuous infusion at a rate of 3 μg/kg/min started simultaneously. Each data point represents the mean ± standard deviation from five patients. (From Fragen RJ, Booij LHDJ, Braak GJJ, et al: Pharmacokinetics of the infusion of alfentanil in man. Br J Anaesth 55:1077–1081, 1983, with permission.)

model,[282] a regimen of alfentanil, 19 μg/kg/min, was given for 20 minutes, followed by 3.5 μg/kg/min. The mean plasma concentration was 1300 ng/ml, higher than expected. This was associated with a reduced plasma clearance of 1.5 ml/kg/min. An alfentanil infusion for cardiac surgery thus appears to be associated with a clearance approximately one-half that which might be suggested from data derived from bolus injection.

Pharmacokinetics in Other Circumstances

The pharmacokinetics of alfentanil are altered by age and obesity (Table 3-10). In children, the half-life is decreased,[286] whereas in the elderly and obese it is prolonged.[287,288] Clearance is not affected by age, but in children the volume of distribution is much smaller. This means that the termination of

effect of alfentanil in children will be elimination dependent and, with large or repeated doses, accumulation will be minimal.

Alfentanil in Short Procedures

It is relevant here to consider noncardiac uses of alfentanil, because the pharmacologic profile of this drug in noncardiac use will give some guidelines to its potential applications in cardiac anesthesia. Since animal data suggest that alfentanil provides analgesia of shorter duration than fentanyl, it has been used as an anesthetic supplement for short surgical procedures. Alfentanil, 5 μg/kg, followed by alfentanil, 2.5 μg/kg every 8 minutes, has been compared with 1 μg/kg of fentanyl and 0.5 μg/kg of fentanyl every 16 minutes as a supplement to methohexital N₂O/O₂ anesthesia.[289] It was found that alfentanil-supplemented anesthesia was associated with more rapid

Table 3-10
Influence of Age and Obesity on Alfentanil Pharmacokinetics

Group	Study	Dose	Elimination Half-life $(T_{1/2}\beta)$	Clearance (ml/kg/min)	Volume of distribution (liters/kg)
Surgical patients	Bovill et al[269]	50 μg/kg	94±8.3	5.1±1.1	1.0±0.32
Young	Meistelman et al[286]	20 μg/kg	40±3	4.7±0.6	0.16±0.11
Old	Helmers et al[288]	50 μg/kg	134±47	4.8±4.07	0.51±0.14
Obese	Bently et al[287]	6838 μg	172	179 (ml/min)	351

recovery of motor coordination than fentanyl. The hemodynamic responses to laryngoscopy and intubation have been studied with larger doses of alfentanil.[290] After oral diazepam premedication and induction of anesthesia with thiopental (4 mg/kg) and succinylcholine (1 mg/kg), intubation following alfentanil (15 μg/kg) was accompanied by an increase in heart rate, but not blood pressure. Alfentanil, 30 μg/kg, or fentanyl, 5 μg/kg, completely suppressed the hemodynamic responses to laryngoscopy and intubation. The duration of action of 30 μg/kg alfentanil was 12 minutes, and 5 μg/kg fentanyl lasted for longer than 15 minutes.[290] These studies demonstrated that, at the lower end of the dosage range, alfentanil has a shorter duration of action than fentanyl, but is equally effective at suppressing hemodynamic responses to stimuli.

Alfentanil as an Induction Agent

Since the duration of action of alfentanil is shorter than fentanyl, various workers have reasoned that it may be possible to use it in an opioid anesthetic technique for noncardiac surgery. Because of the prolonged respiratory depression obtained after anesthetic doses of fentanyl, it is inappropriate to use fentanyl in situations where postoperative ventilation is not anticipated. Alfentanil, on the other hand, may be a suitable agent for induction of anesthesia. In a study of young unpremedicated adults, all American Society of Anesthesiologists Class I (ASA I), the ED_{50} (analogous to MAC of inhalational agents) for alfentanil was found to be 111 μg/kg, and the ED_{95} was 169 μg/kg (Fig. 3-21).[291] The stimulus used was placement of a nasopharyngeal airway, and the alfentanil dose was considered effective if no head, neck, or limb movement occurred in response to this stimulus. Thirty-six percent of patients required naloxone at the end of surgery. Nausea or vomiting occurred in 39 percent of patients, and there was a 75 percent incidence of chest wall rigidity. These complications were independent of dose used. Alfentanil was also assessed as an induction agent for patients with and without cardiac disease.[292] It produced rapid loss of consciousness with an incidence of chest wall rigidity of up to 50 percent. In patients with valvular or coronary artery disease, induction of anesthesia was associated with a small reduction in systolic arterial pressure. In patients without cardiac disease, there were no hemodynamic alterations following induction of anesthesia with alfentanil. Anesthetic induction with alfentanil has been compared with

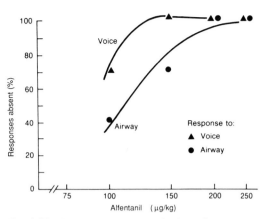

Fig. 3-21. Dose-response curves for loss of response to voice (▲) and insertion of a nasopharyngeal airway (●), 90 seconds following alfentanil in unpremedicated patients. (From McDonnell TE, Bartkowski RR, Williams JJ: ED_{50} of alfentanil for induction of anesthesia in unpremedicated young adults. Anesthesiology 60:136–140, 1984, with permission.)

thiopental, etomidate, and midazolam.[293] Alfentanil (mean dose 173 μg/kg) was superior to the other three induction agents with respect to cardiovascular stability during induction and intubation. The disadvantages were a slower onset of action and an incidence of muscle rigidity (55 percent), which rapidly disappeared after administration of succinylcholine. In contrast, alfentanil, 150 μg/kg, given over 1–3 minutes with succinylcholine, 20 mg, for patients scheduled for thoracotomy was found to produce significant reductions in systemic vascular resistance and mean arterial pressure.[294] Central venous and pulmonary capillary wedge pressures increased, but cardiac index remained unchanged. The fact that cardiac index did not increase despite higher filling pressures suggests an impairment of myocardial performance. Rapid induction of anesthesia with alfentanil and succinylcholine, therefore, appears inappropriate; a nondepolarizing muscle relaxant is to be preferred.

A fixed dose of alfentanil, 120 μg/kg, was compared with thiopental, 5 mg/kg, as an induction agent for female patients premedicated with diazepam and atropine undergoing plastic surgery.[295] In 6 patients, the alfentanil dosage was insufficient and up to 300 μg/kg was required to produce unconsciousness. The authors found that cardiovascular stability was better than with thiopental, but time to unconsciousness was longer and more variable and was often accompanied by muscle rigidity.

Table 3-11

Induction Doses of Alfentanil

Study	Patient type	Number	Age (yr)	Premedication	End point	Dose used (μg/kg)
Nauta et al[292]	General surgical	20	42 ± 10	Atropine	Open eyes on command. Take breath.	119 ± 20
	Mitral valve	9	48 ± 11	Lorazepam and atropine		41 ± 9
	Coronary artery	13	51 ± 9	Lorazepam and atropine		50 ± 10
McDonnell et al[291]	Gynecologic or orthopedic	28	31 ± 7.9	None	Voice response (VR); Nasopharyngeal airway (NP)	Doses used were 100–250 μg/kg. Probit analysis gave ED_{50} VR 92 μg/kg; ED_{50} NP 111 μg/kg
Nauta et al[293]	General surgical	20	44 ± 11	Secobarbital and atropine	Open eyes on command. Take breath.	173 ± 5 μg/kg
Palazzo et al[295]	Plastic surgery	19	31.1 (19–48)	Diazepam	Eyelash reflex	120 μg/kg (inadequate in 6 patients)

The dosage regimens used in these studies are shown in Table 3-11. The induction dose of alfentanil, as with other anesthetic induction agents, depends on the pre-existing disease state, ie, patients with mitral valve disease require less than healthy patients. The dose of alfentanil, 120 μg/kg, given by Nauta et al[292] in their original study has not been found by other workers to reliably produce unconsciousness in healthy patients. The ED_{95} to nasopharyngeal stimulation of 169 μg/kg found by McDonnell et al[291] corresponds well to that subsequently reported by Nauta et al[293] of 173 μg/kg. This appears an effective induction dose for alfentanil in healthy patients. As with other induction agents, however, a lower dose is needed by patients with cardiac disease. Good cardiovascular stability following induction of anesthesia with alfentanil was reported in all studies. It may, therefore, be an appropriate agent to choose for induction of anesthesia for the cardiac patient undergoing both cardiac and noncardiac surgery. The main disadvantage is the occurrence of muscle rigidity. This can easily be prevented by the prior administration of a nondepolarizing muscle relaxant before induction of anesthesia.[296]

Alfentanil Infusions for Noncardiac Surgery

Alfentanil infusions have been used either as fixed-rate regimens or doses determined by patient responses. Fifty patients, scheduled for a variety of surgical procedures, were anesthetized with thiopental, 5 mg/kg, and alfentanil, 30 μg/kg, followed by alfentanil, 3 μg/kg/min, the rate being halved every hour.[297] Good cardiovascular stability was obtained, but one patient became renarcotized in the first hour of recovery. Sudden postoperative respiratory arrest has been reported after a 100 μg/kg bolus of alfentanil followed by 1 μg/kg/min for 2 hours.[298] After a full and rapid recovery, the patient suffered a sudden respiratory arrest. It is possible that this patient hypometabolized alfentanil.

Rather than using a fixed-dosage regimen, other workers have tried to tailor the dose to patient response.[299,300] Twelve patients scheduled for lower abdominal gynecologic surgery were studied. They received 150 μg/kg of alfentanil for induction of anesthesia. Anesthesia was continued with N_2O/O_2, and an infusion of alfentanil that was varied between 0.4 and 2.5 μg/kg/min and supplemented by bolus

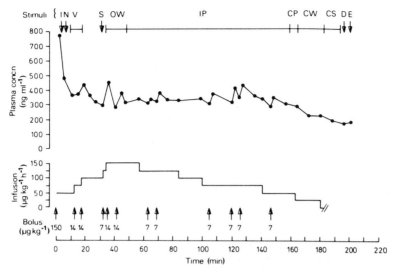

Fig. 3-22. Plasma concentrations, bolus doses (arrows), and infusion rate of alfentanil in relation to procedures producing noxious stimulation in one patient undergoing abdominal gynecologic surgery. The horizontal axis gives the time in minutes. Time zero indicates the start of the induction of anesthesia: I = intubation, N = nasogastric tube, V = vaginal pack and urinary bladder catheter, S = skin incision, OW = opening of abdominal wall, IP = intra-abdominal part of surgery, CP = closing peritoneum, CW = closing of abdominal wall, CS = closing skin, D = discontinuation of nitrous oxide, E = extubation. (From Ausems ME, Hug CC, de Lange S: Variable rate infusion of alfentanil as a supplement to nitrous oxide anesthesia for general surgery. Anesth Analg 62:982–986, 1983, with permission.)

injections of 7 μg/kg (Fig. 3-22).[299] The mean dose of alfentanil required varied from 0.58 to 2.07 μg/kg/min. The plasma concentration needed to suppress somatic and hemodynamic responses was up to 400 ng/ml (Fig. 3-23). Such an anesthetic technique, although generally satisfactory, required the close attention of the anesthesiologist to patient responses. No prolonged recovery or respiratory depression was found in this study.

It has been observed that if a fixed-rate alfentanil infusion is used for all patients, some will receive an excessive dose, leading to prolonged recovery with possible respiratory depression.[297,298] A variable rate infusion would be easier to administer if there were a single indicator of adequate or inadequate anesthesia. Unfortunately, no such indicator exists at present.

Alfentanil for Cardiac Surgery

Initial data obtained in dogs suggested that very large doses of alfentanil (50 μg/kg) could be infused without any cardiac depression.[137] More detailed studies of the effects of alfentanil on canine global ventricular mechanics were undertaken in chronically instrumented dogs, the inotropic state being assessed by computer analysis of the end systolic pressure-length ratio.[301] Alfentanil in a dose of 200 μg/kg given over an unspecified period of time produced significant increases in the slope of the pressure-length relationship and in dP/dt. This suggests that alfentanil, in contrast to the halogenated anesthetics, which are cardiodepressive, causes increased inotropism and may support the failing heart. Alfentanil, 160 μg/kg, has been shown to preserve blood flow to skeletal muscle and maintain peripheral blood flow even in the presence of verapamil.[302]

The exact model and method of administration are critical in interpreting animal studies. In another study in chronically instrumented conscious dogs, alfentanil, 320 μg/kg, given over 20 seconds produced a marked increase in ventricular afterload as well as an increase in calculated systemic vascular resistance.[303] One problem with assessing the cardiac effects of drugs (particularly in humans) is that noxious stimuli that also influence cardiovascular responses are not quantifiable and responses to them before drug administration are not obtainable. In an attempt to overcome these problems, evoked cardio-

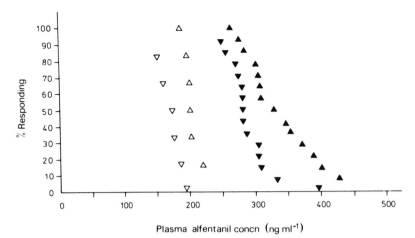

Fig. 3-23. Plasma alfentanil concentrations versus percent of patients responding to surgical stimulation. Open triangles represent responses to microscopic surgery on the fallopian tubes, closed triangles represent responses to intra-abdominal manipulations. ($\triangle$, $\blacktriangle$ = highest concentration associated with a response; ($\triangledown$, $\blacktriangledown$ = lowest concentration without a response). Patients were ventilated with 66% nitrous oxide in oxygen. (From Ausems ME, Hug CC, de Lange S: Variable rate infusion of alfentanil as a supplement to nitrous oxide anesthesia for general surgery. Anesth Analg 62:982–986, 1983, with permission.)

vascular responses to supramaximal electrical stimulation of a cutaneous nerve in the dog have been studied with approximately equipotent doses of alfentanil and fentanyl.[304] Examples of spontaneous and evoked cardiovascular reflexes following fentanyl (100 μg/kg) and alfentanil (500 μg/kg) are shown in Figure 3-24. Both drugs caused similar

reductions in resting heart rate and mean arterial pressure in the absence of stimulation, but the effect of fentanyl lasted longer. Fentanyl, however, produced a greater reduction in the reflex cardiovascular response than did alfentanil. There was a dissociation between the maximum effect and duration of effect of fentanyl and alfentanil on the resting circulation

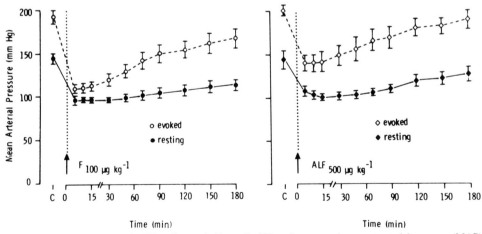

Fig. 3-24. Effect of fentanyl, 100 μg/kg, and alfentanil, 500 μg/kg, on resting mean arterial pressure (MAP) and the maximum values of MAP during electrical stimulation of an exposed radial nerve. Values are mean $\pm$ SEM from 10 dogs. C = control measurements. (From Askitopoulou H, Whitwam JG, Sapsed S, et al: Dissociation between the effects of fentanyl and alfentanil on spontaneous and reflexly evoked cardiovascular responses in the dog. Br J Anesth 55:155–161, 1983, with permission.)

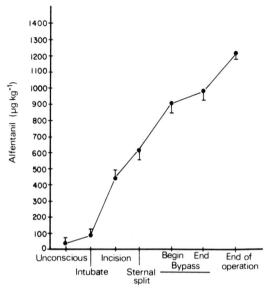

Fig. 3-25. Cumulative doses of alfentanil administered to 15 patients undergoing coronary artery bypass operations. (From de Lange S, Stanley TH, Boscoe MJ: Alfentanil-oxygen anaesthesia for coronary artery surgery. Br J Anaesth 53:1291–1296, 1981, with permission.)

and on evoked cardiovascular responses. These observations may help explain some of the differences in cardiac responses observed between different studies.

Since alfentanil is a very short-acting opioid, it would seem logical to administer it as a continuous infusion when using it as a sole anesthetic agent for cardiac surgery. At the time of the first evaluation of its use for cardiac anesthesia, relatively little of its pharmacology had been determined and the evaluation was carried out using a repeat bolus technique. Alfentanil (3 mg/min) was administered until the patient lost consciousness, and then 2.5–5.0 mg boluses of the drug given whenever systolic blood pressure increased more than 15 percent above preinduction values.[305] A total dosage of 1.2 mg/kg was required to maintain arterial pressure less than 15 percent above preinduction values (Fig. 3-25). Induction of anesthesia was associated with small but significant reductions in arterial pressure, but "breakthrough hypertension" following sternotomy occurred in 73 percent of patients. This probably reflects the inadequate dosage used.

An open evaluation of a fixed-dose infusion technique was carried out for 30 patients undergoing cardiac surgery.[296] After an induction dose of alfentanil, 125 μg/kg, alfentanil was infused at 500 μg/kg/hr until the start of bypass and then the infusion

rate halved until the end of surgery. The patients' lungs were ventilated with air/O_2. Considering the group as a whole, good cardiovascular stability was obtained. However, hypertension was troublesome and 26 patients required supplementation with bolus injections of alfentanil (up to 10 mg). In two patients this was inadequate and vasodilator therapy was required. The total dose requirement for surgery was 1.5 $\pm$ 0.40 mg/kg. In order to define an appropriate infusion regimen for cardiac surgery, plasma concentrations of alfentanil were measured at fixed events during coronary artery surgery during a variable rate alfentanil infusion (up to 50 mg/hr).[306] In 10 of the 14 patients studied, 2.5 mg bolus doses of alfentanil were required to control systolic arterial pressure, but no vasodilators were needed before bypass. Plasma concentrations obtained are shown in Figure 3-26. The average time to return to consciousness after surgery was 3.1 $\pm$ 1.4 hours, when the mean plasma concentration was 270 $\pm$ 130 ng/ml. The total alfentanil dose used in the study was 1030 $\pm$ 240 μg/kg.

The studies described above have been carried out in patients undergoing coronary artery surgery. An infusion of alfentanil (bolus of 125 μg/kg followed by 0.5 mg/kg/hr) has been compared with fentanyl, 100 μg/kg, or sufentanil, 20 μg/kg, by bolus injection as the sole anesthetic for patients undergoing valvular surgery.[307] No differences in hemodynamic effects were found in the study, and it was concluded that all three opioids can provide satisfactory anesthesia for valve replacement surgery.

Alfentanil (5 mg) and fentanyl (0.5 mg) have been compared as a supplement to etomidate (0.3 mg/kg bolus, 0.03 mg/kg/min infusion) anesthesia for cardiac surgery.[308] Using this combination, alfentanil was found to produce greater cardiovascular depression than fentanyl. However, the doses used were not equipotent, 10 times as much alfentanil being used as fentanyl. The potency ratio is closer to 1 to 4; therefore, a relatively much larger dose of alfentanil was given in this study.

It is still undetermined if alfentanil is a suitable agent to use as a sole anesthetic agent for cardiac surgery. It is very short acting and a regimen of repeat bolus injection seems inappropriate.[305] Fixed-rate infusion[296] or variable-rate infusion[306] gave better results, but bolus supplementation was required in both studies. To date, there are limited clinical data on alfentanil infusions. They do not seem to be any better than fentanyl or sufentanil.[307] It is possible that earlier extubation could be achieved, but comparative data with the other opioids is lacking at the present time.

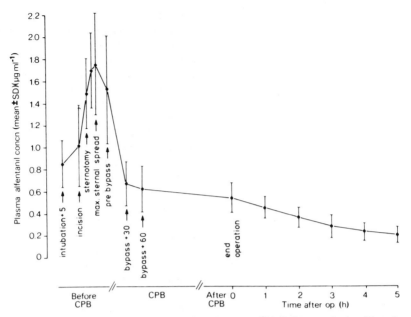

Fig. 3-26. Plasma alfentanil concentrations (mean ± SD) during anesthesia with variable-rate continuous infusion of alfentanil in 14 patients undergoing coronary artery surgery. (From de Lange S, de Bruijn NP: Alfentanil-oxygen anaesthesia: Plasma concentrations and clinical effects during variable-rate continuous infusion for coronary artery surgery. Br J Anaesth 55(Suppl 2):183S–189S, 1983, with permission.)

Metabolic Responses to Alfentanil

Alfentanil anesthesia (in doses of 1 mg/kg) suppresses the catecholamine response to anesthesia and surgery, but not to cardiopulmonary bypass or post-bypass.[309] Cortisol levels also decreased during surgery, but returned to pre-induction levels before the end of surgery. As with sufentanil, but not fentanyl, antidiuretic hormone secretion is suppressed by alfentanil anesthesia.[310]

The reduction in metabolic responses is thus short lived, and it is questionable whether this reduction in metabolic responses will lead to a reduction in morbidity. Alfentanil appears to suppress metabolic responses to the same degree as its congeners, sufentanil and fentanyl, and there is little to choose among them in this regard.

Neurophysiologic Effects of Alfentanil

The electroencephalographic effects of high-dose alfentanil/oxygen/air anesthesia were studied in 10 patients undergoing coronary artery surgery.[257] The dominant feature of the EEG was the presence of high-amplitude, low-frequency delta waves (Fig.

3-27). The EEG response is essentially similar to that obtained after fentanyl, although there is less synchronization with alfentanil than after equivalent doses of fentanyl. Spindle activity was prominent in 70 percent of patients. During this study, the EEG was monitored into the recovery period. No correlation was found between plasma alfentanil concentrations and the EEG during the recovery period. This lack of correlation between alfentanil concentrations and EEG changes can be attributed to the fact that the changes in EEG level occurred when plasma concentrations varied very little.

In other circumstances, it has been possible to correlate alfentanil plasma concentrations with the power spectral edge.[204] Unpremedicated patients received alfentanil, 1500 μg/min, until EEG delta activity occurred. The changes in EEG, as measured by the power spectral edge, were found to lag behind changes in plasma concentration. As can be seen from Figure 3-10, there is some hysteresis; each spectral edge value is associated with two different alfentanil concentrations. The degree of hysteresis seen with fentanyl is greater than that seen with alfentanil (Fig. 3-11). The difference between concentration

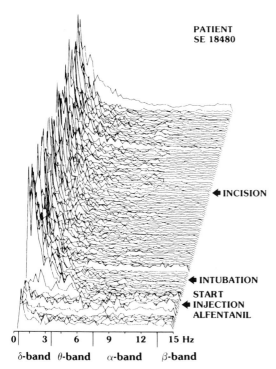

PATIENT
SE 18480

◄ INCISION

◄ INTUBATION
START
◄ INJECTION
ALFENTANIL

0 | 3 | 6 | 9 | 12 | 15 Hz

δ-band θ-band α-band β-band

Fig. 3-27. Compressed spectral array analysis of the EEG from a patient anesthetized with alfentanil, 125 μg/kg, followed by an infusion of alfentanil, 0.5 mg/kg/hr.

and effect may be due to the greater brain-blood partition coefficient for fentanyl. This study suggests that a derivative of the EEG, such as power spectral edge, may be useful in judging depth of opioid anesthesia, but further data is required before EEG monitoring can give assurance of the production and maintenance of unconsciousness.[311]

SUFENTANIL

Of the opioid analgesics currently available for use in humans, sufentanil is the most potent. If the theory is true that the more potent an opioid analgesic the more specific its action and the less the incidence of side effects, then sufentanil should offer various potential advantages for use in cardiac anesthesia. There should be fewer side effects, and there may be greater suppression of hormonal and metabolic responses to surgery. Also, it is possible that by using an opioid more potent than fentanyl, the incidence of perioperative hypertension may be reduced.

Animal Data

In a study of N-4-substituted piperidine derivatives of fentanyl, Van Bever et al discovered that sufentanil (R30730) had a rapid onset of action, was substantially more potent than fentanyl, and was, therefore, selected for further investigation.[312] In the tail withdrawal test in rats, sufentanil is extremely potent, the lowest ED_{50} is 0.71 μg/kg. It has a rapid onset of action, a relatively short duration of action (less than fentanyl), and a very high safety margin. The LD_{50}/ED_{50} ratio for sufentanil in rats is 25,211 compared with 277 for fentanyl and 70 for morphine. In a subsequent evaluation of sufentanil in mice, rats, and dogs, it was found to be more than 2000 times more potent than morphine. The intravenous safety margin of sufentanil in dogs was approximately 1:50,000, and the LD_{50} was approximately 14 mg/kg.[313] All the morphine-like effects of sufentanil were antagonized by nalorphine, thus confirming the mu-receptor specificity of the drug action.

In an attempt to study the anesthetic potency of sufentanil, the effect of increasing concentrations of sufentanil on the MAC of halothane has been studied in rats.[314] Increasing doses of sufentanil produced nonlinear reductions in the MAC of halothane with a sigmoid dose-response curve. An abrupt, steep response, with an additional 62 percent MAC reduction, occurred with doses between 1.10^{-5} mg/kg/min and 1.10^{-4} mg/kg/min. At the higher dose, anesthesia was essentially complete. In a subsequent study from the same group, the tissue concentrations of serotonin in cord, medulla, and hypothalamus were measured in rats given 1 MAC of halothane with no sufentanil, a low-dose infusion of sufentanil ($< 7 \times 10^{-5}$ mg/kg/min), or a high-dose infusion of sufentanil ($> 1 \times 10^{-4}$ mg/kg/min).[315] The low infusion rate reduced the MAC of halothane by 30 percent or less, and the high infusion rate reduced the MAC of halothane by 80 percent or greater. Significant reductions in the tissue concentrations of serotonin in the cord and medulla, but not in the hypothalamus, occurred in the high-dose sufentanil group. No changes in tissue serotonin concentrations occurred in the other two groups. The authors suggested that sufentanil-induced modulation of serotonin release in the cord and medulla may play a role in the analgesic and anesthetic properties of this drug. These studies contrast with data obtained for fentanyl, in which a maximum 65 percent reduction in the MAC of enflurane was found.[217] Since there is a ceiling effect on MAC reduction obtained with fentanyl, but probably not with sufentanil, sufentanil may be more effective as an anesthetic than fentanyl.

The effects of sufentanil, in doses from 5 to 160 μg/kg, on cerebral blood flow (CBF) and cerebral metabolic rate for oxygen (CMR$_{O_2}$) have been studied.[316] Sufentanil decreased CBF by 47 percent and CMR$_{O_2}$ by 36 percent in doses of 80–160 μg/kg. The EEG showed marked depression with low frequencies, high amplitude, and burst suppression. Short periods of epileptoid patterns and spike activities were seen. In order to investigate the influence of sufentanil on subcortical structures, the effects of sufentanil, 40 or 160 μg/kg, on regional cerebral glucose utilization (r-CMRgl) were studied in rats.[317] Both doses of sufentanil reduced regional cerebral glucose utilization in all cortical areas examined. Marked decreases in r-CMRgl (39–54 percent) were found in the caudate nucleus and the ventral thalamic nucleus. However, both doses of sufentanil produced focal areas of increases in r-CMRgl in the limbic structures, the amygdala, and the hippocampus. Associated with the focally increased r-CMRgl in the amygdala was EEG activation suggestive of seizure activity. High doses of sufentanil thus may be associated with subcortical seizure activity.

Since sufentanil is more potent than fentanyl, with a similar or shorter duration of action, and an initial evaluation suggested that it had minimal cardiovascular side effects,[137] various assessments of its cardiovascular effects in animals were carried out. These were prior to its evaluation as a cardiac anesthetic in man. The cardiovascular effects of sufentanil, up to 40 μg/kg, were studied in dogs with and without nitrous oxide.[45] Sufentanil produced minimal changes in cardiovascular dynamics in atropinized dogs. Small decreases in heart rate, mean arterial blood pressure, and cardiac output occurred in dogs without atropine premedication. Addition of nitrous oxide during sufentanil infusion was found, in contrast to most opioids, to have little influence on cardiovascular dynamics. Sufentanil also appears to have minimal effects on the peripheral and central circulation in the dog.[104] Sufentanil, 10 μg/kg, had no adverse effects on peripheral circulation or skeletal muscle surface pH, whereas 4 mg/kg of morphine caused a severe and rapid fall in muscle pH from 7.29 to 7.11. Calculated blood volume also decreased by 20 percent. This effect is presumably histamine mediated.[104] The same dose of sufentanil caused an insignificant decrease in mean arterial pressure; but cardiac index decreased by 30 percent, associated with a similar increase in systemic vascular resistance.[318] In contrast, morphine caused marked cardiovascular depression. The benign effect of sufentanil anesthesia was confirmed in proprano-

lol-pretreated dogs.[319] In the presence of total beta-adrenergic blockade following 2 mg/kg of propranolol, sufentanil did not significantly alter cardiovascular dynamics, whereas morphine again caused marked cardiovascular depression. These studies suggest that in the dog with a normal coronary circulation, sufentanil produces no cardiovascular depression. The effects of sufentanil have also been studied in dogs with a critically constricted left anterior descending coronary artery.[228] Sufentanil, in the absence of nitrous oxide, produced minimal hemodynamic changes, with no evidence of regional dysfunction, even in the presence of significant stenosis. Adding nitrous oxide, in the presence of a critical stenosis, resulted in marked and significant deterioration of function in the area of compromised flow. This suggests that nitrous oxide has a direct detrimental effect on areas of the myocardium supplied by marginal flow. These animal studies suggest that sufentanil with air/oxygen anesthesia is likely to provide stable hemodynamic conditions for cardiac surgery, whereas nitrous oxide is less desirable.

Pharmacokinetics

Unlike fentanyl and alfentanil, the pharmacokinetics of sufentanil have not been extensively studied in humans. The kinetics of sufentanil in volunteers have not been investigated because doses that would produce measurable plasma concentrations, even by sensitive RIA, would be likely to produce respiratory depression. However, the pharmacokinetics of a single bolus injection of 5 μg/kg of sufentanil have been studied in 10 adult surgical patients.[320] The comparative pharmacokinetics of fentanyl and sufentanil are shown in Table 3-9.

The terminal elimination half-life of sufentanil, 164 minutes, is intermediate between that of fentanyl (219 minutes) and alfentanil (90 minutes). The plasma clearance of sufentanil was 935 ml/min, which is very similar to that of fentanyl (956 ml/min). However, the volume of distribution of sufentanil, 2.86 liters/kg, is less than that of fentanyl (4 liters/kg). This explains the more rapid elimination of sufentanil.

The apparent volume of distribution for sufentanil is three times that of the total body water. Sufentanil is highly protein bound, 92.5 percent compared with fentanyl, 84 percent.[146] This combination of high plasma protein binding and a large volume of distribution will result in extensive uptake of sufentanil into tissues. Such a high tissue affinity is in keeping with the highly lipophilic nature of the drug.[146] This

Table 3-12

Induction and Recovery Characteristics of Morphine, Fentanyl, and
Sufentanil in Cardiac Surgical Patients

	Morphine	Fentanyl	Sufentanil
Total dose (μg/kg)	4400±2100	95±30.0	19±6.5
Time to unconsciousness (min)	15+6.9	6±2.2[†]	3±0.7[*‡]
Duration of surgery (hr)	5.7±0.9	5.3±1.7	5.9±1.3
Postoperative time to:			
Respond to commands (hr)	3.0±2.1	2.3±1.6	0.6±0.5[*‡]
Adequate spontaneous ventilation (hr)	13.1±5.5	9.7±3.3	5.6±3.2[*‡]
Tracheal extubation (hr)	18.7±3.1	16.8±3.9	8.9±3.4[*‡]

Source: Data from Sanford TJ, Smith NT, Dec-Silver H, et al: A comparison among morphine,
fentanyl and sufentanil anesthesia for open-heart surgery. Induction, emergence and extubation.
Anesth Analg 65:259–267, 1986, with permission.

Approximately equipotent dilutions of each drug were infused at a standard rate.

Values are mean ± SD: * = P < 0.05 for FvS: † = P < 0.05 for MvF: ‡ = P < 0.05 for MvS.

will allow the drug to penetrate membranes rapidly,
including the blood-brain barrier, and should lead to
rapid onset of the CNS effects of sufentanil, a prediction confirmed by clinical experiences with the drug.

The faster onset of clinical effects was confirmed
by de Lange et al.[209] They found an average time of
induction for fentanyl anesthesia of 4.6 ± 0.5 minutes and for sufentanil of 1.3 ± 0.3 minutes. The
infusion rates used in this study were 300 μg/min for
sufentanil and 400 μg/min for fentanyl. Since sufentanil is approximately 5–10 times as potent as fentanyl, this difference in induction time is not
surprising. In another study, a slower induction of
anesthesia was carried out using approximately equipotent doses.[321] Sufentanil was diluted to 1/5 the
concentration of fentanyl, and a total dose of 18.0 ±
0.5 μg/kg was used for sufentanil and 95.4 ± 30.4
μg/kg for fentanyl during surgery. The mean induction time for sufentanil was 3.0 minutes and for fentanyl, 5.9 minutes. These studies confirm that the
onset of action of sufentanil is somewhat faster than
that of fentanyl. Recovery from anesthesia was also
found to be more rapid (Table 3-12).

HISTAMINE RELEASE

Histamine release has been studied in patients
undergoing cardiac surgery receiving either 100 μg/
kg fentanyl or 15 μg/kg sufentanil as the sole anesthetic.[105] In the 5 minutes after opioid administration,
there were no statistically significant changes in
plasma histamine concentrations in patients receiving
either fentanyl or sufentanil anesthesia. In another
study, Flacke et al studied histamine release after
sufentanil/diazepam anesthesia for cardiac surgery.[322] They confirmed the previous observations

that anesthesia with sufentanil was not associated
with release of histamine, but found that histamine
levels gradually increased following incision and
sternotomy; most steeply after heparinization and
cannulation, and declined slowly after bypass. These
changes roughly paralleled alterations in plasma norepinephrine levels. The authors suggested that,
although histamine release sufficient to cause hemodynamic changes occurred before bypass, the effects
were not obvious because of concomitant release of
norepinephrine.

NONCARDIAC USE OF SUFENTANIL

An initial evaluation of sufentanil, compared
with fentanyl, was carried out for nonstimulating surgery, carotid and vertebral angiography.[323] An initial
dose of 500 μg of fentanyl was compared with 50 μg
of sufentanil. From this study the authors suggested
that sufentanil was approximately 10 times as potent
as fentanyl, and that patients awoke more rapidly and
were more lucid than with fentanyl-supplemented
anesthesia. Using higher doses, 20 μg/kg of fentanyl
and 2 μg/kg of sufentanil in patients anesthetized for
a hysterectomy, no significant differences between
the two drugs were noted with respect to cardiovascular, respiratory, or endocrine responses.[324] In a
double-blind study using much lower doses, no statistically significant differences between fentanyl and
sufentanil were observed.[325] The authors suggested
that sufentanil was 8–9 times as potent as fentanyl.
However, their criteria for supplementation were not
clearly defined.

Various other studies have failed to differentiate
between sufentanil and fentanyl as a supplement to
balanced opioid/nitrous oxide anesthesia for general

surgery. In a comparison of meperidine, morphine, fentanyl, and sufentanil, no differences were found between a total dose of 1000 μg of fentanyl or 100 μg of sufentanil, although both were significantly better than morphine or meperidine.[326] Meperidine caused deleterious effects on objective tests of psychomotor function. Both fentanyl and sufentanil were associated with a more rapid return of mental function than either morphine or meperidine. Faster recovery of alertness and lower pain ratings have been found in patients receiving 2 μg/kg of sufentanil compared with 15 μg/kg of fentanyl.[327] This study did not detect any perioperative differences between the two opioid supplements.

The studies described so far were conducted using intermittent blood pressure measurements. In a carefully controlled study, using continuously recorded blood pressure via an indwelling arterial catheter, and continuous electrocardiograms (ECG) and heart rate monitoring, differences were determined among meperidine, morphine, fentanyl, and sufentanil.[328] Because of increases in blood pressure, heart rate, or both, supplementation with a potent inhalation anesthetic was necessary for patients given meperidine, morphine, or fentanyl. No patients receiving sufentanil required supplementation with a volatile agent. Side effects were common during meperidine anesthesia. Cardiovascular dynamics were most stable and plasma norepinephrine levels were lowest in patients receiving sufentanil. The incidence of postoperative respiratory depression was least in those patients receiving sufentanil. This well-controlled study is the only one in the currently available literature that suggests that sufentanil has marked advantages over fentanyl for supplementation of opioid/N_2O anesthesia.

A potential disadvantage of the use of opioids in large doses is the incidence of chest wall rigidity. It is possible that this can occur after small doses. It has been suggested that chest wall rigidity can occur 3 hours after the administration of sufentanil, 4 μg/kg.[329]

Sufentanil for Cardiac Anesthesia in Humans

The main clinical use for sufentanil has been as an alternative to fentanyl for high-dose opioid anesthesia for patients undergoing cardiac surgery. Sufentanil appears to offer advantages in that anesthesia is more stable with less hemodynamic disturbance than during fentanyl anesthesia. In an initial evaluation of the cardiovascular effects of sufentanil, an induction dose of 15 μg/kg with air/oxygen was used as a complete anesthetic in 40 adult patients.[142] A small decrease in systolic blood pressure after induction and decreases in systolic pressure and systemic vascular resistance before incision occurred. Of the 40 patients, 16 became hypertensive at the time of sternotomy, requiring additional sufentanil. The total dose of sufentanil used in the study was 19.4 μg/kg (range 15–23.4 μg/kg). In a prospective randomized comparison of sufentanil and fentanyl/oxygen anesthesia, sufentanil was found to provide superior conditions.[209] The induction dose of the drug was given by slow infusion, fentanyl at 400 μg/min and sufentanil at 300 μg/min. Additional fentanyl (250 μg bolus) or sufentanil (50 μg bolus) was given whenever systolic blood pressure increased more than 15 percent above control values. The total doses used in the study were 122 μg/kg of fentanyl and 12.9 μg/kg of sufentanil. As with the previously described study, sufentanil and fentanyl anesthesia produced small but significant decreases in systolic pressure on induction. However, there was a marked reduction in the incidence of hypertension during stressful stimulation with sufentanil, particularly in those patients receiving beta-adrenergic blocking agents (Table 3-13). The authors suggested that sufentanil may be a superior opioid to fentanyl for anesthesia for cardiac surgery.

Other studies have supported this initial work and have shown that sufentanil provides stable cardiovascular dynamics during cardiac anesthesia. It is possible that sufentanil produces more hypotension on induction of anesthesia than fentanyl. In a comparative study of the two agents, sufentanil/pancuronium, but not fentanyl/pancuronium, was associated with a decrease in both arterial pressure and systemic vascular resistance.[330] This supports the findings of Sebel and Bovill that sufentanil induction is indeed associated with a small reduction in arterial blood pressure, and there may be a case for volume preloading these patients before induction of anesthesia.[142] Other studies have failed to demonstrate a significant difference between the two drugs. Comparing doses of sufentanil up to 30 μg/kg or fentanyl up to 100 μg/kg, no differences, apart from small reductions in heart rate and mean systemic pressure, could be determined between the two opioids.[331] Another study comparing sufentanil, 20 μg/kg, with fentanyl, 100 μg/kg, failed to detect any clinical differences between the two anesthetic techniques, although sufentanil produced a significantly lower systemic vascular resistance at several times during the study.[210]

Table 3-13

Influence of Preoperative Beta-adrenergic Blockade on Need for Supplementation to
Control Hypertension in Patients Anesthetized with Either Fentanyl or Sufentanil,
Undergoing Coronary Artery Surgery.

	Phentolamine		N_2O	Nitroprusside
	Before bypass	*During bypass*	*After bypass*	*After bypass*
Fentanyl				
All patients (n = 19)	8(42%)	9(47%)	10(53%)	4(21%)
Patients taking beta-adrenergic blocking drugs (n = 12)	3(25%)	3(25%)	4(33%)	2(17%)
Patients not taking beta-adrenergic blocking drugs (n = 7)	5(71%)	3(86%)	6(86%)	2(29%)
Sufentanil				
All patients (n = 18)	1(6%)	2(11%)	2(11%)	1(6%)
Patients taking beta-adrenergic blocking drugs (n = 10)	0(0%)	0(0%)	0(0%)	0(0%)
Patients not taking beta-adrenergic blocking drugs (n = 8)	1(13%)	1(13%)	2(25%)	1(13%)

Source: de Lange S, Boscoe MJ, Stanley TH, et al: Comparison of sufentanil–O_2 and fentanyl–O_2 for coronary artery surgery. Anesthesiology 56:112–118, 1982, with permission.

There is as yet limited information on the effects of sufentanil on myocardial blood flow and metabolism. It appears likely that doses of sufentanil, 10–30 μg/kg, do not adversely affect the coronary circulation.[332] In some patients, however, regional myocardial metabolic imbalances were observed independent of the dose of sufentanil used. The authors suggest that this is associated with a decrease in perfusion pressure. Assessing cardiac effects of the drug by gated nuclear ventriculograms to estimate ejection fraction, sufentanil, 22 μg/kg, was found to produce a greater depression in systolic function than alfentanil or fentanyl.[333] These authors suggested that sufentanil reduces arterial pressure primarily by an effect on contractility.

The studies described so far have used sufentanil doses on the order of 15–30 μg/kg. In a study comparing two dosage regimens, there was a decreased incidence of hypertension following sternotomy in the 30-μg/kg group.[334] However, it should be noted that there were only 6 patients per group in this study. It, therefore, appears that an initial dose of 15 μg/kg of sufentanil provides adequate induction of anesthesia, and the total dose requirement for the whole surgery may be as high as 30 μg/kg.

Sufentanil has also been used for anesthesia in patients undergoing valvular heart surgery. Induction of anesthesia with a 15-μg/kg sufentanil bolus injection produced transient hypotension in 2 of 20 patients.[307] There did not appear to be any advantage in using sufentanil over fentanyl or alfentanil. Sufentanil has also been given by infusion for valvular heart surgery. After an induction dose of 15 μg/kg, a continuous infusion of 0.075 μg/kg/min of sufentanil was given until rewarming on cardiopulmonary bypass.[335] Stable hemodynamics were again obtained. In both of these studies, a lesser incidence of hypertension was noted than in coronary artery patients. This is likely to be related to the underlying pathology as well as the high doses of opioid analgesics used.

Sufentanil Anesthesia for Pediatric Cardiac Surgery

There is as yet limited experience in the use of sufentanil as an anesthetic for pediatric cardiovascular surgery, and the data currently available are somewhat contradictory. Sufentanil/oxygen (5–10 μg/kg) and fentanyl/oxygen (50 and 75 μg/kg) were studied in 40 infants undergoing repair of complex heart defects.[336] Hemodynamic responses to endotracheal intubation were completely blocked, and responses to surgery were partially and variably blocked. Sufentanil appeared to be more effective in blocking responses to surgical stimulation. Induction of anesthesia with both opioids increased transcutaneous oxygen tension, even in cyanotic patients with right-to-left shunts. In contrast, in another study of sufentanil, 5–20 μg/kg, for open heart surgery in children aged 4–12 years, increases in systolic pressure occurred in all groups upon endotracheal intubation.[337] Extubation was impeded by shallow periodic breathing and hypercapnea, and the authors found that sufentanil in bolus form did not provide a reliable degree of anesthesia.

THE METABOLIC EFFECTS OF
SUFENTANIL ANESTHESIA

The metabolic responses seen during sufentanil anesthesia are essentially similar to those seen during fentanyl anesthesia. Induction of anesthesia with sufentanil attenuates the endocrine metabolic response to surgery, including decreases in circulating catecholamines.[251] During cardiopulmonary bypass, however, marked increases in catecholamine concentrations occur. Antidiuretic hormone levels are also increased during bypass, and plasma cortisol increased at the end of surgery. These findings suggest that, although sufentanil attenuates the metabolic response, this attenuation is short lived. Other work comparing sufentanil and alfentanil anesthesia supports these conclusions regarding catecholamine and cortisol responses.[309] However, these workers did not find increases in antidiuretic hormone during sufentanil/oxygen anesthesia.[310] Comparing sufentanil and fentanyl in a double-blind study, no differences between the two agents could be determined for epinephrine or norepinephrine secretion, but sufentanil was more effective in attenuating the increase in plasma renin activity that occurred after skin incision.[338] There were, however, no statistically significant differences between the hemodynamic responses in the fentanyl and sufentanil patients at this time, so the reduction in renin activity is of uncertain physiologic significance.

NEUROPHYSIOLOGIC EFFECTS OF
SUFENTANIL

The electroencephalographic effects of sufentanil are similar to those seen after fentanyl anesthesia. Sufentanil, 15 μg/kg, produces an EEG response characterized by high-voltage, slow delta waves (Fig. 3-16).[256] Although the mean power in the delta band declines with time following sufentanil, the contribution of delta power to total power remains constant until the start of cardiopulmonary bypass (Fig. 3-17). Sharp waves of uncertain neurophysiologic significance were seen with sufentanil, as with fentanyl, but were not associated with clinical signs of epileptic activity. These EEG findings have generally been confirmed by other workers using different techniques of EEG analysis.[258] In this study no sharp waves were seen with either fentanyl or sufentanil anesthesia at any dose or any level. It has been suggested that monitoring the EEG can reduce sufentanil requirements for surgical anesthesia.[339] Sufentanil at a mean dosage of 2.6 μg/kg was found to produce an EEG state consistent with surgical anesthesia. A total dose requirement for coronary artery surgery as low as 10 μg/kg has been reported using EEG monitoring to control sufentanil administration.

Although there have been many studies of the cardiovascular and metabolic effects of sufentanil, most of these have been carried out on small groups of patients. In some studies, patient groups were as small as 6 per group. More extensive clinical experience is required with sufentanil before its relationship to fentanyl can be firmly defined. It appears that the differences between the two drugs, if any, are rather small. Sufentanil anesthesia appears in some studies to produce a lower incidence of hypertension requiring treatment. Other studies have shown a faster time to awakening and extubation after sufentanil, a finding not confirmed by all workers. There does not appear to be any advantage in using sufentanil over fentanyl from the point of view of suppression of metabolic responses. This is surprising because it would seem likely that a more potent opioid analgesic would suppress metabolic responses more than fentanyl. It seems reasonable to conclude at this stage that sufentanil anesthesia probably offers some small advantages over fentanyl used in the same manner. More extensive experience with the drug in routine clinical practice is required to confirm this suggestion.

REFERENCES

1. Jaffe JH, Martin WR: Opioid analgesics and antagonists. *In* Gilman AG, Goodman LS, Rall T, et al (eds): The pharmacological basis of therapeutics, 7th ed. New York, Macmillan, 1985, pp 491–531

2. Janssen PAJ, van der Eycken CAM: The chemical anatomy of potent morphine-like analgesics. *In* Burger A (ed): Drugs affecting the central nervous system, vol 2. New York, Marcel Dekker Inc., 1968, pp 25–60

3. Leysen JE, Laduron PM, Niemegeers CJE: Receptor binding properties in vitro and in vivo of new long acting narcotic analgesics. *In* van Ree, Terenius R (eds): Characteristics and functions of opioids. Amsterdam, Elsevier North-Holland Biomedical Press, 1978, pp 479–482

4. Lasagna L, Beecher HK: The analgesic effectiveness of nalorphine and nalorphine-morphine combinations in man. J Pharmacol Exp Ther 122:356–363, 1965

5. Ariens EF, Simonis AM, Van Rossum JM: Molecular pharmacology: The mode of action of biologically active compounds. New York, Academic Press, 1964

6. Martin WR: Opioid antagonists. Pharmocol Rev 10:452–463, 1967

7. Gilbert PE, Martin WR: The effects of morphine- and nalorphine-like drugs in the nondependent, morphine-dependent and cyclazocine-dependent chronic spinal dog. J Pharmacol Exp Ther 198:66–82, 1976

8. Martin WR, Eades CG, Thompson JA, et al: The effects of morphine- and nalorphine-like drugs in the nondependent and morphine-dependent chronic spinal dog. J Pharmocol Exp Ther 197:517–532, 1976

9. Lord JAH, Waterfield AA, Hughes J, et al: Endogenous opioid peptides: Multiple agonists and receptors. Nature 267:495–499, 1977

10. Schultz R, Wuster M, Herz A: Pharmacological characterisation of the epsilon receptor. J Pharmacol Exp Ther 216:604–606, 1981

11. Lee NM, Leybin L, Chang JK, et al: Opiate and peptide interaction: Effect of enkephalin on morphine analgesia. Eur J Pharmacol 68:181–185, 1980

12. Vaught JL, Rothman RB, Westfall TC: Mu and delta receptors. Their role in analgesia and in the differential effects of opioid peptides on analgesia. Life Sci 30:1443–1455, 1982

13. Pasternak GW: High and low affinity opioid binding sites: Relationship to mu and delta sites. Life Sci 31:1302–1306, 1982

14. Ling GSF, Spiegel K, Nishimura SL, et al: Dissociation of morphine's analgesic and respiratory depressant actions. Eur J Pharmacol 86:487–488, 1983

15. Ward SJ, Takemori AE: Determination of the relative involvement of μ-opioid receptors in opioid-induced depression of respiratory rate, by use of β-funaltrexamine. Eur J Pharmacol 87:1–6, 1983

16. Terenius L: Stereospecific interaction between narcotic analgesics and a synaptic plasma membrane fraction of rat cerebral cortex. Acta Pharmacol Toxicol 32:317–336, 1973

17. Pert CB, Snyder SH: Opiate receptor. Demonstration in nervous tissue. Science 179:1011–1014, 1973

18. Simon EJ, Hiller JM, Edelman I: Stereospecific binding of the potent narcotic analgesic [³H]etorphine in the rat-brain homogenate. Proc Natl Acad Sci USA 70:1947–1949, 1973

19. Snyder SH: Opiate receptors in the brain. N Engl J Med 296:266–271, 1972

20. Hughes J, Smith TW, Kosterlitz HW, et al: Identification of two related pentapeptides from the brain with potent opiate agonist activity. Nature 258:577–579, 1975

21. Rees LH: Brain opiates and corticotrophin-related peptides. J Roy Coll Phys Lond 15:130–134, 1981

22. Benizer AG: Scopolamine-morphine-cocaine anesthesia in surgery. NY J Med 101:1215, 1915

23. Neff W, Mayer EC, Perales M: Nitrous oxide and oxygen anesthesia with curare relaxation. Calif Med 66:67–69, 1947

24. Mushin WW, Rendell-Baker L: Pethidine as a supplement to nitrous oxide anaesthesia. Br Med J 2:472, 1949

25. Eckenhoff JE, Elder JD, King BD: N-allylmorphine in the treatment of morphine or demerol narcosis. Am J Med Sci 222:115, 1951

26. Gray TC, Rees GJ: The role of apnoea in anaesthesia for major surgery. Br Med J 2:891–892, 1952

27. Woodbridge PD: Changing concepts concerning depth of anesthesia. Anesthesiology 18:536–550, 1957

28. Parker EO, Ross AL: Low dose fentanyl. Effects on thiopental requirements and hemodynamic response during induction and intubation. Anesthesiology 57:A322, 1982

29. King BD, Harris LC, Greifenstein FE, et al: Reflex circulatory responses to direct laryngoscopy and tracheal intubation performed during general anesthesia. Anesthesiology 12:556–566, 1951

30. Derbyshire DR, Chmielewski A, Fell D, et al: Plasma catecholamine responses to tracheal intubation. Br J Anaesth 55:855–860, 1983

31. Stoelting RK: Circulatory changes during direct laryngoscopy and tracheal intubation: Influence of duration of laryngoscopy with or without prior lidocaine. Anesthesiology 47:381-383, 1977

32. Prys-Roberts C, Foëx P, Biro GP, et al: Studies of anaesthesia in relation to hypertension V: Adrenergic beta-receptor blockade. Br J Anaesth 45:671–680, 1973

33. Stoelting RK: Attenuation of blood pressure response to laryngoscopy and tracheal intubation

with sodium nitroprusside. Anesth Analg 58:116–119, 1979

34. Davies MJ, Cronin KD, Cowie RW: The prevention of hypertension at intubation. A controlled study of intravenous hydralazine on patients undergoing intracranial surgery. Anaesthesia 36:147–152, 1981

35. Martin DE, Rosenberg H, Aukburg SJ, et al: Low-dose fentanyl blunts circulatory responses to tracheal intubation. Anesth Analg 61:680–684, 1983

36. Atweh SF, Kuhar MJ: Autoradiographic localization of opiate receptors in rat brain. I. Spinal cord and lower medulla. Brain Res 124:53–67, 1947

37. Lowenstein E, Hallowell P, Levine FH, et al: Cardiovascular response to large doses of intravenous morphine in man. N Engl J Med 281:1389–1393, 1969

38. Lowenstein E: Morphine "anesthesia"—A perspective. Anesthesiology 35:563–565, 1971

39. Stanley TH, Gray NG, Stanford W, et al: The effects of high-dose morphine on fluid and blood requirements in open-heart operations. Anesthesiology 38:536–541, 1973

40. Stoelting RK, Gibbs PS: Hemodynamic effects of morphine and morphine-nitrous oxide in valvular heart disease and coronary artery disease. Anesthesiology 38:45–52, 1973

41. McDermott RW, Stanley TH: The cardiovascular effects of low concentrations of nitrous oxide during morphine anesthesia. Anesthesiology 41:89–91, 1974

42. Stanley TH, Bennett GM, Loeser EA, et al: Cardiovascular effects of diazepam and droperidol during morphine anesthesia. Anesthesiology 44:255–258, 1976

43. Stoelting RK, Creasser CE, Gibbs PS: Circulatory effects of halothane added to morphine anesthesia in patients with coronary artery disease. Anesth Analg 53:449–455, 1974

44. Stanley TH, Liu WS: Cardiovascular effects of nitrous oxide-meperidine anesthesia before and after pancuronium. Anesth Analg 56:669–673, 1977

45. Reddy P, Liu WS, Port D, et al: Comparison of haemodynamic effects of anaesthetic doses of alphaprodine and sufentanil in the dog. Can Anaesth Soc J 27:345–350, 1980

46. Welti RS, Moldenhauer CC, Hug CC Jr, et al: High-dose hydromorphone (Dilaudid) for coronary artery surgery. Anesth Analg 63:55–59, 1984

47. Stanley TH, Webster LR: Anesthetic requirements and cardiovascular effects of fentanyl-oxygen and fentanyl-diazepam-oxygen anesthesia in man. Anesth Analg 57:411–416, 1978

48. Lunn JK, Webster LR, Stanley TH, et al: High dose fentanyl anesthesia for coronary artery surgery. Plasma fentanyl concentration and influence of nitrous oxide on cardiovascular responses. Anesth Analg 58:390–395, 1979

49. Bovill JG, Sebel PS, Stanley TH: Opioid analgesics in anesthesia: With special reference to their use in cardiovascular anesthesia. Anesthesiology 61:731–755, 1984

50. Jacobsen AE, May EL, Sargent LJ: Medicinal chemistry, II. New York, Wiley, 1970, pp 1327–1350

51. Janssen PAJ: A review of the chemical features associated with strong morphine-like activity. Br J Anaesth 34:260–268, 1962

52. Horn AS, Rogers JR: The enkephalins and opiates: Structure-activity relation. J Pharm Pharmacol 29:257–260, 1977

53. Osei-Gyimah P, Archer S: Some 14-beta-substituted analogues of N-(cyclo-propylmethyl)normorphine. J Med Chem 24:212–215, 1981

54. Fries DS, Portoghese PS: Stereochemical studies on medicinal agents. J Med Chem 19:1155–1159, 1976

55. Galt RHM: The opiate anomalies—another possible explanation. J Pharm Pharmacol 29:711–714, 1977

56. Thorpe DH: Opiate structure and activity—a guide to understanding the receptor. Anesth Analg 63:143–151, 1984

57. Schlaefke ME: Central chemosensitivity. A respiratory drive. Rev Physiol Biochem Pharmacol 90:171–244, 1981

58. Flórez J, Hurlé MA, Mediavilla A: Respiratory responses to opiates applied to the medullary ventral surface. Life Sci 31:2189–2192, 1982

59. Harper MH, Hickey RF, Cromwell TH, et al: The magnitude and duration of respiratory depression produced by fentanyl and fentanyl plus droperidol in man. J Pharmacol Exp Ther 199:464–468, 1976

60. Kaufman RD, Agleh KA, Belville JW: Relative potencies and duration of action with respect to respiratory depression of intravenous meperidine, fentanyl and alphaprodine in man. J Pharmacol Exp Ther 208:73–79, 1979

61. Kay B, Rolly G: Duration of action of analgesic supplement to anesthesia. Acta Anaesthesiol Belg 28:25–32, 1977

62. McGilliard KL, Takemori AE: Antagonism by naloxone of narcotic-induced respiratory depression and analgesia. J Pharmacol Exp Ther 207:494–503, 1978

63. Freye E: Cardiovascular effects of high doses of fentanyl, meperidine and naloxone in dogs. Anesth Analg 53:40–47, 1974

64. Patschke D, Eberlein HJ, Hess W, et al: Antagonism of morphine with naloxone in dogs. Cardiovascular effects with special reference to the coronary circulation, Br J Anaesth 49:525–532, 1977

65. Azar I, Turndorf H: Severe hypertension and multiple atrial premature contractions following naloxone administration. Anesth Analg 58:524–525, 1979

66. Flacke JW, Flacke WE, William GD: Acute pulmonary edema following naloxone reversal of high-dose morphine anesthesia. Anesthesiology 47:376–378, 1977

67. Andree RA: Sudden death following naloxone administration. Anesth Analg 59:782–784, 1980

68. Azar I, Patel AK, Phau CQ: Cardiovascular responses following naloxone administration during enflurane anesthesia. Anesth Analg 60:237, 1981

69. Estilo AE, Cottrell JE: Hemodynamic and catecholamine changes after administration of naloxone. Anesth Analg 61:349–353, 1982

70. Montastruc JL, Montastruc P, Morales-Olivas F: Potentiation by naloxone of pressor reflexes. Br J Pharmacol 74:105–109, 1981

71. Kraynack BJ, Gintautas JG: Naloxone: Analeptic action unrelated to opiate receptor antagonism. Anesthesiology 56:251–253, 1982

72. Ngai SH, Berkowitz BA, Yang JC, et al: Pharmacokinetics of naloxone in rats and in man. Anesthesiology 44:398–401, 1976

73. Evans JM, Hogg MIJ, Lunn JN, et al: Degree and duration of reversal by naloxone of effects of morphine in conscious subjects. Br Med J 1:589–591, 1974

74. Weinstock M: Acetylcholine and cholinesterases. In Clouet DH (ed): Narcotic drugs: Biochemical pharmacology. New York, Plenum Press, 1971, pp 254–260

75. Dev NB, Loeschke HH: A cholinergic mechanism involved in the respiratory chemosensitivity of the medulla oblongata in the cat. Pfluegers Arch Eur J Physiol 379: 29–36, 1979

76. Weinstock M, Roll D, Erez E: Physostigmine antagonizes morphine-induced respiratory depression but not analgesia in dogs and rabbits. Br J Anaesth 52:1272–1276, 1980

77. Weinstock M, Davidson JT, Rosin AJ, et al: Effect of physostigmine on morphine-induced postoperative pain and somnolence. Br J Anaesth 54:429–434, 1982

78. Snir-Mor I, Weinstock M, Davidson JT, et al: Physostigmine antagonizes morphine-induced respiratory depression in human subjects. Anesthesiology 59:6–9, 1983

79. Magruder MR, Delaney RD, DiFazio CA: Reversal of narcotic-induced respiratory depression with nalbuphine hydrochloride. Anesthesiology Rev 9:34–37, 1982

80. Julien RM: Effects of nalbuphine on normal and oxymorphone-depressed ventilatory responses to carbon dioxide challenge. Anesthesiology 57:A320, 1982

81. Latasch L, Probst S, Dudziak R: Reversal by nalbuphine of respiratory depression caused by fentanyl. Anesth Analg 63:814–816, 1984

82. Tabatabai M, Jaradi P, Tadjziechy M, et al: Effect of nalbuphine hydrochloride on fentanyl-induced respiratory depression and analgesia. Anesthesiology 61:A475, 1984

83. Tran L, Durrani Z, Barabas E, et al: Hemodynamic and endocrine effects of reversal of fentanyl-induced respiratory depression by nalbuphine. Anesthesiology 61:A476, 1984

84. Reitan JA, Stengert KB, Wymore MC, et al: Central vagal control of fentanyl induced bradycardia during halothane anesthesia. Anesth Analg 57:31–36, 1978

85. Liu WS, Bidwal AV, Stanley TH, et al: Cardiovascular dynamics after large doses of fentanyl and fentanyl plus N_2O in the dog. Anesth Analg 55:168–172, 1976

86. Urthaler F, Isobe JH, James TN: Direct and vagally mediated chronotropic effects of morphine studied by selective perfusion of the sinus node of awake dogs. Chest 68:222–228, 1975

87. Prakash O, Verdouw PD, de Jong JW, et al: Haemodynamic and biochemical variables after induction of anaesthesia in patients undergoing coronary artery bypass surgery. Can Anaesth Soc J 27:223–229

88. Smith NT, Eger EI, Stoelting RK, et al: The cardiovascular and sympathetic responses to the addition of nitrous oxide to halothane in man. Anesthesiology 32:410–421, 1970

89. Van de Vusse GJ, Coumans WA, Kruger R, et al: Effect of fentanyl on myocardial fatty acid and carbohydrate metabolism and oxygen utilization during experimental ischemia. Anesth Analg 59:644–654, 1980

90. Goldberg AH, Padget CH: Comparative effects of morphine and fentanyl on isolated heart muscle. Anesth Analg 48:978–982, 1969

91. Strauer B: Contractile responses to morphine, piritramide, meperidine and fentanyl. A comparative study of effects on the isolated ventricular myocardium. Anesthesiology 37:304–310, 1972

92. Sullivan DC, Wong KC: The effects of morphine on the isolated heart during normothermia and hypothermia. Anesthesiology 38:550–556, 1973

93. Bovill JG, Sebel PS: Pharmacokinetics of high-dose fentanyl: A study in patients undergoing cardiac surgery. Br J Anaesth 52:795–801, 1980

94. Sprigge JS, Wynands JE, Whalley DG, et al: Fentanyl infusion anesthesia for aortocoronary bypass surgery: Plasma levels and hemodynamic response. Anesth Analg 61:972–978, 1982

95. Krishna G, Paradise RR: Effect of morphine on isolated human atrial muscle. Anesthesiology 40:147–151, 1974

96. Hug CC Jr: Pharmacokinetics of morphine during cardiac surgery. Anesthesiology 49:305–306, 1978

97. Dahlström B, Bolme P, Feychting J, et al: Morphine kinetics in children. Clin Pharmacol Ther 26:354–365, 1979

98. Stanley TH, Bidwai AV, Lunn JK, et al: Cardiovascular effects of nitrous oxide during meperidine infusion in the dog. Anesth Analg 56:836–841, 1977

99. Zelis R, Flaim SF, Eisele JH: Effects of morphine on reflex arteriolar constriction induced in man by hypercapnia. Clin Pharmacol Ther 22:172–178, 1977

100. Hsu HO, Hickey RF, Forbes AF: Morphine decreases peripheral vascular resistance and increases capacitance in man. Anesthesiology 59:98–102, 1979

101. Rosow CE, Moss I, Philbin DM, et al: Histamine release during morphine and fentanyl anesthesia. Anesthesiology 56:93–96, 1982

102. Philbin DM, Moss J, Rosow CE, et al: The use of H_1 and H_2 histamine antagonists with morphine anesthesia: A double blind study. Anesthesiology 55:292–296, 1981

103. Henny RP, Vasko JS, Brawley RK, et al: The effect of morphine on the resistance and capacitance vessels of the peripheral circulation. Am Heart J 72:242–250, 1966

104. Berthelsen P, Eriksen J, Ahn NC, et al: Peripheral circulation during sufentanil and morphine anesthesia. Acta Anaesth Scand 24:241–244, 1980

105. Rosow CE, Philbin DM, Keegan CR, et al: Hemodynamics and histamine release during induction with sufentanil or fentanyl. Anesthesiology 60:489–491, 1984

106. Rorie DK, Muldoon SM, Tyce GM: Effects of fentanyl on adrenergic function in canine coronary arteries. Anesth Analg 60:21–27, 1981

107. Muldoon S, Otto J, Freas W, et al: The effects of morphine, nalbuphine and butorphanol on adrenergic function in canine saphenous veins. Anesth Analg 62:21–28, 1983

108. Lowenstein E, Whiting RB, Bittar DA: Local and neurally mediated effects of morphine on skeletal muscle vascular resistance. J Pharmacol Exp Ther 180:359–367, 1972

109. Flaim SF, Vismara LA, Zelis R: The effects of morphine on isolated cutaneous canine vascular smooth muscle. Res Commun Chem Pathol Pharmacol 23:542–546, 1977

110. Radnay PA, Brodman E, Mankiker D, et al: The effect of equi-analgesic doses of fentanyl, morphine, meperidine and pentazocine on common bile duct pressure. Anaesthetist 29:26–29, 1980

111. Salik JO, Siegel CI, Mendelhoff AI: Biliary duodenal dynamics in man. Radiology 106:1–11, 1973

112. McCammon RL, Viegas OJ, Stoelting RK, et al: Naloxone reversal of choledochoduodenal sphincter spasm associated with narcotic administration. Anesthesiology 48:437–439, 1978

113. Wang SC: Emetic and anti-emetic drugs. In Root WS, Hofmann FG (eds): Physiological Pharmacology II. Academic Press, New York, 1963, pp 255–328.

114. Niemegeers CJE: The apomorphine antagonism test in dogs. Pharmacology 6:353–364, 1971

115. Jaffe TB, Ramsey FM: Attenuation of fentanyl-induced truncal rigidity. Anesthesiology 58:562–564, 1983

116. Scamman FL: Fentanyl-O_2-N_2O rigidity and pulmonary compliance. Anesth Analg 62:332–334, 1983

117. Christian CM, Waller JL, Moldenhauer CC: Postoperative rigidity following fentanyl anesthesia. Anesthesiology 58:275–277, 1983

118. Sokall MD, Hoyt JL, Georgis SD: Studies in muscle rigidity, nitrous oxide and narcotic analgesic agents. Anesth Analg 51:16–20, 1972

119. Freund FG, Marten WE, Wong KC, et al: Abdominal muscle rigidity induced by morphine and nitrous oxide. Anesthesiology 38:358–362, 1973

120. Hill AB, Nahrwald MD, de Rosayro AM, et al: Prevention of rigidity during fentanyl-oxygen induction of anesthesia. Anesthesiology 55:452–454, 1981

121. Georgis SD, Hoyt JL, Sokoll MD: Effects of Innovar and Innovar plus nitrous oxide on muscle tone and the H-reflex. Anesth Analg 50:743–747, 1971

122. Benthuysen JL, Smith NT, Sanford TT, et al: Physiology of alfentanil-induced rigidity. Anesthesiology 64:440–446, 1986

123. Koffer KB, Berney S, Horrykiewicz O: The role of the corpus striatum in neuroleptic and narcotic-induced catalepsy. Eur J Clin Pharmacol 47:81–86, 1978

124. Moroni F, Peralta E, Cheney DL, et al: On the regulation of gamma-aminobutyric acid neurons in the caudatus, pallidus and nigra. Effects of opioids and dopamine antagonists. J Pharmacol Exp Ther 208:190–194, 1979

125. Cox BM, Ginsberg M, Osman OH: Acute tolerance to narcotic analgesic drugs in rats. Br J Pharmacol Chemother 33:256, 1968

126. Colpaert FC, Niemegeers CJ, Janssen PAJ, et al: The effects of prior fentanyl administration and of pain on fentanyl analgesia. Tolerance to and enhancement of narcotic analgesia. J Pharmacol Exp Ther 213:418–424, 1980

127. Lotti VJ, Lomax P, George R: Acute tolerance to morphine following systemic and intracerebral injection in the rat. J Neuropharmacol 5:36–42, 1966

128. Fennessy MR, Rattray JF: Cardiovascular effects of intravenous morphine in the anaesthetised rat. Eur J Pharmacol 14:1–8, 1971

129. Novack GD, Bullock JL, Eisele JH: Fentanyl: Cumulative effects and development of short-term tolerance. Neuropharmacology 17:77–82, 1978

130. Askitopoulou H, Whitwam JG, Al-Khudhairi D, et al: Acute tolerance to fentanyl during anesthesia in dogs. Anesthesiology 63:255–261, 1985

131. McQuay HJ, Bullingham RES, Moore RA: Acute opiate tolerance in man. Life Sci 28:2513–2517, 1981

132. Shafer A, White PF, Schüttler J, et al: Use of a fentanyl infusion in the intensive care unit. Tolerance to its anesthetic effect? Anesthesiology 59:245–248, 1983

133. Mark JB, Greenberg LM: Intraoperative awareness and hypertensive crisis during high dose fentanyl-diazepam anesthesia. Anesth Analg 62:698–700, 1983

134. Hilgenberg JC: Intraoperative awareness during high-dose fentanyl oxygen anesthesia. Anesthesiology 54:341–343, 1981

135. Mummaneni N, Rao TLK, Montoya A: Awareness and recall with high-dose fentanyl-oxygen anesthesia. Anesth Analg 59:948–949, 1980

136. Janssen PAJ: Potent, new analgesics, tailor-made for different purposes. Acta Anaesth Scand 26:262–268, 1982

137. de Castro J, van de Water A, Wouters L, et al: Comparative study of cardiovascular, neurological and metabolic side-effects of eight narcotics in dogs. Acta Anaesthesiol Belg 30:5–99, 1979

138. Sebel PC, Bovill JG, Wauquier A, et al: The effect of high-dose fentanyl on the electroencephalogram. Anesthesiology 55:203–211, 1981

139. Gommeren W, Leysen JE: Binding properties of [³H] lofentanil at the opiate receptor. Arch Int Pharmacodyn Ther 258:171–173, 1982

140. Leysen JE, Gommeren W, Niemegeers CJE: [³H] Sufentanil, a superior ligand for μ-opiate receptors. Binding properties and regional distribution in rat brain and spinal cord. Eur J Pharmacol 87:209–225, 1983

141. Sebel PS, Bovill JG, Boekhorst RAA, et al: Cardiovascular effects of high dose fentanyl anaesthesia. Acta Anaesth Scand 36:308–315, 1982

142. Sebel PS, Bovill JG: Cardiovascular effects of sufentanil anesthesia. Anesth Analg 61:115–119, 1982

143. Stahl KD, van Bever W, Janssen P, et al: Receptor affinity and pharmacological potency of a series of narcotic analgesics, antidiarrheal and neuroleptic drugs. Eur J Pharmacol 46:199–205, 1977

144. Holford NHG, Sheiner LB: Pharmacokinetic and dynamic modelling in vivo. CRC Crit Rev Bioeng 5:273–322, 1981

145. Bower S, Hull CJ: Comparative pharmacokinetics of fentanyl and alfentanil. Br J Anaesth 54:871–877, 1982

146. Meuldermans WEG, Hurkmans RMA, Heykants JJP: Plasma protein binding and distribution of fentanyl, sufentanil, alfentanil and lofentanil in blood. Arch Int Pharmacodyn Ther 257:4–19, 1982

147. Hug CC Jr, Murphy MR: Tissue redistribution of fentanyl and termination of effect in rats. Anesthesiology 55:369–375, 1981

148. Hug CC Jr, Murphy MR: Fentanyl disposition in cerebrospinal fluid and plasma and its relationship to ventilatory depression in the dog. Anesthesiology 50:342–349, 1979

149. Hess R, Herz A, Friedel K: Pharmacokinetics of fentanyl in rabbits in view of the importance of limiting the effect. J Pharmacol Exp Ther 179:474–484, 1971

150. Hug CC Jr, Murphy MR, Rigel EP, et al: Pharmacokinetics of morphine injected intravenously into the anesthetized dog. Anesthesiology 54:38–47, 1981

151. McClain DA, Hug CC: Intravenous fentanyl kinetics. Clin Pharmacol Ther 28:106–114, 1980

152. Stanski DR, Paalzow L, Edlund PO: Morphine pharmacokinetics: Radioimmunoassay vs gas-liquid chromatography. J Pharmacol Sci 71:314–317, 1982

153. Murphy MR, Hug CC, Jr: Pharmacokinetics of intravenous morphine in patients anesthetized with enflurane-nitrous oxide. Anesthesiology 54:187–192, 1981

154. Craft JB, Coaldrake LE, Bolan JC, et al: Placental passage and uterine effects of fentanyl. Anesth Analg 62:894–898, 1983

155. Eisele JH, Wright R, Rogge P: Newborn and maternal fentanyl levels at Caesarean section. Anesth Analg 61:179–180, 1982

156. Nation R: Meperidine binding in maternal and fetal plasma. Clin Pharmacol Ther 29:472–479, 1981

157. Goromaru T, Matsuura H, Yoshimura N, et al: Identification and quantitative determination of fentanyl metabolites in patients by gas chromatography—mass spectrometry. Anesthesiology 61:73–77, 1984

158. Maruyama Y, Hosoya E: Studies on the fate of fentanyl. Keio J Med 18:59–70, 1969

159. van Rooy HH, Vermeulen NPE, Bovill JG: The assay of fentanyl and its metabolites in plasma of patients using gas chromatography with alkali flame ionisation detection and gas chromatography—mass spectrometry. J Chromatogr 223:85–93, 1981

160. Murphy MR, Olson WA, Hug CC Jr: Pharmacokinetics of ³H-fentanyl in the dog anesthetized with enflurane. Anesthesiology 50:13–19, 1979

161. Mather LE: Clinical pharmacokinetics of fentanyl and its newer derivatives. Clin Pharmacokinet 8:422–446, 1983

162. Fung DL, Eisele JH: Fentanyl pharmacokinetics in awake volunteers. J Clin Pharmacol 20:652–658, 1980

163. Schleimer R, Benjamini E, Eisele J, et al: Pharmacokinetics of fentanyl as determined by radioimmunoassay. Clin Pharmacol Ther 23:188–194, 1978

164. Bently JB, Borel JD, Nenad RE, et al: Age and fentanyl pharmacokinetics. Anesth Analg 61:968–971, 1982

165. Hengstmann JH, Stoeckel H, Schüttler J: Infusion model for fentanyl based on pharmacokinetic analysis. Br J Anaesth 52:1021–1025, 1980

166. Wilkinson GR, Shand DG: A physiological approach to hepatic drug clearance. Clin Pharmacol Ther 18:371–390, 1975

167. Gelman SI: Disturbances in hepatic blood flow during anesthesia and surgery. Arch Surg 111:881–883, 1976

168. Lehman KA, Weski C, Hunger L, et al: Biotransformation von Fentanyl II. Akute Arzneimittelinterakio—Untersuchungen bei Ratten und Mensch. Anaesthetist 31:221–227, 1982

169. Borel JD, Bently JB, Nenad RE, et al: The influence of halothane on fentanyl pharmacokinetics. Anesthesiology 57:A239, 1982

170. Hudson RJ, Thompson IR, Cannon JE, et al: Phar-

macokinetics of fentanyl in patients undergoing abdominal aortic surgery. Can Anaesth Soc J 32:S 60, 1985

171. Koska AJ, Romagnoli A, Kramer WG: Effect of cardiopulmonary bypass on fentanyl distribution and elimination. Clin Pharmacol Ther 29:100–105, 1981

172. Hug CC Jr, Moldenhauer CC: Pharmacokinetics and dynamics of fentanyl infusions in cardiac surgical patients. Anesthesiology 57:A 45, 1982

173. Michiels M, Hendriks R, Heykants J: A sensitive radioimmunoassay for fentanyl. Plasma level in dog and man. Eur J Clin Pharmacol 12:153–158, 1977

174. Henderson GL, Frincke J, Leung CY, et al: Antibodies to fentanyl. J Pharmacol Exp Ther 192:489–496, 1975

175. Schüttler J, White PF: Optimization of the radioimmunoassay for measuring fentanyl and alfentanil in human serum. Anesthesiology 61:315–320, 1984

176. Gillespie TJ, Gandolfi AJ, Maiorino RM, et al: Gas chromatographic determination of fentanyl and its analogues in human plasma. J Anal Toxicol 5:133–137, 1981

177. Reilly CS, Wood AJJ, Wood M: Variability of fentanyl pharmacokinetics in man. Computer predicted plasma concentrations for three intravenous dosage regimens. Anaesthesia 40:837–843, 1985

178. Alvis JM, Reves JG, Govier AV, et al: Computer-assisted continuous infusions of fentanyl during cardiac anesthesia. Comparison with a manual method. Anesthesiology 63:41–49, 1985

179. Murphy MR, Hug CC Jr, McClain DA: Dose-independent pharmacokinetics of fentanyl. Anesthesiology 59:537–540, 1983

180. Greenblatt DJ, Sellers EM, Shader RI: Drug disposition in old age. N Engl J Med 306:1081–1088, 1982

181. Sherlock S, Bearw AG, Belling BH, et al: Splanchnic blood flow in man by the bromsulfalein method: The relation of peripheral plasma bromsulfalein level to calculated flow. J Lab Clin Med 35:923–932, 1950

182. Liddell D, Williams F, Briant R: Phenazone (antipyrine) metabolism and distribution in young and elderly adults. Clin Exp Pharmacol Physiol 2:481–487, 1975

183. Szeto HH, Inturrisi CE, Houde R, et al: Accumulation of normeperidine in patients with renal failure or cancer. Ann Intern Med 86:738–741, 1977

184. Don HF, Dieppa RA, Taylor P: Narcotic analgesics in anuric patients. Anesthesiology 42:745–747, 1975

185. Corall IM, Moore AR, Strunin L: Plasma concentrations of fentanyl in normal surgical patients and those with severe renal and hepatic disease. Br J Anaesth 52:101, 1980

186. Haberer JP, Schoeffler P, Couderc E, et al: Fentanyl pharmacokinetics in anaesthetized patients with cirrhosis. Br J Anesth 54:1267–1270, 1982

187. Hug CC Jr, Murphy MR, Sampson JF, et al: Biotransformation of morphine and fentanyl in anhepatic dogs. Anesthesiology 55:A261, 1981

188. Bently JB, Borel JD, Gillespie TJ, et al: Fentanyl pharmacokinetics in obese and nonobese patients. Anesthesiology 55:A117, 1981

189. Mather LE, Runciman WB, Ilsley AH: Anaesthesia induced changes in regional blood flow: Implications for drug disposition. Regional Anesthesia 7 (Suppl):S24–S33, 1982

190. Runciman WB, Mather LE, Ilsley AH, et al: A sheep preparation for studying interactions between blood flow and drug disposition. III: Effects of general and spinal anaesthesia on regional blood flow and oxygen tensions. Br J Anaesth 56:1247–1258, 1984

191. Cowan RE, Jackson BT, Thompson RPH: The effects of various anaesthetics and abdominal surgery on liver blood flow in man. Gut 16:839, 1975

192. Alfery DD, Benumof JL: Hepatic blood flow alterations during anesthesia and surgery. Contemp Anesth Pract. 4:31–56, 1981

193. Borel JD, Bently JB, Nenad RE, et al: Cimetidine alteration of fentanyl pharmacokinetics in dog. Abstracts, 56th Annual Meeting, International Anesthesia Research Society, San Francisco, California, March 14–18, 1982, pp 149–150

194. Lauven PM, Stoeckel H, Schüttler J, et al: Prevention of fentanyl rebound by administration of cimetidine. Anaesthetist 30:467–471, 1981

195. Hug CC, McClain DB: Ventilatory depression by fentanyl in anesthetized patients, Anesthesiology 53:556, 1980

196. Cartwright P, Prys-Roberts C, Gill K, et al: Ventilatory depression related to plasma fentanyl concentrations during and after anesthesia in humans. Anesth Analg 62:966–974, 1983

197. Andrews CJH, Sinclair M, Dye A, et al: The additive effect of nitrous oxide on respiratory depression in patients having fentanyl or sufentanil infusions. Br J Anaesth 54:1129, 1982

198. Fung DL, Eisele JH: Narcotic concentration-respiratory effect curves in man. Anesthesiology 53:S397, 1980

199. Adams AP, Pybus DA: Delayed respiratory depression after use of fentanyl during anaesthesia. Br Med J 1:278–279, 1978

200. Becker LD, Paulson BA, Muller RD, et al: Biphasic respiratory depression after fentanyl-droperidol or fentanyl alone used to supplement nitrous oxide anesthesia. Anesthesiology 44:291–296, 1976

201. McQuay HJ, Moore RA, Paterson GM, et al: Plasma fentanyl concentration and clinical observations during and after operation. Br J Anaesth 51:543–549, 1979

202. Stoeckel H, Hengstmann JH, Schüttler J: Pharmacokinetics of fentanyl as a possible explanation for recurrence of respiratory depression. Br J Anaesth 51:741–744, 1979

203. Lehmann KA, Freier J, Daub D: Fentanyl-Pharmacokinetik und postoperative Atemdepression. Anaesthetist 31:111–118, 1982

204. Scott JC, Ponganis KV, Stanski DR: EEG quantitation of narcotic effect. The comparative pharmacodynamics of fentanyl and alfentanil. Anesthesiology 62:234–241, 1985

205. Andrews CJH, Sinclair M, Prys-Roberts C, et al: Ventilatory effects during and after continuous infusion of fentanyl or alfentanil. Br J Anaesth 55 (Suppl 2):211S–216S, 1983

206. Hicks HC, Mowbray AG, Yhap EO: Cardiovascular effects of and catecholamine responses to high dose fentanyl-O_2 for induction of anesthesia in patients with ischemic coronary artery disease. Anesth Analg 60:563–568, 1981

207. Waller JL, Hug CC, Nagle DN, et al: Hemodynamic changes during fentanyl-oxygen anesthesia for aortocoronary bypass operations. Anesthesiology 55:212–217, 1981

208. Edde RR: Hemodynamic changes prior to and after sternotomy in patients anesthetized with high-dose fentanyl. Anesthesiology 56:112–118, 1982

209. de Lange S, Boscoe MJ, Stanley TH, et al: Comparison of sufentanil-O_2 and fentanyl-O_2 for coronary artery surgery. Anesthesiology 56:112–118, 1982

210. Howie MB, McSweeney TD, Lingam RP, et al: A comparison of fentanyl-O_2 and sufentanil-O_2 for cardiac surgery. Anesth Analg 64:877–887, 1985

211. Barash PG, Tarabadkar S, Giles R, et al: Preservation of global left ventricular function during intubation in patients with ischemic heart disease. Anesthesiology 55:A6, 1981

212. Barash PG, Kopriva CJ, Giles R: Global ventricular function and intubation: Radionuclear profiles. Anesthesiology 53:S109, 1980

213. Wynands JE, Wong P, Whalley DG, et al: Oxygen-fentanyl anesthesia in patients with poor left ventricular function: Hemodynamics and plasma fentanyl concentrations. Anesth Analg 62:476–482, 1983

214. de Lange S, Stanley TH, Boscoe MJ: Fentanyl-oxygen anesthesia. Comparison of anesthetic requirements and cardiovascular responses in Salt Lake City and Leiden, Holland. Proceedings of 7th World Congress of Anaesthesiologists, Hamburg, 1980, p 313

215. Sonntag H, Larsen R, Hilfiker O, et al: Myocardial blood flow and oxygen consumption during high-dose fentanyl anesthesia in patients with coronary artery disease. Anesthesiology 56:417–422, 1982

216. Zurick AM, Urzua J, Yared JP, et al: Comparison of hemodynamic and hormonal effects of large single-dose fentanyl anesthesia and halothane/nitrous oxide anesthesia for coronary artery surgery. Anesth Analg 61:521–526, 1982

217. Moldenhauer CC, Hug CC: Continuous infusion of fentanyl for cardiac surgery. Anesth Analg 61:206, 1982

218. Wynands JE, Wong P, Townsend GE, et al: Narcotic requirements for intravenous anesthesia. Anesth Analg 63:101–105, 1984

219. Murphy MR, Hug CC Jr: The anesthetic potency of fentanyl in terms of its reduction of enflurane MAC. Anesthesiology 57:485–488, 1982

220. Arndt JO, Mikat M, Parasher C: Fentanyl's analgesic, respiratory, and cardiovascular actions in relation to dose and plasma concentration in unanesthetized dogs. Anesthesiology 61:355–361, 1984

221. Tomicheck RC, Rosow CE, Philbin DM, et al: Diazepam-fentanyl interaction-hemodynamic and hormonal effects in coronary artery surgery. Anesth Analg 62:881–884, 1983

222. Liu W, Bidwai AV, Lunn JK, et al: Urine catecholamine excretion after large doses of fentanyl, fentanyl and diazepam, and fentanyl, diazepam and pancuronium. Can Anaesth Soc J 24:371–379, 1977

223. Reves JG, Kissin I, Fournier SE, et al: Additive negative inotropic effect of a combination of diazepam and fentanyl. Anesth Analg 63:97–100, 1984

224. Eisele JH, Smith NT: Cardiovascular effects of 40% nitrous oxide in man. Anesth Analg 51:956–961, 1972

225. Eisele JH, Reitan JA, Massumi RA, et al: Myocardial performance and N_2O analgesia in coronary-artery disease. Anesthesiology 44:16–20, 1976

226. Motomura S, Kissin I, Aultman DF, et al: Effects of fentanyl and nitrous oxide on contractility of blood-perfused papillary muscle of the dog. Anesth Analg 63:47–50, 1984

227. Moffitt EA, Scovil JE, Barker RA, et al: The effects of nitrous oxide on myocardial metabolism and hemodynamics during fentanyl or enflurane anesthesia in patients with coronary disease. Anesth Analg 63:1071–1075, 1984

228. Philbin DM, Föex P, Lowenstein E, et al: Nitrous oxide causes myocardial dysfunction. Anesthesiology 57:A44, 1983

229. Philbin DM, Föex P, Drummond G, et al: Regional ventricular function with sufentanil anesthesia. The effect of nitrous oxide. Anesth Analg 63:260, 1984

230. Michiels I, Kay H, Barash P: Does nitrous oxide or reduced FIO_2 alter hemodynamic function during high dose fentanyl anesthesia? Anesthesiology 57:A44, 1982

231. Meretoja OA, Takkunen O, Heikkilä H, et al: Haemodynamic response to nitrous oxide during high-dose fentanyl pancuronium anaesthesia. Acta Anaesth Scand 29:137–141, 1985

232. Harrison GA: The cardiovascular effects and some relaxant properties of four relaxants in patients about to undergo cardiac surgery. Br J Anaesth 44:485–494, 1972

233. Heinonen J, Yrjölä H: Comparison of haemodynamic effects of metocurine and pancuronium in patients with coronary artery disease. Br J Anaesth 52:931–937, 1980

234. Salmenperä M, Peltola K, Takkunen O, et al: Cardiovascular effects of pancuronium and vecuronium during high-dose fentanyl anesthesia. Anesth Analg 62:1059–1064, 1983

235. Thomson IR, Putnins CL: Adverse effects of pancuronium during high-dose fentanyl anesthesia for coronary artery bypass grafting. Anesthesiology 62:708–713, 1985

236. Ganz W, Tamura K, Marcus HE, et al: Measurement of coronary sinus blood flow by continuous thermodilution. Circulation 41:181–195, 1971

237. Moffitt EA, Scovil JE, Barker RA, et al: Myocardial metabolism and haemodynamic responses during high-dose fentanyl anaesthesia for coronary patients. Can Anaesth Soc J 31:611–618, 1984

238. Skourtis CT, Nissen M, McGinnis LA, et al: The effect of high-dose fentanyl on cardiac metabolic balance and coronary circulation in patients undergoing coronary artery surgery. Anesthesiology 61:A6, 1984

239. Bovill JG, van Wezel HB, Koolen JJ, et al: Effect of fentanyl on myocardial blood flow and oxygen consumption. Eur J Anaesthesiol (In press)

240. Briggs F, Munson P: Studies on the mechanism of stimulation of ACTH secretion with the aid of morphine as a blocking agent. Endocrinology 57:205–219, 1955

241. George JM, Reier CE, Larense RR, et al: Morphine anesthesia blocks cortisol and growth hormone response to surgical stress in humans. Clin Endocrinol Metab 38:736–741, 1974

242. Glariman NH, Mattie LR, Stephenson WF: Studies on the antidiuretic action of morphine. Science 117:225, 1953

243. Philbin DM, Wilson NE, Sokoloski J, et al: Radioimmunoassay of antidiuretic hormone during morphine anaesthesia. Can Anaesth Soc J 23:290–295, 1976

244. Hall GM, Young C, Holdcroft A, et al: Substrate mobilization during surgery—a comparison between halothane and fentanyl anaesthesia. Anaesthesia 33:924–930, 1978

245. Cooper GM, Patterson J, Ward LD, et al: Fentanyl and the metabolic response to gastric surgery. Anaesthesia 36:667–671, 1981

246. Bent JM, Paterson JL, Mashiter K, et al: Effects of high-dose fentanyl anaesthesia on the established metabolic and endocrine response to surgery. Anaesthesia 39:19–23, 1984

247. Sebel PS, Bovill JG, Schellekens APM, et al: Hormonal responses to high-dose fentanyl anaesthesia. Br J Anaesth 59:941–948, 1981

248. Stanley TH, Philbin DM, Coggins CH: Fentanyl oxygen anaesthesia for coronary artery surgery: Cardiovascular and ADH responses. Can Anaesth Soc J 26:168–172, 1979

249. Walsh ES, Paterson JL, O'Riordan JBA: Effects of high-dose fentanyl anaesthesia on the metabolic and endocrine responses to cardiac surgery. Br J Anaesth 53:1155–1165, 1981

250. Gudelsky GA, Porter JC: Morphine and opioid peptide induced inhibition of the release of dopamine from the tubero-infundibular neurons. Life Sci 25:1697–1702, 1979

251. Bovill JG, Sebel PS, Fiolet JWT, et al: The influence of sufentanil on endocrine and metabolic responses to cardiac surgery. Anesth Analg 62:391–397, 1983

252. Pasternak GW, Gintzler AR, Houghton RA, et al: Biochemical and pharmacological evidence for opioid receptor multiplicity in the central nervous system. Life Sci 33 (Suppl 1):167–173, 1983

253. Spiegel K, Pasternak GW: Meptazinol: A novel Mu-1 selective opioid analgesic. J Pharmacol Exp Ther 228:414–419, 1984

254. Kay NH, Allen MC, Bullingham RES, et al: Influence of meptizanol on metabolic and hormonal responses following major surgery. Anaesthesia 40:223–228, 1985

255. Smith NT, Dec-Silver H, Stanford IJ, et al: EEGs during high-dose fentanyl-, sufentanil-, or morphine-oxygen anesthesia. Anesth Analg 63:386–393, 1984

256. Bovill JG, Sebel PS, Wauquier A, et al: Electroencephalographic effects of sufentanil anaesthesia in man. Br J Anaesth 54:45–52, 1982

257. Bovill JG, Sebel PC, Wauquier A, et al: Influence of high-dose alfentanil anaesthesia on the electroencephalogram: Correlation with plasma concentrations. Br J Anaesth 55 (Suppl 2):199–209, 1983

258. Smith NT, Demetrescu M: The EEG during high-dose fentanyl anesthesia. Anesthesiology 53:S7, 1980

259. de Vos V: Immobilisation of free ranging wild animals using a new drug. Vet Res 103:64–68, 1978

260. Port JD, Stanley TH, Steffey EM: Narcotic inhalation anesthesia. Anesthesiology 57:A344, 1982

261. Cookson RF: Carfentanil and lofentanil. Clinics in Anaesthesiology 1(1): 156–158, 1983

262. Tung AS, Yaksh TL: Evaluation of epidural opiates in the cat. Anesthesiology 55:A155, 1981

263. Bilsback P, Rolly G, Tampubolon O: A double blind epidural administration of lofentanil, buprenorphine or saline for postoperative pain. VIth European Congress of Anaesthesiology. London, Academic Press, Abstract 84:49–50

264. Van den Abeele G, Camu F: Clinical evaluation of the analgesic potency of lofentanil in postoperative pain. Acta Anaesthesiol Belg 34:41–47, 1983

265. Niemegeers CJE, Janssen PAJ: Alfentanil: A particularly short-acting intravenous narcotic analgesic. Drug Devel Res 1:83–88, 1981

266. Brown JH, Pleuvry B, Kay B: Respiratory effects of a new opiate analgesic (R 39209) in the rabbit: Comparison with fentanyl. Br J Anaesth 52:1101–1106, 1980

267. Williams JG, Brown JH, Pleuvry BJ: Alfentanil: a study of its analgesic activity and interactions with morphine in the mouse. Br J Anaesth 54:81–85, 1982

268. Kay B, Pleuvry B: Human volunteer studies of alfentanil (R39209), a new short-acting narcotic analgesic. Anaesthesia 35:952–956, 1980

269. Bovill JG, Sebel PS, Blackburn CL, et al: The pharmacokinetics of alfentanil (R39209). A new opioid analgesic. Anesthesiology 57:439–443, 1982

270. Camu F, Gepts E, Rucquoi M, et al: Pharmacokinetics of alfentanil in man. Anesth Analg 61:657–661, 1982

271. Schuttler J, Stoeckel H: Alfentanil (R39209) a new short action opiate: Pharmacokinetics and preliminary clinical experience. Anaesthetist 31:10–14, 1982

272. Michiels M, Hendriks R, Heykants J: Radioimmunoassay of the new opiate analgesics alfentanil and sufentanil. Pharmacokinetic profile in man. J Pharm Pharmacol 35:86–93, 1983

273. Woestenborghs R, Michielsen L, Heykants J: Rapid and sensitive gas chromatographic method for the determination of alfentanil and sufentanil in biological samples. J Chromatogr 224:122–127, 1981

274. Stanski DR, Hug CC: Alfentanil—a kinetically predictable narcotic analgesic. Anesthesiology 57:435–438, 1982

275. McDonnell TE, Bartkowski RR, Bonilla FA, et al: Nonuniformity of alfentanil pharmacokinetics in healthy adults. Anesthesiology 57:A236, 1982

276. McDonnell TE, Bartkowski RR, Kahn C: Evidence for polymorphic oxidation of alfentanil in man. Anesthesiology 61:A284, 1984

277. Sloan TP, Mahgoub A, Lancaster R, et al: Polymorphism of carbon oxidation of drugs and clinical implications. Br Med J 2:655–657, 1978

278. Fragen RJ, Booij LHDJ, Braak GJJ, et al: Pharmacokinetics of the infusion of alfentanil in man. Br J Anaesth 55:1077–1081, 1983

279. Reitz J, MacKichan JJ, Hoffer L, et al: Reduced plasma clearance of alfentanil associated with prolonged major intra-abdominal surgery. Anesth Analg 63:175–184, 1984

280. Norman J: Editorial. The i.v. administration of drugs. Br J Anaesth 55:1049–1052, 1983

281. Sebel PS, Bovill JG, Lalor JM, et al: Pharmacokinetics of two different infusion regimes of alfentanil. Anesthesiology 63:A371, 1985

282. Wagner JG: A safe method for rapidly achieving plasma concentration plateaux. Clin Pharmacol Ther 16:691–700, 1974

283. Rigg JRA, Wong TY: A method for achieving rapidly steady-state blood concentrations of i.v. drugs. Br J Anaesth 53:1247–1257, 1981

284. Hug CC, de Lange S, Burm AGL: Alfentanil pharmacokinetics in patients before and after cardiopulmonary bypass. Anesth Analg 62:266, 1983

285. de Lange S, de Bruijn NP, Hug CC: Pharmacokinetics of a continuous infusion of alfentanil for coronary artery surgery. Anesthesiology 61:A242, 1984

286. Meistelman C, Saint-Maurice C, Loose JP, et al: Pharmacokinetics of alfentanil in children. Anesthesiology 61:A443, 1984

287. Bently JB, Finley JH, Humphrey LR, et al: Obesity and alfentanil pharmacokinetics. Anesth Analg 62:245–292, 1983

288. Helmers JHJ, Noorduin H, Adam AA, et al: Anaesthesia with alfentanil in the geriatric patient. Anaesthetist 32:228–229, 1983

289. Patrick MR, Eagar BM, Toft DF, et al: Alfentanil supplemented anaesthesia for short procedures: a double blind comparison with fentanyl. Br J Anaesth 56:861–866, 1984

290. Black TE, Kay B, Healy TEJ: Reducing the haemodynamic responses to laryngoscopy and intubation. Anaesthesia 39:883–887, 1984

291. McDonnell TE, Bartkowski RR, Williams JJ: ED_{50} of alfentanil for induction of anesthesia in unpremedicated young adults. Anesthesiology 60:136–140, 1984

292. Nauta J, de Lange S, Koopman D, et al: Anaesthetic induction with alfentanil: A new short-acting narcotic analgesic. Anesth Analg 61:267–272, 1982

293. Nauta J, Stanley TH, de Lange S, et al: Anaesthetic induction with alfentanil: Comparison with thiopental, midazolam and etomidate. Can Anaesth Soc J 30:53–60, 1983

294. Moldenhauer CC, Griesemer RW, Hug CC, et al: Hemodynamic changes during rapid induction of anesthesia with alfentanil. Anesth Analg 62:276, 1983

295. Palazzo MGA, Taylor S, Strunin L: Clinical experience with alfentanil for induction of anaesthesia: A comparison with thiopentone. Can Anaesth Soc J 31:517–522, 1984

296. Sebel PS, Bovill JG, van der Haven A: Cardiovascular effects of alfentanil anaesthesia. Br J Anaesth 54:1185–1190, 1982

297. Lamarch Y, Martin R, Grenier Y: Continuous infusion of alfentanil for surgery. Can Anaesth Soc J 31:564–565, 1984

298. Sebel PS, Lalor JM, Flynn PJ, et al: Respiratory depression after alfentanil infusion. Br Med J 289:1581–1582, 1984

299. Ausems ME, Hug CC, de Lange S: Variable rate infusion of alfentanil as a supplement to nitrous oxide anesthesia for general surgery. Anesth Analg 62:982–986, 1983

300. Ausems ME, Hug CC: Plasma concentrations of alfentanil required to supplement nitrous oxide anaesthesia for lower abdominal surgery. Br J Anaesth 55 (Suppl 2):191S–197S, 1983

301. de Bruijn N, Christian C, Fagraeus L, et al: The effects of alfentanil on global ventricular mechanics. Anesthesiology 59:A33, 1983

302. Berthelsen P, Pedersen J, Strom J, et al: Alfentanil and skeletal muscle circulation, oxygen consumption and P_{50}. Acta Anaesth Scand 28:273–276, 1984

303. Schauble JF, Chen BB, Murray PA: Marked hemodynamic effects of bolus administration of alfentanil in conscious dogs. Anesthesiology 59:A85, 1983

304. Askitopoulou H, Whitwam JG, Sapsed S, et al: Dissociation between the effects of fentanyl and alfentanil on spontaneous and reflexly evoked cardiovascular responses in the dog. Br J Anaesth 55:155–161, 1983

305. de Lange S, Stanley TH, Boscoe MJ: Alfentanil-oxygen anaesthesia for coronary artery surgery. Br J Anaesth 53:1291–1296, 1981

306. de Lange S, de Bruijn NP: Alfentanil-oxygen anaesthesia: Plasma concentrations and clinical effects during variable-rate continuous infusion for coronary artery surgery. Br J Anaesth 55 (Suppl 2):183S–189S, 1983

307. Bovill JG, Warren PJ, Schuller, et al: Comparison of fentanyl, sufentanil, and alfentanil anesthesia in patients undergoing valvular heart surgery. Anesth Analg 63:1081–1086, 1984

308. Spiss CK, Coraim F, Haider W, et al: Haemodynamic effects of fentanyl or alfentanil as adjuvants to etomidate for induction of anaesthesia in cardiac patients. Acta Anaesth Scand 28:554–556, 1984

309. de Lange S, Stanley TH, Boscoe MJ, et al: Catecholamine and cortisol responses to sufentanil-O_2 and alfentanil-O_2 anaesthesia during coronary artery surgery. Can Anaesth Soc J 30:248–254, 1983

310. de Lange S, Boscoe MJ, Stanley TH, et al: Antidiuretic and growth hormone responses during coronary artery surgery with sufentanil-oxygen and alfentanil-oxygen anaesthesia in man. Anesth Analg 61:434–438, 1982

311. Hug CC: Lipid solubility, pharmacokinetics and the EEG: Are you better off today than you were four years ago? Anesthesiology 62:221–226, 1985

312. Van Bever WFM, Niemegeers CJE, Schellekens KHL, et al: N-4 substituted 1-(2-arylethyl)-4-piperidinyl-N-phenylpropanamides, a novel series of extremely potent analgesics with unusually high safety margin. Arzneim Forsch 26:1548–1551, 1976

313. Niemegeers CJE, Schellekens KHL, Van Bever WFM, et al: Sufentanil, a very potent and extremely safe intravenous morphine-like compound in mice, rats and dogs. Arzneim Forsch 26:1551–1556, 1976

314. Hecker BR, Lake CL, DiFazio CA, et al: The decrease of the minimum alveolar anesthetic concentration produced by sufentanil in rats. Anesth Analg 62:987–990, 1983

315. Althaus JS, Miller ED, Moscicki JC, et al: Analgesic contribution of sufentanil during halothane anesthesia. A mechanism involving serotonin. Anesth Analg 64:857–863, 1985

316. Keykhah MM, Smith DS, Carlsson C, et al: Effects of sufentanil on cerebral blood flow and oxygen consumption. Anesthesiology 57:A248, 1982

317. Young ML, Smith DS, Greenberg J, et al: Effects of sufentanil on regional cerebral glucose utilization in rats. Anesthesiology 61:564–568, 1984

318. Eriksen J, Berthelsen P, Ahn NC, et al: Early response in central hemodynamics to high doses of sufentanil or morphine in dogs. Acta Anaesth Scand 25:33–38, 1981

319. Berthelsen P, Strom J, Eriksen J, et al: High-dose analgesic anesthesia with morphine or sufentanil in propranolol-treated dogs. Acta Anaesth Scand 25:447–452, 1981

320. Bovill JG, Sebel PS, Blackburn CL, et al: The pharmacokinetics of sufentanil in surgical patients. Anesthesiology 61:502–506, 1984

321. Sanford TJ, Smith NT, Dec-Silver H, et al: A comparison among morphine, fentanyl and sufentanil anesthesia for open-heart surgery: Induction, emergence and extubation. Anesth Analg 65:259–267, 1986

322. Flacke WE, van Etten AP, Flacke JW, et al: Plasma histamine levels during sufentanil anesthesia for coronary bypass graft surgery. Anesth Analg 62:260–261, 1983

323. Kalenda Z, Scheijgrond HW: Anesthesia with sufentanil-analgesia in carotid and vertebral arteriography. A comparison with fentanyl. Anaesthetist 25:380–383, 1976

324. Rolly G, Kay B, Cockx F: A double blind comparison of high dose fentanyl and sufentanil in man. Influence on cardiovascular, respiratory and metabolic parameters. Acta Anaesthesiol Belg 30:247–254, 1979

325. Van de Walle J, Lauwers P, Adriaensen H: Double blind comparison of fentanyl and sufentanil in anesthesia. Acta Anaesthesiol Belg 27:129–138, 1976

326. Ghoneim MM, Dhanaraj J, Choi WW: Comparison of four opioid analgesics as supplements to nitrous oxide anesthesia. Anesth Analg 63:405–412, 1984

327. Clarke N, Liu WS, Meuleman T, et al: Sufentanil versus fentanyl as a supplement to N_2O anesthesia during general surgery. Anesth Analg 63:175–284, 1984

328. Flacke JW, Bloor BC, Krpke BJ, et al: Comparison of morphine, meperidine, fentanyl and sufentanil in balanced anesthesia: A double-blind study. Anesth Analg 64:897–910, 1985

329. Goldberg M, Ishak S, Garcia C, et al: Postoperative rigidity following sufentanil administration. Anesthesiology 63:199–201, 1985

330. Komatsu T, Shibutani K, Okamoto K, et al: Is sufentanil superior to fentanyl as an induction agent? Anesthesiology 63:A378, 1985

331. Rosow CE, Philbin DM, Moss J, et al: Sufentanil vs. fentanyl: I. Suppression of hemodynamic responses. Anesthesiology 59:A323, 1983

332. Lappas DG, Palacios I, Athanasiadis C, et al: Sufentanil dosage and myocardial blood flow and metabolism in patients with coronary artery disease. Anesthesiology 63:A58, 1985

333. Wellwood M, Teasdale S, Ivanov J, et al: The effects of fentanyl and its analogues (sufentanil and alfentanil) on ventricular function. Anesthesiology 61:A55, 1984

334. Griesemer RW, Moldenhauer CC, Hug CC, et al: Sufentanil anesthesia for aortocoronary bypass surgery: 30 μg/kg vs 15 μg/kg. Anesthesiology 57:A48, 1982

335. Samuelson PN, Reves JG, Kirklin JK, et al: Sufentanil infusion anesthesia in patients undergoing valvular heart surgery. Anesthesiology 63:A74, 1985

336. Hickey PR, Hansen DD: Fentanyl- and sufentanil-oxygen-pancuronium anesthesia for cardiac surgery in infants. Anesth Analg 63:117-124, 1984

337. Moore RA, Yang SS, McNicholas KW, et al: Hemodynamic and anesthetic effects of sufentanil as the sole anesthetic for pediatric cardiovascular surgery. Anesthesiology 62:725-731, 1985

338. Philbin DM, Rosow CE, Moss J, et al: Hormonal responses with fentanyl or sufentanil: A double blind study. Anesth Analg 63:175-284, 1984

339. Zurick AM, Khoury GF, Estafanous FG, et al: Sufentanil requirement of surgical anesthesia (as determined by EEG) and its effect on awakening time. Anesth Analg 62:245-292, 1983

J.G. Reves, M.D.
Paolo Flezzani, M.D.
Igor Kissin, M.D.

4

Pharmacology of Intravenous Anesthetic Induction Drugs

This chapter reviews current information regarding intravenous anesthetics. Emphasis is placed primarily on existing knowledge of cardiovascular pharmacology, and, secondarily, on the pharmacodynamics and pharmacokinetics that are of use to the practicing cardiac anesthesiologist. The chapter is an update of material presented in earlier reviews of the pharmacology of anesthetic drugs.[1,2] New drugs such as diprivan or propofol are discussed and compared with older drugs like ketamine.

There are few studies documenting the effects of cardiac diseases and their variations in cardiac output on the cardiovascular pharmacodynamics of most intravenous anesthetic drugs. The available hemodynamic data for normal patients and for *healthy* patients who have ischemic heart disease are tabulated together. It is valid to categorize the reaction of normal patients together with those who have compensated ischemic heart disease because Slutsky demonstrated almost no differences when these two subgroups are subjected to a variety of physiologic and pharmacologic stresses.[3]

A number of variables influence hemodynamic responses, but their effects are incompletely known and often uncontrolled, ignored, or unreported in the methods of many investigations.[4] Premedication, dose of drug, speed of drug administration, and the

particular disease influence experimental observations. In the discussion of each drug, an attempt has been made to point out any differences in hemodynamic effect caused by the presence of each cardiovascular disease. Unfortunately, investigators group patients only as having congenital, valvular, or ischemic heart disease and seldom distinguish the specific pathology of each disease entity. For example, the difference (if any) of induction with diazepam in patients who have mitral stenosis versus aortic insufficiency is not known. Another important influence on the hemodynamic effect of a drug is the control or baseline experimental conditions. Establishment of baseline values can critically influence the interpretation of hemodynamic data, but there is no consistent definition of the control state among studies. Delineation of the control state is essential, since induction of anesthesia in a calm, comfortable patient may cause only minor hemodynamic alterations, whereas induction in an anxious patient who has been recently *instrumented* in a cold operating room can result in spuriously elevated *control* values that make subsequent drug-associated decreases in hemodynamic variables much more pronounced.[4] It is impossible to correct for these variations in methodology among multiple investigators.

The medications taken by patients preoperatively influence hemodynamic studies as well. Beta-adrenergic blocking drugs and long-acting vasodilators obviously affect the hemodynamics of patients who have heart disease. Another perplexing problem is judging the pharmacologic effect of a drug administered as an intravenous bolus on a patient whose blood and, presumably, cardiac and other tissue levels are decreasing rapidly over time. In this chapter, the effect of a drug is reported as the peak change occurring within 10 minutes of administration. A better assessment of pharmacologic effect of intravenous drugs can be obtained by continuous infusion of the intravenous drug.[5] The duration of the hemodynamic effect is a poorly studied aspect of the clinical pharmacology of intravenous anesthetics. In the literature, the investigative emphasis is on the onset and peak effect rather than on the duration of effect. A final problem with all anesthetic drugs in the intact organism is knowing whether the hemodynamic effects of the drug are a result of the drug itself or secondary to the loss of consciousness. Normal man's hemodynamic values are different during sleep than during the wakeful state; with sleep, mean arterial pressure decreases 9 percent ($p \leq 0.001$), heart rate decreases 8 percent ($p \leq 0.01$), and cardiac output decreases 7 percent ($p \leq 0.01$).[6] Thus, the alteration of consciousness itself is associated with hemodynamic changes that compound those of the anesthetic drugs.

For the most part, the drugs discussed in this chapter are induction agents. They are all hypnotics, but none except ketamine is an analgesic. Therefore, although induction may be accomplished with these drugs, subsequent events such as tracheal intubation (Fig. 4-1) and surgery necessitate administration of other anesthetic drugs. The influence of adjuvant anesthetic drugs on the hemodynamic parameters has been included when the data were available, but this is an area where there remain large gaps in knowledge.

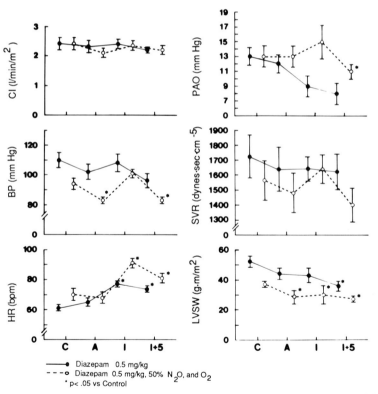

Fig. 4-1. Hemodynamic response (mean ± SDM) of 10 patients anesthetized with diazepam and oxygen and 10 patients anesthetized with diazepam and N_2O/50 percent oxygen. Note that intubation in both groups is associated with a significant elevation in HR. Blood pressure is significantly lower with the addition of N_2O. C = control, A = anesthesia induction, I = intubation, I+5 = intubation plus 5 minutes, PAO = pulmonary artery occluded pressure, LVSW = left ventricular stroke work, CI = cardiac index.

THIOPENTAL

General Characteristics

Thiopental (Pentothal, Abbott Pharmaceuticals, N Chicago, IL) (Fig. 4-2) has survived the test of time as an intravenous anesthetic drug. Since Lundy introduced it in 1934, thiopental has become the most widely used induction agent because of the rapid hypnotic effect (one arm-brain circulation time), highly predictable effect, lack of vascular irritation, and general overall safety.[7] The induction dose of thiopental is lower for older than young healthy patients.[8] Thiopental is biotransformed by the liver and has a relatively low hepatic extraction (25 percent of hepatic blood flow).[9] Recent pharmacokinetic analyses[10-12] confirm the early classic studies of Brodie et al[13] relating the awakening from thiopental to rapid redistribution. Awakening may be delayed in older patients, either because of increased central nervous system (CNS) sensitivity or alterations in metabolism.[14,15] Thiopental has a distribution half-life ($t_{1/2}\alpha$) of 2.5–8.5 minutes, and the total body clearance varies according to sampling times and techniques from 0.15–0.26 liters/kg/hr.[10-12,15,16] The elimination half-life varies from 5 to 12 hours.[10,11,15,16] The young (less than 13 years) patient seems to have a greater total clearance and shorter plasma thiopental clearance than adults, which theoretically might result in earlier awakening, especially after multiple doses.[17]

Because of the affinity of fat for this drug, its relatively large volume of distribution, and its low hepatic clearance, thiopental can accumulate in tissues, especially if given in large doses over a prolonged period of time. Obese patients are likely to have prolonged clearance half-lives of thiopental.[18] Administration by infusion assures relatively constant blood levels, thus maintaining the hypnotic effect with minimal cardiovascular depression.[19] Protein binding is apparently related to the dose of thiopental; the higher the dose, the less the drug binding.[10] This could partially explain the observation that rapid administration of thiopental is more effective than slower administration; however, mass concentration effects and even development of acute tolerance are probably also involved.[20] It is not known if acute tolerance develops to the negative inotropic effects of barbiturates. If not, the clinical implication of acute tolerance is that myocardial depression (which is dose related) may occur if greater doses of thiopental are given to overcome the CNS acute tolerance.

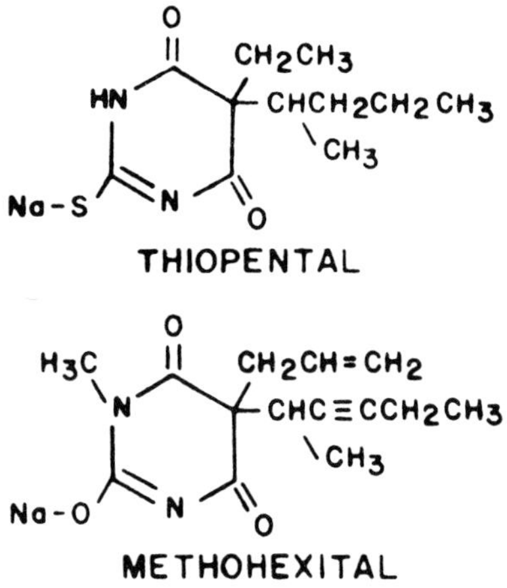

Fig. 4-2. Structural formulae of thiopental and methohexital.

Cardiovascular Effects

The hemodynamic changes produced by thiopental have been studied in normal patients[8,21-27] and in patients who have heart disease[28-33] (Table 4-1). The principal effect is a decrease in contractility,[21,22,34] which is due to reduced availability of calcium to the myofibrils.[35] There is also an increase in heart rate.[8,21-23,26,30,32-34,36] The cardiac index is unchanged[23,28,30,32,33] or reduced,[22,25-27] while the mean blood pressure is maintained[23,24,30,32] or slightly reduced.[25,26,28,30,33,36] Although careful dose-response studies have not been carried out, thiopental infusions and lower doses tend to be accompanied by smaller hemodynamic changes than rapid bolus injections. In the dose range studied, no relationship between plasma thiopental and hemodynamic effect has been found.[8] Early hemodynamic investigations demonstrated that thiopental (100–400 mg) significantly decreased cardiac output (24 percent) and systemic blood pressure (10 percent), presumably by reducing venous return because of an increase in venous capacitance.[25,37] Tracheal intubation after thiopental in normal[26] as well as patients with ischemic heart disease[31,33] is accompanied by marked hypertension and tachycardia. The heart rate (HR) response to intubation can be attenuated by the administration of fentanyl (0.01 mg/kg).[32]

Mechanisms for the decrease in cardiac output include (1) direct negative inotropic action, (2) decreased ventricular filling due to increased capacitance, and (3) transiently decreased sympathetic outflow from the CNS. The increased HR (10–36 percent) that accompanies thiopental administration

Table 4-1
Hemodynamic Changes after Barbiturate Induction

	Thiopental	Methohexital
HR	0 to +36%	+40 to +50%
MBP	−18 to +8%	0 to −10%
SVR	0 to +19%	NR
PAP	Unchanged	NR
PVR	Unchanged	NR
LA/PAO	Unchanged	NR
RAP	0 to +33%	0 to +5%
CI	0 to −24%	0 to −12%
SV	−12 to −35%	NR
LVSWI	0 to −26%	NR
RVSWI	NR	NR
dP/dt	−14%	NR
1/PEP^2	−18 to −28%	NR
References	8,21–28,30–32,34,36,138	48,261,262

HR = heart rate, MBP = mean blood pressure, SVR = systemic vascular resistance, PAP = mean pulmonary artery pressure, PVR = pulmonary vascular resistance, LA/PAO = left atrial or pulmonary artery occluded pressure, RAP = right atrial pressure, CI = cardiac index, SV = stroke volume, LVSWI = left ventricular stroke work index, RVSWI = right ventricular stroke work index, NR = data not reported. All data from normal patients or patients with compensated ischemic heart disease.

probably results from the baroreceptor-mediated sympathetic reflex stimulation of the heart. Thiopental produces dose-related negative inotropic effects that appear to result from a decrease in calcium influx into the cells with a resultant diminished amount of calcium at sarcolemma sites.[38,39] There appears to be little difference in the cardiovascular effects of thiopental in healthy patients versus those who have compensated heart disease. However, a group of patients who had valvular or congenital heart disease and received 4 mg/kg had a greater (18 percent) drop in mean blood pressure than other patients, although the reasons for this were not obvious.[29] The increase in heart rate (11–36 percent) encountered in patients who have coronary artery disease, anesthetized with thiopental, (1–4 mg/kg), is potentially deleterious because of the obligatory increase in myocardial oxygen consumption (MVO_2) that accompanies the increased heart rate.[22,28] Patients who have normal coronary arteries have no difficulty in maintaining adequate coronary blood flow to meet the increased MVO_2;[22] and even patients with ischemic heart disease can maintain normal lactate metabolism with thiopental induction.[36] Despite the well-known potential for cardiovascular depression when given rapidly in large doses, thiopental has minimal hemo-dynamic effects in normal patients and in those who have heart disease when it is given slowly or by infusion. There are no well-documented investigations examining the effects of thiopental in patients who have impaired ventricular function; but significant reductions in cardiovascular parameters in these categories of patients can be predicted. When thiopental is given to hypovolemic patients, there is a significant reduction in cardiac output (69 percent), as well as an important decrease in blood pressure, indicating that patients without adequate compensatory mechanisms may have serious hemodynamic depression with a thiopental induction.[40] This probably explains the disastrous results of thiopental administration at Pearl Harbor.[41] Clearly, thiopental produces greater reductions in blood pressure and heart rate than diazepam when used for induction of ASA class III-IV patients (see diazepam section).

Uses

Thiopental can be used safely for the induction of anesthesia in normal patients and in those who have compensated heart disease. Because of the negative inotropic effects, increased venous capacitance, and dose-related decrease in cardiac output, thiopental should be given cautiously to patients who have left or right ventricular failure, cardiac tamponade, or hypovolemia. The development of tachycardia is a potential problem in patients with ischemic heart disease who are anesthetized with thiopental. No intravenous drug surpasses thiopental, however, as the drug of choice for the induction of anesthesia in fit patients for short procedures. A possible additional use for thiopental infusion is cerebral protection during cardiopulmonary bypass in patients having valvular (open) heart operations.[42] This use may result in myocardial depression requiring additional inotropic support.

METHOHEXITAL

General Characteristics

Methohexital (Brevital, Eli Lilly and Co., Indianapolis, IN) (Fig. 4-2) is an ultra-short–acting methylbarbiturate. It is approximately three times more potent than thiopental and has similar actions and uses. The pharmacokinetics of methohexital have been compared to thiopental in surgical patients.[43] The two barbiturates exhibit a similar distribution half-life, volume of distribution, and protein binding.[44] However, a marked difference exists in elimination half-lives (4 hours for methohexital versus up to 12 hours for thiopental). This difference is due to a threefold increase in the hepatic clearance of methohexital, which explains the more rapid recovery of consciousness. In spite of earlier awakening, the length of time for complete psychomotor recovery does not appear to be different when compared with thiopental.[45]

Cardiovascular Effects

Early claims of less cardiovascular depression with methohexital than with thiopental have not been confirmed.[46] There is little doubt that the cardiovascular depression in patients who have cardiac disease is equal when methohexital or thiopental is administered in equipotent doses.[29,47] In noncardiac patients, methohexital causes a small decrease in cardiac output and a compensatory increase in HR (Table 4-1). The significant increase in HR with methohexital was less than with propanidid, but more than when either althesin or etomidate was used.[48] In hypertensive patients, methohexital caused a greater fall in arterial pressure than did thiopental.[49]

Uses

Methohexital is the only intravenous barbiturate that offers a serious difference from thiopental.[50] It is generally used when early ambulation of patients is required, but appears to have no cardiovascular advantages over thiopental.

DIAZEPAM

General Characteristics

Diazepam (Valium, Roche Laboratories, Nutney, NJ) (Fig. 4-3) is probably the most widely used 1,4-benzodiazepine in the world. Synthesized by Leo H. Steinbach in 1959, diazepam was introduced in the United States in 1963. The presumed mechanism of action of diazepam and other benzodiazepines in the CNS is by potentiation of the inhibitory effect of gamma-amino-butyric acid (GABA) on neuronal transmission.[51] All benzodiazepines have hypnotic, anticonvulsant, muscle relaxant, amnesic, and anxiolytic neuropharmacologic properties.

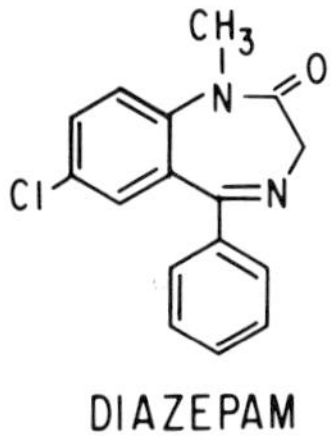

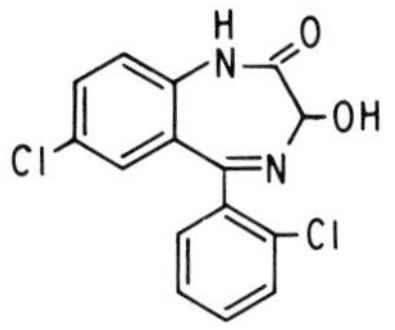

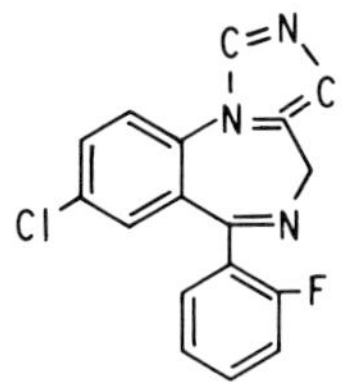

Fig. 4-3. Structural formulas of midazolam, diazepam, and lorazepam.

The biotransformation and pharmacokinetics of diazepam are well known.[52-54] The plasma level of diazepam is a predictor of therapeutic effect.[55] Biotransformed in the liver, diazepam is demethylated to form the active metabolite, desmethyl-diazepam (Nordiazepam), and hydroxylated to form methyloxazepam, which is demethylated to form another active metabolite, oxazepam (Serax, Wyeth Laboratories, Philadelphia, PA).[53] The important pharmacokinetic variables of diazepam are listed in Table 4-2. Of note is diazepam's relatively long $t_{1/2}\alpha$ of 30–66 minutes, suggesting a slow distribution half-life as compared to other benzodiazepines, and, indeed, to most drugs used for induction of anesthesia.[52-54] The elimination $t_{1/2}$ of diazepam is also relatively long at 24–57 hours in normal subjects. The $t_{1/2}\beta$ is longer than that of lorazepam and midazolam, and is even more prolonged by liver disease,[56] older age,[52] and obesity.[57] Diazepam is highly protein bound (96–99 percent), which may account for its moderate volume of distribution (Vd = 0.7–1.7 liter/kg). Clearance of diazepam ranges from 0.24 to 0.53 ml/kg/min in healthy subjects, but clearance of the unbound fraction decreases with age.[52,58] The primary active metabolite of diazepam, desmethyldiazepam, has an extremely long elimination $t_{1/2}$ (41–139 hours),[59-65] and both diazepam and desmethyldiazepam accumulate with chronic ingestion of diazepam. If diazepam is administered during anesthesia to a patient taking it on a chronic basis, higher blood levels will be attained than if there were no previous usage. Also of clinical importance is the administration of diazepam in combination with cimetidine,[66] an hepatic enzyme inhibitor that prolongs plasma clearance of diazepam and extends the hypnotic effect. The administration of heparin significantly increases the free (active) plasma diazepam level as well;[67] this may be important for patients on cardiopulmonary bypass. Whether administration of heparin and other drugs that displace diazepam (or other highly protein-

bound drugs) from protein produces clinically important elevation of the free drug fraction is unknown.

Cardiovascular Effects

The hemodynamic effects of diazepam have been investigated in normal man,[68,69] in patients who have a variety of cardiac disease,[70-84] and in large series of ASA class III and IV patients.[85,86] These studies include sedative doses[70,74,87,88] and doses necessary for induction of anesthesia.[68,69,71,72,75-80,85,86,89] A summary of the reported cardiovascular effects of anesthetic induction with diazepam is presented in Table 4-3. A characteristic of induction with diazepam is hemodynamic stability (Fig. 4-1). Filling pressures and cardiac index remain unchanged,[68,75,76,78-80] with variable but modest changes in heart rate.[68,71,75,76,78-80] Hemodynamic changes do not appear to be dose related, but there are no studies that examine this question. However, if separate studies are used for comparison, for example, in patients who have coronary artery disease given diazepam 0.1 mg/kg[87] or 0.5 mg/kg,[80] there are similar decreases in mean arterial blood pressure of 7 and 18 percent, respectively, and no significant changes in HR, cardiac index (CI), systemic vascular resistance (SVR), stroke index (SI), and left ventricular stroke work index (LVSWI), despite the fivefold difference in dose. Likewise, in an investigation of 60 patients who primarily had valvular heart disease, doses of 0.21, 0.46, and 0.66 mg/kg given over 20 seconds each caused almost identical changes in mean blood pressure and heart rate.[77] The speed of injection does not alter the hemodynamic effect of the induction dose of diazepam (0.5 mg/kg);[90] and there are no differences in hemodynamic effects whether diazepam is given as a bolus (5 seconds) or as a slow infusion (over 10 minutes).

Diazepam's hemodynamic stability makes it suitable as an induction agent in patients who have

Table 4-2

Benzodiazepines: Pharmacokinetic Variables

	Diazepam	Lorazepam	Midazolam
$t_{1/2}\alpha$ (min)	30–66	3–10	6–15
$t_{1/2}\beta$ (hr)	24–57*	14	1.7–2.6
Vd (liters/kg)	0.7–1.7	1.14–1.3	1.1–1.7
Clearance (ml/kg/min)	0.24–0.53	1.05–1.1	6.4–11.1
Protein binding (percent)	96–99	86–93	97
Infusion	No	Yes	?
Active metabolites	Yes	No	No

*Prolonged by liver disease and in elderly. See text for references.

Table 4-3
Hemodynamic Changes after Benzodiazepine Induction

	Diazepam	Lorazepam	Midazolam
HR	−9 to +13%	Unchanged	−14 to +21%
MBP	0 to −19%	−7 to −20%	−12 to −26%
SVR	−22 to +13%	−10 to −35%	0 to −20%
PAP	0 to −10%		Unchanged
PVR	0 to −19%	Unchanged	Unchanged
LA/PAO	Unchanged		0 to −25%
RAP	Unchanged		Unchanged
CI	Unchanged	0 to +16%	0 to −25%
SV	0 to −8%		0 to −18%
LVSWI	0 to −36%		−28 to −42%
RVSWI	0 to −21%		−41 to −57%
dP/dt	Unchanged		0 to −12%
References	68, 71, 75–80, 82, 88	117	26, 80, 138, 139 141–143

HR = heart rate, MBP = mean blood pressure, SVR = systemic vascular resistance, PAP = pulmonary artery pressure, PVR = pulmonary vascular resistance, LA/PAO = left atrial/pulmonary artery occluded pressures, RAP = right atrial pressure, CI = cardiac index, SV = stroke volume, LVSWI = left ventricular stroke work index, RVSWI = right ventricular stroke work index.

ischemic heart disease; there are additional data that demonstrate a nitroglycerin-like effect as well.[87] In the study by Cote et al involving ischemic heart disease, diazepam (0.1 mg/kg) produced a significant reduction in left ventricular end-diastolic pressure (LVEDP), but preserved coronary blood flow and CI in spite of a decrease in systemic perfusion pressure; hence the analogy to nitroglycerin.[87] As with nitroglycerin, diazepam appears to have peripheral arterial and venous effects, unrelated to autonomic nervous system effects.[88] Using the same small dose, other investigators reported an increase in coronary artery blood flow of 73 percent in patients who have ischemic heart disease.[74] Total myocardial oxygen consumption after administration of diazepam is significantly reduced,[87] as would be expected from the abundant studies that show significant decreases in the heart rate-systolic blood pressure product. The cause of these hemodynamic effects is not entirely clear.[2] Diazepam reduces blood levels of circulating catecholamines,[91,92] but there may be other mechanisms responsible for the hemodynamic changes, such as activation of postganglionic sites that control vasoactivity.[93] It is likely that with regard to patients who have ischemic heart disease, the advantage of diazepam is related to a decrease in myocardial oxygen consumption rather than to an increase in blood supply to ischemic regions.

The hemodynamic effects of diazepam have been investigated in patients who have valvular heart disease[70–73,76,77] and elevated filling pressures.[87] In general, the hemodynamic changes are slight in patients with valvular heart disease. Heart rate has been variably decreased by 9 percent,[71] increased by 10 percent, or unchanged[76,77] in patients given diazepam (0.3–0.4 mg/kg). Patients who have valvular heart disease demonstrated no[72,76] or relatively small (15–19 percent)[71,77] reductions in mean arterial blood pressure and no change in cardiac index.[71,76] Since diazepam has negligible effects on contractility in man,[82] and has been demonstrated to reduce elevation of LVEDP in patients who have coronary artery disease,[89] it appears to be a safe and efficacious drug in patients who have valvular heart disease with poor ventricular function. In patients who have mitral valvular disease and pulmonary hypertension, infusion of diazepam, 0.4 mg/kg over 15 minutes reduced the pulmonary artery pressure (PAP) from 47 to 43 mm Hg ($p < 0.05$) and the pulmonary vascular resistance (PVR) from 909 to 820 dynes · sec · cm^{-5}; cardiac output was maintained.[71] A large investigation of ASA class III and IV patients reported in part (400 patients)[85] and in full (800 patients),[86] established the hemodynamic superiority of diazepam over thiopental for induction of anesthesia. In those patients who are undergoing noncardiac surgery, cardiovascular stability (maintenance of blood pressure and cardiac output) was maintained with diazepam (0.2 mg/kg IV) as compared to thiopental, 2 mg/kg. When anesthesia was induced with thiopental, cardiac output decreased by greater than or equal to 15 percent in 85 percent of patients, whereas only 0.75 percent of patients anesthetized with diazepam had a decrease in cardiac output of greater than or equal to 15 percent.[86] Diazepam (0.3 mg/kg) is not as well tolerated as ketamine (1.0 mg/kg) when given to patients with constrictive pericarditis; indeed, in 3 of 10 patients given diazepam serious reductions in cardiac output and hypotension occurred.[83] Presumably, the vasodilation with diazepam caused a reduction in cardiac filling (reflected by a decrease in right atrial pressure [RAP] from 19 to 13 mm Hg).

Although diazepam may be safely combined with other anesthetic drugs, there is some potential for hemodynamic depression.[94] The effect of the combination of diazepam and morphine in patients who have ischemic heart disease (IHD)[91,92] and valvular heart disease[73] has been reported. Administration of diazepam, 0.25–0.35 mg/kg, over 10 minutes to patients who have IHD anesthetized with morphine, 3 mg/kg, did not change HR, pulmonary capillary wedge pressure (PCWP), PAP, PVR, or SVR and produced modest decreases in mean arterial blood pressure (84–73 mg Hg) and cardiac index (2.91–2.36 liters/min/m²). Fentanyl and diazepam may exert a slightly more depressant effect together than alone. Addition of diazepam (10 mg) to patients who have mitral valvular disease anesthetized with fentanyl (up to 50 μg/kg) produced mild but statistically significant hemodynamic depression of cardiac output (21 percent), mean blood pressure (10 percent), and stroke volume (17 percent), while heart rate was unchanged.[95] In another investigation by Tomichek et al, the combination of diazepam (0.125–0.5 mg/kg) and fentanyl (50 μg/kg) was used to induce anesthesia in patients for coronary artery surgery.[96] This combination appeared to depress the cardiovascular system more than either agent alone. Patients who received diazepam before fentanyl showed significant decreases in mean blood pressure and systemic vascular resistance with fentanyl administration. The exact mechanism of this interaction is unclear, but it appears that diazepam may ablate the normal sympathetic tone.[96,97] This mechanism seems to be likely since dogs rendered devoid of sympathetic and parasympathetic tone do not manifest the hemodynamic interaction seen with fentanyl and diazepam.[97] The combination of diazepam with alfentanil or sufentanil also produces vasodilation and hypotension.[98] Induction of anesthesia with the combination of diazepam and 50 percent N_2O in oxy-

gen produces hemodynamic changes similar to those with induction with diazepam alone. The only difference is that N_2O causes a greater decrease in mean arterial blood pressure and LVSWI, which are unchanged with diazepam alone and decreased with N_2O (Fig. 4-1).[79,80]

Uses

Diazepam is used for induction of anesthesia in patients who have multiorgan system disease, as well as those who have heart disease. The relatively prolonged plasma clearance of diazepam means that large doses may produce significant CNS and respiratory depression for a number of hours. The amnesic action prevents recall and facilitates the use of 100 percent oxygen in patients in whom other drugs cause unacceptable cardiovascular depression. It is the practice of some cardiac anesthesiologists to induce anesthesia in adult patients who have congenital, valvular, and ischemic heart disease with diazepam in doses of 0.3–0.5 mg/kg over 5–15 seconds.[79,80] Adjuvant anesthetic and cardiovascular drugs are given to maintain anesthesia, to produce muscle relaxation, and to stabilize hemodynamics in the desired range.[99] Hypovolemia and cardiac tamponade are relative contraindications to the use of diazepam because of the potential for hypotension and further reduction in cardiac output. Diazepam may be better than other benzodiazepines, however, with regard to the maintenance of SVR (Table 4-3).

Undesirable features of induction with diazepam are pain on injection, a significant incidence of thrombophlebitis (which increases with age), variability of response among individual patients, the long half-life, and the tendency for accumulation of the drug with repeated administration in elderly patients and those who have liver disease. The marked hemodynamic stability, amnesic properties, and smooth induction, however, make it a preferred drug for the induction of anesthesia in many cardiac surgical patients.

LORAZEPAM

General Characteristics

Lorazepam (Ativan, Wyeth Laboratories, Philadelphia, PA) (Fig. 4-3) is a 3-hydroxy-1,4-benzodiazepine derivative extensively used as a sedative, hypnotic, and antianxiety agent. These clinical effects make lorazepam an effective premedication.

Lorazepam is a water-soluble compound,

promptly absorbed when given orally, sublingually, and parenterally.[100] Lorazepam is biotransformed by direct conjugation to glucoronic acid, yielding a water-soluble metabolite that is excreted in the urine.[101] No active metabolites have been identified. This metabolic pathway allows the elimination of lorazepam to be independent of age, drug interaction, or renal disease.[102-109] Liver cirrhosis reduces plasma protein binding and prolongs the elimination half-life significantly, but acute viral hepatitis does not change lorazepam pharmacokinetics.[108] The clinical pharmacokinetics of lorazepam are reported in Table 4-2.[100,110] The institution of cardiopulmonary bypass causes a rapid drop in the plasma concentration of lorazepam, probably because of increased dilution and decreased protein binding. After termination of cardiopulmonary bypass, there is a rapid increase in plasma concentration, and the elimination half-life appears to be unchanged from that of nonbypass patients or healthy volunteers.[111]

Cardiovascular Effects

The hemodynamic effects of lorazepam as a premedication have been investigated in healthy volunteers and in patients (ASA I-II) undergoing minor surgery.[112,113] In healthy volunteers, lorazepam in doses ranging from 2.5 to 7.5 mg p.o. did not change HR, cardiac output, or SVR, while causing a dose-related increase in hypnotic states.[113] Lorazepam given orally the night before surgery or parenterally 2 hours prior to surgery did not change hemodynamics.[114-116] Although no human data are yet available, lorazepam shares with diazepam the ability to potentiate the coronary vasodilating effect of adenosine, although it does so to a lesser extent. However, unlike diazepam, lorazepam does not potentiate the negative inotropic effect of adenosine.[112] In patients undergoing coronary artery revascularization, lorazepam, given as a computer-controlled continuous infusion aimed to achieve a central compartment concentration equivalent to 0.1 mg/kg, and in combination with high-dose fentanyl, caused a decrease in mean arterial pressure (MAP) (7–20 percent) and SVR (10–35 percent), with an increase in CO (2–16 percent), ensuring good overall hemodynamic stability (Table 4-3).[117]

Uses

The clinical and pharmacokinetic characteristics of lorazepam make it an excellent premedication. Water solubility, reliable parenteral absorption, short redistribution half-life, and lack of pain or burning upon intramuscular or intravenous injection represent some of the major features.[116] Lorazepam provides good sedation and amnesia, devoid of cardiovascular or respiratory side effects. Its metabolic profile makes it a suitable drug in a patient with impaired liver or renal function. Lorazepam is not commonly used as an induction agent, but it may be used safely and combined with fentanyl.[117] Its characteristics make lorazepam a valuable alternative to diazepam. However, midazolam, in view of its shorter elimination half-life, might be more advantageous when a short, more predictable duration of action is required.

MIDAZOLAM

General Characteristics

Midazolam (Versed, Dormicum) (Fig. 4-3), a water-soluble benzodiazepine, was synthesized in the United States in 1975, in contrast to most new anesthetic drugs, which are synthesized and first tested in European countries. It is unique among benzodiazepines with its rapid onset and short duration of action and relatively rapid plasma clearance.[118] Although controversial, the dose for induction of general anesthesia is between 0.2 and 0.4 mg/kg and depends on the premedication and speed of injection.[119-122] Midazolam is biotransformed in the liver to four known metabolites, all believed to be inactive and short-lived in the plasma.[123]

The pharmacokinetic variables of midazolam reveal that it is cleared significantly more rapidly than diazepam and lorazepam, the other two benzodiazepines commonly used in anesthesia (Table 4-2). The distribution half-life is also brief (6–15 minutes).[124-127] The rapid redistribution of midazolam, as well as high liver clearance, account for its relatively short hypnotic and hemodynamic effects. The elimination half-life is about 2 hours, which is at least 10-fold less than for diazepam.[124-128] The reason for the relatively short $t_{1/2}\beta$ of midazolam is its high total body clearance, which exceeds that of other benzodiazepines.[54] As with other benzodiazepines, however, older patients have a prolonged $t_{1/2}\beta$.[129-131] Major operations also seem to lengthen the $t_{1/2}\beta$ of midazolam.[130] There is a good association between plasma level and therapeutic effect.[132,133] The volume of distribution of midazolam is similar to that of diazepam (0.60–1.7 liters/kg),[124,126,127,134] but is increased in obese subjects.[129] The protein binding resembles that of most other benzodiazepines (greater than 95 percent).[54] The short plasma half-life of midazolam indicates the need for development of a method of administration by infusion to maintain plasma levels for long surgical procedures and for sedation in the intensive care unit. Midazolam may be administered intravenously, orally,[128,129,132,133] or intramuscularly.[127,134] The intramuscular absorption of midazolam is reliable.[135,136]

Cardiovascular Effects

The hemodynamic effects of midazolam have been investigated in normal subjects,[26,136,137] ASA class III patients,[138] and in patients who have ischemic[80,139-145] and valvular[138] heart disease. A summary of the hemodynamic changes after induction of anesthesia with midazolam is presented in Table 4-3. In general, there are only small hemodynamic changes after the intravenous administration of midazolam (0.2 mg/kg) in premedicated patients who have ischemic heart disease.[80,143] Changes of potential importance include a decrease in MAP of 20 percent (from 102 to 81 mm Hg)[143] and an increase in HR of 15 percent (from 55 to 64 beats per minute).[143] The cardiac index is maintained, as are SVR and PVR.[80,143] Filling pressures are either unchanged or decreased in patients who have normal ventricular function,[80,143] but are significantly decreased in patients who have an elevated PCWP (greater than or

equal to 18 mm Hg).[144] There seems to be little effect of differences in dose on hemodynamics since 0.2,[80] 0.25[139] and 0.3 mg/kg[142] all produce similar effects. Sedation with midazolam (0.05 mg/kg) in patients undergoing cardiac catheterization is devoid of any hemodynamic effect.[145] Marty et al recently showed that induction with 0.2 mg/kg produced a 24 percent reduction in coronary blood flow and a 26 percent reduction in myocardial oxygen consumption.[141] As in patients with ischemic heart disease, the induction of anesthesia in patients with valvular heart disease is associated with minimal changes in CI, HR, and MAP after midazolam.[145] When intubation follows anesthesia induction with midazolam, significant increases in HR and blood pressure occur since midazolam is not an analgesic.[26,80,140,142] Adjuvant analgesic drugs are required to block the response to noxious stimuli.

The biggest difference between midazolam and diazepam in terms of hemodynamic effects is the slightly greater decrease in MAP that occurs 4–5 minutes after administration of midazolam (Fig. 4-4).[80] Although CI and SVR remain unchanged, it is possible that midazolam exerts a slightly more negative inotropic effect than diazepam, compensated for by changes in heart rate and filling pressure. In laboratory animals, there is a dose-related decrease in dP/dt MAX with both midazolam and diazepam.[146,147] In humans given midazolam, decreases in

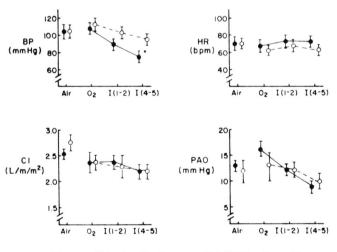

Where ● = Midazolam, O = Diazepam, *P < .05 Midazolam vs Diazepam

Fig. 4-4. Hemodynamic variables in patients with ischemic heart disease anesthetized with midazolam (0.2 mg/kg IV) and diazepam (0.5 mg/kg IV). HR = heart rate, BP = mean blood pressure, CI = cardiac index, PAO = pulmonary artery occluded pressure. Determinations were made breathing room air (air), breathing 100 percent oxygen (O₂), 1 to 2 minutes after induction (I [1–2]), and 4 to 5 minutes after induction (I [4–5]).

LVSWI[80,143] and SI[80,143] may reflect decreases in myocardial contractility and/or decreases in PCWP.[80] In unanesthetized animals, a 40-fold increase in dose (beginning with the subanesthetic dosage of 0.25 mg/kg) causes few reductions in hemodynamic parameters, indicating midazolam's large margin of safety.[147,148] However, in hypovolemic dogs, midazolam produces greater hypotension than during normovolemia.[146,147]

There is a suggestion that midazolam affects the capacitance vessels more than does diazepam, at least during cardiopulmonary bypass, when decreases in venous reservoir volume of the pump are greater with midazolam than with diazepam. In addition, diazepam decreases SVR more than midazolam during cardiopulmonary bypass.[149] The hemodynamic changes after thiopental and midazolam in normal patients are generally similar; both produce decreases in blood pressure and increases in HR,[26,139] but cardiac output is maintained after midazolam, whereas it decreases with thiopental.[138]

Relatively little is known about interactions between midazolam and other drugs. Premedication with morphine and scopolamine decreases induction time.[150] The combination of N_2O (50 percent) with midazolam (0.2 mg/kg) does not cause increased cardiovascular depression.[80] The safe combination of N_2O and midazolam contrasts to the well-known additive depression of N_2O and narcotic agents.[151,152] Midazolam and halothane together are well tolerated,[153] and midazolam (0.15 mg/kg) and ketamine (1.5 mg/kg) have proved to be a safe and useful combination for a rapid-sequence induction for emergency surgery.[24] This was superior to thiopental alone, since it caused less cardiovascular depression, more amnesia, and less postoperative somnolence. If midazolam is given to patients who have received fentanyl, significant hypotension may occur, as seen with diazepam and fentanyl.[96] Administration of midazolam (either 0.075 or 0.15 mg/kg) to patients receiving an infusion of fentanyl (75 μg/kg) produces marked hypotension; thus, the combination of this benzodiazepine with fentanyl must be used with caution.[16]

Uses

Midazolam is distinctly different from the available benzodiazepines because of its rapid onset, short duration, water solubility, and lack of significant thrombophlebitis. Due to its rapid onset and hemodynamic stability, it may be used for emergency induction of anesthesia and sedation of poor-risk patients, and is ideal for such short procedures as cardioversion, cardiac catheterization, and endoscopy. For use in longer operations, the duration of midazolam must be extended by repeated administration, continuous infusion, or combination with other anesthetic drugs. Since midazolam is devoid of analgesic properties, it must be supplemented with analgesic compounds to attenuate hemodynamic responses to stresses like intubation and incision. Because of good absorption by the oral and intramuscular routes, midazolam will be an excellent premedicant. Its use in hypovolemic patients has not been evaluated and should be cautious because of the potential for decreases in blood pressure. Midazolam is useful whenever the neuropharmacologic properties of a benzodiazepine are required rapidly and for a relatively brief period of time. Development of methods of administration by infusion will extend the usefulness of midazolam for longer procedures.

ETOMIDATE

General Characteristics

Etomidate (Hypnomidate, Janssen Pharmaceutica, Belgium; Amidate, Abbott Pharmaceutical, N Chicago, IL) is a carboxylated imidazole derivative (Fig. 4-5) synthesized by Godefroi in 1965.[154] In

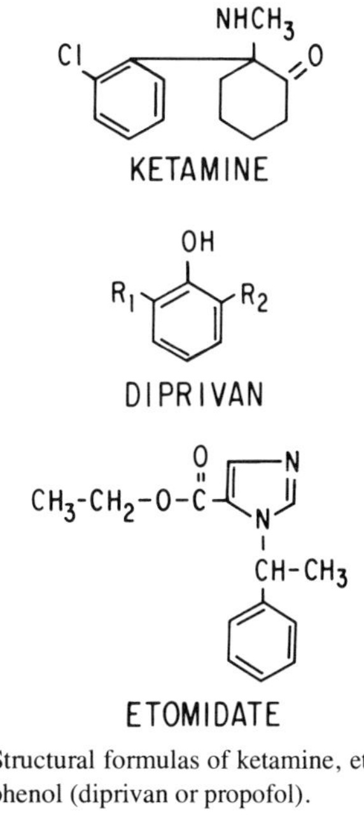

Fig. 4-5. Structural formulas of ketamine, etomidate, and diisopropylphenol (diprivan or propofol).

animal experiments, it was found that etomidate has a safety margin (SM) four times greater than the SM for thiopental.[155] The recommended induction dose of 0.3 mg/kg has pronounced hypnotic effects. Etomidate is moderately lipid soluble[156] and has a rapid onset (10–12 seconds) and brief duration of action.[157-159] It is hydrolyzed primarily in the liver and in the blood as well.[160] The hepatic clearance is extensive, about 50 percent of hepatic blood flow at a rate of about 15 percent of total drug per hour.[161] The metabolites are inactive.[44,162]

Pharmacokinetic investigations reveal that etomidate is rapidly distributed, with a $t_{1/2}\alpha$ of 2.6–2.8 minutes, intermediate $t_{1/2}$ of 28–32 minutes and elimination $t_{1/2}$ of 2.0–4.6 hours.[161,163,164] The rapid and extensive redistribution is reflected by the relatively large apparent volume of distribution (5 liters/kg).[161,163] Etomidate has a relatively low degree of serum albumin binding (77 percent),[165] compared with most hypnotic drugs (greater than or equal to 90 percent). The very short duration of hypnotic effect of etomidate is probably a result of its rapid distribution in peripheral tissue. To maintain sustained plasma levels of etomidate, constant infusions have been employed,[166] without evidence of accumulation.[167] Etomidate's pharmacokinetics can be modified by the concomitant infusion of fentanyl[168] and by the presence of liver disease. It should be emphasized that if large doses are used during constant infusion, etomidate will accumulate since the elimination $t_{1/2}$ is about 5 hours.

The administration of etomidate in a buffered solution was accompanied by a significant incidence of burning (about 40 percent) and myoclonic movements (about 40–50 percent).[157] The myoclonic movements were not associated with an epileptiform pattern on the electroencephalogram (EEG).[156] Pain at the site of intravenous administration from the buffered formulation was reduced by using larger veins, giving the drug slowly, and selecting an analgesic as premedication.[157] The new formulation of etomidate contains 35% propylene glycol (PPG) as the solvent; this appears to have reduced the incidence of both venous pain on injection (10 percent) and myoclonic movements (10–35 percent).[159,169] However, the incidence of thrombophlebitis (18 percent) remains higher than with many other drugs.[170,171] None of these complications is sufficiently severe, however, to prohibit the use of etomidate.

Recent reports have shown that etomidate infusions and single injections directly suppress adrenal cortical function which, in turn, interferes with the normal stress response. The time course and clinical significance of this effect are still under investigation.[172-174] There is an indication that ascorbinic acid can increase cortisol synthesis inhibited by etomidate administration.[175]

Cardiovascular Effects

In comparative studies with other anesthetic drugs, etomidate is usually described as the drug that changes hemodynamic variables the least.[48,169,176-180] Studies in normal patients[48,177-182] and those who have heart disease[30,169,176,179,183,184] document the remarkable hemodynamic stability after administration of etomidate. Hemodynamic changes with etomidate anesthesia are shown in Table 4-4. In normal subjects or patients who have compensated IHD, HR, PAP, PCWP, LVEDP, RAP, CI, SVR, PVR, dP/dt, and systolic time intervals (STI) are not significantly changed after dosages of 0.15–0.30 mg/kg.[30,169,180,182,184] Compared with other anesthetics, etomidate produces the least change in the balance of myocardial oxygen demand and supply (Fig. 4-6). Systemic blood pressure remains unchanged in most series,[48,169,176,178-180] but may be decreased 10–19 percent[179,181,183] in patients who have valvular heart disease. Ammon et al found a modest dose-related decrease in MAP and LVSWI.[169] Doses of 0.3, 0.45, and 0.6 mg/kg caused greater decreases in mean blood pressure (MBP) and LVSWI, but had no effect on HR, PAP, PCWP, CVP, CI, SV, or SVR. Therefore, although there is a small dose-related effect on hemodynamics, the remarkable fact is that there is hemodynamic stability despite the twofold increase in dose. Dose-related changes have been demonstrated in the dog and were attributed to three possible causes: (1) Decreased CNS sympathetic stimulation, (2) autoregulation secondary to decreased regional O_2 consumption, and (3) decreased SV secondary to reduced venous return.[185] A dose-dependent direct negative inotropic effect of etomidate was demonstrated in dogs, although at equianesthetic doses it was half as pronounced as that of thiopental.[186]

Etomidate (0.3 mg/kg IV), used to induce general anesthesia in patients with acute myocardial infarction anesthetized to undergo percutaneous coronary angioplasty, did not alter HR, MAP, and rate pressure product (RPP), demonstrating the remarkable hemodynamic stability of this agent.[187] However, the presence of valvular heart disease may influence the hemodynamic responses to etomidate. Whereas most patients can maintain their blood pressure, patients with both aortic and mitral valvular

Table 4-4
Hemodynamic Changes after Induction with Nonbarbiturate Hypnotics

	Etomidate	Diisopropylphenol	Ketamine
HR	0 to +22%		0 to 59%
MBP	0 to −20%	−20 to 31%	0 to +40%
SVR	0 to −17%	−17%	0 to +33%
PAP	0 to −17%		+44 to +47%
PVR	0 to +27%		0 to +33%
LVEDP/PAO	0 to −11%		Unchanged
RAP	Unchanged		+15 to +33%
CI	0 to +14%	−27 to 29%	0 to +42%
SV	0 to −15%		0 to −21%
LVSWI	0 to −27%		0 to +27%
dP/dt	0 to −18%		Unchanged
STI	Unchanged		NR
References	48, 168–169, 177, 179	260	200–202, 204 216, 217

HR = heart rate, MBP = mean blood pressure, SVR = systemic vascular resistance, PAP = mean pulmonary artery pressure, PVR = pulmonary vascular resistance, LVEDP/PAO = left ventricular end-diastolic pressure or pulmonary artery occluded pressure, RAP = right atrial pressure, CI = cardiac index, SV = stroke volume, LVSWI = left ventricular stroke work index, STI = systolic time interval, NR = unreported data. All data from normal patients or patients with compensated ischemic heart disease.

heart disease had significant decreases of 17–19 percent in systolic and diastolic blood pressure,[179,183] and decreases of 11 and 17 percent in PAP and PCWP, respectively.[183] Cardiac index in patients who had valvular heart disease and received 0.3 mg/kg either remained unchanged[179] or decreased 13 percent.[183] There was no difference in response to etomidate between patients who had aortic valve disease and those who had mitral valve disease.[183]

The cardiovascular effects of etomidate are not significantly altered by the simultaneous administration of other anesthetic drugs, although this has not been systemically studied with all drugs. The administration of 66% N_2O in oxygen has little effect on

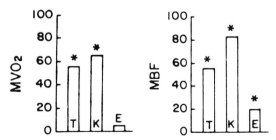

Fig. 4-6. The composite changes in global myocardial oxygen consumption (MVO_2) and myocardial blood flow (MBF) measured after thiopental (T), ketamine (K), and etomidate (E). All data from Sonntag and Kettler.[22,179,209]

changes after induction with etomidate,[177] nor does the presence of basal neuroleptanesthesia (except possibly on contractility). Etomidate (0.3 mg/kg) reduced dP/dt by 18 percent in patients anesthetized with neurolept drugs,[176] and, in cardiac patients anesthetized with fentanyl and alfentanil, decreases were seen in CI (4–17 percent), HR (17–20 percent), SVR (14 percent), MAP (20 percent), and PAP (4–17 percent).[188] In both coronary artery patients and valvular heart disease patients, the association of etomidate and narcotics showed a relatively small margin of safety.[189,190] Systemic blood pressure decreased 14 percent, systemic vascular resistance decreased 17 percent, and dP/dt decreased 9 percent when etomidate (0.3 mg/kg) was given to normal patients anesthetized with 0.3% halothane in 66% N_2O/O_2.[178] Wauquier et al anticipated the widespread clinical use of etomidate in their investigation comparing the effects of etomidate and thiopental in hypovolemic dogs.[191] In a hemorrhagic shock model, dogs were bled to a MAP of 40–45 mm Hg and then given either etomidate (1 mg/kg) or thiopental (10 mg/kg). There was significantly more hemodynamic depression in the thiopental group and increased survival in the etomidate group. Whether this is true in humans is not known, but certainly clinical evidence suggests that etomidate might be useful in hypovolemic patients.

Uses

There are certain situations in which the advantages of etomidate outweigh the disadvantages. Emergency uses include situations in which rapid induction is essential. Patients who have hypovolemia, cardiac tamponade, or low cardiac output probably represent the population for whom etomidate is better than other drugs, with the possible exception of ketamine. The fact that the hypnotic effect is brief means that additional analgesic and/or hypnotic drugs must be administered. Etomidate offers no real advantage over most other induction drugs for fit patients undergoing elective surgical procedures.

KETAMINE

General Characteristics

Ketamine (Ketalar, Parke-Davis, Morris Plains, NJ) (Fig. 4-5) was developed domestically and released in the United States in 1970. It is a phencyclidine derivative whose anesthetic actions differ so markedly from barbiturates and other CNS depressants that Corssen labeled its effect "dissociative anesthesia."[192] The properties of ketamine and its use in anesthesia have been completely reviewed.[193] Although ketamine produces rapid hypnosis and profound analgesia, respiratory and cardiovascular functions are not depressed as much as with most other induction agents. Disturbing psychotomimetic activity (described as vivid dreams, hallucinations, or emergence phenomenon), as well as undesirable increases in myocardial oxygen consumption have limited the use of ketamine.

Ketamine is biotransformed in the liver, and there are four known metabolites.[44,194] Some of the metabolites are active,[44] and their plasma concentration is higher than that of the parent compound after cessation of ketamine administration.[195] Despite the activity of these metabolites, the pharmacodynamic action of ketamine appears to result from the CNS activity of the parent compound.[44,195,196] Pharmacokinetic studies of ketamine reveal that the $t_{1/2}\alpha$ ranges from 17 to 46 minutes[44,196] and the $t_{1/2}\beta$ ranges from 150 to 240 minutes.[44,196,197] The volume of distribution is 3.1 liters/kg and the total clearance is 19.1 ml/kg/min.[196] Thus, ketamine has a relatively large volume of distribution, a short distribution half-life, and a relatively rapid elimination half-life. The pharmacokinetics of ketamine are similar in children and adults.[198] The drug is suitable for development of

pharmacodynamic models; and administration by infusion has been used to maintain therapeutic drug levels.[195,199] Idvall et al administered a loading dose of 2 mg/kg, which was followed during the next 30 minutes by an infusion rate of 58 μg/kg/min and then by an infusion rate of 41 μg/kg/min.[195] During the last 30 minutes, an infusion rate of 17 μg/kg/min maintained a satisfactory therapeutic drug level of greater than 640 ng/ml. Termination of the infusion resulted in the patient's rapid return to consciousness. Although there have been no infusion models tested that are based strictly on the pharmacokinetics of ketamine, this is an area that merits investigation.

Cardiovascular Effects

The hemodynamic effects of ketamine have been examined in normal patients,[179,200-205] critically ill,[206] geriatric,[207] and in patients who have a variety of heart diseases.[72,76,203,208-216] Table 4-4 contains the range of hemodynamic responses to ketamine. One unique feature of ketamine is stimulation of the cardiovascular system. The most prominent hemodynamic changes are significant increases in HR, CI, SVR, and systemic and pulmonary artery pressures. These circulatory changes cause an increase in MVO_2 with an apparently appropriate increase in coronary blood flow.[209,216] Although global increases in MVO_2 occur, there is some evidence that the increased work may be borne primarily by the right ventricle, due to significantly greater rises in PVR than SVR;[217] however, both ventricles certainly demonstrate increased minute work. The hemodynamic changes observed with ketamine are not dose related in the relatively small dose ranges examined; there is no significant difference between changes after administration of 0.5 and 1.5 mg/kg IV.[194] It is interesting that a second dose of ketamine produces hemodynamic effects opposite to those of the first.[213] Thus, the cardiovascular stimulation seen after ketamine induction of anesthesia (2 mg/kg) in a patient who has valvular heart disease is not observed with the second administration, which is accompanied instead by a decrease in the BP, PCWP, and CI.

Ketamine produces similar hemodynamic changes in normal patients and those who have ischemic heart disease.[202] The changes are also qualitatively similar in patients who have congenital and valvular heart disease. Hemodynamic changes after ketamine administration in children with a variety of congenital heart lesions are similar to adults; increases in HR and PAP are most prominent.[214,218,219] There are no significant changes in shunt directions or fraction,[214] or systemic oxygenation after ketamine induction.[215,218] In patients who have elevated PAP (as with mitral valvular disease), ketamine seems to cause a more pronounced increase in PVR than SVR.[211] The presence of a marked tachycardia after administration of ketamine and pancuronium can also complicate the induction of anesthesia in patients who have mitral valvular disease and atrial fibrillation.[220]

The mechanism responsible for ketamine's stimulation of the circulatory system remains enigmatic because of its complexity and the lack of systematic investigation in this area. The flurry of research activity on ketamine's mechanism of action that occurred right after its release has recently been reviewed,[2,194,221,222] but little work is currently under way. There are two certainties: ketamine has a direct-acting negative inotropic effect on the myocardium, and centrally mediated sympathetic responses usually override the depression. Myocardial depression has been demonstrated in isolated rabbit hearts,[223] intact dogs, and isolated dog heart preparations.[224,225] Although the precise site of cardiovascular stimulation is still unknown, Ivankovich et al showed that small doses of ketamine injected directly into the CNS result in immediate hemodynamic stimulation.[226] Ketamine also causes the sympathoneuronal release of norepinephrine (NE), which can be measured in venous blood.[216,227,228] Blockade of this effect is possible with barbiturates, benzodiazepines,[226-229] and droperidol.[216] Animal work supports the hypothesis that the primary hemodynamic effect of ketamine is central and not peripheral.[230-237] The role of ketamine's cocaine-like neuronal inhibition of NE reuptake has yet to be defined in its overall influence on the cardiovascular system.[238,239] It is also unknown whether ketamine exerts the same effect centrally, preventing NE reuptake in the brain.

Stimulation of the cardiovascular system by ketamine is not always desirable, and a number of pharmacologic methods have been used to block the ketamine-induced tachycardia and systemic hypertension. Nishimura et al used adrenergic blocking drugs to attenuate the cardiovascular effects of ketamine, and found that the combination of propranolol (β-blockade) and phenoxybenzamine (α-blockade) was superior to either drug alone and to trimethaphan and chlorpromazine in attenuating the increases in heart rate and blood pressure.[204] The calcium channel blocker and vasodilator, verapamil, also successfully decreased the tachycardia.[240] Droperidol attenuates the hypertensive response to

ketamine, apparently by α-adrenergic blockade as well as central depression of catecholamine release.[216] Probably the most fruitful approach to blocking ketamine-induced hypertension and tachycardia is the prior administration of benzodiazepines. Diazepam, flunitrazepam, and midazolam all successfully attenuate the hemodynamic effects of ketamine.[24,76,199,212,229,241,242] For example, in a study involving 16 patients with valvular heart disease, ketamine (2 mg/kg) did not produce significant hemodynamic changes when preceded by diazepam (0.4 mg/kg).[212] Indeed, HR, MAP, and RPP were unchanged, but there was a slight but significant decrease in CI.[212] The combination of midazolam with ketamine is attractive, since both have relatively similar pharmacokinetic profiles.[24] It is also possible to attenuate the stimulatory effects of ketamine with an infusion of the drug rather than a bolus intravenous injection.[243] Hatano et al reported their experience with 200 cardiac surgical patients in whom the administration of diazepam (0.3–0.5 mg/kg) and then a ketamine infusion (0.7 mg/kg/hr) provided a stable hemodynamic course during induction, intubation, and incision.[199] In fact, the combination of diazepam and ketamine rivals the high-dose fentanyl technique with regard to hemodynamic stability. No patients had hallucinations, although 2 percent had dreams and 1 percent had recall of events in the operating room.[199]

A number of studies have examined the interaction of ketamine with other anesthetic drugs. In general, other anesthetic drugs like benzodiazepines prevent the hemodynamic changes seen during induction with ketamine. Administration of ketamine (2 mg/kg) to healthy patients anesthetized with halothane produced a 10–28 percent reduction in blood pressure,[205,244] but no change in HR.[205,244] Cardiac index, stroke index, and blood pressure decreased when ketamine was administered to patients anesthetized with halothane and enflurane; showing that the hemodynamic depression produced by ketamine is more pronounced in the presence of halothane and enflurane.[244] A plausible explanation for this is that the inhalation drugs block the sympathetic activity normally produced by ketamine, thereby providing no opposition to ketamine's direct myocardial depressive effect. Ketamine, when combined with pancuronium, may be expected to produce tachycardia more than when combined with vecuronium,[242] presumably because of the additive sympathomimetic effects of ketamine and pancuronium.

Ketamine (2 mg/kg IV or 4–6 mg/kg IM) has been combined with heavy premedication (pentobarbital, 5–10 mg/kg; meperidine, 1.0 mg/kg; or scopolamine, 0.01 mg/kg) as the anesthetic for pediatric cardiac catheterization in some institutions, and relatively few complications have been associated with its use. In a retrospective review of 358 patients, in 1981, at the University of Alabama at Birmingham, 4 percent of patients required secondary orotracheal intubation because of excessive coughing or laryngospasm after ketamine administration. Experience with very young (less than or equal to 1 month) and very small (less than or equal to 4 kg) children has shown, however, that ketamine is unsatisfactory in providing immobility and preserving respiratory function. Elective tracheal intubation should be done in these patients (32 percent of the total group). In addition, older patients should receive small doses of diazepam along with ketamine. Using this technique, satisfactory conditions for obtaining high-quality angiographic documentation of cardiac disease can be provided. The most troublesome feature of this technique is the prolonged emergence time in children, which is probably attributable to the combination of all the drugs.

Although ketamine is used for induction and maintenance of anesthesia in many pediatric cardiac surgical centers,[245-248] there is no large series comparing ketamine with other techniques. In a noncontemporaneous, retrospective study of 104 children under 2 years of age, the combination of ketamine, N_2O/O_2, and pancuronium (66 patients) was compared with that of halothane, N_2O/O_2, and curare (38 patients).[247] While the ketamine patients were more stable hemodynamically, there was no difference in either morbidity or mortality between the groups. A concern about the use of ketamine in patients who have congenital heart disease is its effect on elevated pulmonary artery pressure. Santoli et al state that "We have never observed complications related to a drop in pulmonary blood flow caused by a shunt inversion or by an increase in a right-to-left shunt; therefore, we now believe that the use of ketamine is indicated, especially in patients with pulmonary hypertension or bidirectional shunt, as well as in patients with atresia or extremely hypoplastic pulmonary artery and patent ductus arteriosus."[246] This exuberance must be tempered with the realization that ketamine may elevate pulmonary vascular resistance in patients who have congenital lesions,[249,250] and the potential always exists for reversal of a left-to-right shunt if airway obstruction occurs.[250]

Ketamine has been used as the sole agent for adult patients undergoing elective congenital heart operations, and emergency or elective valvular surgery.[251,252] Corssen et al demonstrated ketamine's safety and efficacy in 253 patients undergoing coronary artery bypass graft surgery procedures in 1974.[208] In an early randomized comparison of anesthetic techniques in patients who had valvular [253] and ischemic heart disease,[253,254] there was no significant difference in either morbidity or mortality between ketamine and morphine techniques. Hemodynamic lability was a greater problem with morphine, but sustained tachycardia and hypertension were significantly more troublesome with ketamine. At the present time, neither ketamine nor morphine alone is recommended for patients who have IHD.[254]

Ketamine has been investigated in patients referred to as "poor risks." These patients defy clear definition, but are usually classified as ASA physical status IV or V, and, if conscious, may be candidates for ketamine. Studies have demonstrated the safety and efficacy of induction with ketamine (2 mg/kg) in hemodynamically unstable patients requiring emergency operations.[206,255,256] Most of these patients were hypovolemic because of trauma or massive hemorrhage. Ketamine induction was accompanied in the majority of patients by the maintenance of blood pressure and, presumably, cardiac output as well.[206,255] Waxman et al studied 12 severely ill patients who had unstable cardiovascular dynamics.[257] Ketamine decreased the cardiac index by 10 percent or more in 4 of the 12 patients; 2 of the 4 subsequently died. The data clearly indicate that, in most of these severely ill patients, induction of anesthesia is accomplished with little change in hemodynamics. As would be predicted from animal and isolated heart experiments, however, ketamine may exert a negative inotropic effect. This appears to be particularly the case with patients who have been severely ill for some time and perhaps have depleted their catecholamine stores. In patients who have an accumulation of pericardial fluid, with or without constrictive pericarditis, induction with ketamine (2 mg/kg) maintains CI and increases blood pressure, SVR, and RAP.[83,258] The heart rate in this group of patients is unchanged by ketamine, probably because patients who have cardiac tamponade already have a compensatory tachycardia. Finally, ketamine has been shown to preserve hemodynamic values better than diazepam when used for induction of anesthesia in patients with constrictive pericarditis (Fig. 4-7).

Uses

Ketamine has been available for over 15 years and is widely used for the induction of anesthesia in pediatric patients, partly because of its hemodynamic

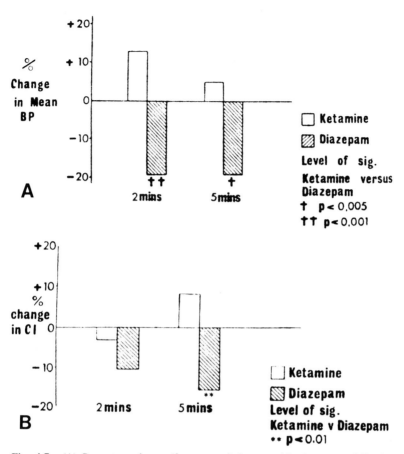

Fig. 4-7. (A) Percentage change (from control) in mean blood pressure following ketamine and diazepam. Change within each group was statistically significant. (B) Percentage change (from control) in cardiac index following ketamine and diazepam. No significant change noted within each group. Doses were ketamine, 1 mg/kg, and diazepam, 0.3 mg/kg.

effects and because of the fact that it may be administered intramuscularly. In adults, ketamine is probably the safest and most efficacious drug for patients who have decreased blood volume or cardiac tamponade. Undesired tachycardia, hypertension, and emergence delirium may be attenuated with benzodiazepines, perhaps making ketamine a good choice for patients who have other cardiovascular diseases.

DIISOPROPYLPHENOL

General Characteristics

2,6-diisopropylphenol (Diprivan, Propofol, ICN Pharmaceuticals, Covina, CA) (Fig. 4-5) is an alkylphenol introduced as a short-acting agent in 1977. The plasma disappearance of this agent fits a two-compartment model and is independent of speed of injection.[259] Distribution half-life is 2–3 minutes, while the elimination half-life is 50–55 minutes when given in doses of 2–4 mg/kg IV. Diisopropylphenol has a very large volume of distribution (50 percent body weight) and a total body clearance (3.5 liters/min) that exceeds liver blood flow. These data suggest that diisopropylphenol is a highly lipophilic drug with elimination pathways other than hepatic metabolism.

Cardiovascular Effects

Induction with a diisopropylphenol infusion combined with 67 percent nitrous oxide in patients free of heart disease decreases MAP (−20 to −31 percent), CI (−27 to −29 percent), and SVR (−17 percent). Heart rate changes minimally so that RPP

Table 4-5
Probable Safety and Efficacy of Anesthetic IV Drugs

	Diazepam	Etomidate	Ketamine	Midazolam	Thiopental
Ischemic heart disease	Yes	Yes	No	Yes	Yes
Valvular heart disease	Yes	Yes	Yes	NR	Yes
Congenital heart disease	Yes	NR	Yes	NR	Yes
Hypovolemic hypotension	NR	Yes	Yes	NR	No
Congestive heart failure	Yes	NR	NR	Yes	No
Cardiac tamponade	NR	NR	Yes	NR	No

Yes = Safety and/or efficacy has been demonstrated; No = safety and/or efficacy has been questioned after investigation or is theoretically unacceptable; NR = not reported and/or investigated.

decreases by approximately 24 percent (Table 4-4). Laryngoscopy and intubation increase MAP (+50 percent) and RPP (+70 percent). Surgical incision causes an increase in MAP (+10 to +12 percent) and a decrease in CI (−30 percent). These results suggest that diisopropylphenol decreases blood pressure and that even with nitrous oxide it will not completely abolish the sympathetic response to perianesthetic stimulation, although this happens to a lesser extent than with methohexital.[260-262]

Uses

Diisopropylphenol has been studied in Europe and the United States as an induction and maintenance anesthetic agent. The major significant advantage over existing intravenous agents is a shorter recovery time due to its relatively short elimination. The decrease in hemodynamics is a potential problem in unstable patients and requires further study.

CONCLUSIONS

The considerable amount of information available about the cardiovascular pharmacology and pharmacokinetics of the intravenous drugs enable more confident prediction of the appropriate drug for each patient. Unfortunately, there are gaps in the knowledge about the steady-state (prolonged maintenance of drug levels) hemodynamic effects, effects of repeated injections, and many of the possible interactions among anesthetic and cardiovascular drugs. Nevertheless, the probable safety and efficacious use of the drugs available or soon to be available in the United States are presented in Table 4-5. This table is controversial, but it is the authors' hope that where disagreement exists, further experimentation into these areas, where often there are more ideas and feelings than scientific evidence, will increase the certainty and knowledge of the indications for particular drugs.

REFERENCES

1. Reves JG, Kissin I: Pharmacology of anesthetic drugs: Intravenous anesthetics. *In* Kaplan JA (ed), Cardiac Anesthesia: Cardiovascular Pharmacology. Orlando, FL, Grune & Stratton, 1983, pp 3–29
2. Reves JG, Kissin I: Drug interactions in anesthesia. *In* Smith T (ed), Intravenous Anesthetics. Philadelphia, Lea and Febiger, 1985
3. Slutsky R: Response of the left ventricle to stress: Effects of exercise, atrial pacing, afterload stress and drugs. Am J Cardiol 47:357–364, 1981
4. Reves JG, Gelman S: Cardiovascular effects of intravenous anesthetic drugs. *In* Covino B, Fozzard J, Rehder K, Strichartz S (eds): American Physiological Society, Clinical Physiology Series, Effects of Anesthesia, 1985, pp 179–193
5. Alvis JM, Reves JG, Govier AV, et al: Computer assisted continuous infusions of fentanyl during cardiac anesthesia. Comparison with a manual method. Anesthesiology 63:41–49, 1985
6. Khatri IM, Freis ED: Hemodynamic changes during sleep. J Appl Physiol 22:867–873, 1967
7. Olesen AS, Huttel MS, Hole P: Venous sequelae following the injection of etomidate or thiopentone I.V. Br J Anaesth 56:171–173, 1984
8. Christensen JH, Andreasen F, Jansen JA: Pharmacokinetics and pharmacodynamics of thiopentone. A

comparison between young and elderly patients. Anaesthesia 37:398–404, 1982

9. Mark LC, Brank L, Kamvyssi S, et al: Thiopental metabolism by human liver *in vivo* and *in vitro*. Nature (Lond) 206:1117, 1965

10. Morgan DJ, Blackman GL, Paull JD, et al: Pharmacokinetics and plasma binding of thiopental. I: Studies in surgical patients. Anesthesiology 54:468–473, 1981

11. Ghoneim MM, Van Hamme MJ: Pharmacokinetics of thiopentone: Effects of enflurane and nitrous oxide anaesthesia and surgery. Br J Anaesth 50:1237–1242, 1978

12. Christensen JH, Andreasen F, Jansen JA: Pharmacokinetics of thiopentone in a group of young women and a group of young men. Br J Anaesth 52:913–918, 1980

13. Brodie BB, Mark LC, Papper EM, et al: The fate of thiopental in man and a method for its estimation in biological material. J Pharmacol Exp Ther 98:85–96, 1950

14. Sear JW, Cooper GM, Kumar V: The effect of age on recovery. A comparison of the kinetics of thiopentone and althesin. Anaesthesia 38:1158–1161, 1983

15. Christensen JH, Andreasen F, Jansen JA: Influence of age and sex on the pharmacokinetics of thiopentone. Br J Anaesth 53:1189–1195, 1981

16. Heikkila H, Jalonen J, Arola M, et al: Midazolam as an adjunct to high-dose fentanyl anaesthesia for coronary artery bypass grafting operation. Acta Anaesthesiol Scand 28:683–689, 1984

17. Sorbo S, Hudson RJ, Loomis JC: The pharmacokinetics of thiopental in pediatric surgical patients. Anesthesiology 61:666–670, 1984

18. Jung D, Mayersohn M, Perrier D, et al: Thiopental disposition in lean and obese patients undergoing surgery. Anesthesiology 56:269–274, 1982

19. Becker KE, Tonnesen AS: Cardiovascular effects of plasma levels of thiopental necessary for anesthesia. Anesthesiology 49:197–200, 1978

20. Aveling W, Bradshaw AD, Crankshaw DP: The effect of speed of injection on the potency of anaesthetic induction agents. Anaesth Intens Care 6:116–119, 1978

21. Seltzer JL, Gerson JI, Allen FB: Comparison of the cardiovascular effects of bolus v. incremental administration of thiopentone. Br J Anaesth 52:527–530, 1980

22. Sonntag H, Hellberg K, Schenk HD, et al: Effects of thiopental (Trapanal) on coronary blood flow and myocardial metabolism in man. Acta Anaesth Scand 19:69–78, 1975

23. Filner BE, Karliner JS: Alterations of normal left ventricular performance by general anesthesia. Anesthesiology 45:610–621, 1976

24. White PF: Comparative evaluation of intravenous agents for rapid sequence induction—thiopental, ketamine and midazolam. Anesthesiology 57:279–284, 1982

25. Flickinger H, Fraimow W, Cathcart RT, et al: Effect of thiopental induction on cardiac output in man. Anesth Analg 40:694–700, 1961

26. Nauta J, Stanley TH, deLange S, et al: Anaesthetic induction with alfentanil. Comparison with thiopental, midazolam, and etomidate. Can Anaesth Soc J 30:53–60, 1983

27. Christensen JH, Andreasen F, Kristoffersen MB: Comparison of the anaesthetic and haemodynamic effects of chlormethiazole and thiopentone. Br J Anaesth 55:391–396, 1983

28. Reiz S, Balfors E, Friedman A, et al: Effects of thiopentone on cardiac performance, coronary hemodynamics, and myocardial oxygen consumption in chronic ischemic heart disease. Acta Anaesth Scand 25:103–110, 1981

29. Lyons SM, Clarke RSJ: A comparison of different drugs for anaesthesia in cardiac surgical patients. Br J Anaesth 44:575–582, 1972

30. Tarabadkar S, Kopriva CJ, Sreenivasan N, et al: Hemodynamic impact of induction in patients with decreased cardiac reserve. Anesthesiology 53:S43, 1980

31. Fischler M, Dubois C, Brodaty D, et al: Circulatory responses to thiopentone and tracheal intubation in patients with coronary artery disease. Br J Anaesth 57:493–496, 1985

32. Tarnow J, Hess W, Klein W: Etomidate, althesin and thiopentone as induction agents for coronary artery surgery. Can Anaesth Soc J 27:338–344, 1980

33. Milocco I, Löf BA, William-Olsson G, Appelgren LK: Haemodynamic stability during anaesthesia induction and sternotomy in patients with ischaemic heart disease. Acta Anaesthesiol Scand 29:465–473, 1985

34. Toner W, Howard PJ, McGowan WAW, et al: Another look at acute tolerance to thiopentone. Br J Anaesth 52:1005–1008, 1980

35. Frankl WS, Poole-Wilson PA: Effects of thiopental on tension development, action potential, and exchange of calcium and potassium in rabbit ventricular myocardium. J Cardiovasc Pharmacol 3:554–565, 1981

36. Reiz S, Balfors E, Friedman A, et al: Effects of thiopentone on cardiac performance, coronary hemodynamics and myocardial oxygen consumption in chronic ischemic heart disease. Acta Anaesth Scand 25:103–110, 1981

37. Eckstein JW, Hamilton WK, McCammond JM: The effect of thiopental on peripheral venous tone. Anesthesiology 22:525–528, 1961

38. Kissin I, Motomura S, Aultman DF, et al: Inotropic and anesthetic potencies of etomidate and thiopental in dogs. Anesth Analg 62:961–965, 1983

39. Komai H, Rusy BF: Differences in myocardial depressant action of thiopental and halothane. Anesth Analg 63:313–318, 1984

40. Pedersen T, Engbaek J, Klausen NO, et al: Effects of low-dose ketamine and thiopentone on cardiac per-

formance and myocardial oxygen balance in high-risk patients. Acta Anaesth Scand 26:235–239, 1982

41. King E: The treatment of army casualties in Hawaii. Army Med Bull 61:18–20, 1942

42. Nussmeier NA, Slogoff S: Neuropsychiatric complications after cardiopulmonary bypass. Cerebral protection by a barbiturate. Anesthesiology 64:165–170, 1986

43. Hudson, RJ, Stanski DR, Burch PG: Pharmacokinetics of methohexital and thiopental in surgical patients. Anesthesiology 59:215–219, 1985

44. Ghoneim MM, Kortilla K: Pharmacokinetics of intravenous anaesthetics. Implications for clinical use. Clin Pharmacokinet 2:344–372, 1977

45. Kortilla K, Linnoila M, Ertama P, et al: Recovery and simulated driving after intravenous anesthesia with thiopental, methohexital, propanidid, or alphadione. Anesthesiology 43:291–299, 1975

46. Dundee JW, Moore J: Thiopentone and methohexital. A comparison as main anesthetic agents for a standard operation. Anaesthesia 16:50–60, 1961

47. Conway CM, Ellis DB: The hemodynamic effects of short-acting barbiturates. Br J Anaesth 41:534–542, 1969

48. Lamalle D: Cardiovascular effects of various anesthetics in man. Four short-acting intravenous anesthetics: althesin, etomidate, methohexital and propanidid. Acta Anaesth Belg 27:208–224, 1976

49. Prys-Roberts C, Greene LT, Meloche T, et al: Studies of anaesthesia in relation to hypertension. II. Haemodynamic consequences of induction and endotracheal intubation. Br J Anaesth 43:533–541, 1971

50. Dundee JW: Intravenous anaesthetic agents. Curr Top Anaesth 1: 5–7, 1979

51. Richter JJ: Current theories about the mechanisms of benzodiazepines and neuroleptic drugs. Anesthesiology 54:66–72, 1981

52. Greenblatt DJ, Allen MD, Harmatz JS, et al: Diazepam disposition determinants. Clin Pharmacol Ther 27:301–312, 1980

53. Mandelli M, Tognoni G, Gratattini S: Clinical pharmacokinetics of diazepam. Clin Pharmacokinetic 3:72–91, 1978

54. Reves JG: Benzodiazepines. In Prys-Roberts C, Hug C (eds): Pharmacokinetics of Anesthesia. Oxford, Blackwell, 1984, pp 157–187

55. Ellinwood EH, Nikaido A, Heatherly D: Diazepam. Prediction of pharmacodynamics from pharmacokinetics. Psychopharmacology 83:297–298, 1984

56. Klotz U, Antonin KH, Brugel H, et al: Disposition of diazepam and its major metabolite desmethyldiazepam in patients with liver disease. Clin Pharmacol Ther 21:430–436, 1977

57. Abernethy DR, Greenblatt DJ, Divoll M, et al: Prolonged accumulation of diazepam in obesity. J Clin Pharmacol 23:369–376, 1983

58. Macklon AF, Barton M, James O, et al: The effect of age on the pharmacokinetics of diazepam. Clin Sci 59:479–483, 1980

59. Allen MD, Greenblatt DJ, Harmatz JS, et al: Single-dose kinetics of prazepam, a precursor of desmethyldiazepam. J Clin Pharmacol 19:445–450, 1979

60. Bertler A, Lindgren S, Malmgren H: Pharmacokinetics of dipotassium chlorazepate in patients after repeated 50 mg oral doses. Psychopharmacology 71:165–167, 1980

61. Carrigan PJ, Chao GC, Barker WM, et al: Steady state bioavailability of two clorazepate dipotassium dosage forms. J Clin Pharmacol 17:18–28, 1977

62. Hillestad L, Hansen T, Melsom H: Diazepam metabolism in normal man. II. Serum concentration and clinical effect after oral administration and cumulation. Clin Pharmacol Ther 16:485–489, 1974

63. Klotz U, Reimann I: Influence of cimetidine on the pharmacokinetics of desmethyldiazepam and oxazepam. Eur J Clin Pharmacol 18:517–520, 1980

64. Rey E, d'Athis P, Giraux P, et al: Pharmacokinetics of clorazepate in pregnant and non-pregnant women. Eur J Clin Pharmacol 15:175–180, 1979

65. Smith MT, Evans LEJ, Eadie MJ, et al: Pharmacokinetics of prazepam in man. Eur J Clin Pharmacol 16:141–147, 1979

66. Klotz U, Reimann I: Delayed clearance of diazepam due to cimetidine. N Engl J Med 302:1012–1014, 1980

67. Routledge PA, Kitchell BB, Bjornsson TD, et al: Diazepam and n-desmethyldiazepam redistribution after heparin. Clin Pharmacol Ther 27:528–532, 1980

68. Rao S, Sherbaniuk RW, Prasad K, et al: Cardiopulmonary effects of diazepam. Clin Pharmacol Ther 14:182–189, 1973

69. Fox GS, Wynands JE, Bhambhami M: A clinical comparison of diazepam and thiopentone as induction agents to general anesthesia. Can Anaesth Soc J 15:281–289, 1968

70. Dalen JE, Evans GL, Banas JS, et al: The hemodynamic and respiratory effects of diazepam (Valium). Anesthesiology 30:259–263, 1969

71. D'Amelio G, Volta SD, Stritoni P, et al: Acute cardiovascular effects of diazepam in patients with mitral valve disease. Eur J Clin Pharmacol 6:61–63, 1973

72. Lyons SM, Clarke RSJ, Dundee JW: Some cardiovascular and respiratory effects of four non-barbiturate anaesthetic induction agents. Eur J Clin Pharmacol 7:275–279, 1974

73. Stanley TH, Bennett GM, Loeser EA, et al: Cardiovascular effects of diazepam and droperidol during morphine anesthesia. Anesthesiology 44:255–258, 1976

74. Ikram H, Rubin AP, Jewkes RF: Effect of diazepam on myocardial blood flow of patients with and without coronary artery disease. Br Heart J 35:626–630, 1973

75. Prakash R, Thurer R, Vargas A, et al: Cardiovascular effects of diazepam induction in patients for aortocoronary saphenous vein bypass grafts. Abstracts of Scientific Papers, San Francisco, CA, ASA Annual Meeting, 1976

76. Jackson APF, Dhadphale PR, Callaghan ML, et al: Haemodynamic studies during induction of anaesthesia for open-heart surgery using diazepam and ketamine. Br J Anaesth 50:375–378, 1978

77. Clarke RSJ, Lyons SM: Diazepam and flunitrazepam as induction agents for cardiac surgical operations. Acta Anaesth Scand 21:282–292, 1977

78. McCammon RL, Hilgenberg JC, Stoelting RK: Hemodynamic effects of diazepam and diazepam-nitrous oxide in patients with coronary artery disease. Anesth Analg 59:438–441, 1980

79. Samuelson PN, Lell WA, Kouchoukos NT, et al: Hemodynamics during diazepam induction of anesthesia for coronary artery bypass grafting. South Med J 73:332–334, 1980

80. Samuelson PN, Reves JG, Kouchoukos NT, et al: Hemodynamic responses to anesthetic induction with midazolam or diazepam in patients with ischemic heart disease. Anesth Analg 60:802–809, 1981

81. Falk Jr RB, Denlinger JK, Nahrwold ML, et al: Acute vasodilation following induction of anesthesia with intravenous diazepam and nitrous oxide. Anesthesiology 49:149–150, 1978

82. Dhadphale PR, Behrendt DM, Jackson PF, et al: The effect of diazepam on contractility in the intact human heart. Abstracts of Scientific Papers, New Orleans, LA, ASA Annual Meeting, 1977

83. Kingston HGG, Bretherton KW, Holloway AM, et al: A comparison between ketamine and diazepam as induction agents for pericardiectomy. Anaesth Intens Care 6:66–70, 1978

84. Markiewicz W, Hunt S, Harrison DC, et al: Circulatory effects of diazepam in heart disease. J Clin Pharmacol 16:637–644, 1976

85. Knapp RB, Dubow HS: Diazepam as an induction agent for patients with cardiopulmonary disease. South Med J 63:1451–1453, 1970

86. Knapp RB, Dobow H: Comparison of diazepam with thiopental as an induction agent in cardiopulmonary disease. Anesth Analg 49:722–726, 1970

87. Cote P, Gueret P, Bourassa MG: Systemic and coronary hemodynamic effects of diazepam in patients with normal and diseased coronary arteries. Circulation 50:1210–1216, 1974

88. Cote P, Noble J, Bourassa MG: Systemic vasodilation following diazepam after combined sympathetic and parasympathetic blockade in patients with coronary heart disease. Cath Cardiovasc Diagn 2:369–380, 1976

89. Knight PR, Kroll DA, Nahrwold ML, et al: Comparison of cardiovascular responses to anesthesia and operation when intravenous lidocaine or morphine sulfate is used as adjunct to diazepam-nitrous oxide

90. Alvis JM, Flezzani P, Jacobs JR, et al: Diazepam pharmacokinetics and pharmacodynamics during induction of anesthesia in CAGB patients, in Society of Cardiovascular Anesthesiologists Annual Meeting, Montreal, 1986

91. Melsom MM, Andreassen P, Melsom H, et al: Diazepam in acute myocardial infarction. Clinical effects and effects on catecholamines, free fatty acids, and cortisol. Br Heart J 38:804–810, 1976

92. Hoar PF, Nelson NT, Mangano DT, et al: Adrenergic response to morphine-diazepam anesthesia for myocardial revascularization. Anesth Analg 60:406–411, 1981

93. Abel RM, Reis RL, Staroscik RN: The pharmacological basis of coronary and systemic vasodilator actions of diazepam (Valium). Br J Pharmacol 39:261–274, 1970

94. Bailey PL, Stanley TH: Pharmacology of intravenous narcotic anesthetics. In Miller RD (ed): Anesthesia, 2nd ed, London, Churchill Livingstone, 1986, pp 745–798

95. Stanley TH, Webster LR: Anesthetic requirements and cardiovascular effects of fentanyl-oxygen and fentanyl-diazepam-oxygen anesthesia in man. Anesth Analg 57:411–416, 1978

96. Tomichek RC, Rosow CE, Schneider RC, et al: Cardiovascular effects of diazepam-fentanyl anesthesia in patients with coronary artery disease. Anesth Analg 61:217–218, 1982

97. Flacke JW, Davis JD, Flacke WE, et al: Effects of fentanyl and diazepam in dogs deprived of autonomic tone. Anesth Analg 64:1053–1059, 1985

98. Silbert BS, Rosow CE, Keegan CR, et al: The effect of diazepam on induction of anesthesia with alfentanil. Anesth Analg 65:71–77, 1986

99. Reves JG, Samuelson PN, Lell WA, et al: Myocardial damage in coronary artery bypass surgical patients anaesthetized with two anaesthetic techniques: A random comparison of halothane and enflurane. Can Anaesth Soc J 27:238–247, 1980

100. Greenblatt DJ, Divoee M, Harmatz JS, et al: Comparisons of sublingual lorazepam with intravenous, intramuscular and oral lorazepam. J Pharm Sci 71:248–252, 1982

101. Shader RI, Greenblatt DJ: The use of benzodiazepines in clinical practice. Br J Clin Pharmacol 11:55–95, 1981

102. Ruffalo RL, Thompson JF, Segal J: Cimetadine-benzodiazepine drug interaction. Am J Hosp Pharm 38:1365–1366, 1981

103. Oehs HR, Greenblatt DJ, Verburg-Oehs B: Propranolol interactions with diazepam, lorazepam, and alprazolam. Clin Pharmacol Ther 36:451–455, 1984

104. Sellers EM, Giles MG, Greenblatt DJ, et al: Different effects on benzodiazepine disposition by disulfi-

ram and ethanol. Arzneim-Forsch/Drug Res 30:882–886, 1980

105. Desmond PV, Roberts RK, Wood ATJ, et al: Effect of heparin administration on plasma binding of benzodiazepines. Br J Clin Pharmacol 9:171–175, 1980

106. Morrison G, Chang ST, Koepke HH, et al: Effect of renal impairment and hemodialysis on lorazepam kinetics. Clin Pharmacol Ther 35:646–652, 1984

107. Greenblatt DJ, Shader RI, Franke K, et al: Pharmacokinetics and bioavailability of intravenous, intramuscular and oral lorazepam in humans. J Pharmacol Sci 68:1320–1322, 1979

108. Kraus JW, Desmond PV, Marshall JP, et al: Effects of aging and liver disease on disposition of lorazepam. Clin Pharmacol Ther 24:411–418, 1985

109. Greenblatt DJ, Shader RI: Effects of age and other drugs on benzodiazepine kinetics. Arzneim-Forsch/Drug Res 30:886–890, 1980

110. Johnson RF, Schenker S, Roberts RK, et al: Plasma binding of benzodiazepines in humans. J Pharmacol Sci 68:1320–1322, 1979

111. Aaltonen L, Kanto J, Arola M, et al: Effect of age and cardiopulmonary bypass on the pharmacokinetics of lorazepam. Acta Pharmacol Toxicol 51:126–131, 1982

112. Kenakin TP: The potentiation of cardiac responses to adenosine by benzodiazepines. J Pharmacol Exp Ther 222:752–758, 1981

113. Elliott HW, Nomof N, Navarro G, et al: Central nervous system and cardiovascular effects of lorazepam in man. Clin Pharmacol Ther 12:668–681, 1970

114. Verschraegen R, Rolly G: The influence of lorazepam (Temesta) on anesthesia. Acta Anaesthesiol Belgica 3:256–263, 1973

115. Knapp RB, Flerrol: Evaluation of the cardiopulmonary safety and effects of lorazepam as a premedicant. Anesth Analg 53:122–124, 1974

116. Newton DW, Narducci WA, Leet WA, et al: Lorazepam solubility in and sorption from intravenous admixture solutions. Am J Hosp Pharm 40:424–427, 1983

117. Ruff R: The hemodynamic interaction of lorazepam and fentanyl for anesthetic induction during aortocoronary bypass surgery. Submitted for presentation at the Duke University Spring Cardiovascular Symposium, Durham, NC, April 1986

118. Reves JG, Fragen RJ, Vinik HR, et al: Midazolam: Pharmacology and uses. Anesthesiology 62:310–324, 1985

119. Reves JG, Kissin I, Smith LR: The effective dose of midazolam. Anesthesiology 55:82–86, 1981

120. Reves JG, Samuelson PN, Vinik HR: Consistency of midazolam. Anesth Analg 61:545–546, 1982

121. Dundee JW, Kwar P: Consistency of action of midazolam. Letter to Editor. Anesth Analg 61-545–546, 1982

122. Gross JB, Caldwell CB, Edwards MW: Induction dose-response curves for midazolam and ketamine in premedicated ASA Class III and IV patients. Anesth Analg 64:795–800, 1985

123. Woo GK, Kolis SJ, Schwartz MA: In vitro metabolism of an imidazobenzodiazepine. Pharmacologist 19:164, 1977

124. Brown CR, Sarnquist FH, Canup CA, et al: Clinical electroencephalographic, and pharmacokinetic studies of a water-soluble benzodiazepine, midazolam maleate. Anesthesiology 50:467–470, 1979

125. Puglisi CV, Meyer JC, D'Arconte L, et al: Determination of water soluble imidazo-1, 4-benzodiazepines in blood by electron-capture gas-liquid chromatography and in urine by differential pulse polarography. J Chromatogr 145:81–96, 1978

126. Greenblatt DJ, Locniskar A, Ochs HR, et al: Automated gas chromatography for studies of midazolam pharmacokinetics. Anesthesiology 55:176–179, 1981

127. Allonen H, Ziegler G, Klotz U: Midazolam kinetics. Clin Pharmacol Ther 30:653–661, 1981

128. Heizmann P, Eckert M, Ziegler WH: Pharmacokinetics and bioavailability of midazolam in man. Br J Clin Pharmacol 16:43S–49S, 1983

129. Greenblatt DJ, Abernethy DR, Lockniskar A, et al: Effect of age, gender and obesity on midazolam kinetics. Anesthesiology 61:27–35, 1984

130. Harper KW, Collier PS, Dundee JW, et al: Age and nature of operation influence the pharmacokinetics of midazolam. Br J Anaesth 57:866–871, 1985

131. Smith MT, Heazlewood V, Eadie MJ, et al: Pharmacokinetics of midazolam in the aged. Eur J Clin Pharmacol 26:381–388, 1984

132. Crevoisier C, Ziegler WH, Eckert M, et al: Relationship between plasma concentration and effect of midazolam after oral and intravenous administration. Br J Clin Pharmacol 61:51S–61S, 1983

133. Kanto J, Allonen H: Pharmacokinetics and the sedative effect of midazolam. Int J Clin Pharmacol Ther Toxicol 21:460–463, 1983

134. Smith MT, Eadie MJ, Brophy TO: The pharmacokinetics of midazolam in man. Eur J Clin Pharmacol 19:271–278, 1981

135. Fragen RJ, Funk DI, Avram MJ, et al: Midazolam versus hydroxyzine as intramuscular premedicants. Anesthesiology 55:A278, 1981

136. Forster A, Gardaz JP, Suter PM, et al: I.V. midazolam as an induction agent for anesthesia: A study in volunteers. Br J Anaesth 52:907–911, 1980

137. Lebowitz PW, Cote ME, Daniels AL, et al: Comparative cardiovascular effects of midazolam and thiopental in healthy patients. Anesth Analg 61:771–775, 1982

138. Lebowitz PW, Cote ME, Daniels AL, et al: Cardiovascular effects of midazolam and thiopentone for induction of anaesthesia in ill surgical patients. Can Anaesth Soc J 30:19–23, 1983

139. Massaut J, d'Hollander A, Barvais L, et al: Haemodynamic effects of midazolam in the anaesthetized

patient with coronary artery disease. Acta Anaesth Scand 27:299-302, 1983

140. Schulte-Sasse U, Hess W, Tarnow J: Haemodynamic responses to induction of anaesthesia using midazolam in cardiac surgical patients. Br J Anaesth 54:1053-1058, 1982

141. Marty J, Nitenberg A, Blancet F, et al: Effects of midazolam on the coronary circulation in patients with coronary artery disease. Anesthesiology 64:206-210, 1986

142. Kwar P, Carson IW, Clarke RSJ, et al: Haemodynamic changes during induction of anaesthesia with midazolam and diazepam (Valium) in patients undergoing coronary artery bypass surgery. Anaesthesia 40:767-771, 1985

143. Reves JG, Samuelson PN, Lewis S: Midazolam maleate induction in patients with ischaemic heart disease. Haemodynamic observations. Can Anaesth Soc J 26:402-409, 1979

144. Reves JG, Samuelson PN, Linnan M: Effects of midazolam maleate in patients with elevated pulmonary artery occluded pressure. *In* Aldrete JA, Stanley TH (eds): Trends in Intravenous Anesthesia. Chicago, Year Book, 1980, pp 253-257.

145. Fragen RJ, Meyers SN, Barresi V, et al: Hemodynamic effects of midazolam in cardiac patients. Anesthesiology 51:S103, 1979

146. Adams P, Gelman S, Reves JG, et al: Midazolam pharmacodynamics and pharmacokinetics during acute hypovolemia. Anesthesiology 63:140-146, 1985

147. Jones DJ, Stehling LC, Zauder HL, et al: Cardiovascular responses to diazepam and midazolam maleate in the dog. Anesthesiology 51:430-434, 1979

148. Reves JG, Mardis M, Strong S: Cardiopulmonary effects of midazolam. Ala J Med Sci 15:347-351, 1978

149. Samuelson PN, Reves JG, Smith LR, et al: Midazolam versus diazepam: Different effects on systemic vascular resistance. Arzneim Forsch/Drug Res 31(II):2268-2269, 1981

150. Reves JG, Samuelson PN, Vinik HR: Midazolam. *In* Brown BR (ed): Contemporary Anesthesia Practice. (Submitted)

151. Lappas DG, Buckley MJ, Laver MB, et al: Left ventricular performance and pulmonary circulation following addition of nitrous oxide to morphine during coronary artery surgery. Anesthesiology 43:61-69, 1975

152. Lunn JK, Stanley TH, Eisele J, et al: High dose fentanyl anesthesia for coronary artery surgery. Plasma fentanyl concentrations and influence of nitrous oxide on cardiovascular responses. Anesth Analg 58:390-395, 1979

153. Melvin MA, Johnson BH, Quasha AL, et al: Induction of anesthesia with midazolam decreases halothane MAC in humans. Anesthesiology 57:238-242, 1982

154. Godefroi EF, Janssen PAJ, Van Der Eycken CAM, et al: DL-1-(1-arylalkyl) imadazole-5-carboxylate esters. A novel type of hypnotic agent. J Med Chem 8:220-223, 1965

155. Kissin I, McGee T, Smith LR: The indices of potency for intravenous anesthetics. Can Anaesth Soc J 28:585-589, 1981

156. Ghoneim MM, Yamada T: Etomidate: A clinical and electroencephalographic comparison with thiopental. Anesth Analg 56:479-485, 1977

157. Shuermans V, Dom J, Dony J, et al: Multinational evaluation of etomidate for anesthesia induction. Anaesthesist 27:52-59, 1978

158. Horrigan RW, Moyers JR, Johnson BH, et al: Etomidate vs thiopental with and without fentanyl—a comparative study of awakening in man. Anesthesiology 52:362-364, 1980

159. Fragen RJ, Caldwell N: Comparison of a new formulation of etomidate with thiopental—side effects and awakening times. Anesthesiology 50:242-244, 1979

160. Thoneim MM, Van Hamme MJ: Hydrolysis of etomidate. Anesthesiology 50:227-229, 1979

161. Van Hamme MJ, Ghoneim MM, Ambre JJ: Pharmacokinetics of etomidate, a new intravenous anesthetic. Anesthesiology 49:274-277, 1978

162. Heykants JJ, Meuldermans WE, Michiels LJ, et al: Distribution, metabolism and excretion of etomidate, a short acting hypnotic drug in the rat. Comparative study of (R)-$(+)$ and (S)-$(-)$-etomidate. Arch Int Pharmacodyn Ther 216:113-219, 1975

163. Ambre JJ, Van Hamme MJ, Ghoneim MM, et al: Pharmacokinetics of etomidate, a new intravenous anesthetic. Fed Proc 36:997, 1977

164. Hebron BS, Edbrooke DL, Newby DM, et al: Pharmacokinetics of Etomidate associated with prolonged IV infusion. Br J Anaesth 55:281-287, 1983

165. Meuldermans WEG, Heykants JJP: The plasma protein binding and distribution of etomidate in dog, rat and human blood. Arch Int Pharmacodyn Ther 221:150-162, 1976

166. Van De Walle J, Demeyere R, Vanacker B, et al: Total i.v. anesthesia using a continuous etomidate infusion. Acta Anaesthesiol Belg 30:117-122, 1979

167. Sear JW: General kinetic and dynamic principles and their application to continuous infusion anesthesia. Anesthesiology 58:10-25, 1983

168. Schuttle J, Lavken PM, Schwildenh H, et al: Alterations of the pharmacokinetics of etomidate caused by fentanyl. Anesthetist, abstract 700. Volume of Summaries, London, 1981

169. Ammon JR, Fogdall RP, Garman JK: Hemodynamic effects of etomidate and thiopental in patients undergoing cardiac surgery. (Unpublished contribution)

170. Korttila K, Aromaa U: Venous complications after intravenous injection of diazepam, flunitrazepam, thiopentone and etomidate. Acta Anaesth Scand 24:227-230, 1980

171. Clarke RSJ: Adverse effects of intravenously administered drugs used in anaesthetic practice. Drugs 22:26–41, 1981

172. Wagner RL, White PF: Etomidate inhibits adrenocortical function in surgical patients. Anesthesiology 61:647–651, 1984

173. Fragen RJ, Shanks CA, Molteni A, et al: Effects of etomidate on hormonal responses to surgical stress. Anesthesiology 61:652–656, 1984

174. Wanscher M, Tonnesen E, Hüttel M, et al: Etomidate infusion and adrenocortical function: A study in elective surgery. Acta Anaesthesiol Scand 29:483–485, 1985

175. Boidin MP: Steroid response to ACTH and to ascorbinic acid during infusion of etomidate for general surgery. Acta Anaesth Belg 36:15–22, 1985

176. Hempelmann G, Piepenbrock S, Hempelmann W, et al: Influence of althesin and etomidate on blood gasses (continuous PO_2-monitoring) and hemodynamics in man. Acta Anaesth Belg 25:402–412, 1974

177. Firestone S, Kleinman CS, Jaffe CC, et al: Human research and noninvasive measurement of ventricular performance. An echocardiographic evaluation of etomidate and thiopental. Anesthesiology 51:S22, 1979

178. Patschke D, Pruckner JB, Eberlein JH, et al: Effects of althesin, etomidate and fentanyl on haemodynamics and myocardial oxygen consumption in man. Can Anaesth Soc J 24:57–69, 1977

179. Kettler D, Sonntag H, Wolfram-Donath U, et al: Haemodynamics, myocardial function, oxygen requirement, and oxygen supply of the human heart after administration of etomidate. In Doenick A (ed): Anaesthesiology and Resuscitation. Berlin, Springer-Verlag, 1977, pp 91–97

180. Doenicke A, Gabanyi D, Lemcke H, et al: Circulatory behaviour and myocardial function after the administration of three short-acting i.v. hypnotics: etomidate, propanidid, and methohexital. Anaesthetist 23:108–115, 1974

181. Criado A, Maseda J, Navarro E, et al: Induction of anaesthesia with etomidate. Haemodynamic study of 36 patients. Br J Anaesth 52:803–806, 1980

182. Gooding JM, Corssen G: Effect of etomidate on the cardiovascular system. Anesth Analg 56:717–719, 1977

183. Colvin MP, Savege TM, Newland PE, et al: Cardiorespiratory changes following induction of anaesthesia with etomidate in patients with cardiac disease. Br J Anaesth 51:551–556, 1979

184. Gooding JM, Weng JT, Smith RA, et al: Cardiovascular and pulmonary responses following etomidate induction of anesthesia in patients with demonstrated cardiac disease. Anesth Analg 58:40–41, 1979

185. Prakash O, Dhasmana M, Verdouw PD, et al: Cardiovascular effects of etomidate with emphasis on regional myocardial blood flow and performance. Br J Anaesth 53:591–599, 1981

186. Kissin I, Motomura S, Aultman DF, et al: Inotropic and anesthetic potencies of etomidate and thiopental in dogs. Anesth Analg 62:961–965, 1983

187. Kates RA, Stack RS, Hill RF, et al: General anesthesia for patients undergoing percutaneous transluminal coronary angioplasty during acute myocardial infarction. Anesth Analg 65:815–818, 1986

188. Spiss CK, Carim F, Harper W, et al: Haemodynamic effects of fentanyl or alfentanil as adjuvants to etomidate for induction of anaesthesia in cardiac patients. Acta Anaesthesiol Scand 28:554–556, 1984

189. Karliczek GF, Brenken U, Schokkenbrook R, et al: Etomidate–analgesic combination for the induction of anaesthesia in cardiac patients. Part I. Anaesthetist 31:51–60, 1982

190. Karliczek GF, Brenken U, Schokkenbrook R, et al: Etomidate–analgesic combinations for the induction of anaesthesia in cardiac patients. Part II. Anaesthetist 34:213–220, 1982

191. Wauquier A, Hermans C, Van den Broeck W, et al: Resuscitative drug-effects in hypovolemic-hypotensive animals. Part I. Comparative cardiovascular effects of an infusion of saline, etomidate, thiopental or pentobarbital in hypovolemic dogs. (Unpublished observations)

192. Corssen G, Domino EF: Dissociative anesthesia: Further pharmacologic studies and first clinical experience with the phencyclidine derivative CI-581. Anesth Analg 45:29–40, 1966

193. White PF, Way WL, Trevor AJ: Ketamine—Its pharmacology and therapeutic uses. Anesthesiology 56:119–136, 1982

194. Zsigmond EK, Domino EF: Clinical pharmacology and current uses of ketamine. In Aldrete JA, Stanley TH (eds): Trends in Intravenous Anesthesia. Chicago, Year Book Medical Publishers, 1980, pp 283–330

195. Idvall J, Ahlgren I, Aronsen KF, et al: Ketamine infusions: Pharmacokinetics and clinical effects. Br J Anaesth 51:1167–1173, 1979

196. Clements JA, Nimmo WS: Pharmacokinetics and analgesic effect of ketamine in man. Br J Anaesth 53:27–30, 1981

197. Clements JA, Nimmo WS, Grant IS: Bioavailability, pharmacokinetics, and analgesic activity of ketamine in humans. J Pharmaceutical Sciences 71:539–542, 1982

198. Grant IS, Nimmo WS, McNicol LR, et al: Ketamine disposition in children and adults. Br J Anaesth 55:1107–1111, 1983

199. Hatano S, Keane DM, Boggs RE, et al: Diazepam-ketamine anaesthesia for open heart surgery: A "micro-mini" drip administration technique. Can Anaesth Soc J 23:648–656, 1976

200. Virtue RW, Alanis JM, Mori M, et al: An anesthetic agent: 2-orthochlorophenyl, 2-methylamino cyclo-

hexanone HCl (CI-581). Anesthesiology 28:823–833, 1967

201. Tweed WA, Minuck M, Mymin D: Circulatory responses to ketamine anesthesia. Anesthesiology 37:613–619, 1972

202. Tweed WA, Mymin D: Myocardial force-velocity relations during ketamine anesthesia at constant heart rate. Anesthesiology 41:49–52, 1974

203. Stanley V, Hunt J, Willis KW, et al: Cardiovascular and respiratory function with CI-581. Anesth Analg 47:760–768, 1968

204. Nishimura K, Kitamura Y, Hamai R, et al: Pharmacological studies of ketamine hydrochloride in the cardiovascular system. Osaka City Med J 19:17–26, 1973

205. Stanley, TH: Blood-pressure and pulse-rate responses to ketamine during general anesthesia. Anesthesiology 39:648–649, 1973

206. Lippman M, Appel PL, Mok MS, et al: Sequential cardiorespiratory patterns of anesthetic induction with ketamine in critically ill patients. Crit Care Med 11:730–734, 1983

207. Stefansson T, Wickström I, Haljamae H: Hemodynamic and metabolic effects of ketamine anesthesia in the geriatric patient. Acta Anaesth Scand 26:371–377, 1982

208. Corssen G, Moustapha IF, Varner E: The role of dissociative anaesthesia with ketamine in cardiac surgery—a preliminary report based on 253 patients. 4th Asia-Australian Congress of Anaesthesiologists, Singapore, 1974

209. Sonntag H, Heiss HW, Knoll D, et al: Coronary blood flow and myocardial oxygen consumption in patients during induction of anesthesia with droperidol/fentanyl or ketamine. Z Kreislaufforsch 61:1092–1105, 1972

210. Hobika GH, Evers JL, Mostert JW, et al: Comparison of hemodynamic effects of glucagon and ketamine in patients with chronic renal failure. Anesthesiology 37:654–658, 1972

211. Spotoft H, Korshin JD, Sorensen MB, et al: The cardiovascular effects of ketamine used for induction of anaesthesia in patients with valvular heart disease. Can Anaesth Soc J 26:463–467, 1979

212. Dhadphale PR, Jackson APF, Alseri S: Comparison of anesthesia with diazepam and ketamine vs morphine in patients undergoing heart-valve replacement. Anesthesiology 51:200–203, 1979

213. Savege TM, Colvin MP, Weaver EJM, et al: A comparison of some cardiorespiratory effects of althesin and ketamine when used for induction of anaesthesia in patients with cardiac disease. Br J Anaesth 48:1071–1081, 1976

214. Morray JP, Lynn AM, Stamm SJ, et al: Hemodynamic effects of ketamine in children with congenital heart disease. Anesth Analg 63:895–899, 1984

215. Greeley WJ, Bushman GA, Davis DP, et al: Comparative effects of two induction techniques on arterial

oxygen saturation during pediatric cardiovascular surgery. (Abstract) Submitted to SCA, 1985

216. Balfors E, Häggmark S, Nyhman H, et al: Droperidol inhibits the effects of intravenous ketamine on central hemodynamics and myocardial oxygen consumption in patients with generalized atherosclerotic disease. Anesth Analg 62:193–197, 1983

217. Gooding JM, Dimick AR, Tavakoli M, et al: A physiologic analysis of cardiopulmonary responses to ketamine anesthesia in noncardiac patients. Anesth Analg 56:813–816, 1977

218. Coppel DL, Dundee JW: Ketamine anesthesia for cardiac catheterization. Anaesthesia 27:25–31, 1972

219. Faithfull NS, Haider R: Ketamine for cardiac catheterization: An evaluation of its use in children. Anaesthesia 26:318–323, 1971

220. McIntyre JWR, Dobson D, Aitken G: Ketamine with pancuronium for induction of anesthesia. Can Anaesth Soc J 21:475–481, 1974

221. Zsigmond EK, Domino EP: Ketamine clinical pharmacology, pharmacokinetics and current clinical uses. Anesthesiology Rev 7:13–33, 1980

222. White PF, Way WL, Trevor AJ: Ketamine—its pharmacology and therapeutic uses. Anesthesiology 56:119–136, 1982

223. Dowdy EG, Kaya K: Studies of the mechanism of cardiovascular responses to CI-581. Anesthesiology 29:931–943, 1968

224. Valicenti JF, Newman WH, Bagwell EE, et al: Myocardial contractility during induction and steady-state ketamine anesthesia. Anesth Analg 52:190–194, 1973

225. Urthaler F, Walker AA, James TN: Comparison of the inotropic action of morphine and ketamine studied in canine cardiac muscle. J Thorac Cardiovasc Surg 72:142–149, 1976

226. Ivankovich AD, Miletich DJ, Reimann C, et al: Cardiovascular effects of centrally administered ketamine in goats. Anesth Analg 53:924–933, 1974

227. Zsigmond EK, Kothary SP, Matsuki A, et al: Diazepam for prevention of the rise in plasma catecholamines caused by ketamine. Clin Pharmacol Ther 15:223–224, 1974

228. Zsigmond EK: Guest discussion. Anesth Analg 53:931–933, 1974

229. Kumar SM, Kothary SP, Zsigmond EK: Plasma free norepinephrine and epinephrine concentrations following diazepam-ketamine induction in patients undergoing cardiac surgery. Acta Anaesth Scand 22:593–600, 1978

230. Slogoff S, Allen GW: The role of baroreceptors in the cardiovascular response to ketamine. Anesth Analg 53:704–707, 1974

231. Clanachan AS, McGrath JC, Mackenzie JE: Cardiovascular effects of ketamine in the pithed rat, rabbit and cat. Br J Anaesth 48:935–939, 1976

232. Traber DL, Wilson RD, Priano LL: Differentiation

of the cardiovascular effects of CI-581. Anesth Analg 47:769–778, 1968

233. Traber DL, Wilson RD: Involvement of the sympathetic nervous system in the pressor response to ketamine. Anesth Analg 48:248–252, 1969

234. Traber DL, Wilson RD, Priano LL: Blockade of the hypertensive response to ketamine. Anesth Analg 49:420–426, 1970

235. Traber DL, Wilson RD, Priano LL: The effect of beta-adrenergic blockade on the cardiopulmonary response to ketamine. Anesth Analg 49:604–613, 1970

236. Traber DL, Wilson RD, Priano LL: A detailed study of the cardiopulmonary response to ketamine and its blockade by atropine. South Med J 63:1077–1081, 1970

237. Traber DL, Wilson RD, Priano LL: The effect of beta-adrenergic blockade on the cardiopulmonary response to ketamine. Anesth Analg 50:737–742, 1971

238. Hill GE, Wong KC, Shaw CL, et al: Interactions of ketamine with vasoactive amines at normothermia and hypothermia in the isolated rabbit heart. Anesthesiology 48:315–319, 1978

239. Miletich DJ, Ivankovich AD, Albrecht RF, et al: The effect of ketamine on catecholamine metabolism in the isolated perfused rat heart. Anesthesiology 39:271–277, 1973

240. Johnstone M: The cardiovascular effects of ketamine in man. Anesthesia 31:873–882, 1976

241. Freuchen I, Ostergaard J, Kuhl JB, et al: Reduction of psychotomimetic side effects of ketalar (ketamine) by rohypnol (flunitrazepam). Acta Anaesth Scand 20:97–103, 1976

242. Pedersen T, Engbaek J, Ording H, et al: Effect of vecuronium and pancuronium on cardiac performance and transmural myocardial perfusion during ketamine anaesthesia. Acta Anaesth Scand 28:443–446, 1984

243. Chodoff P, Stella JG: Use of CI-581, a phencyclidine derivative for obstetric anesthesia. Anesth Analg 45:527–530, 1966

244. Bidwal AV, Stanley TH, Graves CL, et al: The effects of ketamine on cardiovascular dynamics during halothane and enflurane anesthesia. Anesth Analg 54:588–592, 1975

245. Radnay PA: Anesthetic management of surgery requiring cardiopulmonary bypass. *In* Radnay PA, Nagashima H (eds): Anesthetic Considerations for Pediatric Cardiac Surgery. International Anesthesiology Clinics. Boston, Little, Brown, 1980, pp 95–122

246. Santoli FM, Pensa PM, Azzolina G: Anesthesia in open-heart surgery for correction of congenital heart diseases in children over one year of age. *In* Weichmann V (ed): Anesthesia for Open-Heart Surgery. International Anesthesiology Clinics. Boston, Little, Brown, 1976, pp 165–201

247. Levin RM, Seleny FL, Streczyn MV: Ketamine-pancuronium-narcotic technique for cardiovascular surgery in infants—a comparative study. Anesth Analg 54:800–805, 1975

248. Vaughan RW, Stephen CR: Ketamine for corrective cardiac surgery in children. South Med J 66:1226–1230, 1973

249. Gassner S, Cohen M, Aygen M, et al: The effect of ketamine on pulmonary artery pressure. Anaesthesia 29:141–146, 1974

250. Hickey PR, Hansen DD, Cramolini GM, et al: Pulmonary and systemic hemodynamic responses to ketamine in infants with normal and elevated pulmonary vascular resistance. Anesthesiology 62:287–292, 1985

251. Lippmann M, Cleveland RJ: Emergency closed mitral commissurotomy using ketamine anesthesia: Report of a case. Anesthesiology 35:543–544, 1971

252. Posner MA, Reves JG, Lell WA: Aortic valve replacement in a hemodialysis-dependent patient: Anesthetic considerations—a case report. Anesth Analg 54:24–28, 1975

253. Reves JG, Kravetz RA, McCracken LE, et al: Comparison of morphine and ketamine anesthetic techniques for open heart surgery. A prospective randomized study. Abstracts of Scientific Papers, Chicago, IL, ASA Annual Meeting, 1975

254. Reves JG, Lell WA, McCracken LE Jr, et al: Comparison of morphine and ketamine anesthetic techniques for coronary surgery: A randomized study. South Med J 71:33–46, 1978

255. Corssen G, Reves JG, Carter JR: Neuroleptanesthesia, dissociative anesthesia, and hemorrhage. Int Anesthesiol Clin 12:145–161, 1974

256. Nettles DC, Herrin TJ, Mullen JG: Ketamine induction in poor-risk patients. Anesth Analg 52:59–64, 1973

257. Waxman K, Shoemaker WC, Lippman M: Cardiovascular effects of anesthetic induction with ketamine. Anesth Analg 59:355–358, 1980

258. Patel K, Gelman S, McElvein R: Ketamine in patients with pericarditis: Hemodynamic effects. In press.

259. Adam MK, Briggs LP, Bamar M, et al: Pharmacokinetic evaluation of ICI 35 868 in man. Br J Anaesth 55:47–103, 1983

260. Prys-Robert C, Davis JR, Calverley RK, et al: Haemodynamic effects of infusions of Diisopropylphenol (ICI35868) during nitrous oxide anaesthesia in man. Br J Anaesth 55:105–111, 1983

261. Fahmy NR, Alkhouli HM, Sunder N, et al: Diprivan: A new intravenous induction agent. Anesthesiology 63:A363, 1985

262. Williams JP, McArthur JD, Walker WE, et al: The cardiovascular effects of propofol in patients with impaired cardiac function. Anesth Analg 65:S166, 1986

Ralph P.F. Scott, B.Sc., M.B.Ch.B., F.F.A.R.C.S.
John J. Savarese, M.D.

5

New Muscle Relaxants and the Cardiovascular System

In the early 1980s the most commonly used muscle relaxants in anesthetic practice in the United States were succinylcholine, tubocurarine, metocurine, pancuronium and, to a lesser extent, gallamine. However, these agents have certain cardiovascular side effects that limit their use. These effects are generally due to stimulation or inhibition of peripheral autonomic sites, to the release of histamine and possibly other vasoactive substances from vascular mast cells, or to increases in serum potassium levels secondary to motor end-plate depolarization. A major reason for developing new neuromuscular blocking agents is to produce drugs that avoid these well-known side effects. A careful examination of the advantages and disadvantages of the above agents will lead to the conclusion that a nondepolarizing muscle relaxant such as pancuronium, without cardiovascular side effects, would provide a significant improvement.

The accumulated knowledge of structure-activity relationships in the field of neuromuscular blockade allows chemists to produce effective neuromuscular blocking drugs more predictably, with less reliance on chance, than is the case with any other class of drugs. Consequently, most kinds of unwanted activity can be avoided by appropriate molecular design; and new compounds that produce unwanted effects can be discarded at an early stage in preclinical testing. The development of atracurium and vecuronium has marked an exciting stage in the production of drugs with improved cardiovascular stability. These two drugs fall into the intermediate duration class, but research is continuing to find agents of similar cardiovascular stability with shorter and longer durations of action.

PHARMACOLOGY OF THE AUTONOMIC NERVOUS SYSTEM

In order to understand the autonomic responses to existing muscle relaxants and the developmental pharmacology of new agents, it is important to have a working knowledge of the autonomic nervous system, and, in particular, the possible sites of interaction between muscle relaxants and cholinoceptors.

Acetylcholine acts on both muscarinic and nicotinic receptors (Table 5-1). Muscarinic receptors are present in various smooth muscles, cardiac muscle, and exocrine glands. They are termed "muscarinic" because muscarine, a quaternary amine alkaloid, has

CARDIAC ANESTHESIA, SECOND EDITION
ISBN 0-8089-1848-6

Table 5-1
Cholinoceptive Sites

Site	Activator or Substrates	Inhibitor
Nicotinic receptors Neuromuscular junction	Nicotine, tetramethylammonium, succinylcholine, decamethonium	d-tubocurarine All nondepolarizing neuromuscular blocking agents
Autonomic ganglia	Dimethylphenylpiperazinium	Hexamethonium, d-tubocurarine
Muscarinic receptors, (bowel, bladder, bronchi, sinus node of the heart, pupillary sphincter)	Muscarine	Atropine, gallamine, pancuronium
Esteratic receptors Active site of acetylcholinesterase	Acetylcholine, methacholine	Neostigmine, pyridostigmine, benzoquinonium
Active site of plasmacholinesterase	Benzoylcholine, butyrylcholine, succinylcholine	Hexaflurenium, tetrahydroaminacrine, pancuronium

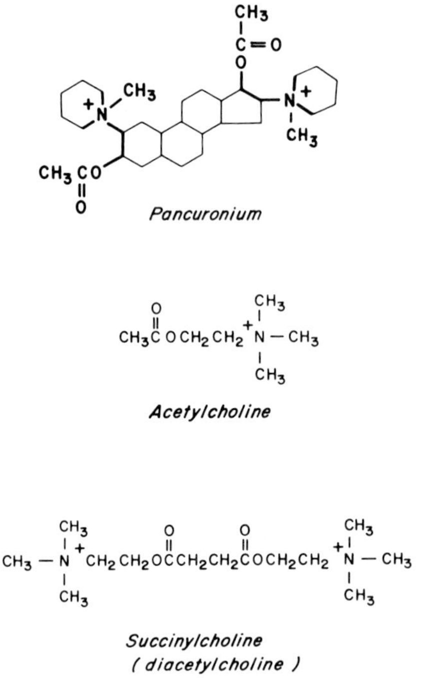

Fig. 5-1. Structural relationship of acetylcholine to two neuromuscular blocking agents. Succinylcholine (diacetylcholine) is simply two molecules of acetylcholine linked through the acetate methyl groups. Pancuronium may be viewed as two acetylcholine-like fragments (outlined in dark print) properly orientated conformationally on a bulky, rigid, inflexible steroid nucleus.

actions similar to those of acetylcholine at the sites indicated. The muscarinic receptor is blocked by atropine and related drugs. The nicotinic receptors of acetylcholine are located in autonomic ganglia and at the skeletal neuromuscular junction. They are termed "nicotinic" because nicotine also acts on these receptors. However, the nicotinic receptors in the autonomic ganglia and skeletal muscle are not identical. The effect of acetylcholine on autonomic ganglia is blocked by tubocurarine and related compounds. Further cholinoceptive sites are found on the esteratic receptors of acetylcholinesterase and plasma cholinesterase. Crystalographic analysis of acetylcholine and related agonists provides a tentative answer to the nature of the cholinergic receptor. Acetylcholine is a flexible molecule, and rotation is possible at two different bonds (Fig. 5-1). Muscarinic and nicotinic drugs differ from acetylcholine in the degree of rotation at the sites of torsion. Thus, acetylcholine has both muscarinic and nicotinic effects, whereas the purely muscarinic or nicotinic congeners have constraints imposed on them by conformational factors. In order for neuromuscular blocking drugs to interact with the recognition sites of the cholinoceptors at the neuromuscular junction, the drugs must bear some chemical relationship to acetylcholine. Consequently, there is the possibility that they might compete with or mimic acetylcholine at other sites (eg, cholinesterases, nicotinic autonomic ganglionic receptors, and muscarinic receptors).

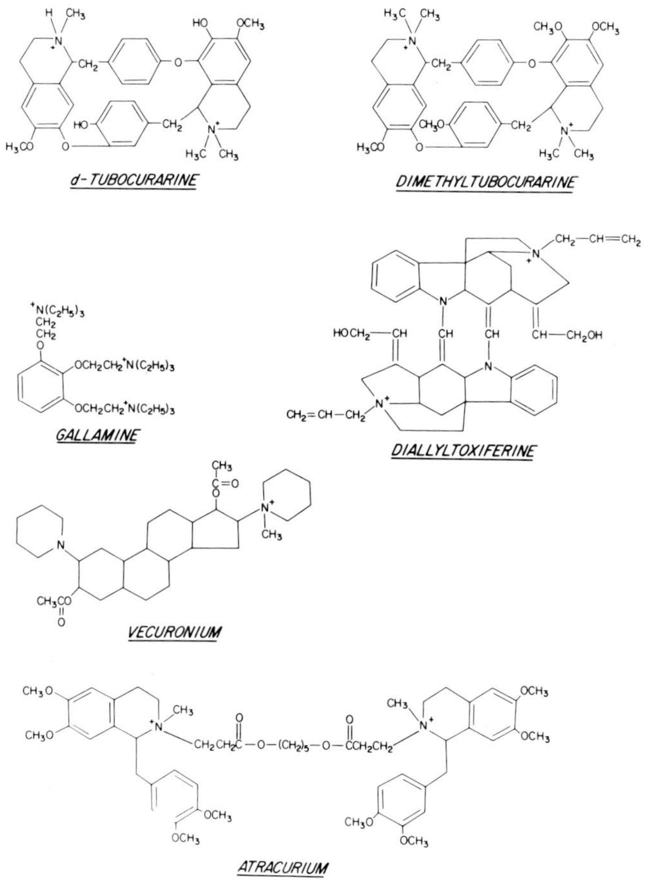

Fig. 5-2. The chemical structure of some common nondepolarizing neuromuscular blocking agents.

Interaction of Neuromuscular Blocking Agents at Different Cholinoceptive Sites

AUTONOMIC GANGLIA

Tubocurarine (Fig. 5-2) blocks ganglionic nicotinic receptors and produces some ganglionic blockade in a dose range similar to that required to produce neuromuscular blockade. It may have a slightly more powerful action on parasympathetic than on sympathetic ganglia.[1] Autonomic reflexes arising in the course of surgical operations may be impaired by the ganglionic blocking action, and this action may contribute to hypotension.[2,3] Recent evidence, however, suggests that the role of ganglionic blockade in the hypotensive action of tubocurarine is possibly less important than its ability to release histamine.[4]

Metocurine (dimethyltubocurarine) and alcuronium (diallyltoxiferine) are weaker ganglionic blockers; and other neuromuscular blocking drugs (eg, gallamine, pancuronium, atracurium, and vecuronium) have no ganglionic blocking activity in the doses used clinically (Fig. 5-2). Succinylcholine has a weak autonomic ganglion stimulant action that may have some clinical importance, since a hypertensive response is occasionally observed (Fig. 5-3).[5]

MUSCARINIC RECEPTORS

Evidence has accumulated in recent years that muscarinic receptors are probably not a homogeneous group.[6] By definition they are all stimulated by muscarine and they are all blocked by atropine, but they may differ with respect to their interactions with

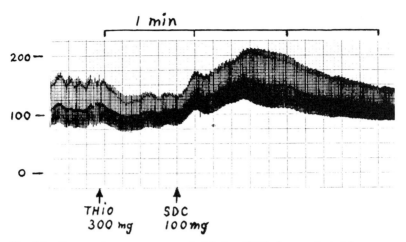

Fig. 5-3. Hypertensive response to succinylcholine (SDC). Increased arterial pressure after succinylcholine administration may represent a clinical manifestation of its ganglion stimulating action. This patient had a hypertensive response to succinylcholine. There was no other anesthetic or surgical intervention.

other agonists and antagonists. Figure 5-4 is a diagrammatic representation of the main components of the autonomic nervous system with respect to the heart. For the purpose of the diagram, the muscarinic cholinoceptors have been labeled "M1," "M2," and "M3" receptors, but this is not a strict classification and is probably an oversimplification.[7]

The first indication that muscarinic receptors may not all be identical in character came from Riker and Wescoe[8] who showed that gallamine, although generally free from atropine-like activity in smooth muscle, nevertheless blocked muscarinic receptors in the cat heart, and, consequently, inactivated the car-

diac vagus nerve. In Figure 5-4 the cardiac muscarinic receptors are included in the "M2" group to distinguish them from the more usual type labeled "M1." Other workers have since shown that pancuronium,[9] fazadinium,[10] alcuronium,[11] and stercuronium[12] also block the cardiac muscarinic receptors in doses approximating those required to produce muscle relaxation. Tubocurarine, metocurine, vecuronium, and atracurium block cardiac muscarinic receptors and other muscarinic receptors only in doses that greatly exceed the neuromuscular blocking dose.[13-15]

Arterioles also have muscarinic receptors, but

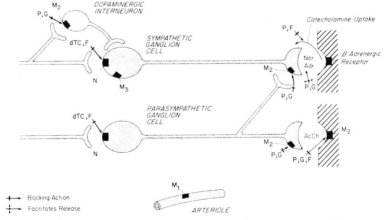

Fig. 5-4. Diagrammatic representation of the autonomic nervous system with respect to the heart, and sites of action of some neuromuscular blocking drugs on this system. The muscarinic receptors have been divided into three subclasses (M_1, M_2, M_3). By permission of the authors. N = nicotinic receptor, P = pancuronium, G = gallamine, F = fazadinium, dTc = d-tubocurarine.

these receptors are not innervated. They resemble most of the noncardiac muscarinic receptors in their agonist and antagonist selectivity, and are labeled "M1" in Figure 5-4. The vasopressor response to methacholine, although blocked by atropine, is not affected by pancuronium, showing that the muscarinic receptors involved in the arterioles are not the same type as those in the sinoatrial node.

Experiments have shown that cardiac muscarinic receptors are not the only muscarinic receptors that are blocked by certain neuromuscular blocking drugs. Stimulation of the vagus nerve has been shown to reduce the release of norepinephrine from concomitantly stimulated sympathetic nerves to the heart.[16] It is, therefore, believed that vagus nerve terminals impinge not only on the nodal and atrial cells of the heart, but also on the sympathetic nerve endings where they act to inhibit the release of norepinephrine. The cholinergic receptors on the sympathetic nerve endings are of the muscarinic type, and there is indirect evidence that they are blocked by gallamine and pancuronium, but much less effectively by vecuronium.[17] This effect would enhance the tachycardia arising from blockade of the cardiac muscarinic receptors. Because the muscarinic receptors on the sympathetic terminals resemble the cardiac muscarinic receptors in being blocked by gallamine and pancuronium, they have both been labeled "M2," but the evidence of similarity is not very strong.

Another location of muscarinic cholinoceptors that are blocked by pancuronium and gallamine and are, therefore, indicated as "M2" receptors in Figure 5-4 is on the small dopaminergic interneurons on sympathetic ganglia. These cells are activated through muscarinic receptors stimulated by acetylcholine that is released from collaterals of the preganglionic cholinergic nerve fibers. Dopamine released from these cells onto the ganglion cells hyperpolarizes them and, therefore, suppresses ganglionic transmission.[18] Blockade of these inhibitory cells by gallamine or pancuronium may, therefore, at appropriate stimulation frequencies, facilitate transmission through the ganglia by inactivating the inhibitory modulating influence of the dopaminergic cell loop.[19]

Transmission through sympathetic ganglia is mediated by acetylcholine acting on nicotinic receptors. There are, however, muscarinic cholinoceptors present on sympathetic ganglia whose physiological function is as yet unknown. These are labelled "M3" receptors in Figure 5-4. They differ from those labeled "M2" in that they are not blocked by gallamine or pancuronium; and, they differ from those

labeled "M1" and "M2" in that they are especially sensitive to certain unusual muscarinic agonists.[20] It should be noted that gallamine causes norepinephrine release in guinea pig and cat atria and in anesthetized cats by a mechanism that may be quite independent of muscarinic blockade.[21] Similarly, very large concentrations of pancuronium produce norepinephrine release in isolated guinea pig atria under conditions in which parasympathetic block could not be involved.[22] Pancuronium and fazadinium have also been shown to block norepinephrine reuptake into sympathetic nerve endings both in cardiac muscle and in smooth muscle in guinea pigs and rats.[22-24] In the cat, the main mechanism through which certain neuromuscular blocking drugs depress cardiovagal activity is by blocking postjunctional muscarinic cholinoceptors as described above. However, Lee Son and Waud calculated that the concentrations of pancuronium and gallamine that block responses to postjunctional vagal stimulation are too low to exert significant blocking action on the postjunctional muscarinic receptors; they concluded that the main site of action of these two drugs in blocking the guinea pig cardiac vagus is on the postganglionic nerve terminals.[25]

It can be concluded from the foregoing discussion that a combination of any of the above actions of gallamine, pancuronium, and fazadinium may account for the cardiovascular effects of these drugs. There is considerable species difference with regard to the relative importance of these effects. It is not known which effect is the most predominant in humans, but it is likely that the relative importance varies from patient to patient according to such factors as the pre-existing autonomic balance, the type of premedication, the anesthetic, and any concurrent drug therapy.

The Demonstration of Autonomic Effects of Neuromuscular Agents in Whole Animals

There are no appropriate means for testing the autonomic effects of relaxants in man, and most of the knowledge of these actions is derived from experiments performed in isolated organ systems or in whole animals such as the cat. In the cat, measurements of neuromuscular and autonomic functions may be accomplished simultaneously. Neuromuscular function is assessed by recording the twitch response of the tibialis anterior (or other appropriate muscle) evoked indirectly via the sciatic or peroneal nerve. Vagal function is determined by quantitation

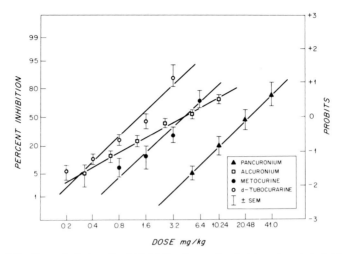

Fig. 5-5. Sympathetic (ganglionic) inhibition by nondepolarizing relaxants in the cat. (JJ Savarese, unpublished data).

of the bradycardia and hypotension elicited by stimulation of the nerve. Sympathetic ganglionic responses (Fig. 5-5) are assayed by preganglionic stimulation of the sympathetic trunk, central to the superior cervical ganglion, and recording the evoked contraction of the nictitating membrane (Fig. 5-6).

The separation of neuromuscular blocking action from autonomic effects can be described for each drug as its *autonomic margin of safety*. This indicates the number of multiples of a dose of relaxant, producing 95 percent neuromuscular blockade, that must be administered in order to produce side effects. The higher the autonomic margin of safety, the lower the probability of occurrence of a side effect. The following quotients are used:

1. $\dfrac{ED_{50} \text{ (Ganglion block)}}{ED_{95} \text{ (Neuromuscular block)}}$

2. $\dfrac{ED_{50} \text{ (Cardiac vagal block)}}{ED_{95} \text{ (Neuromuscular block)}}$

3. $\dfrac{ED_{50} \text{ (Histamine release)}}{ED_{95} \text{ (Neuromuscular block)}}$

Calculation of autonomic margins of safety for neuromuscular blocking drugs in man is not possible because suitable methods for quantitating autonomic responses in humans are not available. There is considerable indication, however, that when a neuromuscular blocking drug produces an autonomic effect in the cat within or near the neuromuscular dose range, the neuromuscular blockade in humans

will be accompanied by cardiovascular changes corresponding to those autonomic actions (Table 5-2).

The ED_{95} for neuromuscular blockade for some of the nondepolarizing relaxants in humans, under nitrous oxide, has been determined. These values, together with the ED_{50} for ganglion and vagal block derived in the cat (since these cannot be determined in humans), were used to calculate the values in the table. The ED_{50} for histamine release can, however, be calculated in humans, using an isotope radioenzymatic assay. The relative importance of ganglion block, vagal block, and histamine release for each of the nondepolarizing relaxants is outlined in Table 5-3.

Anesthesiologists encounter both immunologically mediated reactions and chemically mediated reactions associated with the administration of muscle relaxants. Immunological reactions to muscle relaxants have never attracted as much attention as those to intravenous induction agents. These reactions are rare but no less dangerous in their manifestations, since many have been severe enough to necessitate cardiopulmonary resuscitation. Reactions to succinylcholine are more common than with any other muscle relaxant.

Chemically mediated reactions happen much more frequently and occur when the injected substance acts directly on tissue cells and basophil leukocytes, leading to the release of histamine without antibody or complement involvement. Most organic bases can release histamine, and most neuromuscular blocking drugs have been shown to produce this effect when sufficiently large doses or concentrations

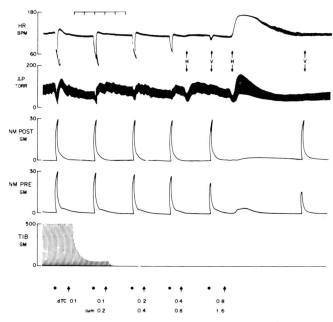

Fig. 5-6. Simultaneous recording of autonomic and neuromuscular function in a cat anesthetized with chloralose. Recordings are (top to bottom) of heart rate, femoral arterial pressure, contractions of the left and right nictitating membranes elicited preganglionically and postganglionically, and tibialis anterior muscle twitch. At times indicated by dots below the graphs, stimulation of the right vagus nerve and both sympathetic trunks (left postganglionically, and right preganglionically) was applied at 20 Hz for 10 seconds. At times indicated by arrows below graphs, *d*-tubocurarine in doses indicated (mg/kg) was given intravenously. Lower figures indicate cumulative dosage. Note that vagal response (bradycardia and hypotension), ganglionic response (preganglionically stimulated nictitating membrane) and neuromuscular response are all inhibited at a cumulative dose of 0.8 to 1.6 mg/kg. Marker H between the upper two graphs indicates cardiovascular changes suggestive of histamine release. Marker V indicates points of vagal stimulation with little or no response. (From Savarese JJ: The autonomic margins of safety of metocurine and d-tubocurarine in the cat. Anesthesiology 50:40, 1979, with permission.)

Table 5-2

Autonomic Margin of Safety of Nondepolarizing Relaxants in Man

Drug	Neuromuscular Block* ED_{95} in Man	Autonomic Margin of Safety Ganglion block	Vagal block	Margin of safety for histamine release
d-tubocurarine	0.51	2.94	0.59	1
Metocurine	0.28	18.6	2.86	2
Pancuronium	0.07	328.6	2.86	High
Alcuronium	0.25	18.0	1.84	High
Vecuronium	0.056	89.2	40.6	High
Atracurium	0.28	35.7	8.7	3

*ED_{95} in humans (mg/kg)

$$\text{Autonomic margin of safety} = \frac{ED_{50} \text{ for autonomic inhibition in the cat}}{ED_{95} \text{ for neuromuscular block in man}}$$

$$\text{Margin of safety for histamine release} = \frac{ED_{50} \text{ for histamine release in man}}{ED_{95} \text{ for neuromuscular block in man.}}$$

157

Table 5-3
Effects of 1.5–2 × ED$_{95}$ Blocking Dose of Nondepolarizing Muscle Relaxants in Humans Under Halothane Anesthesia

	Ganglion block	(Muscarinic) vagal block	Histamine release	Under Anesthesia			
				SVR	CO	BP	HR
Tubocurarine	*	–	***	↓	↓	↓	–
Metocurine	–	–	*	↓	–	↓	–
Pancuronium	–	**	–	–	↑	↑	↑
Gallamine	–	***	–	–	↑	↑	↑
Alcuronium	*	*	–	↓	↑	↓	↑
Fazadinium	**	**	–	↓	↑	↓	↑
Vecuronium	–	–	–	–	–	–	–
Atracurium	–	–	(– to *)	(– or ↓)	(– or ↑)	(– or ↓)	–

SVR = Systemic Vascular Resistance, CO = Cardiac Output, BP = Blood Pressure (Mean arterial pressure), HR = Heart Rate

   * = Mild
  ** = Moderate
*** = Major

are used.[26] It is important to know, however, whether the effect is likely to occur with the dosage used in clinical practice. It has been recognized that tubocurarine is a potent liberator of histamine, and this is possibly the major cause of the hypotension occurring in most patients given clinical doses.

Recent work has demonstrated that the release of histamine by muscle relaxants in humans is dose-dependent (Fig. 5-7), and that the release is well-correlated with significant hemodynamic effects

(Fig. 5-8).[4] Further studies, however, have shown that there are clinical strategies, such as slowing the injection rate (Fig. 5-7), or administering histamine receptor blockers (H1 and H2), that can blunt these effects in humans.[27]

The ability of atracurium to release histamine relative to its neuromuscular blocking potency is approximately one-half that of dimethyltubocurarine, and about one-third that of tubocurarine.[28] Succinylcholine has a histamine-liberating activity about 1

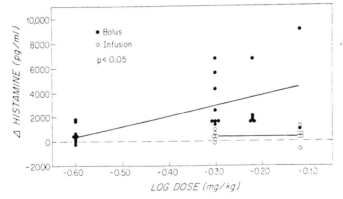

Fig. 5-7. Slowing the injection rate of *d*-tubocurarine minimizes histamine release. In a study with *d*-tubocurarine, Moss et al found dose-related increases in plasma histamine occurring 2 minutes after injection in the groups receiving boluses, but not in those receiving a slow (60–90 sec) infusion. (From Moss J, Rosow CE, Savarese JJ, et al: Role of histamine in the hypotensive action of d-tubocurarine in humans. Anesthesiology 55:19, 1981, with permission.)

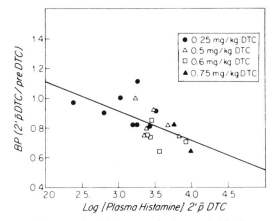

Fig. 5-8. Relationship between the decrease in blood pressure and plasma histamine concentration 2 minutes after the administration of indicated doses of *d*-tubocurarine in 21 patients. (From Moss J, Rosow CE, Savarese JJ, et al: Role of histamine in the hypotensive action of d-tubocurarine in humans. Anesthesiology 55:19, 1981, with permission.)

percent that of tubocurarine, while gallamine, pancuronium, and vecuronium have minimal potential for releasing histamine in clinical doses.

STRUCTURE-ACTIVITY RELATIONSHIPS

The natural transmitter at the neuromuscular junction, acetylcholine, has a positively charged ammonium group, which is attracted to the negatively charged cholinergic receptor sites. This feature is also common to the neuromuscular blocking drugs that contain at least one quaternary ammonium group (Figs. 5-1 and 5-2).

The neuromuscular blocking agents show certain structural similarities to acetylcholine. Succinylcholine is essentially two molecules of acetylcholine linked through the acetate-methyl groups. Depolarizing agents, such as succinylcholine, generally stimulate nicotinic and muscarinic receptors in imitation of the role of acetylcholine. The depolarizing action of succinyl choline is due to the presence in the molecule of the trimethyl ammonium group and the carboxyl groups in a linear flexible chain (Fig. 5-1). The separation of the quaternary ammonium functions from the carboxyl groups by a distance of 4.5 Å, as occurs with acetylcholine, also contributes to the agonist (depolarizing) action of succinylcholine.[29] Removal of the carboxyl groups of succinylcholine results in decamethonium, which has much weaker

autonomic stimulating properties than succinylcholine.[30]

The shape and flexibility of the molecule is important. Most agonists such as succinylcholine are flexible, long, and slender. Bulky molecules such as pancuronium with a rigid ring system cannot activate or stimulate the receptors themselves, but block the approach of acetylcholine, and, therefore, produce a nondepolarizing block by antagonism or receptor inhibition.

Tubocurarine (Fig. 5-2) has now been shown to have only one quaternary ammonium group and a tertiary amine group in equilibrium with a proton at physiological pH.[31] The new formula supports the autonomic ganglionic properties of tubocurarine as a monoquaternary structure, which is more likely to produce ganglionic blockade than a bisquaternary compound. The histamine-releasing properties of tubocurarine are probably due to the presence of the tertiary amine.[32] In general, bisquaternary compounds do not possess strong ganglionic blocking or histamine-releasing properties. Methylation of tubocurarine to produce metocurine or dimethyltubocurarine (a bisquaternary compound) reduces the histamine-releasing and ganglion-blocking activities associated with tubocurarine, and results in a muscle relaxant that is three times less potent than tubocurarine in blocking sympathetic and parasympathetic ganglia.[11,13] Gallamine (a trisquaternary compound) has marked vagolytic properties probably due to the presence of the three positively charged nitrogen atoms.[8,11]

THE DEVELOPMENTAL CHEMISTRY OF THE NEW DRUGS

In 1973, a model of the perfect relaxant was described by Savarese and Kitz[33] as a drug having a brief, noncumulative, nondepolarizing neuromuscular blocking action with a rapid onset and recovery. It should be readily reversible by an appropriate antagonist, cause neither histamine release nor ganglionic blockade, and give rise to minimal cardiovascular side effects. It should be highly potent and its metabolites should neither accumulate nor have any pharmacologic activity or toxicity.

In 1851, coincidentally in the same year that Claude Bernard first described the action of curare on the neuromuscular junction, A.W. Hofmann described his method of degrading quaternary ammonium compounds, now known as "Hofmann elimination," which required strong alkaline conditions and

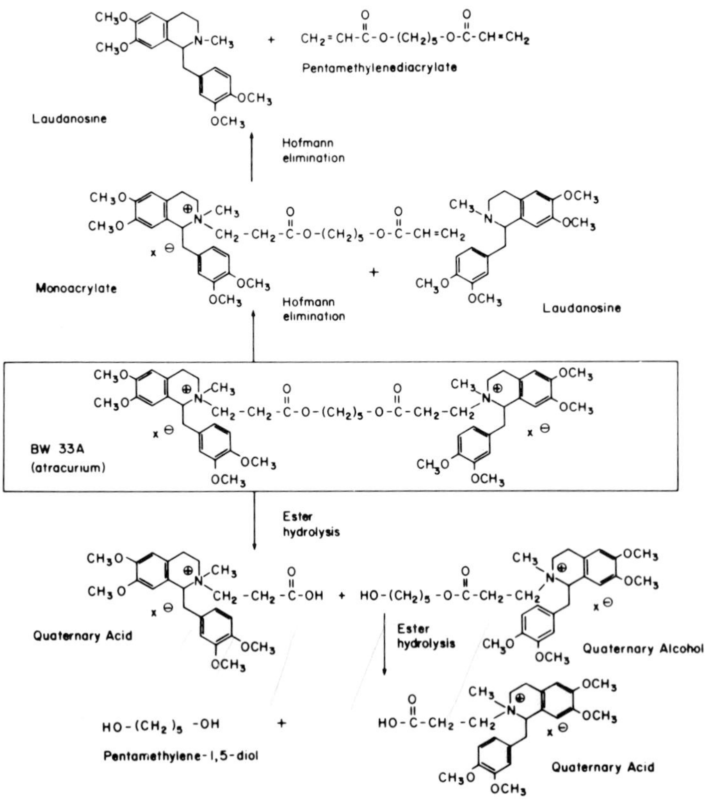

Fig. 5-9. Proposed pathways of inactivation of atracurium by Hofmann elimination reaction and ester hydrolysis. (From Basta SJ, Ali HH, Savarese JJ, et al: Clinical pharmacology of atracurium besylate (BW 33A): A new non-depolarizing muscle relaxant. Anesth Analg 61:723, 1982, with permission.)

very high temperatures. More than 100 years later these two apparently unrelated events were brought together and led to the development of atracurium. Professor J.B. Stenlake of the University of Strathclyde, Glasgow, had the novel idea of incorporating these features into the chemical structure of a neuromuscular blocking agent that would allow the Hofmann elimination to proceed under physiological conditions at body pH and temperature.[34] The idea was that the incorporation of this self-destructing mechanism would provide a drug that was not dependent on hepatic or renal function for the termination of its action. This nonenzymatic biodegradation mechanism (Fig. 5-9) is promoted by the combined electron-withdrawing properties of the two beta-linked estercarbonyl groups and the positively charged nitrogens of the quaternary ammonium groups. Nucleophylic attack by hydroxyl ions occurs readily at physiological pH and temperature. It results in the destruction of the bisquaternary struc-

ture essential for neuromuscular blocking activity through molecular fragmentation to laudanosine and other products without significant neuromuscular or cardiovascular effects.[35] Hydrolysis of the ester groupings is similarly promoted by the electron-withdrawing effects of the positively charged quaternary ammonium groups. Hofmann elimination is, therefore, accompanied by ester hydrolysis, which further fragments the molecule to inactive components. Breakdown and loss of potency of atracurium in human plasma is independent of plasma esterase activity. The time course of action is unaffected by hepatic metabolism or renal function.

The rates of Hofmann elimination and ester hydrolysis of atracurium control the stability and life of the intact molecule both in vivo and in vitro. Both reactions are base-catalyzed so that potency and duration of the full block are reduced and recovery is hastened by alkalosis. Ester hydrolysis is also acid catalyzed, but Hofmann elimination is increasingly inhibited with the decreasing pH. Stability of the molecule, as a whole, is, therefore, achieved at about pH 3.5, and aqueous injection solutions at this pH stored under refrigerated conditions have a shelf life adequate for clinical use. It follows that artificial lowering of body temperature in vivo as in open heart surgery may, therefore, slow the inactivation of atracurium to advantage; whereas rewarming should enhance this decomposition and hasten recovery.

Hofmann elimination was originally postulated to be the major route of in vivo degradation of atracurium, although a recent in vitro study in human plasma has demonstrated that ester hydrolysis is possibly of more importance as the major metabolic pathway.[36] If these findings can be confirmed, the hypothetical potential adverse effects from the acrylate end-products of Hofmann elimination would be lessened. A further hypothetical side effect of an atracurium metabolite is the known convulsant effect of laudanosine. This, however, occurs at blood levels unlikely to be achieved even by prolonged atracurium administration.[37]

Savage et al are responsible for the manipulation of the steroid nucleus that resulted in the development of many neuromuscular blocking drugs, the most successful being the bisquaternary compound, pancuronium (Fig. 5-1).[38] In order to provide a nondepolarizing neuromuscular blocker with a more rapid onset of action and a shorter duration of action, the monoquaternary vecuronium bromide (Fig. 5-2) was developed from a continuation of the research that originally resulted in pancuronium. Extensive studies of many analogues of pancuronium identified the importance of retaining an intact ring D-acetylcholine-like fragment to ensure high neuromuscular blocking activity.[39] However, when the acetylcholine moiety involving ring A is modified, resulting in a tertiary nitrogen atom at position 2, the remaining monoquaternary derivative, vecuronium bromide, exhibits an unusually high selectivity for the postjunctional cholinoceptors at the neuromuscular junction. It is considered that the high selectivity for the postjunctional cholinoceptors that vecuronium and pancuronium display can be attributed to the unique hydrogen-bonded, cagelike structure of this particular ring D-acetylcholine fragment.

Although vecuronium differs from pancuronium only in the nature of its 2-piperidine nitrogen atom, which is tertiary, as distinct from quaternary, this single apparently minor molecular modification results in a drug molecule that is significantly different in both physical and chemical properties and in chemical reactivity. Although both vecuronium and pancuronium are hydrophilic, vecuronium is slightly more lipophilic because it is a monoquaternary rather than a bisquaternary compound. Increased lipophilicity should enhance penetration into membranes and could alter vecuronium's route of elimination, as compared with pancuronium, which has proved to be the case. In short, vecuronium is a significantly different chemical entity from pancuronium.

COMPARATIVE PHARMACOLOGY OF VECURONIUM AND ATRACURIUM

Potency

When dose-response curves are constructed, the ED_{95} (ie, the mean dose of neuromuscular blocking drug that depresses twitch tension by 95 percent) can be derived. This dose usually provides adequate relaxation in an anesthetized patient. The ED_{90} and ED_{95} reported by different investigators[40-49] have varied because of several factors, including the anesthetic and the method of peripheral nerve stimulation used (eg, single twitch tension, train of four). However, an approximate ED_{95} value for atracurium is 0.28 mg/kg, for vecuronium, 0.056 mg/kg, and for pancuronium, 0.07 mg/kg. Vecuronium is the most potent muscle relaxant currently available for use in clinical practice. The log dose-response curves for vecuronium, pancuronium, and atracurium are essentially parallel (Fig. 5-10).

Volatile anesthetic agents will enhance a nondepolarizing neuromuscular block more than a nitrous oxide-narcotic technique. Studies have shown that enflurane is the most potent volatile agent, followed by isoflurane, and then halothane in enhancing neuromuscular blockade.[50] The potencies of atracurium and vecuronium appear to be influenced less by the choice or concentration of volatile anesthetic than are the potencies of tubocurarine and pancuronium. Enflurane and isoflurane augment tubocurarine and pancuronium neuromuscular blockade about twice as much as does an equipotent concentration of halothane.[51-53] In contrast, the augmentation of a vecuronium- or atracurium-induced neuromuscular blockade by enflurane or isoflurane is only 20–30 percent greater than the augmentation produced by halothane or nitrous oxide-narcotic anesthesia.[54-56] Changes in the end-tidal concentration of inhaled anesthetics also have a lesser influence on neuromuscular blockade produced by vecuronium or atracurium than those produced by other nondepolarizing neuromuscular blockers. The reasons for vecuronium

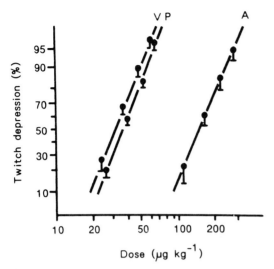

Fig. 5-10. The log dose-response curves for vecuronium (V), pancuronium (P), and atracurium (A). (From Gramstad L, Lilleaason P, Minsaas B: Comparative study of atracurium, vecuronium (Org NC 45) and pancuronium. Br J Anaesth 55(Suppl 1):95S, 1983, with permission.)

and atracurium being less influenced by the specific anesthetic and its dose or concentration are unknown.

Pharmacokinetics

Both vecuronium and atracurium have distinct pharmacokinetic properties as compared with currently used nondepolarizing muscle relaxants. For example, unlike pancuronium, metocurine, tubocurarine, or gallamine, neither vecuronium nor atracurium depends heavily on the kidney for elimination. Because atracurium is metabolized nearly completely through Hofmann elimination and ester hydrolysis, it should be excreted either in the urine or bile mostly in the form of metabolites. Although urinary and biliary excretion have not been determined in humans, the elimination half-life has been shown to be about 20–30 minutes.[57-58] Further confirmation of rapid metabolism is the appearance of laudanosine in the blood within 5–20 minutes.[57]

Only 10–25 percent of an injected dose of vecuronium is excreted in the urine.[59-61] The predominant route of elimination is almost certainly the bile.[59] Although vecuronium should be metabolized into its 3-hydroxy, 17-hydroxy, and 3,17-hydroxy metabolites as is pancuronium, only small amounts of these metabolites have been detected by methods such as thin layer chromatography.[60] The precise extent to which vecuronium is metabolized has not yet been determined, although most of the drug

seems to be excreted unchanged in the urine and bile.[59] The proposed metabolites have little or no cardiovascular or neuromuscular effects, and, therefore, are of little concern.[62-63] In humans, vecuronium has a more rapid clearance (5.2 ml/kg/min) and a shorter elimination half-life (71 min) than pancuronium (1.8 ml/kg/min; 140 min).[64] These two characteristics probably account for the shorter duration of action of vecuronium compared to pancuronium.

Although atracurium and vecuronium produce neuromuscular blockade of similar duration, calculated values for their pharmacokinetic variables are quite different. For example, the elimination half-life is about 22 minutes for atracurium, and 71 minutes for vecuronium.[64] It appears that the inter-relationship between pharmacokinetic variables and neuromuscular blockade differs for these two drugs. All previous pharmacokinetic models, including that for vecuronium, assume that elimination of a drug occurs from only one compartment. This approach is obviously inappropriate for atracurium because Hofmann elimination can occur from all body compartments.

Onset Time and Priming

The onset time (time from administration of muscle relaxant to its peak effect) is similar for both vecuronium and atracurium. The doses of atracurium and vecuronium that depress twitch height less than 100 percent have onset times ranging from 4 to 8 minutes, and the speed of onset of these intermediate-duration muscle relaxants is dose dependent.[41,48,49] By using high doses of these intermediate-duration drugs it is possible to achieve a more rapid onset without the excessively prolonged duration of action that may be observed following high doses of the longer-acting agents. For example, four times the ED$_{95}$ of vecuronium has an onset time of 1.3 minutes.[65] When three times the ED$_{95}$ of atracurium was given, onset times were 1.2[48] and 1.3[66] minutes. The onset times of atracurium and vecuronium, however, although similar in equipotent doses, are significantly slower than succinylcholine in the clinical dose range.[67]

Several authors have recently shown that it is possible to accelerate the onset of the nondepolarizing block by administering a small "priming" dose about 3–6 minutes before the full dose in order to more rapidly produce intubating conditions. Foldes et al advocate administration of 0.015 mg/kg of vecuronium or 0.08 mg/kg of atracurium 6 minutes before giving 0.05–0.06 mg/kg of vecuronium or 0.25–0.3 mg/kg of atracurium, respectively, for intubation.[68] They claim that intubation can be easily accomplished within 60–90 seconds using this priming principle. Later studies, however, most of them still in progress, indicate that in order to ensure good intubating conditions within 90 seconds, the doses given for intubation should be at least twice as large as recommended by Foldes et al, ie 0.5–0.6 mg/kg of atracurium or 0.12–0.15 mg/kg of vecuronium. There is no doubt that priming will become an important maneuver, but for a rapid sequence induction, succinylcholine is still the drug of choice.

Duration and Recovery of Action

When equipotent doses are compared, both vecuronium and atracurium have a similar duration of action, about one-third to one-half that of pancuronium.[41,42,44,45,47,49] For doses depressing twitch tension less than 100 percent, duration of action is about 15–30 minutes.[40,41,44,45,47,49] When three times the ED_{95} of these drugs is given, duration of action is between 50 and 76 minutes.[41,48,49] In contrast, when only two times the ED_{95} of pancuronium was given, the time from administration of the muscle relaxant to only 25 percent recovery of control twitch tension was 158 minutes. Recovery time (time from 25 to 75 percent recovery of control twitch tension) is also 30–50 percent shorter for vecuronium and atracurium than for pancuronium;[40,42,46,47,49] these times range from 9 to 12 minutes for both atracurium and vecuronium.[40–42,44,45,49]

After a single dose of vecuronium or pancuronium, plasma concentration falls rapidly because of redistribution from the central to the peripheral compartment. With subsequent doses, muscle relaxant in the peripheral compartment limits this distribution phase, and the decrease in plasma concentration results from elimination or metabolism. Thus, both pancuronium and, to a lesser extent, vecuronium can be demonstrated to have cumulative effects. This is not the case for atracurium. For although biphasic pharmacokinetic models have been described, there is not a distinct distribution phase with a rapid decrease in plasma concentration. Recovery from the effects of atracurium depends predominantly upon elimination (in this case metabolism by Hofmann elimination and ester hydrolysis) rather than redistribution. As a result, recovery from the neuromuscular effects of atracurium is similar for the first and all subsequent doses. This lack of accumulation makes atracurium the ideal agent for use as an infusion. Gargarian et al found that a mean infusion rate of 8.4 μg/kg/min produced excellent muscle relaxation and maintained 90–99 percent suppression of the single twitch.[69] There was no difference in recovery rates following a single bolus administration or continuous infusion.

Hepatic and Renal Failure

Because of its unique degradation pathways, the pattern of neuromuscular blockade produced by atracurium has been shown to be remarkably little affected by renal or hepatic failure.[70] Hofmann elimination is a nonbiological process, so atracurium is not dependent on the liver or kidney for its removal from the body and does not accumulate even in renal or hepatic failure, where its behavior is much the same as in normal patients. Atracurium is therefore the nondepolarizing relaxant of choice in these patients because of this advantage.

Vecuronium is the first and only relaxant to be eliminated mainly via the liver. Most of this elimination seems to be as the unchanged molecule with the kidney a secondary route. Some authors have postulated spontaneous deacetylation of vecuronium to account for its relative lack of cumulative property, but this is not yet proven. Since vecuronium is excreted mainly by the liver, it is a good second choice in renal failure where the pharmacokinetic profile of a single bolus is very similar to the profile in normal subjects.[61] There is a small cumulative effect after 1½ to 2 hours of vecuronium administration to patients in renal failure. Although statistically significant, this cumulative effect is probably of minor clinical importance. In cirrhotic patients, however, the duration is approximately double.[71]

THE CARDIOVASCULAR EFFECTS OF THE NEW MUSCLE RELAXANTS

Atracurium

Dose-response curves for atracurium obtained from results in anesthetized cats, dogs and rhesus monkeys (Fig. 5-11) demonstrate that there is a wide separation between the doses required for neuromuscular paralysis and those that inhibit autonomic mechanisms.[72,73] In cats, significant hypotension and slight bradycardia were evident after 4 mg/kg IV, but this dose was 16 times that required for full neuromuscular paralysis. Similar results were found in rhesus monkeys. In dogs, atracurium, 2 mg/kg, reduced mean arterial pressure to 53 percent of the control value, but this dose was 8 times that required for full neuromuscular paralysis. Atracurium at high concen-

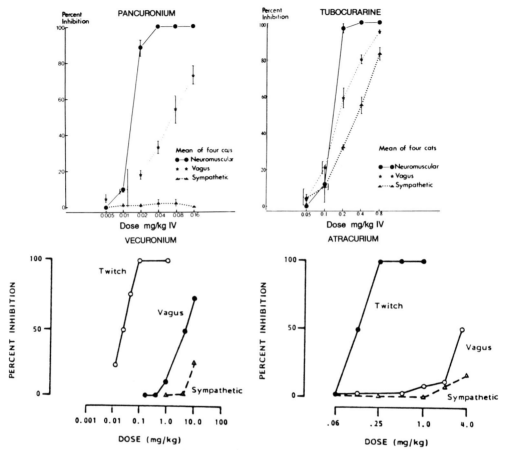

Fig. 5-11. Dose-response curves for neuromuscular and autonomic function inhibition in cats following pancuronium, tubocurarine and vecuronium; and in monkeys following atracurium. Note that vecuronium and atracurium cause insignificant autonomic inhibition at doses considerably in excess of that required to produce 100 percent depression of the single twitch. (Data modified from Durant NW, Marshall IG, Savage DS, et al: The neuromuscular and autonomic blocking activities of pancuronium, ORG NC 45, and other pancuronium analogues in the cat. J Pharm Pharmacol 31:831, 1979, and from Hughes R, Chapple DJ: The pharmacology of atracurium, a new competitive neuromuscular blocking agent. Br J Anaesth 53:31, 1981, with permission.)

trations had no inotropic or chronotropic effects on spontaneously beating guinea pig atria.

Cardiovascular studies in man have been carried out under halothane, enflurane and isoflurane anesthesia. During halothane anesthesia (0.7–0.9 percent end-tidal), maximum changes in mean arterial blood pressure and mean heart rate following intravenous doses of 0.2 and 0.4 mg/kg of atracurium were 6 and 8 percent, respectively, in one study;[74] and changes averaged less than 5 percent in another study.[75] Hilgenberg et al investigated the hemodynamic effects of 0.2 and 0.4 mg/kg of atracurium during enflurane anesthesia (1.0 to 1.25 percent inspired) and found no change in heart rate, cardiac index, stroke index, central venous pressure, or systemic mean arterial pressure.[76] Systemic vascular resis-

tance was decreased by 7 percent, compared with the control value, following both doses of atracurium. Similarly, Ramsey et al found no significant changes in heart rate and arterial blood pressure during enflurane anesthesia (1.16 end-tidal) after administration of 0.36 mg/kg of atracurium.[55] During isoflurane anesthesia (1.25 percent), Sokoll et al reported that there were no clinically significant changes in mean arterial blood pressure, mean heart rate, systemic vascular resistance, cardiac index, or central venous pressure after 0.2 and 0.4 mg/kg doses of atracurium.[77]

In man, under nitrous oxide/narcotic anesthesia, mean arterial pressure and heart rate first showed significant changes from control values at 0.6 mg/kg, double the full paralyzing dose (Fig. 5-12).[28] Maxi-

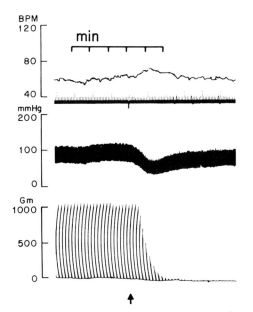

Fig. 5-12. The transient hemodynamic response occasionally observed following a bolus of 0.6 mg/kg of atracurium. Illustrated are the heart rate (by tachograph), intra-arterial blood pressure, and the single twitch at 0.15 Hz. Atracurium, 0.6 mg/kg, was injected as a rapid bolus at the arrow mark to a patient under balanced anesthesia.

mum heart rate and arterial pressure changes occurred 1–2 minutes after drug injection, and returned to normal within approximately 5 minutes. These changes have been shown to be due to a dose-dependent release of histamine, and the increase in plasma histamine levels correlates with the heart rate and arterial pressure changes. Scott et al have shown that these changes can be abolished by either slowing the rate of injection of atracurium to 75 seconds or by intravenous pretreatment with H1 and H2 blockers (chlorpheniramine and cimetidine) (Fig. 5-13).[78] A subsequent study by the same group has shown that doses as high as 0.8 mg/kg of atracurium can be administered safely, with hemodynamic stability, provided the injection rate is slowed.[79] Although atracurium will release histamine when high doses are bolused intravenously, it is important to keep this side effect in perspective. The ability of atracurium to release histamine relative to its neuromuscular blocking potency is only one-half that of dimethyltubocurarine, and less than one-third that of tubocurarine.[28]

Vecuronium

Since initial testing with vecuronium, it has been apparent that the margin between the neuromuscular

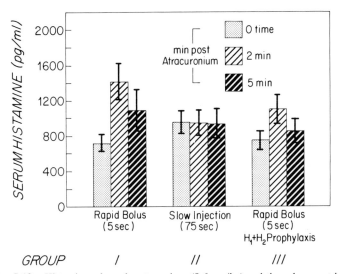

Fig. 5-13. Histamine release by atracurium (0.6 mg/kg) and the subsequent hemodynamic response is prevented by administering this dose slowly over 75 seconds. Pretreatment with intravenous H_1 and H_2 antagonists does not prevent histamine release but does attenuate the hemodynamic response. (From Scott RPF, Savarese JJ, Basta SJ, et al: Atracurium: Clinical strategies for preventing histamine release and attenuating the haemodynamic response. Br J Anaesth 57:550, 1985, with permission.)

blocking dose of this drug and the dose producing cardiovascular and autonomic effects is very wide. Results obtained in anesthetized cats and dogs (Fig. 5-11) have demonstrated that vecuronium, even in doses 20 times greater than those required for neuromuscular blockade, has no effect on heart rate, arterial pressure, autonomic ganglia, alpha- or beta-adrenoreceptors, or baroreceptor reflex activity.[72,80] Studies in pithed rats and guinea pig atria have further shown that vecuronium has little effect on cardiac muscarinic receptors or on norepinephrine reuptake mechanisms.[80] In contrast to its analogue, pancuronium, vecuronium appears to have far less indirect sympathomimetic activity.[81]

Eighteen adult patients studied under nitrous oxide-narcotic anesthesia demonstrated no significant changes in heart rate or arterial pressure with doses of vecuronium up to 150 μg/kg, which is nearly 3 times the 95 percent blocking dose.[82] Equipotent doses of pancuronium and vecuronium were compared in 20 patients receiving halothane anesthesia. Pancuronium (0.08 mg/kg) caused a significant increase in heart rate, insignificant change in arterial pressure, and significant changes in systolic time intervals.[83] The roughly equipotent dose of vecuronium, 0.057 mg/kg, caused no significant changes in heart rate, arterial pressure, or systolic time intervals. In both experimental animals and in humans, vecuronium has shown minimal potential for histamine release.[82,83]

In a clinical study that measured skin redness and induration caused by the intradermal injection of tubocurarine, metocurine, pancuronium, and vecuronium, vecuronium caused the smallest reaction, and tubocurarine and metocurine the largest. These results indicate that vecuronium had the least tendency to release histamine of the drugs tested. In a comparative study with tubocurarine, metocurine, and atracurium, Basta demonstrated that following 0.2 mg/kg of vecuronium (2 times the normal intubating dose) the heart rate, mean arterial pressure, and serum histamine levels were not altered.[84]

CARDIAC SURGERY AND CARDIOPULMONARY BYPASS

Since they have little or no cardiovascular effects, vecuronium and atracurium may be appropriate neuromuscular blocking drugs for cardiac surgery or noncardiac surgery on patients with cardiac dis-

ease. Very large doses of vecuronium (eg, 0.28 mg/kg) can be given with no cardiovascular effects.[85] As already indicated, however, large doses of atracurium may occasionally cause hypotension. Pokar and Brandt administered atracurium in doses of 0.6–1.0 mg/kg into right atrial catheters in patients who had undergone coronary artery bypass surgery.[86] Of the 9 patients, 4 had a decrease of more than 10 percent in arterial blood pressure. In a further study, when atracurium, 0.3 mg/kg, was given to 8 patients about to undergo elective coronary artery surgery, 1 patient had a decrease in mean arterial pressure (from 70 to 55 mm Hg) and other signs consistent with histamine release.[87] It is possible that prior diuretic therapy had made this patient more susceptible to even the slight histamine release associated with atracurium administration.

The hemodynamic stability of vecuronium may be a disadvantage when high-dose fentanyl or sufentanil anesthesia is used. The vagolytic action of pancuronium often protects against the tendency of the narcotics to produce bradycardia. When vecuronium is used with high-dose narcotic anesthesia, however, the heart rate often decreases.[88] This effect may be more apparent in patients who are receiving beta-blocker therapy during anesthesia for cardiac surgery.

Hypothermia and cardiopulmonary bypass can also affect the amount of atracurium or vecuronium required for neuromuscular blockade. Flynn et al found that 43 percent less atracurium was required to maintain a 90–95 percent neuromuscular blockade during the hypothermic cardiopulmonary bypass period.[89] They attributed the apparent increased potency of atracurium to the fact that hypothermia reduces the rate of Hofmann degradation. Buzello et al compared pancuronium and vecuronium before and after cardiopulmonary bypass.[90] Before bypass, pancuronium acted about twice as long as vecuronium. However, during hypothermic bypass, the durations of action of pancuronium and vecuronium increased 1.8-fold and 5-fold, respectively. It thus appears that during hypothermic bypass, pancuronium and vecuronium have similar durations of action. It may therefore be concluded that hypothermic cardiopulmonary bypass is associated with a marked increase in the duration of the neuromuscular blockade of both atracurium and vecuronium.[91] This point is, however, largely academic as the majority of patients requiring cardiopulmonary bypass will be ventilated postoperatively for a period longer than the duration of any muscle relaxant.

EFFECTS OF MUSCLE RELAXANTS ON CARDIAC RHYTHM

Nondepolarizing Agents

The nondepolarizing agents generally do not produce cardiac dysrhythmias. In fact, there is evidence that tubocurarine increases the dose threshold for the production of epinephrine-induced dysrhythmias in dogs under halothane and nitrous oxide anesthesia.[92,93]

Dysrhythmias after administration of pancuronium and gallamine may occur as a result of the following factors:

1. A sudden shift of autonomic balance towards the adrenergic side due to the vagal blocking effect of these drugs
2. A possible indirect sympathomimetic effect
3. A relatively greater inhibition of the AV node than the sinus node

These mechanisms may manifest themselves clinically as single or multifocal premature ventricular contractions, ventricular tachycardia, or nodal (junctional) tachycardia. In the case of gallamine, there is a higher incidence of ventricular dysrhythmias under light halothane or cyclopropane anesthesia probably because of the lowering of the threshold for ventricular excitability caused by these anesthetics.[94] In patients with sinus node disease, a vagolytic effect might cause a relatively greater increase in the spontaneous rate of activity of the atrioventricular node than the sinus node, the result being nodal tachycardia.

Succinylcholine

In man, succinylcholine is probably the only neuromuscular blocking agent that may itself precipitate cardiac dysrhythmias during anesthesia. It stimulates all cholinergic autonomic receptors, nicotinic receptors in both sympathetic and parasympathetic ganglia, and muscarinic receptors in the sinus node of the heart. The development of cardiac dysrhythmias is a clinical manifestation of this generalized autonomic stimulation; and sinus bradycardia, junctional rhythms, and ventricular dysrhythmias ranging from unifocal premature ventricular contractions to ventricular fibrillation have all been documented. However, many authors have noted these dysrhythmias in the presence of intense autonomic stimuli, most notably including tracheal intubation; and it is not always clear whether the cardiac irregularities are

due to the action of succinylcholine alone or to the presence of extraneous autonomic stimulation.

Sinus bradycardia after succinylcholine occurs most commonly in nonatropinized, relatively sympathotonic individuals (eg, children), and is due to stimulation of cardiac muscarinic receptors in the sinus node.[95] Sinus bradycardia has also been noted in adults, and appears more commonly after a second dose of the drug given approximately 5 minutes after the first.[96,97] It has been suggested that the higher incidence of bradycardia after a second dose of succinylcholine may be due to the hydrolysis products sensitizing the heart.[98] Thiopental, atropine, ganglion-blocking drugs, and nondepolarizing relaxants have all been used to prevent the bradycardia.

Nodal rhythms commonly occur as bradycardias and are probably due to the relatively greater stimulation of the sinus node than the atrioventricular node. The result is suppression of the sinus mechanism and the emergence of the atrioventricular node or even a ventricular focus as the pacemaker. The incidence of a junctional rhythm is higher after a second dose of succinylcholine, but is prevented by prior administration of tubocurarine.[96,99,100]

Succinylcholine lowers the threshold of the ventricle to catecholamine-induced dysrhythmias in the monkey[101] and the dog[92] under stable anesthetic conditions. Other autonomic stimuli, such as endotracheal intubation, hypoxia, hypercarbia, and surgery are probably additive to the effect of succinylcholine and may provoke ectopic activity. Ventricular escape may also occur after severe sinus and atrioventricular nodal slowing, secondary to succinylcholine administration.

The depolarizing nature of the drug encourages ventricular dysrhythmias by releasing potassium from skeletal muscle.[102] The rise of potassium in normal people following a 1-mg/kg dose of the drug is about 0.5 mEq/l.[102] However, marked increases may occur within 1–2 minutes of succinylcholine administration in the following groups:

1. Burned patients[99]
2. Patients with extensive denervation of skeletal muscle due to injury or disease of the central nervous system
3. Massively traumatized patients[103]
4. Patients with severe intra-abdominal infection[104]

The period of danger in these groups begins within a few days in the burned and denervated patients, and within a few hours in the traumatized patient. Studies in baboons have shown that hyperkalemia following surgical denervation begins as early as 4 days after the establishment of the lesion, and reaches a peak within 14 days.[105] Whether the hyperkalemic response to succinylcholine in these 4 groups represents a permanent lesion is not known. Uremic patients and patients at least 6 months past complete healing of burns are probably not at risk.[106] A study in dogs has suggested that immobilization atrophy does not seem to provoke the hyperkalemic response either.[107] The use of succinylcholine is probably contraindicated in these various groups. A modest dose of a nondepolarizing relaxant (6 mg of tubocurarine, 40 mg of gallamine, 3 mg of metocurine, or 1 mg of pancuronium) administered 3 minutes before succinylcholine may attenuate but will not guarantee the absence of the hyperkalemic response.

DRUG INTERACTIONS WITH THE CARDIOVASCULAR EFFECTS OF THE RELAXANTS

Succinylcholine lowers the threshold of the ventricle to catecholamine-induced dysrhythmias. To this must be added the possible influence of drugs such as digitalis, tricyclic antidepressants, monoamine-oxidase inhibitors, catecholamines, and anesthetic drugs such as halothane and cyclopropane, all of which may lower the ventricular threshold for ectopic activity or increase the dysrhythmogenic effect of the catecholamines.

The nondepolarizing agents may also produce cardiovascular effects upon interaction with other drugs. Edwards et al showed that simultaneous administration of pancuronium and imipramine caused a tachycardia in an additive manner.[108] An 80-μg/kg dose of pancuronium produced premature ventricular contractions and ventricular tachycardia, which rapidly progressed to ventricular fibrillation in 2 of the 10 dogs given imipramine, 8 mg/kg/day, and 4 of 10 dogs given 16 mg/kg/day. The authors concluded that severe ventricular dysrhythmias may occur as a result of administration of pancuronium in dogs anesthetized with halothane and chronically receiving imipramine. Since vecuronium is much less potent than pancuronium in blocking norepinephrine uptake, the possibility of ventricular dysrhythmias arising during halothane anesthesia in patients on tricyclic antidepressants would presumably be reduced.

In another study, neither pancuronium nor tubo-

curarine affected the dysrhythmogenic dose of epinephrine during halothane anesthesia in dogs.[109] This finding indicates that the usual guidelines for the administration of adrenaline during halothane anesthesia are not affected by concomitant administration of these two nondepolarizing muscle relaxants. Gallamine and tubocurarine may decrease the incidence of epinephrine-induced dysrhythmias, in contrast to succinylcholine, which may enhance epinephrine's effects.[92]

Occasionally, drug interactions may be advantageous. Combinations of pancuronium and metocurine not only potentiate neuromuscular blockade,[110] but minimize the heart rate change associated with pancuronium on its own. At twice the ED_{95}, the heart rate increased significantly more in the pancuronium group than in the pancuronium/metocurine combination group.

THE CARDIOVASCULAR EFFECTS OF THE ANTAGONISTS

Cardiovascular complications have been associated with the use of anticholinesterase drugs as antagonists of nondepolarizing neuromuscular blockade. Dysrhythmias and cardiac arrest following the administration of neostigmine and atropine have been reported.[111,112] As a result, various techniques have been described to improve the safety of reversal. These include hyperventilation to produce mild respiratory alkalosis, simultaneous injection of atropine and neostigmine, slow administration of neostigmine and atropine in a ratio of 2.5:1, and maintenance of adequate oxygenation throughout the period of reversal.[113,114]

The cardiac arrests have been attributed to cholinergic (muscarinic) stimulation of the heart by neostigmine combined with insufficient atropine. The relationship of dysrhythmias such as inverted P waves, Wenckebach phenomena, premature atrial contractions, junctional rhythms, atrioventricular dissociation, premature ventricular contractions, and bigeminy to atropine, neostigmine, or their combination is less clear.[115-118] Many of these reports occurred during emergence from anesthesia when changing anesthetic concentrations, surgical stimulation, and ventilation may have caused the dysrhythmias. However, dysrhythmias may occur even when these variables are held constant.[119] A decrease in the amount of atropine or replacement of it with another anticholinergic drug, such as glycopyrrolate, have been used to attenuate the tachycardia and reduce the frequency of dysrhythmias.[120]

Patients receiving glycopyrrolate with neostigmine have smaller changes in heart rate than those who receive atropine.[121] Glycopyrrolate also decreases the frequency of dysrhythmias when combined with neostigmine, pyridostigmine, or edrophonium.[119,120,122] Although a greater frequency of dysrhythmias occurs with atropine, there is insufficient evidence to implicate it as the etiological agent. It is possible that glycopyrrolate blocks the dysrhythmogenic stimulus of the anticholinesterase agents more effectively than atropine.

In view of this, the antagonist that requires the least amount of vagal blockade to prevent a bradycardia may provide an advantage clinically in terms of dysrhythmias. Edrophonium has two distinct advantages:[123] It has a shorter onset time than neostigmine or pyridostigmine; and it requires about half as much atropine to block adverse cardiac muscarinic effects as neostigmine. In order to minimize changes in heart rate, the rapidly acting edrophonium and atropine should be given together, and the slower acting neostigmine and glycopyrrolate together. Edrophonium has fewer muscarinic actions than neostigmine, and its predominant mechanism of action is probably presynaptic.

4-Aminopyridine has no muscarinic properties.[124] When it is combined with neostigmine or pyridostigmine, approximately 5 μg/kg of atropine is required to prevent bradycardia.[125] The atropine dose must be increased to 15 μg/kg when either neostigmine or pyridostigmine is used alone. 4-Aminopyridine is devoid of anticholinesterase activity and acts by increasing the amount of acetylcholine released by nerve impulses. However, the facilitatory actions of 4-aminopyridine are not confined to the neuromuscular junction. Transmission is also facilitated at autonomic, adrenergic, and cholinergic junctions including sympathetic ganglia and central synapses. In animal studies, 4-aminopyridine produced increases in left ventricular systolic pressure and dP/dt$_{max}$, right atrial pressure, stroke volume, myocardial blood flow, myocardial oxygen consumption, external cardiac work, arterial oxygen content, and blood hemoglobin.[126] These effects were attributed to facilitation of sympathetic transmission to the blood vessels, heart and spleen. Heart rate was not greatly affected because facilitation of vagal transmission to the sinoatrial node counteracted the increased sympathetic effect. While 4-aminopyridine may be useful in certain relatively rare conditions of neuromuscular transmission failure, such as

botulism, myasthenia gravis, and Eaton-Lambert syndrome, its actions are too widespread for routine use as an antagonist to nondepolarizing drugs.

Reversal of neuromuscular blockade after prolonged tricyclic antidepressant therapy can also lead to electrocardiographic disturbances. Results of one study demonstrated that minor ST-T wave and myocardial conduction changes observed in cats under chloralose anesthesia during chronic amitriptyline treatment markedly intensified during reversal of tubocurarine blockade with neostigmine alone or with a mixture of neostigmine and atropine.[127] This is probably due to the effect of neostigmine on the heart, coupled with the quinidine-like activity and direct action of tricyclic drugs on the myocardium.

Because of the relatively rapid recovery pattern of the new intermediate duration drugs, it may be possible in many cases to avoid the necessity of antagonism of residual blockade if dosing is carefully judged, properly timed, and monitored. When the new drugs have been employed, reversal should be done on clinical indication rather than as a routine. Anticholinesterases need not be administered, particularly if patients show no fade on train of four, are ventilating adequately, are responsive, and can demonstrate adequate head lift or grip strength.

MUSCLE RELAXANTS OF THE FUTURE

Pipecuronium

Pipecuronium bromide is an analogue of pancuronium with the quaternary nitrogen groups situated at the more remote nitrogen of the piperazine groups substituted at the 2 and 16 positions of the androstane skeleton (Fig. 5-14). In contrast to pancuronium it has no acetylcholine-like fragments, and the interonium distance is considerably larger than in pancuronium.

In isolated nerve-muscle preparations (rat phrenic-nerve diaphragm and chick biventor cervicis muscle), pipecuronium produced a pure nondepolarizing type of neuromuscular blockade, showing a relative potency of 1.7–3 times that of pancuronium under similar experimental conditions.[128] The nondepolarizing mode of action has been further demonstrated in experiments in vivo in cats, rabbits, and dogs.[128] Further observations in animals suggest that this new compound possesses remarkable cardiovascular stability.[129]

The initial clinical data on pipecuronium has been generated and reported mainly in Hun-

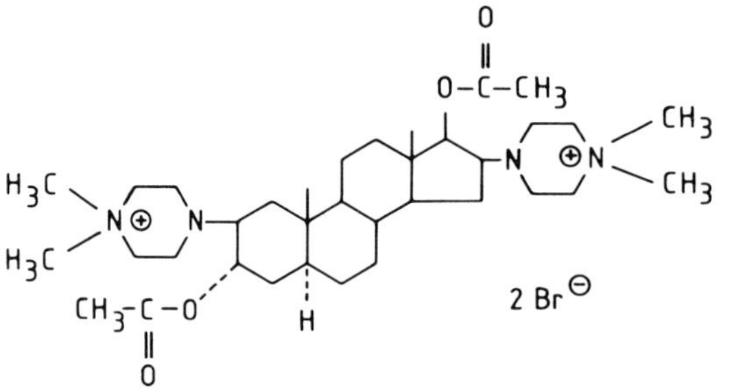

Fig. 5-14. The structural formula of pipecuronium bromide. (From Agoston S, Richardson FJ: Pipecuronium bromide—a new long-acting nondepolarizing neuromuscular blocking drug. Clin Anesthesiol 3:361, 1985, with permission.)

gary.[130,131] In many respects pipecuronium is similar to pancuronium. In man, neuromuscular blocking potency is equal to or slightly greater than that of pancuronium and, consequently, its routine use in clinical practice should follow the existing pattern for pancuronium. A dose of 0.05 mg/kg after intubation with succinylcholine will provide adequate muscle relaxation for 40–50 minutes. For intubation, however, the dose should be increased to 0.08–0.1 mg/kg, which will give satisfactory intubating conditions in 2.5–3 minutes and adequate surgical relaxation for 80–120 minutes. As with pancuronium, cumulative effects after repeated doses and potentiation of inhalational anesthetic agents, particularly enflurane, can be expected.

Pipecuronium appears to be free from histamine-releasing properties. The most important advantage of this compound in comparison with other long-acting drugs like pancuronium or alcuronium is that it is devoid of circulatory effects. Pipecuronium does not cause a tachycardia as does pancuronium, and in patients undergoing abdominal surgery there was no significant changes in blood pressure, central venous pressure, pulmonary capillary wedge pressure, or cardiac index.[132]

Pipecuronium, like vecuronium, has a minor disadvantage in that it has to be dissolved in solvent before use. The ampules currently used contain 4 mg of the agent that should be dissolved in 2 ml of solvent. Pipecuronium should be stored in a refrigerator at 4°C and should be used shortly after dissolving the powder.

BWB109OU

For a number of years, workers have been investigating a series of nondepolarizing bulky diester compounds that are metabolized by plasma cholinesterase. In 1979, BW785U, a short-acting nondepolarizing ester neuromuscular blocking agent was described. During a brief clinical trial, neuromuscular blocking activity of BW785U was indeed found to be very short.[133] A hypotensive response, however, first noted in animals and apparently due to histamine release, was found to be much more prominent in humans and forced the cancellation of further trials. BWA444U was another compound in the benzylisoquinolinium series.[134] Pharmacodynamically this agent's neuromuscular blocking effect was very similar in duration to that of atracurium, but its margin of safety for histamine release was somewhat less, so that it was withdrawn from further studies. Additional structure activity studies have since led to the development of BWB109OU.

BWB109OU (Fig. 5-15) is another short-acting nondepolarizing benzylisoquinolinium ester. The duration of action in the rhesus monkey was found to be about one-third that of atracurium and vecuronium. Its safety margin for histamine release was found to be about 10 times as great as that of BW785U. In initial clinical studies, the ED_{95} has been estimated to be approximately 0.08 mg/kg. The duration of action (injection to 95 percent return of twitch) is 25–30 minutes at 0.15–0.25 mg/kg, doses that produce 100 percent block. Spontaneous recovery time (5–95 percent) averages 14–15 minutes for all doses above 0.10 mg/kg. There is no significant

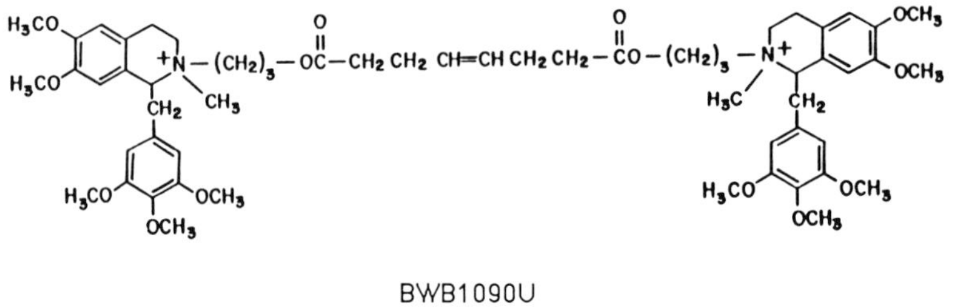

BWB109OU

Fig. 5-15. Chemical structure of BWB109OU.

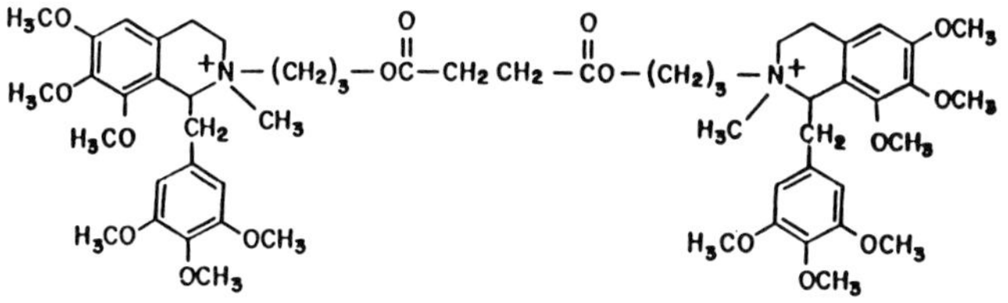

BWA938U

Fig. 5-16. Chemical structure of BWA938U.

difference in recovery times between single bolus doses or after 1–3 hour infusions. Neuromuscular blockade is readily reversed with neostigmine. In a further trial of 53 ASA class I and II patients, the cardiovascular effects and histamine-releasing properties of large doses were studied.[135,136] Brief decreases in arterial pressure after 2.5 and 3.1 times the ED_{95}, given as a rapid bolus, corresponded with elevations in plasma histamine levels. Cardiovascular changes were less after a second identical dose of BWB109OU or after slower bolus administration. The cardiovascular effect of BWB109OU, therefore, seems attributable to a relatively weak histamine-releasing property. The safety margin for this side effect is 2.5 to 3 times greater than that of tubocurarine or roughly similar to that of atracurium (2.5 to 3 times ED_{95}).

BWA938U

BWA938U (Fig. 5-16) is another benzylisoquinolinium ester.[137] Preclinical pharmacological studies in cats, dogs and rhesus monkeys showed that BWA938U is a very potent and rather safe nondepolarizing neuromuscular blocking agent. Compared with BWB109OU and atracurium, BWA938U is more potent, has a longer onset time, and longer duration of action. The ED_{95} for BWA938U in the monkey is estimated to be 0.017 mg/kg; the ED_{95} in man is 0.025–0.03 mg/kg. Bolus doses of 9 times the ED_{95} of BWA938U produced no significant cardiovascular effects in dogs. In patients under balanced anesthesia, doses of 0.08 mg/kg (three times ED_{95}) produced no significant cardiovascular effect.

In summary, BWA938U is a very potent, long-acting nondepolarizing neuromuscular blocking agent, about three times as potent as pancuronium. Preclinical data suggests that two properties of BWA938U may significantly distinguish it from other long-acting agents. These properties are a lack

of cardiovascular effects at several multiples of the ED_{95} dose for neuromuscular blockade, and a lack of cumulative effects following repeated dosing. These properties have been confirmed recently in volunteer studies and clinical trials evaluating the safety and efficacy of this drug. This agent has a small advantage over pipecuronium in that it is stable in solution and may be stored at room temperature.

CONCLUSIONS

The history and development of neuromuscular blocking agents have been characterized by a progressive reduction in side effects and improvement in pharmacodynamic profiles. Atracurium and vecuronium have set new standards in this field, and several of the older drugs would be unlikely to pass the animal testing stage today. This is certainly true in terms of cardiovascular side effects

Most of the commonly used nondepolarizing muscle relaxants can be classified as either steroids (pancuronium, vecuronium) or benzylisoquinolinium compounds (tubocurarine, metocurine, atracurium); and further research is continuing with both of these groups of substances. In the future, there will probably be more published about pipecuronium, a pancuronium analogue with a similar duration to its parent compound but without the tachycardia. Research with the benzylisoquinoliniums is also producing a number of interesting new agents. This group of compounds has a wide variety of pharamacodynamic profiles (BWB109OU and BWA938U). Work on the structure-activity relations on both types of compounds has resulted in three new drugs reaching full-scale clinical trials; with successful completion of human studies, the new drugs should be available for general use in the United States within 2–3 years.

REFERENCES

1. Guyton AC, Reeder RC: Quantitative studies on autonomic actions of curare. J Pharmacol Exp Ther 98:188, 1950

2. Burstein CL, Jackson A, Bishop HF, et al: Curare in the management of autonomic reflexes. Anesthesiology 11:409, 1950

3. McDowell SA, Clarke, RSJ: A clinical comparison of pancuronium with d-tubocurarine. Anesthesia 24:581, 1969

4. Moss J, Philbin DM, Rosow CE, et al: Histamine release by neuromuscular blocking agents in man. Klin Wochenschr. 60:891, 1982

5. Paton WDM: The effects of muscle relaxants other than muscle relaxation. Anesthesiology 20:453, 1959

6. Bowman WC: Pharmacology of neuromuscular function. University Park Press, Baltimore, 1980, p 103

7. Birdsall NJM, Hulme EC: Biochemical studies on the muscarinic acetylcholine receptor. J Neurochem 27:7, 1976

8. Riker WF, Wescoe WC: The pharmacology of flaxedil with observations on certain analogs. Ann NY Acad Sci 54:573, 1951

9. Saxena PR, Benta IL: Mechanism of selective cardiac vagolytic action of pancuronium bromide. Specific blockade of cardiac muscarinic receptors. Eur J Pharmacol 11:332, 1970

10. Marshall IG: The ganglion blocking and vagolytic actions of three short-acting neuromuscular blocking drugs in the cat. J Pharm Pharmacol 25:530, 1973

11. Hughes R, Chapple DJ: Effects of non-depolarizing neuromuscular blocking agents on peripheral autonomic mechanisms in cats. Br J Anaesth. 48:59, 1976

12. Li CK, Mitchelson F: The effects of stercuronium on cardiac muscarinic receptors. Eur J Pharmacol 51:251, 1978

13. Hughes R, Chapple DJ: Cardiovascular and neuromuscular effects of dimethyltubocurarine in anaesthetized cats and rhesus monkeys. Br J Anaesth 48:847, 1976

14. Hughes R, Chapple DJ: The pharmacology of atracurium: a new competitive neuromuscular blocking agent. Br J Anaesth. 53:31, 1981

15. Durant NW, Marshall IG, Savage DS, et al: The neuromuscular and autonomic blocking activities of pancuronium, ORG NC 45, and other pancuronium analogues in the cat. J Pharm Pharmacol 31:831, 1979

16. Loffelholz K, Muscholl E: Inhibition by parasympathetic nerve stimulation of the release of adrenergic transmitter. Naunyn-Schmiedebergs Arch Pharmacol 267:181, 1970

17. Vercruysse P, Bossuyt P, Hanegreefs G, et al: Gallamine and pancuronium inhibit prejunctional and post-junctional muscarinic receptors in canine saphenous veins. J Pharmacol Exp Ther 209:225, 1979

18. Greengard P, Kebabian JW: Role of cyclic AMP in synaptic transmission in the mammalian peripheral nervous system. Fed Proc 33:1059, 1974

19. Gardier RW, Tsevdos EJ, Jackson DB, et al: Distinct muscarinic mediation of suspected dopaminergic activity in sympathetic ganglia. Fed Proc 37:2422, 1978

20. Marshall RJ: A new muscarinic agent: 1,4,5,6-tetrahydro-5-phenoxy pyrimidine (AH 6405). Br J Pharmacol 39:191, 1970

21. Brown BR, Crout JR: The sympathomimetic effect of gallamine on the heart. J Pharmacol Exp Ther 172:266, 1970

22. Marshall RJ, Ojewole JAO: Comparison of autonomic effects of some currently used neuromuscular blocking agents. Br J Pharmacol 66:77, 1979

23. Quintana A: Effect of pancuronium bromide on the adrenergic reactivity of the isolated rat vas deferens. Eur J Pharmacol 46:275, 1977

24. Salt PJ, Barnes PK, Conway CM: Inhibition of neuronal uptake of noradrenalin in the isolated perfused rat heart by pancuronium and its homologues ORG 6368, ORG 7268 and ORG NC45. Br J Anaesth 52:315, 1980

25. Lee Son S, Waud BE: Effects of non-depolarizing neuromuscular blocking agents on the cardiac vagus nerve in the guinea pig. Br J Anaesth 52:981, 1980

26. Walts LF: Complications of muscle relaxants: In Katz RL (ed): Muscle Relaxants. Monographs in Anesthesiology, New York, American Elsevier, 1975, pp 209

27. Moss J, Rosow CE, Savarese JJ, et al: Role of histamine in the hypotensive action of d-tubocurarine in humans. Anesthesiology 55:19, 1981

28. Basta SJ, Savarese JJ, Ali HH, et al: Histamine-releasing potency of atracurium, di-methyltubocurarine and tubocurarine. Br J Anaesth 55:105S, 1983

29. Danilov AF, Kvitko IJ, Laurenteiva VV: Action of some bisquaternary derivatives of phtalic acids and related substances on neuromuscular transmissions. Br J Pharmacol 44:765, 1972

30. Paton WDM, Zaimis EJ: Methonium compounds. Pharmacol Rev 4:219, 1952

31. Everett AJ, Cowe LA, Wilkonson S: Revision of the structures of (+) tubocurarine chloride and (+) chrondrocurine. Chem Commun 1020, 1970

32. Paton WDM: Histamine release by compounds of single chemical structure. Pharmacol Rev 9:269, 1957

33. Savarese JJ, Kitz RJ: The quest for a short-acting non-depolarizing neuromuscular blocking agent. Acta Anaesthesiol Scand 53:43, 1973

34. Stenlake JB: Ions-cyclic nucleotides-cholinergy. In Stoclet JP (ed): Advances in Pharmacology and Therapeutics. Oxford, Pergamon 1979, p 303

35. Chapple DJ, Clark JS: Pharmacological action of

breakdown products of atracurium and related substances. Br J Anaesth 55 (Suppl 1):11S, 1983

36. Stiller RL, Cook DR, Chakrauoriti S: In vitro degradation of atracurium in human plasma. Br J Anaesth 57:1085, 1985

37. Mercier J, Mercier E: Action de quelques alcalvides secondaires de l'opium sur l'electrocorticogramme du chien. C R Soc Biol 149:760, 1955

38. Savage DS, Sleigh T, Carlyle I: The emergence of Org N.C. 45 from the pancuronium series. Br J Anaesth 52 (Suppl 1):3S, 1980

39. Durant NN, Marshall IG, Savage DS, et al: The neuromuscular and autonomic blocking activities of pancuronium Org NC 45 and other pancuronium analogues in the cat, J Pharm Pharmacol 31:831, 1979

40. Fahey MR, Morris RB, Miller RD, et al: Clinical pharmacology of ORG NC45 (Norcuron): a new nondepolarizing muscle relaxant. Anesthesiology 55:6, 1981

41. Agoston S, Salt P, Newton D, et al: The neuromuscular blocking action of Org NC45, a new pancuronium derivative, in anaesthetized patients. A pilot study. Br J Anaesth 52(Suppl 1):53S, 1980

42. Crul JF, Booij LHDJ: First clinical experiences with Org NC 45. Br J Anaesth 52(Suppl 1):49S, 1980

43. Baird WLM, Herd D: A new neuromuscular blocking drug, Org NC 45. A pilot study in man. Br J Anaesth 52 (Suppl 1):61S, 1980

44. Buzello W, Bischoff G, Kuhls E, et al: The new nondepolarizing muscle relaxant Org NC 45 in clinical anaesthesia: Preliminary results. Br J Anaesth 52(Suppl 1):62S, 1980

45. Krieg N, Curl JF, Booij LHDH: Relative potency of Org NC 45, pancuronium, alcuronium and tubocurarine in anaesthetized man. Br J Anaesth 52:783, 1980

46. Walts LF, Stirt JA, Katz RL: A comparison of neuromuscular blocking effects of norcuron and pancuronium. Anesthesiology 55:A210, 1981

47. Gramstad L, Lilleaasen P, Minsaas B: Comparative study of atracurium, vecuronium (Org NC 45) and pancuronium. Br J Anaesth 55(Suppl 1):95S, 1983

48. Payne JP, Hughes R: Evaluation of atracurium in anaesthetized man. Br J Anaesth 53:45, 1981

49. Basta SJ, Ali HH, Savarese JJ, et al: Clinical pharmacology of atracurium besylate (BW 33A): A new non-depolarizing muscle relaxant. Anesth Analg 61:723, 1982

50. Miller RD, Savarese JJ: Pharmacology of muscle relaxants, their antagonists and monitoring of neuromuscular function. In Miller R (ed): Anesthesia, New York, Churchill Livingstone, 1981, p 487

51. Fogdall RP, Miller RD: Neuromuscular effects of enflurane, alone and combined with d-tubocurarine, pancuronium, and succinylcholine, in man. Anesthesiology 42:173, 1975

52. Miller RD, Eger EI II, Way WL, et al: Comparative neuromuscular effects of Forane and halothane alone and in combination with d-tubocurarine in man. Anesthesiology 35:38, 1971

53. Miller RD, Way WL, Dolan WM, et al: Comparative neuromuscular effects of pancuronium, gallamine, and succinylcholine during Forane and halothane anesthesia in man. Anesthesiology 35:509, 1971

54. Rupp SM, Miller RD, Gencarelli PJ: Vecuronium-induced neuromuscular blockade during enflurane, halothane and isoflurane in humans. Anesthesiology 60:102, 1984

55. Ramsey FM, White PA, Stuliken EH, et al: Enflurane potentiation of neuromuscular blockade by atracurium. Anesthesiology 57,A255, 1982

56. Foldes FF, Bencini A, Newton D: Influence of halothane and enflurane on the neuromuscular effects of Org NC 45 in man. Br J Anaesth 52(Suppl 1):64S, 1980

57. Fahey MR, Rupp SM, Fisher DM, et al: The pharmacokinetics and pharmacodynamics of atracurium in patients with and without renal failure. Anesthesiology, 61:699, 1984

58. Ward S, Neill EAM, Weatherley BC, et al: Pharmacokinetics of atracurium besylate in healthy patients (after a single i.v.) bolus dose. Br J Anaesth 55(Suppl 1):113, 1983

59. Upton RA, Nguyen TL, Miller RD, et al: Renal and biliary elimination of vecuronium (ORG NC 45) and pancuronium in rats. Anesth Analg 61:313, 1982

60. Sohn YJ, Bencini A, Scaf AHJ, et al: Pharmacokinetics of vecuronium in man. Anesthesiology 57:A256, 1962

61. Fahey MR, Morris RB, Miller RD, et al: Pharmacokinetics of Org NC45 (Norcuron) in patients with and without renal failure. Br J Anaesth 53:1049, 1981

62. Marshall IG, Gibb AJ, Durant NN: Neuromuscular and vagal blocking actions of pancuronium bromide, its metabolites, and vecuronium bromide (Org NC 45) and its potential metabolites in the anaesthetized cat. Br J Anaesth 55:703, 1983

63. Booij LHDJ, Vree TB, Hurkmans F, et al: Pharmacokinetics and pharmacodynamics of the muscle relaxant drug Org NC-45 and each of its hydroxy metabolites in dogs. Anaesthetist 30:329, 1982

64. Cronnelly R, Fisher DM, Miller RD, et al: Pharmacokinetics and pharmacodynamics of vecuronium (ORG NC45) and pancuronium in anaesthetized humans. Anesthesiology 58:405, 1983

65. Viby-Mogensen J, Jorgensen BC, Engback J, et al: On Org NC 45 and halothane anaesthesia. Preliminary results. Br J Anaesth 52(Suppl 1):67S, 1980

66. Savarese JJ, Basta SJ, Ali HH, et al: Neuromuscular and cardiovascular effects of BW 33A (atracurium) in patients under halothane anesthesia. Anesthesiology 57:A262, 1982

67. Scott RPF, Goat VA: Atracurium: its speed of onset. A comparison with suxamethonium. Br J Anaesth 54:909, 1982

68. Foldes FF, Schwartz S, Ilias W, et al: Rapid tracheal intubation with vecuronium: the priming principle, Anesthesiology 61:A294, 1984

69. Gargarian MA, Basta SJ, Savarese JJ, et al: The efficacy of atracurium by continuous infusion. Anesthesiology 61:A291, 1984

70. Ward S, Neill EAM: Pharmacokinetics of atracurium in acute hepatic failure (with acute renal failure), Br J Anaesth 55:1169, 1983

71. Duvaldestin P, Lebrault C, Terestchenko MC, et al: Vecuronium in patients with liver disease. Proceedings of the symposium on clinical experiences with Norcuron, Geneva, Amsterdam, Excerpta Medica, 1983, p 180

72. Sutherland GA, Squire IB, Gibb AJ, et al: Neuromuscular blocking and autonomic effects of vecuronium and atracurium in the anaesthetized cat. Br J Anesth 55:1119, 1983

73. Hughes R, Chapple DJ: The pharmacology of atracurium, a new competitive neuromuscular blocking agent. Br J Anaesth 53:31, 1981

74. Savarese JJ, Basta SJ, Ali HH, et al: Neuromuscular and cardiovascular effects of BW33A (atracurium) in patients under halothane anesthesia, Anesthesiology. 57:A262, 1982

75. Stirt JA, Murray AL, Katz AL et al: Atracurium during halothane anesthesia in humans, Anesth Analg 62:207, 1983

76. Hilgenberg JC, Stoelting RK, Harris WA: Systemic vascular responses to atracurium during enflurane-nitrous oxide anesthesia in humans. Anesthesiology 58:242, 1983

77. Sokoll MD, Gereis SD, Mehta M, et al: Haemodynamic effects of atracurium in surgical patients under nitrous oxide, oxygen and isoflurane anaesthesia. Br J Anaesth 55:77S, 1983

78. Scott RPF, Savarese JJ, Basta SJ, et al: Atracurium: Clinical strategies for preventing histamine release and attenuating the haemodynamic response. Br J Anaesth 57:550, 1985

79. Scott RPF, Savarese JJ, Basta SJ, et al: The clinical pharmacology of high dose atracurium. Anesth Analg 65:S137, 1986

80. Marshall RJ, McGrath TC, Miller RD, et al: Comparison of the cardiovascular actions of ORG NC45 with those produced by other non-depolarizing neuromuscular blocking agents in experimental animals. Br J Anaesth 52:21S, 1980

81. Bowman WC: Non-relaxant properties of neuromuscular blocking drugs. Br J Anaesth. 54:147, 1982

82. Crul JF, Booij LHDJ: First clinical experiences with ORG NC45. Br J Anaesth. 52:49S, 1980

83. Engbaek J, Ording H, Sorensen B, et al: Cardiac effects of vecuronium and pancuronium during halothane anaesthesia. Br J Anaesth. 55:501, 1983

84. Basta SJ. Release of endogenous histamine by non-depolarizing neuromuscular blocking agents. Proceedings of the International Symposium on Clinical Neuromuscular Pharmacology. Boston, Harvard Medical School, 1983

85. Morris RB, Cahalan MK, Miller RD, et al: The cardiovascular effects of vecuronium (ORG NC45) and pancuronium in patients undergoing coronary artery bypass grafting. Anesthesiology 58:438, 1983

86. Pokar H, Brandt L: Haemodynamic effects of atracurium in patients after cardiac surgery. Br J Anaesth 55 (Suppl 1):139S, 1983

87. Philbin DM, Machaj VR, Tomichek RC, et al: Hemodynamic effects of bolus injection of atracurium in patients with coronary artery disease. Br J Anaesth. 55:131S, 1983

88. Salmenpera M, Peltola K, Takkunen O, et al: Cardiovascular effects of pancuronium and vecuronium during high-dose fentanyl anesthesia. Anesth Analg 62:1059, 1983

89. Flynn PJ, Hughes R, Walton B: The use of atracurium in cardiopulmonary bypass with induced hypothermia. Anesthesiology 59:A262, 1983

90. Buzello W, Schluermann D, Schindler M, Spillner F: Hypothermic cardiopulmonary bypass and neuromuscular blockade by pancuronium and vecuronium. Anesthesiology 1986, in press

91. Miller RD, Rupp SM, Fisher D et al: Clinical pharmacology of vecuronium and atracurium. Anesthesiology 61:444, 1984

92. Tucker WA, Munson ES: Effects of succinylcholine and d-tubocurarine on epinephrine-induced arrhythmias during halothane anesthesia in dogs. Anesthesiology 42:41, 1975

93. Wong KC, Wyte SR, Martin WE: Antiarrhythmic effects of skeletal muscle relaxants. Anesthesiology 34:458, 1971

94. Walts LF, McFarland W: Effect of vagolytic agents on ventricular rhythm during cyclopropane anesthesia. Anesth Analg 44:429, 1965

95. Leigh MD, McCoy DD, Belton KM: Bradycardia following intravenous administration of succinylcholine chloride to infants and children. Anesthesiology 18:698, 1957

96. List WFM: Succinylcholine-induced cardiac arrhythmia. Anesth Analg 50:361, 1971

97. Cooperman LH: Succinylcholine-induced hyperkalemia in neuromuscular disease. JAMA 213:1867, 1970

98. Schoenstadt DA, Whitcher CE: Observation on the mechanism of succinylcholine-induced cardiac arrhythmia. Anesthesiology 24:358, 1963

99. Bush GH, Graham HAP, Littlewood ANM: Danger of suxamethonium and endotracheal intubation in anaesthesia for burns. Br Med J 2:1081, 1962

100. Mathias JA, Evans-Prosser CDG, Churchill-Davidson HC: The role of non-depolarizing drugs in the prevention of suxamethonium bradycardia. Br J Anaesth 42:609, 1970

101. Galindo AHF, Davis TB: Succinylcholine and cardiac excitability. Anesthesiology 23:32, 1962

102. Bali IM, Dundee JW, Daggart JR: The source of increased plasma potassium following succinylcholine. Anesth Analg 54:680, 1975

103. Mazze RI, Escue HM, Houston JB: Hyperkalemia and cardiovascular collapse following succinylcholine injection in the traumatized patient. Anesthesiology 33:328, 1970

104. Kohlschutter B, Baur H, Roth F: Suxamethonium induced hyperkalemia in patients with severe intraabdominal infection. Br J Anaesth 48:557, 1976

105. John DA, Tobey RE, Homer LD: Onset of succinylcholine induced hyperkalemia following denervation. Anesthesiology 45:294, 1976

106. Koide M, Waud BE: Serum potassium concentrations after succinylcholine in patients with renal failure. Anesthesiology 36:142, 1972

107. Gronert GA, Theye RA: Effect of succinylcholine on skeletal muscle with immobilization atrophy. Anesthesiology 40:268, 1974

108. Edwards RP, Miller RD, Roizen MF: Cardiac responses to imipramine and pancuronium during anesthesia with halothane or enflurane. Anesthesiology 50:421, 1979

109. Schick LM, Chapin JC, Munson ES: Pancuronium, d-tubocurarine and epinephrine induced arrhythmias during halothane anesthesia in dogs. Anesthesiology 52:207, 1980

110. Lebowitz PW, Ramsey FM, Savarese JJ, et al: Potentiation of neuromuscular blockade in man produced by combination of pancuronium and metocurine or pancuronium and d-tubocurarine. Anesth Analg 59:604, 1980

111. Bain WH, Broadbent JZ: Death following neostigmine. Br Med J 1:1137, 1949

112. Clutten-Brock J: Death following neostigmine. Br Med J 1:1007, 1949

113. Pooler HE: Atropine, neostigmine and sudden death. Anesthesia 12:198, 1957

114. Riding JE, Robinson JC: The safety of neostigmine. Anesthesia 16:346, 1961

115. Gottlieb JD, Sweet RB: The antagonism of curare: the cardiac effects of atropine and neostigmine. Can Anaesth Soc J 10:114, 1963

116. Baraka A: Safe reversal: atropine-neostigmine mixture. Br J Anaesth 40:30, 1968

117. Ovassapian A: The effects of administration of atropine and neostigmine in man. Anesth Analg 48:219, 1969

118. Tan CK, Balasaraswathi K, El-Etr AA: Neostigmine-induced Wenckebach phenomenon. Anesthesiol Rev 7:28, 1980

119. Fogdall RP, Miller RD: Antagonism of d-tubocurarine and pancuronium induced neuromuscular blockades by pyridostigmine in man. Anesthesiology 39:504, 1973

120. Ramamurthy S, Shaker MH, Winnie AP: Glycopyrrolate as a substitute for atropine in neostigmine reversal of muscle relaxant drugs. Can Anaesth Soc J 19:399, 1972

121. Cozanitas DA, Dundee SW, Merrett JD: Evaluation of glycopyrrolate and atropine as adjuncts to reversal of non-depolarizing neuromuscular blocking agents in a "true to life" situation. Br J Anaesth 52:85, 1980

122. Klingenmaier CH, Bullard R, Thompson D, et al: Reversal of neuromuscular blockade with a mixture of neostigmine and glycopyrrolate. Anesth Analg 51:468, 1972

123. Miller RD, Cronnelly R: A new look at an old drug. Editorial: Anesthesiology 59:84, 1983

124. Randall LO: Anti-curare activity of phenolic quaternary ammonium salts. J Pharmacol Exp Ther 100:83, 1950

125. Miller RD, Booij LHD, Agoston S: 4-aminopyridine potentiates neostigmine and pyridostigmine in man. Anesthesiology 50:416, 1979

126. Bowman WC, Marshall RJ: Actions of 4-aminopyridine on the cardiovascular systems of anaesthetised cats and dogs. Br J Anaesth 53:555, 1981

127. Glissen SN, El-Etr AA: Reversal of neuromuscular blockade and tricyclic antidepressants. Anesthesiology 51:575, 1979

128. Agoston S, Richardson FJ: Pipecuronium bromide— a new long-acting non-depolarizing neuromuscular blocking drug. Clin Anesthesiol 3:361, 1985

129. Karpati E, Biro K: Pharmacological study of a new competitive neuromuscular blocking steroid, pipecuronium bromide. Arzneimittel Forschung/Drug Research 30:346, 1980

130. Boros M, Szenobradszky J, Kertesz A, et al: Clinical experiences with pipecuronium bromide. Acta Chirurgica Hungarica 24:207, 1983

131. Tassony I, Szabo G, Vimlati L: The use of pipecuronium bromide in anesthesiology. Handbook of experimental pharmacology. In press.

132. Szenohradszky J, Marosi G, Keresz A, et al: Clinical experience with pipecuronium bromide. Sixth European Congress of Anesthesiologists, London, 1982

133. Rosow CW, Basts SJ, Savarese JJ, et al: BW785U: Correlation of cardiovascular effects with increases in plasma histamine, Anesthesiology 53, S270, 1980

134. Basta SJ, Moss J, Savarese JJ, et al: Cardiovascular effects of BWA444U: Correlation with plasma histamine levels, Anesthesiology 50, A198, 1981

135. Basta SJ, Savarese JJ, Ali HH, et al: The neuromuscular pharmacology of BWB109OU in anaesthetized patients. Anesthesiology 63:A318, 1985

136. Savarese JJ, Basta SJ, Ali HH, et al: Cardiovascular effects of BW109OU in patients under nitrous oxide-oxygen-thiopental-fentanyl anesthesia. Anesthesiology 63:A319, 1985

137. Basta SJ, Savarese JJ, Ali HH, et al: The neuromuscular and cardiovascular effects of BWA938U in anaesthetised patients. 1987, In press

PART II

Monitoring

Joel A. Kaplan, M.D.

6

Hemodynamic Monitoring

In patients with severe cardiovascular disease, adequate hemodynamic monitoring should be available at all times. Continuous measurements and recordings of all vital physiological parameters can be obtained with modern catheters and electronic monitoring equipment. The development of acute hemodynamic events can be observed and corrected before they proceed to sudden catastrophic cardiac arrests; thus, the number of major cardiovascular complications should be reduced.

Many devices are currently available to monitor the cardiovascular system. These devices range from those that are totally noninvasive, such as the blood pressure cuff and electrocardiogram (ECG), to those that are extremely invasive, such as the pulmonary artery catheter (PAC). In order to use the invasive monitors, the potential benefit to be gained from the information must heavily outweigh the risk of the procedure. In many patients with cardiac disease, the benefit obtained does outweigh the risks, which explains the increasing utilization of invasive monitoring.

Standard monitors such as blood pressure, ECG, central venous pressure (CVP), urine output, temperature, and arterial blood gases are used in all patients undergoing cardiac surgery. Increasing use is being made of PACs, left atrial pressure (LAP) catheters,

cardiac output measurements, echocardiography, invasive measurements of myocardial contractility, such as pressure development (dP/dt), and indices of myocardial oxygenation. All of these measurements and their derivatives can be obtained and recorded; however, interpretation of the complex data requires an astute clinician fully aware of the patient's overall condition and the problems inherent with the monitors. Wider application of computer technology will help with some of the correlations of data.

A modern anesthesia department utilizing sophisticated monitoring equipment requires the services of a complex electronic laboratory. Technicians and engineers are needed to modify and service the equipment at frequent intervals. An acute-care laboratory in the operating room area is also needed to provide rapid information concerning arterial blood gases, electrolytes (Na^+, K^+, Ca^{++}), hematocrit, blood sugar, and oncotic pressure.

ARTERIAL BLOOD PRESSURE

The arterial blood pressure is a quantitative measurement used for assessment of the status of the cardiovascular system. The mean arterial pressure is

CARDIAC ANESTHESIA, SECOND EDITION
ISBN 0-8089-1848-6

the average pressure during a cardiac cycle and is dependent on the cardiac output and peripheral resistance.[1] This relationship is expressed by the following formula:

$$MAP = CO \times SVR$$

which is the cardiovascular equivalent of Ohm's law of electricity:

$$E = I \times R$$

where MAP is mean arterial pressure, CO is cardiac output, SVR is systemic vascular resistance, E is voltage, I is current, and R is resistance. The MAP can be obtained by electrical integration or by calculation with the following formula:

$$MAP = DP + 1/3(SP - DP)$$

where DP is diastolic pressure and SP is systolic pressure. The arterial pulse pressure is the difference between the systolic and diastolic pressure and is dependent on the stroke volume and arterial capacitance.

Indirect Measurement of Blood Pressure

Today the anesthesiologist depends primarily on techniques developed over 80 years ago, utilizing the Riva-Rocci occlusive cuff and auscultation of Korotkoff sounds. The cuff is inflated above systolic pressure and slowly deflated at 2–3 mm Hg per beat for the most accurate measurement of blood pressure. The systolic pressure may be obtained by observation of oscillations, by palpation of pulsations distal to the cuff, or by auscultation of the Korotkoff sounds. Van Bergen et al found that the oscillatory method correlated better with direct pressure measurements than did the standard Korotkoff sounds;[2] however, blood pressure is most often obtained by the auscultatory method. The systolic blood pressure is the point at which Korotkoff sounds are first heard (phase 1). The diastolic blood pressure is more controversial and may be taken either at the end of phase 4 when the sounds disappear or between phases 3 and 4 when the sounds change quality.[3]

There are four major techniques for automated indirect blood pressure measurements: (1) detection of oscillation of pressure, which occurs as the cuff pressure approaches the blood pressure (eg, Dinamap); (2) electronic auscultation of Korotkoff sounds under the cuff (eg, Infrasonde); (3) ultrasonic detec-

tion of arterial wall motion under the cuff (eg, Arterisonde); and (4) blood flow detection distal to the cuff by Doppler ultrasound, photoelectric plethysmography (eg, Penaz finger cuff), or palpation techniques.[4]

Several studies have compared noninvasive techniques using the above methods with direct intraarterial pressures in adults and infants. The results in general have been quite good ($r > 0.9$);[5,6] however, the blood pressure values obtained by invasive and noninvasive techniques are not identical, since they are measured in a totally different manner.[7] Recently, Braissoulis compared automatic oscillometric pressures with direct arterial pressure in infants and found that 4–9 percent of the indirect measurements were more than 10 mm Hg different from direct pressures.[8] This finding is significant, since it is in this pediatric group that indirect pressure measurements are most often used during induction of anesthesia for cardiac surgery. The oscillometric devices have been shown to underestimate systolic and mean pressures at high arterial pressures and to overestimate them at low pressures.[9] Other situations in which discrepancies have been found include obesity, hypertension, hypothermia, and shock.

Direct Measurements of Blood Pressure

Invasive arterial monitoring of blood pressure has become routine in recent years with the increased complexity of surgery and intensive care of critically ill patients. Catheters are placed in various arteries of the body for continuous beat-to-beat blood pressure monitoring and for multiple arterial blood gas measurements. Anesthetic procedures in which an arterial catheter may be indicated include the following: (1) cardiac surgery with cardiopulmonary bypass (CPB); (2) major central or peripheral vascular surgery; (3) pulmonary resections; (4) intracranial operations; (5) major trauma procedures; (6) deliberate hypotension; and (7) deliberate hypothermia.

Surgical procedures in patients with any of the following abnormalities may also require an arterial catheter for careful monitoring: (1) significant pulmonary disease; (2) cardiovascular disease; (3) severe metabolic derangements; and (4) obesity.

SITES AND METHODS OF DIRECT
MONITORING

Radial artery. The radial artery is the most commonly used artery for continuous blood pressure monitoring because it is easy to cannulate, readily accessible during surgery, and the collateral circulation is usually adequate and easy to check. The collateral circulation of the hand is formed by an arterial arcade on the palm of the hand where the radial and ulnar arteries come together. This collateral circulation is checked by performing an Allen's test prior to cannulation.[10] This test demonstrates that if the radial artery becomes thrombosed, adequate ulnar collateral flow is present to safely perfuse the hand. Palm showed that if there is adequate ulnar collateral flow, circulatory perfusion pressure to the fingers is also adequate following radial artery catheterization.[11] The Allen's test is performed by occluding both the radial and ulnar arteries and having the patient squeeze his or her fist until the hand blanches. Then the ulnar artery is released with the patient's hand open, and the color of the hand is observed. If the circulation is normal, color returns to the hand in less than 5 seconds. If the hand does not regain its color in 15 seconds, it is considered relatively contraindicated to cannulate that radial artery. It is important to prevent the patient from overextending the wrist; otherwise, a false abnormal result will be produced by occlusion of the transpalmar arch under the flexor retinaculum.[12] Some investigators have recommended the use of the Doppler finger pulse transducer or the plethysmograph to check for adequate ulnar artery collateral circulation in anesthetized patients in whom an unanticipated radial artery catheter is needed.[13]

When selecting an artery for cannulation, it is preferable not to use a radial artery distal to a brachial artery cutdown site from a previous cardiac catheterization, since distorted pressures and early occlusion of these vessels may result.[14] Other factors that affect selection of a radial artery include the following:

1. Site of surgery: for descending thoracic aortic aneurysms, the right radial artery should be used, since the left subclavian artery may be occluded by the surgeons, and the left radial artery pressure may be misleading
2. Dissection of an internal mammary artery: use of the Favaloro retractor may obstruct the arterial circulation on the ipsilateral side
3. Prior surgery on the hand
4. The nondominant hand is the preferred side
5. Preference of the surgeon and/or anesthesiologist

Good technique is necessary to obtain a high degree of success in arterial catheterization.[15] The wrist should be sharply dorsiflexed over a pack of sponges and immobilized on a short arm board. It is helpful to draw the course of the artery for 1 in. and to be comfortably seated. A wheal of local anesthetic is raised over the artery, and a small skin nick is made with an 18-gauge needle. A short, 20-gauge, nontapered Teflon catheter is used, without a syringe attached, to make the puncture. The angle between the needle and the skin should be shallow (30° or less), and the needle should be advanced parallel to the course of the artery. When the artery is entered, the angle between the needle and skin is reduced to 10°, and the outer catheter is threaded off the needle while watching that blood continues to drip out of the needle hub (Fig. 6-1). The back wall of the artery should not be punctured. If the blood stops dripping, the needle has penetrated the back wall. The needle should be removed; and then the catheter should be pulled back until a brisk spurt of blood occurs, and then it should be advanced slowly up the artery. After

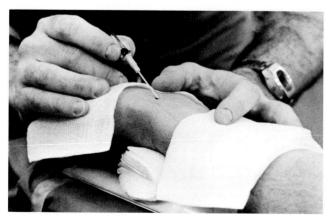

Fig. 6-1.   Placement of a percutaneous 20-gauge radial artery catheter. The artery has been entered and the catheter-needle unit is being gently threaded up the vessel. Note the position of the hand. The back wall of the artery has not been punctured.

insertion of the catheter, the wrist should be taken out of the dorsiflexed position, since continued dorsiflexion can lead to median nerve damage by stretching of the nerve over the wrist.

The catheter is attached via nondistensible tubing to the pressure transducer. A stopcock should not be placed directly on the catheter for at least two reasons: (1) it may easily become disconnected; and (2) constant manipulation of it will traumatize the artery. The tubing is connected to a manifold that holds a series of pressure transducers and extension tubes. The mechanical characteristics of this connecting system can markedly influence the fidelity of the arterial pressure tracing, and, thus, the systolic and diastolic digital displays. Most commonly, artifactual arterial traces are caused by "ringing" or "resonance" in the connecting system as it interacts with the mechanical characteristics of the transducer. Almost all the "ringing" artifacts are "false highs." Rarely, ringing, resonance, or damping can lead to a false low reading.

The level of analysis necessary to understand the above-mentioned problems with the connecting system is quite complex. In general, most pressure systems can be made better by (1) using the transducer with the highest frequency response (usually one of the modern small transducers); (2) keeping the tubing as short as possible (ideally, 3–6 in.); and (3) keeping the tubing, stopcocks, and domes completely free of bubbles.

The major problems with a catheter pressure system are (1) improper zeroing and drift; (2) improper transducer or monitor calibration; and (3) inadequate dynamic response.[16] Zero drift can occur from (1) changes in patient position; (2) membrane-dome coupling problems; or (3) transducer electrical zero change. Many of these problems can be eliminated by use of disposable pressure transducers. A fast-flush test can be used to determine if the recorded waveforms are accurate.[17] Opening the flush valve on a continuous flush system generates a square wave that permits assessment of the dynamic response of the system (Fig. 6-2). Factors leading to a poor dynamic response include air bubbles, kinked tubing, too long or compliant tubing, or a clot on the catheter.

Testing the fidelity of the arterial pressure tracing can also be done by using the simple return-to-flow method. The blood pressure cuff on the same arm is pumped up until the pulsatile trace disappears, and then air is slowly bled from the cuff, reducing the pressure in the conventional manner and noting the pressure (on the mercury or dial manometer) at which the first pulsatile trace reappears on the oscilloscope

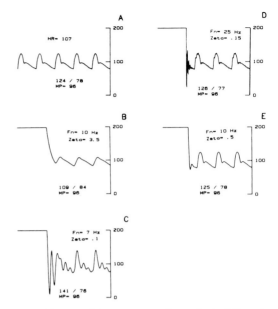

Fig. 6-2. Arterial pressure waveforms obtained from the same patient. (A) Patient's actual arterial pressure waveform as if recorded with a catheter-tipped transducer (MP, mean pressure). (B) The same patient's arterial waveform recorded with an overdamped system. Note that the fast-flush signal (upper left) returns slowly to the patient waveform. Systolic pressure is underestimated, diastolic is overestimated, and MP is unchanged. (C) An underdamped condition with low Fn (natural frequency). Systolic pressure is overestimated, diastolic is slightly underestimated, and MP is correct. (D) An underdamped condition with high Fn. Waveform is only slightly distorted, and systolic, diastolic, and mean pressures are close to the actual ones. (E) An ideally damped pressure monitoring system. The undershoot after the fast flush is small, and the original patient waveform is adequately reproduced. (From Gardner RM: Direct blood pressure measurement—Dynamic response requirements. Anesthesiology 54:227–236, 1981, with permission.)

screen. This is the best systolic pressure and should be very close to the same pressure at which the Korotkoff sounds are heard.

The arterial catheter should be kept patent with a continuous infusion of heparinized solution (1–3 ml/hr). The infusion minimizes thrombus formation and helps prolong the usefulness of the catheter.[18] Gardner et al showed that pressure errors resulting from this flush system are clinically insignificant, averaging less than 2 percent.[19] In the operating room, the catheter should also be flushed intermittently with a small volume (2–3 ml) of heparinized solution (1 unit of heparin per milliliter of saline). Larger volumes may produce central arterial embolization and cerebral vascular accidents and thus must be avoided.[20]

A large amount of information can be obtained from a direct arterial blood pressure tracing in addition to the blood pressure itself. The heart rate and rhythm can be ascertained as can their hemodynamic significance. An estimation can be made of myocardial contractility by looking at the upstroke (dP/dt) of the arterial tracing, and the SVR can be estimated by looking at the downslope of the tracing. A rapid upstroke implies good contractility, and a steep downslope indicates a low SVR. The size of the pulse pressure can be used to estimate blood volume and stroke volume. Hypovolemia can be detected by a large fluctuation in the beat-to-beat blood pressure associated with positive pressure ventilation. This can sometimes be an early and very useful sign of hypovolemia.

Thrombosis of the radial artery after cannulation is a common complication. The thrombi appear to be induced by the presence of the catheter itself, since the incidence of thrombosis increases with increasing duration of cannulation. In a study by Bedford and Wollman, 18-gauge catheters in place for less than 20 hours induced a 25 percent incidence of thrombosis, while catheters in for longer durations (20–40 hours) resulted in 50 percent thrombosis.[21] The onset of thrombosis was frequently found to be delayed until some days after decannulation. There was a 10 percent incidence of minor vascular problems but no major complications, and 100 percent of the thrombosed vessels eventually recanalized. In other stud-

ies, nontapered 20-gauge Teflon catheters have had the lowest incidence of thrombosis (about 20 percent).[22] Bedford showed that the incidence of postcannulation radial artery occlusion could be decreased significantly by using 20-gauge cannulae instead of 18-gauge cannulae.[23] Tapered catheters tend to obstruct more of the vessel with their shoulders and therefore further reduce flow past the catheter. Teflon catheters appear to be less thrombogenic than polypropylene catheters.[24,25] Downs et al found 90 percent occlusion with polypropylene and only 29 percent with Teflon.[24] Bedford also found that the incidence of radial artery occlusion was related to the radial artery diameter, with small vessels having a higher rate of occlusion.[26] Wrist circumference can be used as a predictor of radial artery occlusion. Forty-seven percent of patients with a circumference of less than 18 cm sustained occlusion, while only 21 percent with a circumference greater than 18 cm had occlusion. Slogoff et al found that abnormal flow after radial artery cannulation was more common in patients with hematomas at the site and in women.[27] In their study of 1699 patients, they concluded that radial artery cannulation was a low-risk method of monitoring.

It appears to be possible to remove some radial artery thrombi during decannulation. Bedford reported the technique of applying suction with a syringe to the hub of the radial artery catheter while it is being withdrawn.[28] In 9 of 19 patients with marked thrombus, the clot was successfully removed by aspiration (Fig. 6-3). Feeley reported four cases of cathe-

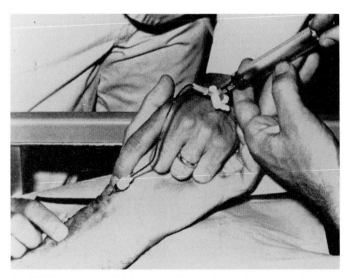

Fig. 6-3. Withdrawal of arterial thrombus. Note occlusion of vessel proximal and distal to cannulation site. (From Bedford RF: Removal of radial artery thrombi following percutaneous cannulation. Anesthesiology 46:430–432, 1977, with permission.)

ter thrombectomy to reestablish flow in thrombosed radial arteries.[29] A No. 3 French embolectomy catheter was inserted through an 18-gauge arteriotomy and the thrombus was removed. Then an 18-gauge catheter was reinserted through the same arteriotomy and monitoring was continued. The new catheters worked satisfactorily for 32–72 hours in the four patients. This technique may be useful in long-term monitoring when the radial artery is felt to be the best site for blood pressure and gas measurements.

Numerous other complications of radial artery catheterization have been reported, including ecchymosis and hematoma formation at the puncture site, hand and wrist discomfort, arteriovenous fistulae or aneurysms, localized ischemia of digits, and embolic phenomena. Cases of proximal skin necrosis after radial artery catheterization have also been reported.[30,31] These have occurred secondary to interference by the catheter and/or thrombus with the local cutaneous branches of the radial artery. Wyatt et al suggested cannulating as far distal as possible with a 20-gauge catheter to try to avoid this unfortunate complication.[30] The radial artery catheter may also be the source of bacterial contamination. An outbreak of flavobacterium sepsis was traced to contaminated blood gas syringes, which in turn contaminated the stopcock and arterial catheter and ultimately led to positive blood cultures in 14 patients.[32]

Another technique of radial artery catheterization allows percutaneous insertion of a long catheter in order to obtain a central aortic tracing of arterial blood pressure. Gardner et al reported on 495 insertions of a 100-cm-long Teflon catheter through an 18-gauge thin-walled needle.[33] Ninety-two percent of the catheters were successfully placed in the radial artery, and only 2.9 percent could not be advanced into the subclavian artery. The advantages of a central arterial trace are that beat-to-beat determinations of stroke volume can be made by the pulse contour method (see below) and that the aortic pressure is more reliable than the radial artery pressure in patients with low-flow states or after CPB.[34] After CPB, the radial artery pressure can be 10–100 mm Hg lower than the central aortic pressure due to vasoconstriction. The main disadvantage of the central arterial catheter is the increased incidence of complications. In the series reported by Gardner et al, 3 patients required thrombectomies for complete arterial occlusion, and 1 patient required surgical removal of a catheter that was sheared off by the needle.[33] The risk of retrograde arterial dissection by the catheter is also present during insertion up the arm.

Ulnar artery. The ulnar artery may occasionally be cannulated instead of the radial artery. In a small percentage of patients, the regular Allen's test is inadequate, but when it is *reversed,* with the radial artery being released, the hand fills adequately. This shows radial artery dominance and, in this instance, it is preferable to cannulate the ulnar artery. This finding can be further confirmed with Doppler flow measurements over the radial and ulnar arteries. The same technique and equipment are used to cannulate the ulnar artery as for the radial artery.

Brachial or axillary arteries. The brachial or axillary arteries can also be cannulated for pressure measurements in the operating room or intensive care unit. The brachial artery has been shown to have a 17 percent incidence of obstruction after cardiac catheterization, with two thirds being asymptomatic;[35] however, Barnes et al reported that complications resulting from brachial artery pressure monitoring are lower than those following cardiac catheterization.[36] Fifty-four patients had 18-gauge Teflon brachial artery catheters placed for monitoring during cardiac surgery without any of the patients developing evidence of obstruction of the brachial artery or distal ischemic symptoms during the 1–3 days of cannulation. About 10 percent of the patients in this group had a low-output syndrome requiring inotropic therapy. Three patients developed localized obstruction of the radial or ulnar artery, however, probably secondary to embolic phenomena in spite of a continuous heparin infusion through the arterial catheter. None of these 3 patients developed ischemic symptoms in the hand.

The axillary artery has been recommended for long-term arterial pressure monitoring in the intensive care unit.[37] It allows freedom of the patient's hands and permits a large catheter to be placed in a central artery. Using the Seldinger technique, a 6- or 8-in. 18-gauge Teflon catheter can be inserted via the axillary artery into the aortic arch.[38] The left axillary artery is preferred to reduce the possibility of cerebral embolization off the catheter. The main complications reported have been related to axillary sheath hematomas with brachial plexus compression. This potential complication makes axillary artery cannulation relatively contraindicated prior to heparinization for CPB.

Femoral artery. Femoral artery catheterization may be used intraoperatively or in the postoperative period. This is a relatively simple technique in which the catheter may remain patent for a prolonged period of time. A 6- or 8-in. 18-gauge catheter is advanced up the artery without difficulty in most cases. If an obstruction is encountered in patients with arteriosclerosis, a small J-wire can be used to bypass the obstruction with a high degree of success. Ersoz et al reported prolonged femoral artery catheterization in 64 patients with no major complications during 1–10 days of monitoring.[39] Twelve patients had minor complications, including decreased distal pulses and hematoma formation. None of the catheter sites became infected, but three of the catheter tips had positive cultures upon removal. The femoral artery is also a useful monitoring site during descending thoracic aorta aneurysm surgery. Using either partial left heart bypass or femoral-femoral bypass with the aorta cross-clamped, it is useful to monitor the blood pressure in the lower circulation to assess renal and spinal cord perfusion. Some surgeons are now using the Gott external shunt instead of CPB in these cases. It is necessary to measure pressure distal to the shunt, since kinking and partial occlusion of flow is a frequent problem with this technique[40] (see Chapter 18).

Dorsalis pedis artery. The two main arteries to the foot are the dorsalis pedis artery, which is a continuation of the anterior tibial artery extending from the ankle to the great toe, and the lateral plantar artery off the posterior tibial artery. These two vessels form an arterial arch on the foot that is similar to the one formed by the radial and ulnar arteries in the hand. The presence of collateral flow to the foot from the lateral plantar artery should be checked prior to cannulation of the dorsalis pedis artery. The test is performed by occluding both arteries and blanching the great toe by compressing it. The lateral plantar artery is released, and the toe should rapidly flush with color. It is not safe to cannulate the dorsalis pedis artery if color does not return to the toes within 10 seconds. The circulation may alternatively be checked using a Doppler flow meter. It is recommended to catheterize this vessel with a 20-gauge Teflon catheter in a manner similar to that of the radial artery.

The dorsalis pedis artery appears to be a reasonable alternative to radial artery catheterization in patients undergoing surgical procedures in which the anesthesiologist is located along the patient's side; however, the vessel may not be palpable or present in 5–12 percent of patients.[41] This vessel probably should not be used in patients with diabetes or other peripheral vascular diseases. Youngberg and Miller demonstrated the safety of cannulating this artery.[42] In 26 patients who had catheters in the dorsalis pedis artery for 2–25 hours, the incidence of thrombosis was lower than that reported for radial artery catheters, and no major complications were observed.

The pressure measured in the peripheral dorsalis pedis artery is different from a more central pressure, since the arterial pressure contour becomes progressively more distorted as the wave is transmitted down the arterial system. The high-frequency components such as the incisura disappear, the systolic peak increases while the diastolic value decreases, and there is a transmission delay. These changes are due to decreased arterial compliance in the periphery and reflection and resonance of previous waves.[43] The systolic pressure is usually 10–20 mm Hg higher in the dorsalis pedis artery than in the radial or brachial arteries, while the diastolic pressure is 15–20 mm Hg lower.[42,44]

VENOUS PRESSURE MONITORING

Central Venous Pressure

The CVP is usually measured as an indication of right atrial and right ventricular pressures. The catheter must lie within the thorax in a major vein or be in the right side of the heart; a reproducible landmark, such as the midaxillary line, must be used for repeated reference to the zero level; and the monitoring system has to be reliable. Electronic monitoring is preferable to a simple water manometer (1 cm H_2O = 1.36 mm Hg) because it allows observation and diagnosis from the venous waves; respiratory fluctuations can be observed; and it is quickly responsive to changes in pressure.[45]

The normal venous tracing has three positive waves (a, c, and v) and two negative ones (x and y).[46] These waveforms have a fixed relationship to the ECG and phonocardiogram (PCG) (Fig. 6-4). The a wave is produced by right atrial contraction and begins before the first heart sound. When the atrium relaxes, the venous pulse descends and is interrupted by the second positive wave, the c wave. This is produced by the bulging of the tricuspid valve into the right atrium during the onset of ventricular contraction and occurs right after the first heart sound and QRS complex of the ECG. The x descent results from further atrial relaxation and downward displacement of the ventricle and tricuspid valve during ventricular systole. The v wave is formed by right atrial filling with a closed tricuspid valve, and the y descent is formed by opening of the tricuspid valve with blood flow into the right ventricle.

The a wave will be absent in patients with atrial fibrillation. Large a waves occur when there is

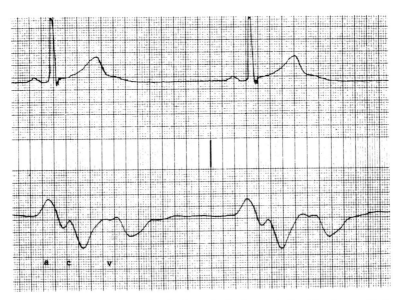

Fig. 6-4. A normal CVP tracing is shown in the bottom half of the figure with its corresponding ECG in the top half. The a, c, and v waves on the venous pressure tracing are labeled. The x descent occurs between the c and v waves, while the y descent occurs after the v wave.

increased resistance to right atrial emptying, as in tricuspid stenosis, right ventricular hypertrophy, pulmonary stenosis, or pulmonary hypertension. If the right atrium contracts when the tricuspid valve is still closed, a giant a wave or cannon wave will occur. This is frequently seen during anesthesia when a nodal rhythm occurs and may produce a drop in blood pressure varying from 5 to 20 percent (Fig. 6-5). Cannon waves may also be seen during ventricular dysrhythmias and heart block. In patients with tricuspid regurgitation, the x descent disappears and is replaced by a large v wave.

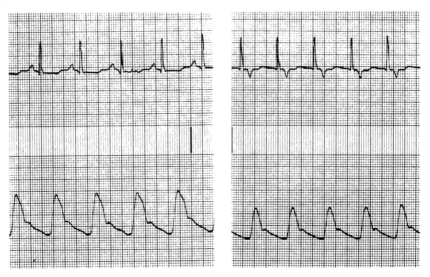

Fig. 6-5. The ECG in the top panel and the arterial tracing in the bottom panel are from a patient receiving enflurane anesthesia. The tracings on the left side show a blood pressure of 140/80 mm Hg when the patient is in a sinus rhythm. The tracings on the right side show a blood pressure of 110/60 mm Hg when the patient loses his atrial kick and is in a nodal rhythm. The CVP tracing at this time showed a cannon wave.

The CVP is a useful monitor if the factors affecting it are realized and its limitations are understood. The CVP reflects the patient's blood volume, venous tone, and right ventricular performance. It is also affected by central venous obstructions and alterations of intrathoracic pressure, such as positive end-expiratory pressure. Serial measurements are more useful than an individual number, and the response of the CVP to a volume infusion is a useful test of right ventricular function. A rapid infusion of 100–200 ml of fluid can be used to judge hemodynamic performance by observing how much of an increment it produces in the CVP and blood pressure. It must be remembered that the CVP reflects *right* heart performance and not left ventricular function; therefore, it is possible to have a patient develop pulmonary edema with a normal CVP. Thus, the combination of the CVP to monitor right atrial pressure and the esophageal stethoscope to monitor left atrial pressure (ie, rales and S_3) is still a useful monitoring technique in patients with good left ventricular function. The CVP does not give any direct indication of left heart filling pressure; however, it can be used as a crude estimate of left-sided pressures in patients with good left ventricular function. Mangano showed a good correlation between CVP and left-sided filling pressures during a change in volume status in patients with coronary artery disease and ejection fractions over 0.4.[47]

CVP monitoring is indicated in (1) all cardiac surgical procedures (measured by itself or along with pulmonary artery pressure); (2) surgical procedures in which large volume shifts may occur (eg, Whipple procedure); (3) potentially hypovolemic patients (eg, those with bowel obstruction); (4) patients in shock; (5) massively traumatized patients; and (6) some patients with preexisting cardiovascular disease undergoing surgery (others will require a PAC).

The CVP should be monitored in all patients during CPB. When the catheter tip is in the superior vena cava, it indicates both right atrial pressure and cerebral venous pressure. Significant increases in the cerebral venous pressure can produce critical drops in the cerebral perfusion pressure. This is often caused by a superior vena cava cannula for CPB obstructing the innominate vein and must be corrected by the surgeon to avoid cerebral edema and poor cerebral perfusion.

A CVP catheter may even be preferred over a PAC in certain types of cardiac surgical patients (ie, those with tricuspid valve disease, atrial septal defects, and other congenital lesions, or those in whom autologous blood may need to be removed from the CVP catheter). Other indications for a CVP catheter include neurosurgical operations done in the sitting position with the possibility of air embolization, patients with poor peripheral veins, hyperalimentation, and rapid administration of fluid. Temporary transvenous cardiac pacemakers may also be placed using a central venous cannulation technique.

Many methods and routes of central venous catheterization have been described, together with their frequent and sometimes bizarre complications. Anesthesiologists should become experts in the introduction of these catheters via various techniques in order to give their patients the best possible care. They must understand and appreciate the risks of these techniques in order to avoid them and see the benefits of this method of monitoring (Table 6-1).

INTERNAL JUGULAR VEIN

Cannulation of the internal jugular vein (IJV) was first described by English et al in 1969; since then, it has steadily increased in popularity to its present position as one of the methods of choice for CVP monitoring.[48] The technique is contraindicated in the hands of people not familiar with the anatomy, in anticoagulated patients, and in patients with prior surgery of the neck. Advantages of this technique are (1) ease of cannulation as a result of the constant

Table 6-1

CVP Techniques

	IJV	EJV	Subclavian	Arm
Success rate	1	3	2	4
Safety	3	2	4	1
Complications	2	3	1	4
Ease of later insertion of PAC or pacemaker	1	2	3	4

Key: 1, highest; 4, lowest. IJV = internal jugular vein; EJV = external jugular vein.

relationships of the anatomic structures leading to a high success rate; (2) a short, straight course to the right atrium that almost assures right atrial or superior vena cava localization of the catheter tip; (3) easy access from the head of the table; and (4) fewer complications than subclavian catheterization.

The IJV is located under the medial border of the lateral head of the sternocleidomastoid muscle (Fig. 6-6). The carotid artery is consistently deep and medial to the IJV. The right IJV is preferred, since this vein leads straight into the superior vena cava, the right cupula of the lung is lower than the left, and the thoracic duct is on the left side. The anatomy is demonstrated more easily in the awake patient who can make the sternocleidomastoid muscle stand out by momentarily lifting his head and tensing it. The cannulation is no more uncomfortable than starting a peripheral venous line and is well-tolerated by awake, premedicated patients. The neck is extended and turned sharply to the left while the patient is placed in a 15° Trendelenberg position. The muscle borders should be identified and the location of the carotid artery noted (Fig. 6-7).

Three main routes of cannulation of the IJV have been described,[49] but the central route, which is described below, is preferred.[50] After the skin is prepared, a wheal of local anesthetic is raised at the apex of the triangle formed by the two heads of the sterno-

cleidomastoid muscle. This point is two to three fingerbreadths above the clavicle and well above the cupula of the right lung. The initial identifying venipuncture is made with a 1½-in. 22-gauge needle on a 5-ml syringe containing 1 ml of 1 percent lidocaine. With the skin tensed, the needle is advanced in a caudad direction at a 30° angle to the skin, away from the midline, and under the lateral head of the sternocleidomastoid muscle (Fig. 6-7). The needle tip should not enter the medial half of the sternocleidomastoid triangle where the carotid artery is located. Constant aspiration is maintained on the syringe as the needle is advanced into the vein at a depth of ½–1½ in. If the vein is not found, a Valsalva maneuver by the patient will help distend it to a size of 2–3 cm and make location easier. After the vein is located, the skin is infiltrated with 1 ml of lidocaine and the needle removed. The skin should continue to be tensed by the left hand so that the underlying anatomy does not change position. An 18-gauge, 1¾-in. thin-walled needle–catheter unit is then inserted at the same angle and depth into the vein (Fig. 6-8). The needle and catheter should be slowly advanced down the IJV until the catheter is fully threaded into the vein. The needle is removed, and a syringe is placed directly on the catheter, being sure that venous blood can be easily aspirated. The guidewire's straight or J flexible end is passed

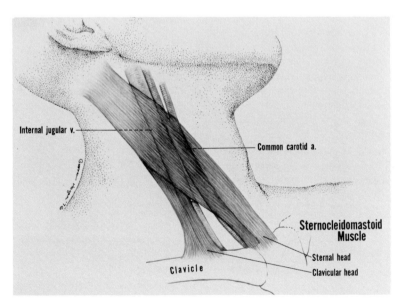

Fig. 6-6. A diagrammatic representation of the anatomy of the major structures in the region of the right IJV. Note that the IJV runs under the medial border of the clavicular head (lateral) of the sternocleidomastoid muscle. The carotid artery is deep under the sternal head (medial) of the sternocleidomastoid muscle.

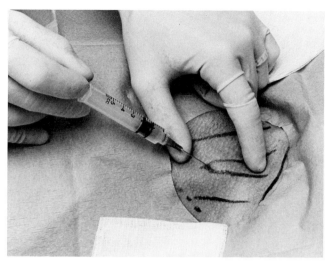

Fig. 6-7. The IJV is located with a 22-gauge needle on a 5-ml syringe. The skin puncture is made at the apex of the sternocleidomastoid triangle, which is usually two to three fingerbreadths above the clavicle (1½–2 in.) and lateral to the carotid pulse. The needle is advanced in a caudad direction at a 30° angle to the skin under the lateral head of the muscle while aspirating on the syringe.

through the 18-gauge catheter into the superior vena cava, and the 18-gauge catheter is removed. The wire should easily advance through the catheter without much resistance. The skin hole around the guidewire should be enlarged with a scalpel blade and the 16-gauge, 8-in. CVP catheter threaded over the guidewire by a twisting motion into the IJV (Fig. 6-9). The guidewire should then be removed, and venous blood should easily be aspirated through the CVP catheter. The catheter is then attached to the pressure monitoring system and is taped along the anterior border of the ear in a stable manner. The tip

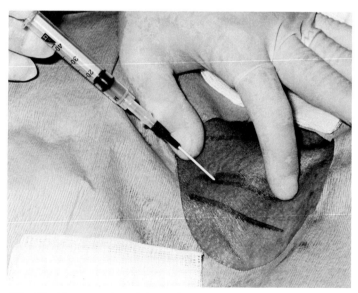

Fig. 6-8. The 18-gauge catheter is inserted at the same angle as the finder needle. It is slowly advanced to the same depth, where the IJV should be identified. Venous blood should be easily aspirated as the catheter is slowly advanced down the vein.

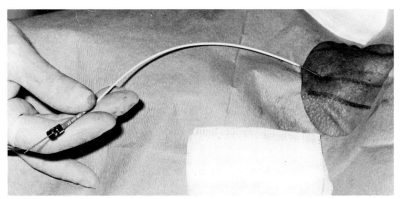

Fig. 6-9. The CVP catheter is positioned over the guidewire prior to advancement into the central circulation.

of the 8-in. catheter is usually located at the junction of the superior vena cava and right atrium in the average adult. Using this technique, over a 90 percent success rate of catheterization of the IJV has been obtained with only a 1–2 percent incidence of carotid puncture.

Two other approaches described for cannulating the IJV are the posterior and anterior routes. In the posterior route, the needle is introduced under the sternocleidomastoid muscle near the junction of the middle and lower thirds of its lateral border and is advanced toward the suprasternal notch.[51] In this technique, the needle is aimed in the direction of the carotid artery, and, therefore, the incidence of carotid artery puncture may be higher. In the anterior approach, the needle is inserted at the midpoint of the sternocleidomastoid muscle on its medial border and aimed toward the ipsilateral nipple.[52]

Another technique of IJV catheterization was introduced in Canada by Boulanger et al in 1976.[53] The needle is introduced much higher on the medial border of the sternocleidomastoid muscle, at the level of the superior border of the thyroid cartilage. The needle is directed inferiorly and laterally under the posterior aspect of the muscle and meets the IJV at its widest diameter. The technique differs from those previously described by its high entry point, which further reduces the possibility of a pneumothorax, and its lateral, superficial path away from the carotid artery. The authors reported a 94 percent success rate, with a 2 percent incidence of carotid artery puncture.

Some authors have recommended additional techniques for cannulating the IJV in order to reduce the incidence of carotid artery puncture. Civetta et al recommended placing a 22-gauge spinal needle through a 14-gauge intracath needle,[54] and Petty recommended leaving a small identifying needle in place while advancing the larger needle.[55] Jobes et al recommended attaching a 20-gauge catheter to a transducer prior to passing the guidewire and observing the pressure and waveform.[56] In a prospective study of 1284 patients, 10 episodes of arterial catheterization were diagnosed by this technique of pressure monitoring when they were not suspected by other signs.

Many studies have verified the high degree of success in cannulating the IJV in the hands of experienced personnel. Vaughan and Weyjandt reported a failure rate of only 2 patients in 227 adults (less than 1 percent) and of 6.2 percent when children 1–2 years of age were included.[57] Kuramoto and Sakav reported successful CVP catheterization via the right IJV in 96 percent of their adult patients and overall in 88 percent of IJV catheterizations versus only 70 percent using the basilic vein.[58] The success rate has been lower in children, but with experience and proper equipment, it can be quite reasonable. Prince et al reported successful CVP catheterization in 68 percent of children 6 weeks to 2 years of age and in 82 percent in the 2–14-year-old group.[59] The rate of success was higher in infants weighing more than 10 kg and in patients with CVPs above 10 cm H_2O.

EXTERNAL JUGULAR VEIN

Cannulation of the external jugular vein (EJV) is the alternate method of choice when the right IJV cannot be cannulated. This vein contains valves that can make passing a catheter into the central circulation very difficult; however, Blitt et al introduced a J-wire EJV catheterization technique that makes this approach a reasonable alternative to the IJV.[60] This technique is based on the J-wire principle used for retrograde catheterization of tortuous vessels during radiologic studies.[61] An 18-gauge, 1¾-in. over-the-needle Teflon catheter is introduced into the EJV. The needle is removed, and a 35-cm-long flexible J-wire is inserted through the catheter and rotated past venous valvular obstructions into the central circulation. Then a 14- or 16-gauge, 8-in. CVP catheter is introduced over the J-wire. This technique avoids insertion of a needle deep into the neck, and more than a 90 percent success rate of central venous catheter placement has been reported.

BASILIC AND CEPHALIC VEINS

When a neck vein is not available, one of the arm veins can be cannulated and an attempt made to advance the catheter into the central venous circulation. The disadvantages of using the arm veins are the unreliability of obtaining a truly central catheter; the need for x-ray confirmation if right atrial location is required (eg, in the sitting position); and the time delay in determining if the catheter is central.

A number of studies have examined the results of blind insertion of CVP catheters through the arm. Kellner and Smart found that 25 percent of the catheters were outside the central veins, with most of these passing up one of the jugular veins.[62] Fluctuation with respiration was found not to be a reliable sign of central location, since it was present in 21 percent of noncentral catheters. False high CVP readings of 2–6 mm Hg were found in the noncentral catheters. Webre and Arens found that only 59 percent of arm catheters passed into the central circulation.[63] In the basilic vein, 65 percent of catheters passed central, while only 45 percent of those in the cephalic vein reached the central veins. Of the incorrectly placed catheters, 45–67 percent lay in the IJVs.[64] Burgess et al have shown that turning the head of the patient toward the arm of insertion and placing the chin onto the ipsilateral shoulder during the threading of the catheter reduces the incidence of catheter passage up the IJV instead of into the central circulation.[65] Eighteen percent of catheters entered the IJV with the head in the midline, but only 4 percent entered when the head was turned. Central placement was successful in 80 percent of patients who had their heads turned during catheterization.

SUBCLAVIAN VEIN

The subclavian vein is readily available and has frequently been used for CVP catheterization in the past.[66] It has fallen into disfavor, however, because of the high incidence of major complications. It can be cannulated either from a supraclavicular or infraclavicular approach. Both methods have a high incidence of pneumothorax and the possibility of subclavian artery laceration.

COMPLICATIONS

All the methods of CVP monitoring mentioned above have the following potential complications: (1) local and systemic infection; (2) thrombophlebitis; (3) mediastinal fluid infusion producing hydrothorax; (4) hematomas; (5) air embolism; (6) catheter shearing; (7) nerve injuries; and (8) pericardial tamponade.

Specific complications of internal jugular and subclavian venipuncture include[67]

1. Carotid or subclavian artery puncture: This can lead to significant hemorrhage from the subclavian artery into the chest, since it is difficult to compress this artery under the clavicle. Puncture of the carotid artery rarely causes problems if recognized immediately and compressed until the bleeding ceases in 10–15 minutes; however, large hematomas can develop and endanger the airway. An arteriovenous fistula has been reported as a complication, as has a chronic hematoma requiring surgical removal.[68,69]

2. Pneumothorax: This is much more common after subclavian puncture. It has been reported in 2–16 percent of attempted subclavian venipunctures but only rarely after jugular puncture; however, a tension pneumothorax after IJV catheterization and general anesthesia has been reported.[70]

3. Nerve damage: If the needle is directed too far laterally in the neck, it is possible to injure the brachial plexus. A Horner's syndrome has also been reported after puncture of the IJV.[71]

4. Thoracic duct injury: This can occur if the left IJV is used, and it is the main reason for preferring the right IJV. This can be a major complication requiring surgical intervention.[72]

Left Atrial Pressure

In patients with left-sided heart disease, the CVP cannot be reliably used as an estimate of left ventricular filling pressure. In these patients, it is necessary to monitor LAP directly with a catheter in the left atrium or indirectly with a PAC in the pulmonary artery using the pulmonary capillary wedge pressure (PCWP) as an approximation of LAP. Measurement of left-sided filling pressure is indicated in patients with mitral and aortic valvular disease, coronary artery disease with poor left ventricular function, or certain types of congenital heart disease, and in any patient in whom difficulty is encountered upon discontinuing CPB.

A 16-gauge, 12-in. Teflon catheter is placed by the surgeon through a 14-gauge intracath needle or the previous vent site into the right superior pulmonary vein and advanced into the left atrium. A Teflon-pledgetted purse-string stitch is placed around the catheter to provide a surface for clotting upon removal of the catheter (Fig. 6-10). The catheter is brought out through the skin in the epigastric area and sutured in place. It is important to maintain positive airway pressure during insertion of the catheter in order to avoid the possibility of air entry into the pulmonary vein, and, thus, into the left side of the heart, where it could embolize to the systemic circulation.

The left atrial catheter is an extremely informative monitor, but it is also quite risky and requires extreme caution in its use. The possibility of air embolism to the coronary or cerebral circulation is always present. This problem exists both on insertion and during its continued use postoperatively in the intensive care unit. There is also the risk of clot formation on the catheter and subsequent embolization when the catheter is flushed or removed; therefore, a continuous heparin infusion is necessary in an effort to avoid thrombus formation on the catheter tip in the postoperative period. There is also the risk of bleeding when the LAP catheter is removed postoperatively. It should therefore be removed while the chest tubes are still in place to diagnose and treat this problem.

In the past, CVP catheters were used to monitor patients with left-sided heart disease; however, the CVP has been shown to have a very poor correlation with the LAP in these patients. In 200 patients with mitral valve disease undergoing cardiac catheterization, the correlation coefficient of LAP and CVP was only 0.48.[73] Rapid changes in LAP induced by volume expansion, tachycardia, or vasoactive drugs frequently were not reflected in the CVP. When volume was infused in some of the patients, the LAP and CVP moved in opposite directions. This is supported by Sarnoff and Berglund's work showing that there is not a consistent relationship between right atrial pressure and left ventricular stroke work.[74] Other studies have shown the disparity between left and right ventricular function both in medical patients with coronary artery disease and in surgical patients.[47,75-78] The relationship of the various filling pressures is shown below.[79]

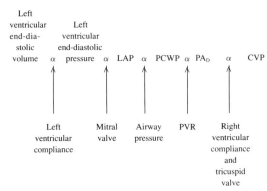

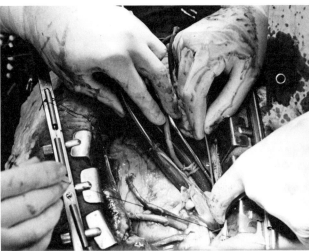

Fig. 6-10. At the end of CPB, a 12-in. 16-gauge catheter is placed by the surgeons into the right superior pulmonary vein and advanced into the left atrium for continuous measurement of LAP. The three aortocoronary bypass grafts can be seen as can the cannulae for CPB.

Pulmonary Artery Pressure

One of the major advances in recent years in the care of the cardiac patient has been the introduction and extensive use of the PAC.[80] This catheter allows measurement of pulmonary artery systolic (PA_s), diastolic (PA_d), and mean pressures (PAP); PCWP, which is also called the pulmonary artery occluded pressure (PA_o); CVP; and cardiac output, using the thermodilution technique. The PCWP has been shown to have a good correlation with direct LAP monitoring and, thus, can be used as a measure of the left ventricular filling pressure. The PCWP was within ±4 mm Hg of LAP in 95 percent of 1620 simultaneous measurements in 43 patients after cardiac surgery.[81] Lappas et al showed an even better correlation, with the LAP–PCWP difference exceeding ±1 mm Hg in only 10 percent of patients;[82] however, the relationship between LAP and PCWP may not be as close when the LAP exceeds 15 mm Hg.[83] The PCWP also may not correlate as well with the LAP in patients on positive end-expiratory pressure (PEEP) of more than 10 cm H_2O. Lorzman et al showed a good correlation when PEEP was 5 cm H_2O or less ($r = 0.83$) but no significant correlation when PEEP was 10 cm H_2O or greater.[84] This may be a significant handicap in the postoperative care of these critically ill patients. When the catheter cannot be placed in a wedge position, the PA_D can also be used as an estimate of LAP; however, the PA_D–PCWP gradient often increases after CPB by as much as 5 mm Hg.[85]

The use of the PAC by anesthesiologists has been a tremendous advance. It allows measurements of left-sided hemodynamics in the awake patient, during and after anesthetic induction, and in the prebypass period, as well as after CPB and postoperatively when the LAP is easily measured. This has contributed significantly to the understanding and care of these cardiac patients. It is impressive to observe large changes in the PAP and PCWP with almost no reflection in the CVP. Connors et al prospectively analyzed 62 consecutive pulmonary artery catheterizations.[86] They found that less than half of a group of clinicians correctly predicted the PCWP or cardiac output, and over 50 percent made at least one change in therapy based on data from the PAC. Waller et al demonstrated that a group of experienced cardiac anesthesiologists and surgeons who were "blinded" to the information from the PAC during coronary artery bypass graft (CABG) surgery were unaware of any problem during 65 percent of severe hemodynamic abnormalities.[87] Similarly, Iberti and Fisher showed that a group of physicians was unable to accurately predict hemodynamic data on clinical grounds and that 60 percent made at least one change in therapy and 33 percent changed their diagnosis based on PAC data.[88]

The indications for catheterization of the pulmonary artery in the operating room are still evolving and vary from hospital to hospital. Indications for the use of the PAC can be divided into noncardiac and cardiac surgical cases. Noncardiac surgical indications for pulmonary artery catheterization are as follows:

1. Major surgery with large volume shifts in patients with known significant heart disease
2. Patients with severe coronary artery disease (eg, recent infarction) for all surgical procedures
3. Sepsis with an unstable circulation
4. Patients requiring inotropes, vasodilators, or the intra-aortic balloon pump for heart failure
5. Massive trauma cases
6. Patients in shock
7. Surgery of the aorta requiring cross-clamping
8. Patients in respiratory failure undergoing surgery
9. Patients with suspected or diagnosed pulmonary emboli
10. Cirrhotic patients undergoing portal systemic shunts

Cardiac surgical indications for pulmonary artery catheterization are as follows:

1. Patients undergoing coronary revascularization who have
   a. poor left ventricular function, eg, EF less than 0.4 or left ventricular end-diastolic pressure (LVEDP) greater than 18 mm Hg
   b. significant abnormality of left ventricular wall motion
   c. a recent acute myocardial infarction
   d. a complication such as acute mitral insufficiency, ventricular septal rupture, or a ventricular aneurysm
2. Mitral or aortic valve replacement
3. Pulmonary hypertension
4. Combined lesions (ie, coronary stenosis and valvular heart disease)
5. Complex lesions (ie, idiopathic hypertrophic subaortic stenosis)

There is a variety of equipment available to catheterize the pulmonary artery. For adult patients, the PAC comes in 5-Fr, 7-Fr, and 7½-Fr sizes. Most PACs are now heparin bonded to reduce thrombosis

Table 6-2
Intracardiac Pressures

| Cardiac Location | Normal Pressures (mm Hg) | |
	Mean	Range
RA	5	1–10
RV	25/5	15–30/0–8
PA S/D	23/9	15–30/5–15
PAP	15	10–20
PCWP	10	5–15
LAP	8	4–12
LVEDP	8	4–12

RA = right atrial; PA S/D = pulmonary artery (systolic/diastolic)

and emboli.[89] A variety of special catheters are available including PACs with an extra infusion lumen (VIP), pacing electrodes (multipurpose PAC),[90] a pacing lumen with separate ventricular pacing wire (Paceport), and capability of measuring the mixed venous oxygen saturation.[91] There are also small catheters available for percutaneous use in children or for surgical use in which the catheters are brought out through the chest wall. All of these catheters may be introduced by a variety of techniques: (1) venous cutdown in the antecubital fossae: this is the original technique, but it is rarely necessary any longer; (2) percutaneously via a large intravenous catheter: the 7-Fr PAC will fit through a 10-gauge cannula; or (3) percutaneously in a central vein using a dilator set and a modified Seldinger technique.[38]

It is also necessary to have high-frequency pressure transducers, a calibrated oscilloscopic display, and, preferably, a recorder for observation of waveforms during the passage of the catheter through the right side of the heart. The normal intracardiac pressures are shown in Table 6-2.[92] The waveforms observed during passage of the PAC are shown in Figure 6-11. The right atrial trace is seen at 25–35 cm, the right ventricle at 35–45 cm, the pulmonary artery at 45–55 cm, and the PCWP at 50–60 cm using the right IJV approach.

The preferred method of insertion of a PAC utilizes the right IJV and a modified Seldinger technique. This technique has the advantages of speed of insertion and a high success rate. The time for the entire procedure averages about 15 minutes after a little practice. The PAC should be inserted prior to the induction of anesthesia. Studies by Waller et al[93] and Quintin et al[94] showed that after premedication and with continuation of all preoperative cardiac

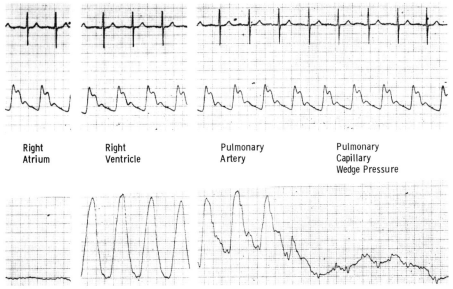

Right Atrium   Right Ventricle   Pulmonary Artery   Pulmonary Capillary Wedge Pressure

Fig. 6-11. The ECG and arterial pressure tracings are shown on the top panel, and the venous pressure tracing as the PAC is advanced is shown in the bottom panel. Starting from the left, the catheter enters the right atrium and the pressure changes to a large pulsatile tracing when the catheter enters the right ventricle. Notice that the right ventricular end-diastolic pressure is very low, as is the right atrial pressure. When the catheter enters the pulmonary artery, the pulmonary artery diastolic pressure is elevated because of the interposition of the valve. This is frequently the key sign that the pulmonary artery has been entered. The catheter is then advanced into the PCWP.

medications, awake insertion produced no changes in hemodynamics. Patients scheduled for elective CABG had no changes in blood pressure, heart rate, or rate–pressure product in those studies (Fig. 6-12). No patient experienced angina or ECG changes indicative of myocardial ischemia during PAC insertion. Nicolson et al also showed that the right IJV was the preferred approach in pediatric cardiac patients, with an 86 percent success rate.[95]

The patient is first attached to an ECG, and an arterial catheter is inserted for continuous blood pressure monitoring throughout the procedure. The anatomy of the neck is defined, and a surgical prep and draping is performed. The right IJV is identified with a 22-gauge needle as in the CVP cannulation technique (see above). Then an 18-gauge, thin-walled, 1 3/4-in. Teflon catheter is placed into the vein and threaded down the vessel for a short distance (Fig. 6-13A–C).[96] This is a key step to be sure that the catheter threads easily and that blood can be freely aspirated from the vein. The reason this step is so important is that the rest of the procedure is blind, and the introducer can inadvertently be passed into other structures if this step is incorrectly performed. A catheter introducer set is used at this point. The guidewire's flexible end is passed through the 18-gauge catheter into the superior vena cava, and the 18-gauge catheter is removed (Fig. 6-13D). The wire must advance easily without too much resistance or the next step should not be performed. The skin hole

around the guidewire is enlarged with a scalpel blade to allow introduction of the dilator set. The dilator set consists of an internal vessel dilator and an external 10-gauge catheter sheath. This combination is passed into the IJV over the guidewire by a twisting motion until the catheter sheath is in the superior vena cava (Fig. 6-13E). Then the PAC, which has been filled with fluid and attached to a transducer, is passed through the sheath into the superior vena cava, with the tip pointed up toward the pulmonary outflow tract (Fig. 6-13F). The PAC is advanced about 20 cm into the superior vena cava, and then 1 ml^3 of air is put into the balloon to allow it to float into the right ventricle. When it reaches the right ventricle, 1.5 ml^3 of air is put into the balloon to totally cover the tip of the catheter in an effort to reduce ventricular dysrhythmias. The location of the catheter tip is determined by the venous pressure tracing as shown above. If multiple premature ventricular contractions (PVCs) or runs of ventricular tachycardia occur with the catheter in the right ventricle, lidocaine (50–100 mg) can be used to suppress them. In some instances, the augmented stroke volume after the PVC will float the balloon into the pulmonary artery. A large inspiration by the patient can also be used to augment the stroke volume and help pass the catheter into the pulmonary artery. If the catheter does not enter the pulmonary artery by 60 cm, it should be brought back into the right atrium and another pass made. Excessive coiling of the catheter in the right ventricle

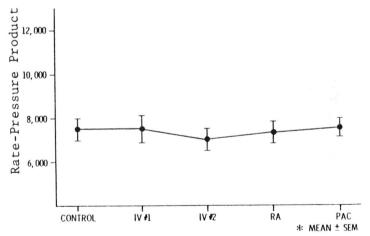

Fig. 6-12. Rate–pressure product in patients undergoing CABG at the following times: control; IV #1: time of insertion of first peripheral IV; IV #2: time of insertion of second peripheral IV; RA: radial artery catheter inserted; and PAC: PAC inserted. No significant change is seen from control, indicating safety of performing these procedures under local anesthesia. (From Waller JL, Zaidan JR, Kaplan JA, et al: Hemodynamic response to preoperative vascular cannulation in patients with coronary artery disease. Anesthesiology 56:219–221, 1982, with permission.)

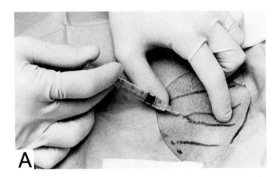

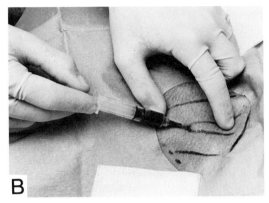

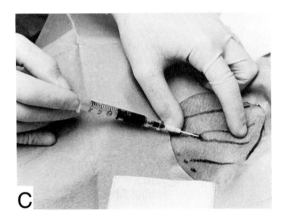

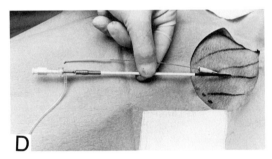

should be avoided to prevent catheter knotting. When the pulmonary artery is entered, the tracing will change and the diastolic pressure will become elevated. The catheter is further advanced into the wedge position with 1.5 ml^3 of air in the balloon; letting the air out of the balloon will show a pulmonary arterial tracing. The balloon should be left deflated and should be inflated only for short periods of time to measure the PCWP. The pulmonary artery oscilloscopic tracing should be constantly monitored to make sure the catheter does not float out into a constant wedge position and possibly infarct an area of the lung. The catheter sheath should be left in the IJV and the sidearm used for drug and fluid infusion. The PAC is covered by a sterile sheath, and often the PAC has to be pulled back a short distance as extra catheter in the right ventricle floats out into the pulmonary artery (Fig. 6-13G).

A chest x-ray should be obtained postoperatively in all patients to check the position of the PAC. Benumof et al found that most catheters pass into the

right middle or lower lobes (Fig. 6-14).[97] The catheters seem to work best if located proximally in either of these lobes and worst if located in the left lung because of the inherent curvature of the PAC. For the PAC to present accurate information, its tip must not be in a zone 1 region of the lung where it will reflect airway pressure rather than LAP. The most ideal position is to have the tip in the right middle or lower lobe, within 5–6 cm of where it is seen crossing the catheter that passes through the right atrium on the chest x-ray (Fig. 6-15). This places the tip of the catheter in the proximal third of the right lung on the chest x-ray.

Johnston et al have shown that PACs migrate a great distance during cardiac surgery toward the periphery of the lung.[98] They showed that migration of the catheters averaged 4.9 ± 0.6 cm, with a range of 2.1–8.4 cm, during CPB. They recommended that the PAC be pulled back 5 cm prior to the onset of CPB to reduce this migration and to maintain function after CPB. Murray et al, however, have recently

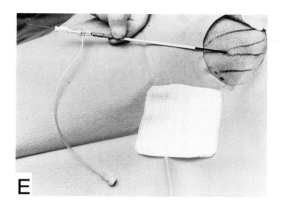

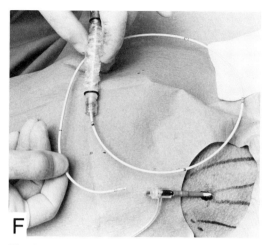

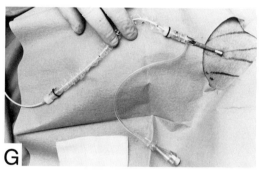

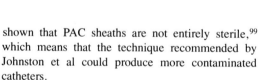

Fig. 6-13. Insertion of a PAC. (A) Skin wheal of local anesthetic placed at apex of the triangle of the sternocleidomastoid muscle. (B) IJV identified with 22-gauge finder needle. (C) An 18-gauge catheter re-identifies the IJV and is advanced down the vein. (D) The guidewire has been passed into the IJV and is pulled back beyond the length of the introducer set; the 18-gauge catheter is then removed. (E) The dilator set is advanced over the guidewire into the IJV. (F) The PAC is passed into the catheter introducer after having the sterile sheath placed on it. (G) The PAC is properly positioned in the pulmonary artery. The sidearm is filled with heparinized saline and has a three-way injection adapter on it. The sterile sheath is extended to cover 70 cm of the PAC. The introducer will be sewn into place to prevent accidental withdrawal.

shown that PAC sheaths are not entirely sterile,[99] which means that the technique recommended by Johnston et al could produce more contaminated catheters.

As would be expected, many problems can be anticipated with the use of right heart catheterization with the PAC. The following complications have been reported.[100–104]

IMMEDIATE COMPLICATIONS

Supraventricular and ventricular dysrhythmias on insertion. Katz et al reported a 17 percent incidence of PVCs on passing the catheters and one case of ventricular tachycardia and fibrillation.[105] Geha et al reported a persistent supraventricular dysrhythmia on insertion of a PAC.[106]

Heart block. Abernathy reported a case of third-degree heart block and death.[107] Tomson et al reported the development of a right bundle branch

block on insertion and complete heart block in the presence of a left bundle branch block.[108] Nikolic and French reported an alternate-beat Wenckebach block on PAC insertion.[109]

Other complications associated with cannulation of central veins. These include arterial puncture, air emboli, etc. (see CVP above).

LONG-TERM COMPLICATIONS

Balloon rupture. This is not uncommon when the catheters have been left in place for more than a few days or when the balloon is inflated with more than 1.5 ml³ of air. Small volumes of air injected into the pulmonary artery will be of no consequence, and rupture can be diagnosed if the injected air cannot be withdrawn. In patients with right-to-left shunts, carbon dioxide can be used for inflation; great care must be taken not to rupture the balloon, with the attendant possibility of systemic gas embolization.

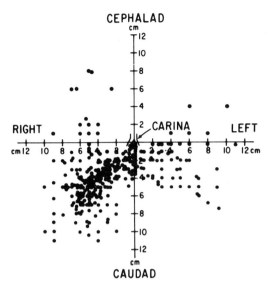

Fig. 6-14. Intrathoracic distribution of locations of PAC tips. (From Benumof JL, Saidman LJ, Arkin DB, et al: Where pulmonary artery catheters go: Intrathoracic distribution. Anesthesiology 48:336–338, 1977, with permission.)

Pulmonary infarction. Foote et al reported a 7.2 percent incidence of ischemic infarction of the lung in 125 patients with PACs.[110] This incidence can be markedly reduced by continuously monitoring the pulmonary artery trace for inadvertent wedging and by frequent checks of the catheter tip position by chest x-ray. The largest pulmonary infarctions can be induced by leaving the balloon inflated; therefore, this should be avoided (Fig. 6-16).

Pulmonary artery rupture. Rapid inflation of the balloon can damage the pulmonary artery wall and lead to production of hemoptysis or hemorrhage.[111] This can be avoided by proper inflation of the balloon to the minimum volume necessary to wedge it (see Chapters 20 and 32).

Knotting. This is more likely with the smaller 5-Fr catheters, which are very flexible.[112] Knotting has been reported and is more common if the catheter is advanced excessively in the right ventricle when it is unable to be passed out into the pulmonary artery.[113] The catheter should not be advanced further than 60 cm from the right IJV or more than 15 cm once it enters the right ventricle if it does not pass into the pulmonary artery.

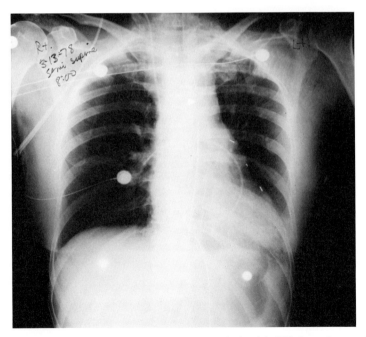

Fig. 6-15. The PAC is shown to have passed through the right IJV, down the superior vena cava, through the right atrium and right ventricle, and out into the right pulmonary artery. Note that the tip is slightly beyond the point where the catheter crosses the superior vena cava. This is ideal positioning of the PAC.

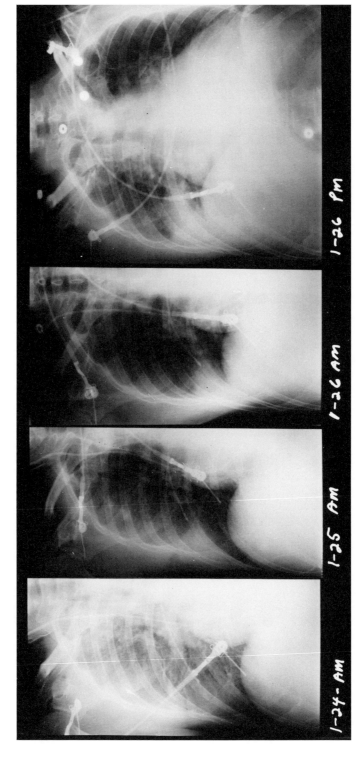

Fig. 6-16. This series of x-rays demonstrates a pulmonary infarction over a 2-day period of time that occurred because the PAC was too far out in the periphery of the right lung. The second panel, labeled 1-25, shows a triangular-shaped pulmonary infarction. The next two films show evolution of this infarction in a severely ill patient.

199

Formation of thrombotic endocardial vegetations. These were found in 33 percent of patients in one series and in 5 of 413 patients in another series.[114,115]

Infections. Both local and generalized systemic infections have been reported in patients with PACs in place.[116,117] Such infections require removal of the catheter.

Electrode detachment. Macander et al reported detachment of pacing electrodes from a multipurpose PAC 60 hours after insertion,[118] while Heiselman et al described displacement upon withdrawal of the pacing catheter.[119]

Vascular obstruction. Hypotension secondary to balloon inflation has been reported in a patient after a pneumonectomy where the balloon obstructed the pulmonary circulation.[120] Coronary sinus obstruction has also been reported from a PAC with the appearance of systemic pressures.[121]

Erroneous diagnosis from malfunctioning catheters. Malfunctions of the catheter and balloon can lead to spurious numbers for the PCWP and incorrect treatment of the patient. Shin et al reported the problem of eccentric inflation of the balloon, with the catheter tip impinging on the pulmonary artery wall.[122] This causes "pseudowedging" of the catheter and an incorrect estimate of LAP. This can be avoided, to some degree, by always being sure the PCWP is less than the PAP and similar to the PA_D pressure. Large errors have also been reported in measuring cardiac output by the Fick technique with incorrect blood sampling via the PAC.[123]

Erroneous diagnosis from misinterpretation of the data. Three recent reviews have pointed out many of the problems with clinical use of the PAC.[124-126] These include errors in interpretation due to ventilation modes, compliance changes (Fig. 6-17), ventricular interdependence, and associated technical problems.

NEW DEVELOPMENTS IN PULMONARY
ARTERY CATHETERIZATION

Continuous S_vO_2 monitoring. A major development in PACs has been the addition of fiberoptic bundles for light transmission, allowing continuous measurements of oxygen saturation of the mixed

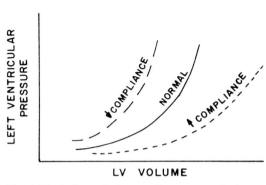

Fig. 6-17. Left ventricular compliance curves. A change in compliance can lead to an erroneous diagnosis (eg, a decrease in compliance can produce an increase in the left ventricular filling pressure, which may be diagnosed as hypervolemia).

venous blood (S_vO_2) by an oximeter. According to the Fick equation,

$$C_vO_2 = CaO_2 - VO_2/CO$$

If dissolved O_2 is neglected, S_vO_2 can be substituted for C_vO_2:

$$S_vO_2 = SaO_2 - VO_2/CO \times Hg \times 1.34$$

Four mechanisms can account for a decreased S_vO_2: (1) decreased SaO_2; (2) decreased cardiac output; (3) increased oxygen consumption (VO_2); and (4) decreased hemoglobin. The S_vO_2 measurement allows determination of the adequacy of cardiac output for the patient and his or her cardiovascular status.[127] The S_vO_2 can also be used as an early indicator of when to obtain a thermodilution cardiac output (when S_vO_2 decreases by 5 or more percent).[91] The S_vO_2 has been shown to correlate with cardiac index during CABG surgery when oxygen consumption is constant (Fig. 6-18)[91] but not to correlate with cardiac index when oxygen consumption is changing, such as during shivering after anesthesia.[128] The S_vO_2 provides valuable information in regard to the adequacy of the cardiac output for tissue demands but requires considerable interpretation. Guffin et al showed that shivering after CABG led to a marked decrease in S_vO_2 due to an increased VO_2, which could not be compensated for by changes in cardiac output (Fig. 6-19).[128] Table 6-3 shows some of the oxygen transport parameters with normal values.

Multipurpose pacing catheters. The multipurpose PAC with five pacing electrodes is now widely available. This catheter can be used for atrial, ventricular, or atrioventricular (AV) sequential pacing in

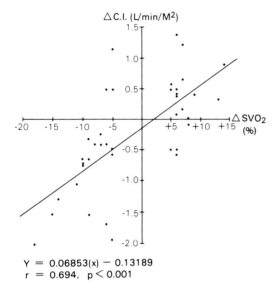

$$Y = 0.06853(x) - 0.13189$$
$$r = 0.694, \quad p < 0.001$$

Fig. 6-18. The change in cardiac index (ΔCI) is plotted against change in pulmonary arterial oxygen saturation (ΔS_vO_2). A highly significant correlation between the two is seen, ie, a decrease in S_vO_2 indicates a decrease in CI. (From Waller JL, Kaplan JA, Bauman DI, et al: Clinical evaluation of a new fiberoptic catheter oximeter during cardiac surgery. Anesth Analg 61:676–679, 1982, with permission.)

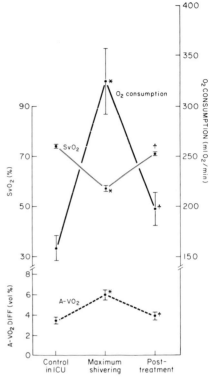

Fig. 6-19. Postoperative shivering in a group of patients after CABG produced a decrease in S_vO_2 due to a huge increase in O_2 consumption. This was corrected after treatment with meperidine or pancuronium. (From Guffin A, Girard D, Kaplan JA: Shivering following cardiac surgery: Hemodynamic changes and reversal. J Cardiothorac Anesth 1:24, 1987, with permission.)

a patient who requires a PAC for hemodynamic monitoring. With proper precautions, the catheter can also be used to record an intracardiac ECG (see Chapter 7). Indications for the pacing PAC are as follows:

1. Intermittent third-degree heart block
2. Second-degree heart block (Mobitz II)
3. Left bundle branch block
4. Digitalis toxicity
5. Severe bradycardia
6. Need for AV sequential pacing
7. Need for an intracardiac electrogram

Zaidan and Freniere reported a high success rate with the multipurpose PAC in patients during and after cardiac surgery, as opposed to poorer experiences reported in medical patients.[129] Atrial pacing was possible in 80 percent of patients, ventricular pacing in 93 percent, and AV sequential pacing in 73 percent. A new PAC with an additional RV port 19 cm from the catheter tip has been introduced (Paceport). This additional lumen allows the introduction of a thin wire for emergency RV pacing.

Right ventricular ejection fraction (RVEF). Assessment of RV function is made difficult by the complex geometry and shape of the RV (see Chapter 27). The thermodilution technique used to measure cardiac output with the PAC can also determine RVEF if a fast-response thermistor is used.[130] There are numerous situations when decreased RV function (eg, pulmonary hypertension) precludes adequate right heart output to a normal left ventricle. In these situations, RV function must be optimized before systemic perfusion improves. The RVEF catheter allows for easily repeatable measurements of RVEF, cardiac output, right ventricular end-diastolic volume (RVEDV), and right ventricular end-systolic volume (RVESV). Since the RV is very sensitive to increases in afterload, RV function can be evaluated by comparing RVEF with a measure of RV afterload, such as PVR. Ventricular function curves can be derived for both the right and left ventricles in patients with both cardiac and pulmonary disease. Hines and Barash recently reported a case of RV ischemia with

Table 6-3

O_2 Delivery Parameters

Formula*	Units	Normal Value
Arterial O_2 content $CaO_2 = 1.39 \times Hbg \times SaO_2 + 0.0031 \times PaO_2$	ml/dl	18–20
Mixed venous O_2 content $C_vO_2 = 1.39 \times Hbg \times S_vO_2 + 0.0031 \times P_vO_2$	ml/dl	13–16
Arteriovenous O_2 content difference $avDO_2 = CaO_2 - C_vO_2$	ml/dl	4–5.5
Pulmonary capillary O_2 content $C_AO_2 = 1.39 \times Hbg \times SaO_2 + 0.0031 \times PaO_2$	ml/dl	20
Pulmonary shunt $Qs/Qt = 100 \times C_AO_2 - CaO_2 / C_AO_2 - C_vO_2$	%	2–8
O_2 transport $O_2 \text{ trans} = 10 \times CO \times CaO_2$	ml/min	960 ± 80
O_2 consumption $VO_2 = 10 \times CO \times (CaO_2 - C_vO_2)$	ml/min	224 ± 40

Source: Reprinted from McGrath R: Invasive bedside hemodynamic monitoring. Prog Cardiovasc Dis 29: 129–144, 1986, with permission.

*Hbg = Hemoglobin; $avDO_2$ = arterial-venous oxygen content difference; C_AO_2 = arterial O_2 content; Qs/Qt = pulmonary shunt

dysfunction diagnosed by a decrease in RVEF when all other parameters were normal and treatment with nitroglycerin.[131]

CARDIAC OUTPUT MEASUREMENT

The cardiac output is the amount of blood pumped to the peripheral circulation by the heart each minute. It is a measurement that reflects the status of the entire circulatory system, not just the heart, since it is governed by autoregulation from the tissues. It is an insensitive guide to evaluation of left ventricular function. Cardiac output is affected by a number of peripheral factors, but severe cardiac dysfunction may serve to limit it. The cardiac output equals the stroke volume (SV) per beat times the heart rate (HR) per minute:

$$CO = SV \times HR$$

Normal average values are a cardiac output of 5–6 l/min in a 70-kg man, with a stroke volume of 60–90 ml per beat and a heart rate of 80 beats each minute. In order to compare patients of different body sizes, the cardiac output may be corrected in relation to body surface area; this is called the cardiac

index (CI), which equals the cardiac output divided by the body surface area (BSA):

$$CI = \frac{CO}{BSA}$$

The normal value for a 70-kg man is 3–3.5 l/min/m².[132] A normal person has a tremendous reserve capacity in the ability to increase the cardiac output, with some people attaining outputs of 25–30 l/min. Factors controlling the cardiac output include venous return to the heart, SVR, peripheral tissue oxygen need, blood volume, body position, pattern of respiration, heart rate, and myocardial contractility. The heart rate is affected by the central and autonomic nervous systems, and the stroke volume is affected by preload, afterload, and myocardial contractility.

Cardiac output monitoring during and after cardiac surgery has become routine. Serial measurements are used to assess the general status of the circulation, determine the appropriate hemodynamic therapy, and evaluate the response to the intervention. This is especially important in patients requiring treatment with inotropes, vasodilators, and aortic counterpulsation. Connors et al[86] and Iberti and Fisher[88] showed that cardiac output values cannot be predicted by clinical signs in patients in an intensive care unit.

The measured cardiac output value is important, but equally useful are the parameters that may be determined once the cardiac output is known. These parameters include the SVR, PVR, SV, and left ventricular stroke work (LVSW). These values can then be used to determine ventricular function by deriving Starling curves (see below). Formulas for these parameters, units, and normal values are shown in Table 6-4. These parameters can be rapidly calculated in the operating room or in the intensive care unit and used to help manage the patient. A programmable calculator can be useful in managing patients. This can be programmed to give SV, SI, CI, right ventricular stroke work index (RVSWI), left ventricular stroke work index (LVSWI), left ventricular minute work index (LVMWI), Starling point, PVR, and SVR when the HR, MAP, PAP, PCWP, CO, and BSA are entered.

There are many techniques currently available to measure cardiac output. The thermodilution method, employing the PAC, is the method of choice for measuring cardiac output in the clinical setting. With this technique, multiple outputs can be obtained at frequent intervals; arterial blood withdrawal and reinfusion are not required; the indicator is inert 5% dextrose in water; and, in addition, the catheter allows measurement of filling pressures of both the right and left sides of the heart. Calibration for measurements by this technique is simple to perform and highly reproducible and does not require blood withdrawal. Also, the technique is suitable to computer

analysis, since there is little recirculation of the indicator.

Ganz et al and Forrester et al introduced their catheter for the thermodilution method in 1971 and first documented the accuracy and reproducibility of the system.[133,134] They found that thermodilution-measured flow was accurate to within 2.2 percent of known pump flow in vitro, with a correlation coefficient of 0.993. In 20 patients, they found the standard deviation of triplicate measurements was 4.6 percent in the range of 2–8 l/min. Weisel et al compared the thermodilution method to the indocyanine green method in 83 subjects and found an excellent correlation ($r = 0.990$).[135] Kohanna and Cunningham also found a high correlation between dye and thermodilution cardiac output in patients after cardiac surgery ($r = 0.90$).[136] They felt that the thermodilution method was more accurate at low outputs (less than 2.0 l/min), since there is no recirculation of indicator and the indicator curve is sharp and well defined. Hillis et al also showed that thermodilution was more accurate than the dye technique at cardiac outputs less than 2.0 l/min and in the presence of aortic or mitral insufficiency.[137]

The theory and calculations of the thermodilution technique assume[138] (1) complete mixing of the indicator with blood; (2) a constant flow rate; (3) the indicator passes the thermistor only one time; and (4) the indicator was injected as a bolus (less than 4 seconds). If the PAC is "partly wedged" and there is no flow or reduced flow past it, unreliable cardiac output measurements will be obtained.

In order to get the high rate of reproducibility

Table 6-4

Derived Parameters

Formula	Units	Normal Value
$CI = \dfrac{CO}{BSA}$	l/min/m^2	2–5
$SV = \dfrac{CO}{HR} \times 1000$	ml/beat	60–90
$SI = \dfrac{SV}{BSA}$	ml/beat/m^2	40–60
$LVSWI = \dfrac{1.36\,(MAP - PCWP)}{100} \times SI$	gram-meters/m^2	45–60
$RVSWI = \dfrac{1.36\,(PAP - CVP)}{100} \times SI$	gram-meters/m^2	5–10
$SVR = \dfrac{MAP - CVP}{CO} \times 80$	dynes·sec·cm^{-5}	900–1500
$PVR = \dfrac{PAP - PCWP}{CO} \times 80$	dynes·sec·cm^{-5}	50–150

reported above, the technique of measurement must be standardized. The injectate temperature and volume, as well as the speed of injection, should be carefully controlled and duplicated. The most reproducible results have been obtained using injections of 10 ml of room-temperature 5% dextrose in water. Iced injectate is not required for accuracy or reproducibility[139] and may even lead to complications such as dysrhythmias.[140] An error of 0.5 ml in the injectate volume will cause a 5–10 percent error in the measurement. Loss of injectate via the sidearm or rapid fluid administration during the measurement will also produce errors. If the volume of the injectate is less than the value entered into the computer, the area under the curve will be reduced and the cardiac output overestimated. All measurements should be made in duplicate or triplicate during expiration for reproducibility.[141] Needed equipment includes a sterile system for injecting the indicator, a cardiac output computer, and precise temperature measurements of the injectate and the patient. Additional pieces of equipment that may be used are a mechanical injector for greater reproducibility and a recorder for observation and calculation of the curves.

The thermodilution PAC contains two fine wires that extend the length of the catheter and terminate in a thermistor embedded in the catheter wall just proximal to the balloon. The principle of measurement is similar to the dye dilution method of cardiac output measurements except that room-temperature fluid acts as the indicator. A known change in the temperature of the blood is induced at one point in the circulation, and the resulting change in temperature is detected at a point downstream. The baseline pulmonary artery body temperature is recorded in the computer. The solution is then injected via the CVP port into the right atrium, and the resulting temperature change is detected by the thermistor in the pulmonary artery. The thermodilution principle is described by the Stewart-Hamilton equation:

$$Q = \frac{V_I(T_B - T_I)K_1K_2}{T_B(t)dt}$$

where Q is cardiac output; V_I is injectate volume; T_B is blood temperature; T_I is injectate temperature; K_1 is density factor; K_2 is computation constant; and $T_B(t)dt$ is the change in blood temperature as a function of time. Solution of this equation is performed by the computer, which integrates the area under the curve. Cardiac output is inversely proportional to the area under the curve. A typical thermodilution temperature time curve, which is similar to a dye dilution curve except for the absence of recirculation and a more protracted downslope, is shown in Figure 6-20. The thermistor in the PAC has a linear relationship between temperature and electrical resistance. It acts as a variable resistor in a Wheatstone bridge, which is balanced before each measurement. The change in temperature alters the resistance and thus the output from the bridge, which is amplified and recorded, and the cardiac output is calculated by the computer.[142]

Thermodilution cardiac outputs may also be used in pediatric cardiac surgery. A 4-Fr double-lumen catheter may be passed by the surgeon into the pulmonary artery through the right atrium or ventricle. Another technique involves placing a small 2.5-Fr thermistor in the pulmonary artery and injecting through a separate 3.5-Fr right atrial catheter. A standard cardiac output computer can be used with a 2-ml aliquot of 5% dextrose in water. Colgan and Stewart found a correlation coefficient of 0.976 between this technique and dye dilution in eight infants and children.[143] The thermodilution technique measures right-sided cardiac outputs. This is very important because the technique cannot be used for

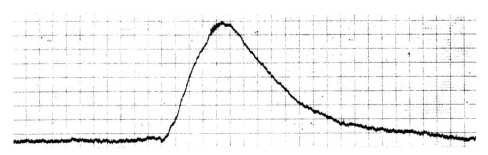

Fig. 6-20. A typical thermodilution cardiac output curve is demonstrated. Note that there is no recirculation peak.

patients with intracardiac shunts—totally erroneous data will be obtained. For example, a patient with a ventricular septal defect and a left-to-right shunt will have a falsely elevated cardiac output measured by this technique.

Other methods with which to measure cardiac output include the standard Fick and dye dilution techniques, aortic pulse contour measurements, direct flowmeter techniques, and ultrasound measurements (Doppler and echocardiography). The Fick technique is the standard for steady-state measurements of cardiac output and is said to be accurate to within ±10 percent, while the other methods have error rates of 15–20 percent. The Fick principle states that

$$CO = \frac{VO_2}{A - VO_2}$$

where CO is cardiac output in milliliters per minute; VO_2 is uptake of oxygen each minute in milliliters per minute; and $A - VO_2$ is the arteriovenous oxygen difference in milliliters per milliliter of blood. The technique is complex and cumbersome, however, involving both the collection of expired gases and right heart catheterization to obtain mixed venous blood, and it is usually used only in the catheterization laboratory.

The indicator dilution method using indocyanine green dye had been the most popular technique of cardiac output measurement prior to the thermodilution method. This technique consists of rapid injection of a precise amount of dye into the central venous circulation, where the indicator passes rapidly through the heart and lungs and into the arterial circulation and is detected by sampling arterial blood and passing it through a densitometer. Recirculation of the indicator is one of the main problems with the technique, since it makes calculation of the area under the primary circulation curve more difficult. A typical dye dilution curve with the recirculation hump is shown in Figure 6-21. Central shunting can be diagnosed by alterations of the dye dilution curve. Left-to-right shunts produce a decrease in the peak concentration of the dye, a prolonged disappearance time, and absence of the recirculation peak. In contrast, right-to-left shunts produce an early appearing hump on the dye curve.

The area under the curve must be calculated to derive the cardiac output. This may be done by the following methods:

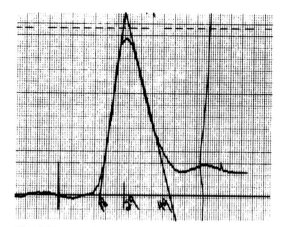

Fig. 6-21. A typical dye dilution curve is shown. There is a recirculation peak. Also, some of the lines have been drawn over it for calculation of the cardiac output by the fore-n-aft triangle method.

1. Exponential extrapolation using the method of Hamilton, where

$$CO = \frac{I \times 60}{A \times Cal\ f}$$

   where I is the amount of dye injected; Cal f is the calibration factor converting the recorder deflection to the concentration of dye; and A is the area plotted on semilogarithmic paper.

2. The fore-n-aft triangle method, where

$$CO = \frac{I \times 51.4}{PC \times T_{50} \times Cal\ f}$$

   where $PC \times T_{50}$ is the area; PC is the peak concentration of the dye in millimeters; and T_{50} is the time span in seconds from PC_{50} on the ascent to PC_{50} on the descent of the curve. Bradley and Barr found that this rapid method of calculation gave very good correlation with the laborious Hamilton method.[144]

3. Cardiac output computer methods to give on-line computation of the dye dilution curves. Carey et al studied two commercially available computers and compared them with arithmetic calculation.[145] They found that net errors ranged from +11 percent to −22 percent.

Another method of cardiac output measurement using computers is the aortic pulse contour analysis, which requires a central aortic catheter. This allows on-line measurement of stroke volume; however, this technique makes assumptions concerning the distensibility of the systemic arterial bed that may not be valid with certain therapeutic interventions (eg, sodium nitroprusside). Poor correlation was found between the pulse contour method and thermodilution measurements when SVR changed by more than 30 percent.[146] This technique has been questioned by some, therefore, and has not gained great popularity. It also carries the risk of dissection of the brachial or radial artery as the catheter is advanced centrally.

A reliable noninvasive method for monitoring changes in cardiac output would be very useful in the operating room and intensive care units. Estimation of cardiac output by Doppler ultrasound is noninvasive, rapid, and reliable (see Chapter 8).[147] All Doppler ultrasound systems employ an emitting and receiving transducer in one unit placed in the suprasternal notch (ascending aorta) or in the esophagus (descending aorta).[148] A significant frequency difference arises from the movement of red blood cells in the continuous wave ultrasound beam either toward or away from the transducer. The ultrasound beam must be almost in line ($\pm 20°$) with the blood flow. The stroke volume in the vessel is proportional to the area under the systolic Doppler curve, and cardiac output is determined by multiplying by the heart rate. The technique requires measuring the area of the vessel by A-mode echo, as well, or estimating it. The final equation for measuring cardiac output is[149]

$$CO = \text{vessel area} \times \text{systolic velocity interval} \times HR$$

where the systolic velocity interval is the area under the Doppler systolic curve.

A number of studies have found a good correlation between the aortic ultrasound technique and other cardiac output systems. Rose et al compared thermodilution and ultrasound cardiac outputs in patients undergoing vasodilator therapy and found a correlation coefficient of 0.92 before and 0.88 after vasodilation.[150] The technique has been compared with thermodilution in adult[151] and pediatric[152] intensive care unit patients with excellent results. Recent studies in the operating room during CABG have also shown an excellent correlation with thermodilution cardiac outputs.[153]

MEASUREMENTS OF VENTRICULAR FUNCTION

Two categories of measurement techniques are included in this section: (1) ventricular function curves, and (2) contractility measurements; however, it is necessary to review some cardiac physiology prior to describing these techniques.[154,155]

Preload is determined by the intraventricular *volume*. In the intact heart, the preload of the left ventricle can be measured as the left ventricular end-diastolic volume (LVEDV) (Fig. 6-22). This is the initial stretch on the ventricular muscle. The LVEDV is difficult to measure clinically, however, and measurement is only beginning to be possible with techniques such as echocardiography. Transesophageal echocardiography has been extensively used to measure the left ventricular end-diastolic area as an approximation of left ventricular volume; however, it is limited by its two-dimensionality and therefore is not a totally adequate measure of the true LVEDV (see Chapter 8). LVEDP can be measured

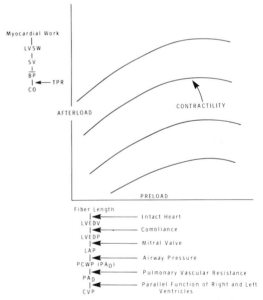

Fig. 6-22. The Frank–Starling family of curves is demonstrated. The horizontal axis represents the preload of the heart and the various factors used to estimate preload are shown. The vertical axis represents the myocardial work, and the various factors used to represent this are shown. The vertical axis is also affected by the afterload of the heart. See text for details. (Abbreviations: LVSW, left ventricular stroke work; SV, stroke volume; BP, mean blood pressure; TPR, total peripheral resistance; CO, cardiac output; LVEDV, left ventricular end-diastolic volume; LVEDP, left ventricular end-diastolic pressure; LAP, left atrial pressure; PCWP, pulmonary capillary wedge pressure; PA$_o$, pulmonary artery occluded pressure; PA$_D$ pulmonary artery diastolic pressure; CVP, central venous pressure.) (Modified from Bonner J: Advances in monitoring. Anesthesiol Rev July: 26–29, 1977.)

clinically as an approximation of the LVEDV. This assumes that left ventricular compliance is entirely normal, which is not a valid assumption in many patients with cardiac disease (Fig. 6-23). With ischemic heart disease or aortic stenosis, the left ventricular compliance curve is frequently shifted to the left, where small increases in volume can produce large increases in left ventricular filling pressure (decreased compliance). With aortic insufficiency or relief of myocardial ischemia with vasodilator drugs, compliance increases and large volumes can be placed in the left ventricle with minimal increases in pressure. Therefore, LVEDP is not always a good reflection of LVEDV.[156] The LVEDP can be measured with a catheter in the left ventricle, but this is usually done only at cardiac catheterization and not during surgery, because a high incidence of ventricular dysrhythmias exists with this technique.

During cardiac surgery, the preload of the left heart is frequently measured by inserting a catheter into the left atrium and measuring LAP, which gives a good approximation of the LVEDP, as long as there is a normal mitral valve.[81] The CVP is the poorest approximation of LVEDP, but it is often used to estimate the LVEDP in patients with good function of both the right and left ventricles. When cardiac disease is characterized by disparate right and left ventricular function, however, the CVP may be misleading when quantitating left ventricular filling pressure. The CVP can be higher or lower than the LVEDP, depending on the underlying pathology; however, the CVP is a reasonably good reflection of right ventricular preload. It accurately reflects RVEDV in most cases, unless a change in right ventricular compliance occurs with events such as a right ventricular infarction.

Factors affecting the preload of the heart include the total blood volume, body position, intrathoracic pressure, intrapericardial pressure, venous tone, pumping action of skeletal muscles, and the atrial contribution to ventricular filling.[157] Large increases in heart rate decrease the duration of diastole and hence can lower preload. Synchronous atrial contraction makes a significant contribution to left ventricular preload. This is best seen when a patient develops a nodal rhythm. There is often a 10–30 percent decrease in blood pressure and cardiac output with loss of atrial contraction (Fig. 6-5). The hemodynamic effect of loss of this contribution to preload is most severe in patients with decreased left ventricular compliance (aortic stenosis or idiopathic hypertrophic subaortic stenosis).

There is probably a descending limb of the Starling curve in humans, which can be explained by Laplace's law, $P = T/R$, where P is the pressure developed by a particular level of wall tension, T, and R is the radius of the chamber. This formula states that if the diastolic volume is markedly increased, a greater myocardial tension is needed to develop a particular level of intraventricular pres-

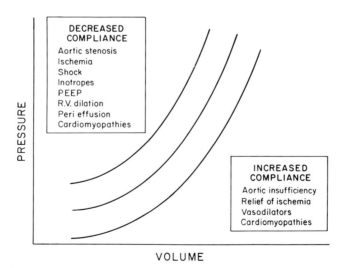

Fig. 6-23. The left ventricular compliance is the relationship between the LVEDP and the LVEDV. An increased compliance shifts the curve down and to the right, while a decreased compliance shifts it up and to the left. Examples of increased and decreased compliance are shown in the boxes.

sure. In other words, overdistention of the ventricle produces a need for greater wall tension and work of the ventricle in order to eject blood at an adequate pressure.

The vertical or work axis on the Starling curve would ideally reflect myocardial work, but this value cannot be derived clinically. Variables often placed on this axis instead of work are blood pressure (BP), cardiac output, stroke volume, and LVSW. The afterload, as expressed by total peripheral resistance (TPR) or SVR, also has an effect on this axis.

Afterload of the left ventricle is the wall stress faced by the myocardium during left ventricular ejection; therefore, it depends on a complicated relationship of left ventricular size, shape, pressure, and wall thickness. Afterload, however, can be thought of as the impedance to left ventricular ejection, which, in the absence of aortic stenosis, depends on the distensibility of the large arteries and the SVR.[158] Clinically, SVR is calculated to assess the afterload of the left heart. Right ventricular afterload or impedance is less easily derived than left ventricular afterload because of the physics and physiology of the pulmonary circulation. The PVR is calculated as the right ventricular afterload and is an important variable in patients with right ventricular failure, backward failure of the left heart affecting the right ventricle (eg, mitral stenosis), and pulmonary insufficiency from many causes. McGregor and Sniderman have pointed out the problem in using PVR for right ventricular afterload, since the value is altered by changes in flow without any change in the opposing forces.[159]

When preload and afterload are held constant, stroke volume is a function of the contractile state of the myocardium. This is an intrinsic property of the myocardium and reflects its ability to do mechanical work at any given level of preload. A true measure of contractility must be made with a constant preload, afterload, and heart rate, since all of these factors affect the heart's function. Therefore, this is a difficult parameter to measure clinically.

The relationship between myocardial activation and contraction is dependent on the presence of calcium.[160] Excitation of the cell membrane and depolarization are accompanied by a rapid entry of extracellular calcium into the cell, and the spread of electrical activity by way of the sarcoplasmic tubules causes the release of intracellular calcium and activation of contraction. For the cardiac muscle to relax, intracellular calcium must be recaptured by the sarcoplasmic reticulum or mitrochondria. Myocardial contraction is initiated when the ionic calcium reaches the reactive sites on the myofilaments. The present concept of myocardial contraction is based on the fact that, in diastole, the troponin–tropomyosin complex inhibits the interaction between the two major contractile proteins, actin and myosin. The presence of ionic calcium released from the sarcoplasmic reticulum causes a confirmational change in the troponin-tropomyosin complex so that it no longer inhibits the actin-myosin interaction, and myocardial contraction results.

The behavior of the left ventricle during diastole depends on properties of ventricular relaxation affecting early diastolic filling and on ventricular stiffness, mainly affecting mid-diastolic and late-diastolic filling.[161] Ventricular relaxation is an energy-dependent process that can be altered separately from contraction and is probably dependent on the rate of sequestration of calcium ion by the sarcoplasmic reticulum and mitochondria after systole.[162] Relaxation of the ventricle is enhanced by beta$_1$-adrenergic stimulation and can be impaired by heart failure, myocardial ischemia, hypercalcemia, and tachycardia. In these conditions, early diastolic filling can be impaired.

Ventricular Function Curves

Multiple measurements of cardiac output and its derivatives, along with ventricular filling pressures, allow the construction of Starling ventricular function curves to aid in patient care. The Frank-Starling mechanism of the heart relates the filling volume of the heart (preload) to the stroke work of the corresponding ventricle. Stroke volume is a function of the diastolic fiber length, with increases in fiber length causing increases in stroke volume up to a certain point. It is possible to overdistend the ventricular muscle and then decrease the stroke volume (descending limb of the curve). A typical Starling curve is shown in Figure 6-24. Preload can be expressed on the horizontal axis as PCWP, and ventricular work can be expressed on the vertical axis as LVSWI. These are both measurements of left ventricular function. They could be replaced by CVP and RVSWI to measure right ventricular function. It is not accurate, however, to mix one measurement from each side of the heart, eg, CVP and LVSWI. Interventions that increase contractility shift the curve up and to the left. Disease states or drugs that depress the heart shift the curve down and to the right.[163]

Ventricular performance curves have been used to define the status of the cardiovascular system and

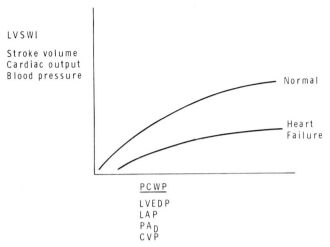

Fig. 6-24. A typical Starling curve is shown. The normal curve is shown above with a hypofunctioning curve below (heart failure).

to define the level of the contractile state in a number of studies. Crexells et al found optimal ventricular performance at a PCWP of 14–18 mm Hg after acute myocardial infarction.[164] Forrester et al have used performance curves to divide patients into subsets, after infarction, with different therapies and results according to the subset.[165] Weisel et al[135] and Gudwin et al[166] recommended using left ventricular function curves for the management of critically ill medical and surgical patients. The use of serial hemodynamic measurements, including Starling curves, is very useful in a number of situations in the operating room and the intensive care unit.

TREATMENT OF PATIENTS IN HEART FAILURE

Heart failure in patients can occur postoperatively in the intensive care unit or intraoperatively either before or after CPB (Fig. 6-25). A patient may be at point 1 with the following hemodynamics: BP, 80/40 mm Hg; HR, 90; CI, 2.0 l/min/m²; and SVR, 3500 dynes·sec·cm⁻⁵. If the patient is given an ino-

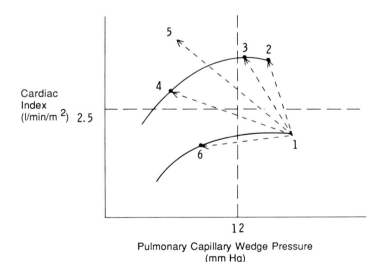

Fig. 6-25. This figure demonstrates a patient at point 1 on a hypofunctioning Starling curve. Therapeutic interventions are labeled 2, 3, 4, 5, and 6. See text for full explanation.

tropic drug, such as dopamine (5–10 μg/kg/min), he or she will probably move up and to the left (point 2) with an increase in BP and CI. However, the measurements are needed to document the therapeutic response. A vasodilator, such as nitroprusside, will decrease the SVR, reducing the afterload, and the patient will move up and to the left (point 3) with an increase in BP and CI. If too much nitroprusside is given, however, the patient will lose too much preload and move to point 6 without an increase in BP and CI. A volume infusion will increase the preload and move the patient from point 6 back to point 3, but this obviously requires close monitoring. Some patients will get the best response from a combination of an inotrope and a vasodilator and move the furthest up and to the left to point 5. It is necessary to add one drug at a time, measure the response, and then add the next drug in this complex pharmacologic scheme of treatment (see Chapter 26). This technique of treatment maximizes contractility while minimizing the afterload.[167]

GUIDING THERAPY WITH THE INTRA-AORTIC BALLOON PUMP (IABP)

Serial hemodynamic measurements during aortic counterpulsation have been very helpful.[168] These patients are frequently receiving inotropes, vasodilators, and positive pressure ventilation along with the balloon support (see Chapter 28). Specific serial measurements are necessary to be able to judge the effects of each therapy. The measurements are also useful in helping to decide if the patient needs the IABP preoperatively or if he or she is a reasonable risk for anesthesia without counterpulsation (eg, a patient with four-vessel coronary artery disease, an EF of 0.2, and an LVEDP of 30 mm Hg at cardiac catheterization). Hemodynamics are obtained before deciding if the IABP is indicated. If BP is 90/60 mm Hg, CI is 2.0 l/min/m^2, PCWP is 7 mm Hg, SVR is 2000 dynes·sec·cm^{-5}, and the patient is at point 4 on the above curve, volume is used to improve hemodynamics and not the IABP. If BP is 90/60 mm Hg, but CI is 1.5 l/min/m^2 and SVR is 3500 dynes ·sec·cm^{-5}, and the patient is at point 1, the IABP or a vasodilator should be considered before the surgical procedure.

GUIDING THERAPEUTIC DECISIONS COMING OFF CARDIOPULMONARY BYPASS

Patients are frequently hypotensive at the end of CPB. Additional hemodynamic measurements can take the guesswork out of this difficult situation. For example, if the BP is 80/50 mm Hg, HR is 85, and PCWP is 15 mm Hg, what is the problem? Is the patient dilated with a low SVR or is the heart not working well? The cardiac output and derived values can give the answer. If cardiac output is 5.0 l/min, SVR will be under 1000 dynes·sec·cm^{-5}, and the patient needs an inotrope or vasopressor.

GUIDING THERAPY DURING ANESTHESIA

It is useful to know the patient's left ventricular function at many critical times during surgery because the anesthetic management will vary depending on this factor. Two examples will help to explain:

1. A patient becomes hypertensive during CABG surgery with fentanyl and nitrous oxide anesthesia. If cardiac output and ventricular function are good, then a myocardial depressant, such as halothane, is a proper choice to control the blood pressure. If cardiac output is low and SVR is high, however, a vasodilator, such as nitroglycerin, is a better choice.
2. During aortic aneurysm surgery, hypotension often occurs after releasing the aortic cross-clamp. Measurements of hemodynamics can rapidly assess whether this is secondary to vasodilation or myocardial depression and guide appropriate therapy for each individual patient.

Measurements of Contractility

The contractile state of the heart is only one of several determinants of its ability to eject blood. The cardiac output and the heart's contractile state cannot be related to one another in a simple manner. Measurements of cardiac output alone are of limited value in deducing myocardial contractility. It is important to realize the difference between cardiac output and myocardial contractility and not to equate the two.[169]

Considerable controversy exists over the definition and measurement techniques of myocardial contractility. Many techniques have been proposed to measure this elusive factor, and all have had their problems, since most of the techniques are also affected by changes in preload, afterload, and heart rate. Some of these techniques are highly invasive, while others are totally noninvasive.

INVASIVE TECHNIQUES

Force–velocity curve. The force–velocity curve is the basic measurement based on Hill's model of contraction of an isolated muscle. There is an inverse relationship between force and velocity in cardiac muscle. Velocity decreases as the total load (preload and afterload) increases. The maximum velocity of shortening is called V_{max} and is a good measurement of contractility. It is derived by extrapolating the curve to zero load. Positive inotropic interventions shift the curve up and to the right and raise V_{max};[170] however, even V_{max} has been questioned as to its validity as a pure measure of contractility.[171]

Walton–Brodie strain gauge arch. The strain gauge arch can be sutured to the surface of the ventricle to measure contractile force. This technique was used by Morrow and Morrow to measure the effects of halothane on the intact human heart while on CPB.[172]

Rate of pressure development (dP/dt). The rate at which ventricular pressure rises (the first derivative of the ventricular pressure) is called dP/dt and is expressed in millimeters of mercury per second. The normal range is 800–1700 mm Hg/sec.[173] This num-

ber can be obtained during cardiac surgery or catheterization using catheters with microtransducers at their tip, which are inserted into the left ventricle and attached to an external differentiating circuit. Many studies have shown that when contractility is augmented, dP/dt increases. Examples of left ventricular pressure and dP/dt tracings are shown in Figure 6-26. However, dP/dt is also affected by changes in preload, afterload, and heart rate; increases in any of these three factors also increase dP/dt.[174] This problem has been partially solved by using a series of correction factors. The best measurement is dP/dt/ CPIP, where CPIP is the common peak isovolemic pressure. This is the peak pressure common to both the control measurement and the measurement after the intervention. This factor corrects any differences in afterload but not in preload or heart rate, which still must be held relatively constant.[175]

Catheter tip flowmeters. Tomlin et al have found a good correlation between indices derived from velocity and flow of blood compared with dP/dt.[176] Nobel et al have shown that the maximum

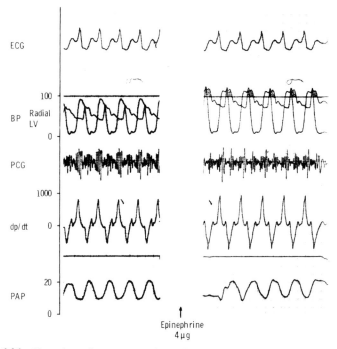

Fig. 6-26. Hemodynamic responses of a patient during cardiac surgery are demonstrated. The panel on the left was before the administration of 4 μg of epinephrine, and the panel on the right is after administration. Note that the dP/dt changed from 800 to about 950 mm Hg/sec. This was associated with an increase in the radial artery and left ventricular blood pressures to about 110–120 mm Hg. Also shown are the PCG, and pulmonary artery pressure tracings.

acceleration of aortic blood flow is a good measurement of contractility, which is relatively independent of preload and afterload.[177]

Angiography. Left ventriculography is an important part of a cardiac catheterization and can provide useful information about ventricular function.[178] The EF is a measurement of overall systolic function and is the difference between the end-diastolic volume (EDV) and the end-systolic volume (ESV):

$$EF = \frac{EDV - ESV}{EDV}$$

Normal ventricles eject more than 55 percent of their volume (EF = 0.55). In addition, abnormalities of left ventricular wall motion can also be observed at catheterization. Inward motion of a wall segment may be totally impaired (akinetic) or partially impaired (hypokinetic). Segments that bulge outward during systole are called dyskinetic. Potential reversibility of these abnormal wall segments is often tested for with nitroglycerin or post-extrasystolic potentiation. These measurements are more sensitive measures of myocardial function than is the resting cardiac output, and they are therefore frequently seen to be abnormal in patients with normal cardiac outputs.

NONINVASIVE TECHNIQUES

Systolic time intervals (STIs).   STIs measure the phases of left ventricular systole in humans and are determined from simultaneous high-speed recordings of the ECG, phonocardiogram, and an arterial pressure tracing (Fig. 6-27). Total electromechanical systole (QS_2) is the interval from the onset of the QRS complex on the ECG to the first major deflection of the second heart sound. The left ventricular ejection time (LVET) is the phase of systole when the ventricle ejects blood into the aorta; it is measured from the beginning of the arterial upstroke to the dicrotic notch. The preejection period (PEP) is the interval from onset of ventricular depolarization to the beginning of ejection and is derived by subtracting the LVET from the QS_2.[179] These intervals vary with heart rate; Weissler et al developed correction factors to adjust for this fact.[180] An ECG lead showing a clear onset of the QRS complex is selected. A chest phonocardiogram is used over the upper precordium

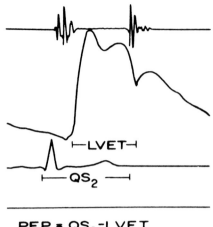

$$PEP = QS_2-LVET$$
Derived Intervals
$$PEP/LVET$$
$$1/PEP^2$$
$$EF = 1.125 - 1.250 \; PEP/LVET$$

Fig. 6-27. High-speed recordings of the phonocardiogram, arterial pressure tracing and ECG are demonstrated. Measurement of the QS$_2$ and LVET is shown. The PEP is derived by subtracting the LVET from the QS$_2$. Further derived intervals are shown at the bottom of the figure.

when possible. During cardiac surgery, an esophageal phonocardiogram is used. Tonneson et al showed a good correlation between the time intervals recorded using an esophageal phonocardiogram versus a chest microphone.[181] Central aortic, carotid, or subclavian arterial tracings are preferred, but more peripheral arterial tracings have been used in some studies.

The PEP has been found to be the best of the measured STIs as an estimate of contractility. It changes inversely to the dP/dt measurement, and there is a direct correlation between the externally derived STIs and internal measures of left ventricular function.[182,183] The PEP/LVET ratio shows an even better relation to internal measurements. Increases in contractility decrease the PEP, increase the LVET, and decrease the PEP/LVET ratio from its normal value of 0.35. With decreased left ventricular performance, the PEP increases, LVET shortens, and PEP/LVET increases. These correlate closely with a decreased stroke volume, cardiac output, and EF. The closest correlation ($r = 0.90$) was found between PEP/LVET and the EF. Garrard et al even proposed a regression formula for noninvasively deriving the ejection fraction from the STIs:[184]

$$EF = 1.125 - 1.25 \ PEP/LVET$$

Another indirect index of contractility using the PEP along with PCWP was described by Diamond et al.[185] The mean electromechanical $\Delta P/\Delta T$ is derived as follows:

$$\frac{\Delta P}{\Delta T} = \frac{DP - PCWP}{PEP}$$

where DP is diastolic blood pressure. This index had a correlation with dP/dt of 0.96 in a study of 18 patients.

Several studies have shown that the STIs, especially PEP, are influenced by changes in preload and afterload. The PEP is lengthened by increased afterload and shortened by increased preload. PEP/LVET is somewhat less affected by these changes but is still altered. Reitan et al proposed the use of $1/PEP^2$, which correlated well with peak ascending aortic blood flow.[186] Peak blood flow acceleration is minimally affected by changes in loading conditions, and, therefore, $1/PEP^2$ may be the STI least affected by these factors.

The STIs have been used to study patients with coronary artery disease, acute infarctions, and valvular heart disease. They have also been used in clinical studies of drug effects and comparisons of anesthetic agents.[187] Table 6-5 summarizes the factors affecting STIs. Attempts have also been made to use STIs as on-line monitors of ventricular function during anesthesia and surgery.[188]

Ballistocardiogram (BCG). The BCG is a complex apparatus designed to record body motion produced by cardiovascular phenomena. The BCG was studied extensively by Starr, and Harrison et al showed a good correlation between the IJ wave of the BCG and dP/dt.[189] In recent years, however, there has arisen a fair amount of skepticism and criticism concerning the merits and uses of this technique.[190] In anesthesia, the BCG has been used by one group of investigators to measure contractility during

Table 6-5
Systolic Time Intervals: Influencing Factors

	QS_2	PEP	LVET	PEP/LVET
1. Tachycardia				
a. Spontaneous	↓	↓	↓	
b. Atrial pacing	↓	→	↓	
c. Vagal blockade	↓	→	↓	
d. Adrenergic stimulation	↓	↓	↓	
2. Increased afterload	↑	↑	↑	
3. Increased preload	→	↓	↑	↓
4. Inotropes	↓	↓	↓↑	
5. Beta blockade	→	↑	↓↑	↑
6. Decreased left ventricular performance	→	↑	↓	↑
7. AS and/or AI without CHF	↑	↓	↑	↓
AS and/or AI with CHF	→	↑	↓	↑
AS and/or MI with CHF	→	↑	↓	↑
8. Chronic hypertension without CHF	→	→	→	
Chronic hypertension with CHF	→	↑	↓	↑
9. Acute myocardial infarction with CHF	↓	↑	↓	↑
10. LBBB	→	↑	→	↑
RBBB	→	→	→	
11. Advanced age	↑	↑	↑	
12. Upon assuming an erect posture	↓	↑	↓	↑
13. 4–8 P.M. diurnal cycle	↓	→	↓	↑

Code: ↑, increased time interval; ↓, decreased time interval; →, unchanged time interval.

AS = aortic stenosis; AI = aortic insufficiency; CHF = congestive heart failure; MI = myocardial infarction; LBBB = left bundle branch block; RBBB = right bundle branch block.

hemodynamic studies of anesthetic agents in volunteers.[191]

Echocardiography. Echocardiography has become extremely popular in cardiology and is finally beginning to be applied to the field of anesthesiology. It has already proven very useful in studies of anesthetic agents and ventricular function. The echocardiogram is useful for measuring right or left ventricular function (ejection fraction or wall motion),[192] analyzing valve function,[193,194] and detecting pericardial effusions (see Chapter 8).

Controversy exists as to the accuracy and reliability of M-mode echocardiographic measurements (single dimension) for quantifying ventricular volume, stroke volume, and cardiac output. Because of the limitations of the M-mode echocardiogram, many investigators are using two-dimensional echocardiography (2D-Echo) as a continuous monitor of cardiac function. The major advantage of the technique is its ability to visualize an entire cross-sectional slice of the ventricle as opposed to a single linear dimension. It is possible to measure areas of structures seen in cross-sectional image, which allows for estimation of ventricular volumes. In addition, areas of poorly functioning ventricles (eg, hypokinetic areas) or abnormal anatomy (eg, myxomas) can be visualized. For example, Dubroff et al used a hand-held 2D-Echo probe directly on the epicardium during cardiac surgery in 44 adult patients.[195] Ejection fraction was measured by a short-axis area change. The ejection fraction derived by this method was fairly well correlated ($r = 0.85$) with angiographic values.

Transesophageal echocardiography (TEE) provides a readily accessible location for continuous cardiac monitoring. The location is stable, monitoring does not interfere with the operation, and the technique can be used before the chest is open and after it is closed. With TEE, recordings can be made at the same location throughout the entire operation, and the quality of the image and resolution of the posterior left ventricular wall are better than those obtained via the chest wall. Another advantage of TEE is that it allows visualization of all structures on the right side of the heart.

Two-dimensional TEE (2D-TEE) with a phased-array transducer was first introduced in 1982 by Schluter et al from West Germany.[196] They attached a transducer to a standard gastroscope, allowing complete control of the tip of the scope. Good diagnostic pictures were obtained without complications, and the authors suggested using the 2D-TEE as an intraoperative monitor of cardiac function. Since then, numerous investigators have utilized the 2D-TEE probe during studies in anesthetized patients. Intraoperative monitoring with the 2D-TEE is a safe and simple procedure that permits continuous assessment of left ventricular area, contractility, and wall motion. Provided that the probe is not moved, relative changes in the left ventricular image can be easily detected. Left ventricular area at the level of the papillary muscles in the short-axis view is easily measured, but the calculation of left ventricular volume assumes symmetry, which may not always be present. Therefore, fractional shortening of areas, rather than true ejection fractions, are often calculated as follows:

$$EFA = \frac{(EDA - ESA)}{EDA}$$

where EFA is the ejection fraction area, EDA is the end-diastolic area, and ESA is the end-systolic area. Konstadt et al have recently validated these measurements as derived by TEE with on-heart echo values.[197] Ejection fraction showed a correlation coefficient of 0.92, and there was good reproducibility between observers.

Anesthetic agents, myocardial ischemia, surgical events, and changes in left ventricular preload or afterload can profoundly affect intraoperative cardiovascular function. Rathod et al demonstrated the effects of inhaled anesthetic agents on echocardiographic measurements.[198] Kremer et al showed with 2D-TEE that changes in left ventricular function occurred in 80 percent of patients without heart disease undergoing abdominal surgery.[199] The less-invasive 2D-TEE offers several advantages over a PAC in patients undergoing surgery. The true preload of the left ventricle (LVEDV) can be estimated rather than using the PCWP, and a measurement of contractility (ejection fraction area) can be obtained instead of using only the Frank-Starling curve.

The relation between pressure and volume in the beating ventricle was first studied in the 1800s. Recently, interest has been revived by Sagawa, who has shown it can be used as an excellent measure of contractility that is not affected by preload or afterload.[200] The pressure–volume relationship can be used to assess myocardial contractility in humans relatively noninvasively by using 2D-Echo to record left ventricular volume and arterial pressure tracings to estimate left ventricular pressure.[201] It can also be performed with direct measurements of left ventricular pressure and estimates of left ventricular volume using epicardial markers and radiographic volume measurements.[202]

Figure 6-28 shows a hypothetical left ventricular pressure–volume relationship (see Chapters 8 and 16). The ventricular volume is on the abscissa, while the pressure is on the ordinate. The end-diastolic point (EDP) represents the preload or left ventricular volume and pressure at the end of diastole. The upward limb describes the isovolumic contraction (pressure increase without a change in volume) leading to the opening of the aortic valve and ejection. At the end-systolic point (ESP), the ventricle terminates its contraction and a relaxation phase begins. Stroke volume is the difference between the end-diastolic volume and end-systolic volume:

$$SV = EDV - ESV$$

The ejection fraction equals the stroke volume divided by the end-diastolic volume.[203]

$$EF = SV/EDV$$

For a given contractile state, all end-systolic pressure points will fall on the same line. Figure 6-29 shows three hypothetical cardiac cycles in which the afterload was modified, generating different end-systolic pressures, end-systolic volumes, and stroke volumes; however, a linear relationship is seen between the end-systolic pressures and end-systolic volumes. This shows that the relationship of pressure to volume is independent of afterload changes when used to assess contractility.[204,205] When preload remains constant, the stroke volume is inversely proportional to the end-systolic pressure. The greater the end-systolic pressure, the smaller the stroke volume.

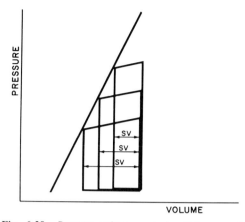

Fig. 6-29. Pressure–volume analysis of three cardiac cycles starting at the same EDV that generate different end-systolic pressures when afterload is modified. All three cycles fall on the same contractility line. (From Thys D: Pulmonary artery cauterization: past, present, and future. Mt Sinai J Med 51-582, 1984, with permission.)

The end-systolic pressure–volume relationship (ESPVR) is also preload independent. If preload is decreased or increased, the relation between end-systolic pressure and end-systolic volume remains the same as long as contractility has not changed.[206] Positive inotropic interventions will result in a shift to the left of the end-systolic pressure–volume slope, whereas myocardial depression produces a rightward displacement of the slope (Fig. 6-30). A change in slope, therefore, means a change has occurred in the intrinsic contractile properties of the ventricle.[207] An increase in stroke volume accompanies the increase in contractility. Any combinations of pressure and

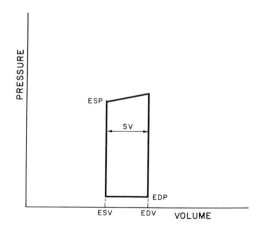

Fig. 6-28. The left ventricular pressure–volume relationship. See text for explanation.

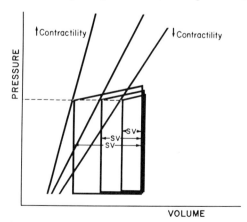

Fig. 6-30. The effect of changes in contractility is shown as an alteration of the slope of the E_{max} line. (From Thys D: Pulmonary artery cauterization: past, present, and future. Mt Sinai J Med 51:582, 1984, with permission.)

volume that would fall on the new line defined by the new slope would represent the new contractile state. Studies have shown that changes in the inotropic state of the heart can markedly affect the slope.[208] Pharmacologic interventions also preserve the ESPVR while increasing or decreasing the slope in a predictable fashion.

Radioisotopic techniques. Measurements of ventricular function, including the ejection fraction, can be obtained using radiopharmaceuticals, such as labeled albumin, and a scintillation counter. The use of mobile scintillation counters and computers makes these measurements available at the bedside of the sickest patient. Using these techniques, Poliner et al demonstrated an altered diastolic filling rate,[209] and Coriat et al demonstrated a decreased EF after anesthesia in patients with coronary artery disease.[210] Thallium scans are widely used during exercise stress testing to detect areas of poor myocardial perfusion,[211] and MUGA scans are used to evaluate right and left ventricular function (see Chapter 10).

Nuclear magnetic resonance (NMR) (or magnetic resonance imaging [MRI]). MRI is being widely investigated in regard to cardiovascular applications.[212,213] The technique can be used to measure regional myocardial blood flow and metabolism, characterize diseases affecting the myocardium, and analyze function of the cardiovascular system. The most promising aspect of MRI is the potential for metabolic imaging. Studies of high-energy phosphate metabolism in intact hearts have demonstrated the cyclical changes in the concentration of the phosphates from diastole to systole and during regional and global ischemia.

HEMODYNAMIC MEASUREMENTS OF MYOCARDIAL ISCHEMIA

There is a delicate balance between the myocardial oxygen supply and the oxygen demand in patients with coronary artery disease (Fig. 6-31). The myocardial oxygen supply depends on the following factors:

1. Coronary blood flow (CBF)
   a. Patency of coronary arteries
   b. Aortic diastolic blood pressure
   c. Intracavitary end-diastolic pressure
   d. Diastolic filling time

2. Oxygen content of coronary artery blood
   a. Hemoglobin content
   b. Arterial oxygen tension (PaO_2)
   c. Position of the hemoglobin-dissociation curve

Determinants of the myocardial oxygen demand (myocardial oxygen consumption [MVO_2]) include[214,215]

1. Systolic wall tension
   a. Aortic systolic blood pressure
   b. Left ventricular end-diastolic pressure
   c. Ventricular volume
2. Contractile state of the myocardium
3. Heart rate
4. Other less important factors
   a. Basal cost—oxygen use of the nonbeating heart
   b. Oxygen cost of depolarization
   c. Direct metabolic cost of catecholamines
   d. Activation cost of calcium
   e. Energy of maintenance of the active state
   f. Fenn effect—cost of shortening against a load

CORONARY BLOOD FLOW

CBF is regulated by the following equation:

$$Q = \frac{\Delta P}{R}$$

where Q is coronary blood flow; ΔP is the driving pressure across the coronary vascular bed; and R is total coronary resistance.

Total coronary resistance is made up of (1) basal resistance tone in diastole; (2) autoregulatory resistance, which is the major factor affecting the tone of the vessels and is under the control of the autonomic nervous system and local metabolites; and (3) compressive resistance, which is caused by compression of the coronary vessels by intracavitary pressure; this is especially important in the subendocardium during systole when the vessels are obstructed secondary to this pressure.[216]

Coronary artery disease with its stenotic resistance obviously must also be considered. Flow through stenotic areas is reduced only with severe stenosis (above 60–70 percent) and is compensated, to some degree, by a decreased autoregulatory resistance. Stenosis of the vessel is critical when about 90 percent of the lumen is occluded and CBF markedly

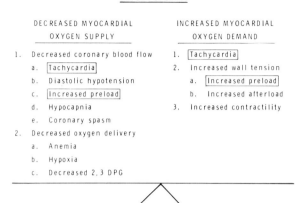

Fig. 6-31. Detrimental changes in the myocardial oxygen balance. Tachycardia and increased preload adversely affect both sides of the balance.

falls. Coronary collateral blood flow may also compensate for decreased CBF to an area of the heart. Collateral flow may be either (1) intercoronary, ie, it may connect capillary beds of two different coronary arteries; or (2) intracoronary, ie, it may connect vessels within the same capillary bed. The rapidity of coronary occlusion appears to play a role in the development of these collateral channels.

There are regional differences in myocardial blood flow that make studies of CBF more difficult. Subendocardial ischemia and infarctions are seen earlier and more commonly than transmural damage, probably because of the coronary flow pattern relative to the needs of the myocardium. In patchy diseases, such as coronary artery disease, the disorders of blood flow are typically regional; thus, measurement of CBF should measure total as well as regional CBF. Methods of measuring *total* CBF include the following:[217]

1. Venous sampling techniques: these techniques are based on the Fick principle using inert gases, where

$$CBF = \frac{\text{myocardial inert gas uptake}}{\text{arteriovenous difference of the inert gas}}$$

Commonly used gases include nitrous oxide, krypton, xenon, hydrogen, and helium. Kety and Schmidt first used this technique with nitrous oxide for measurement of cerebral blood flow. The gases are inhaled, and blood levels of the gases are measured in arterial and coronary sinus blood. CBF for normal patients is 70–90 ml/min/100 gm, while patients with coronary artery disease have values averaging 58 ml/min/100 gm.[218,219]

2. Precordial counting technique: this is analogous to the above technique and is based on the residue detection of a radioisotope indicator rather than on outflow detection in the coronary sinus. The indicator, xenon, is injected directly into the coronary artery.

3. Coronary sinus thermodilution: Ganz et al designed a 7-Fr catheter for percutaneous insertion into the coronary sinus to measure total CBF.[220] The principle and operation are similar to the thermodilution cardiac output measurements. In 14 patients studied, the coronary sinus outflow averaged 122 ml/min. This predominantly represents flow from the left coronary system. This technique has been extensively used to study the effects of anesthetic agents on the coronary circulation (see Chapters 1 and 3).[221]

4. Absolute flow of the entire heart with isotope counting: radioactive isotopes of potassium or rubidium are injected into the left atrium and detected by a scinticamera. The advantage of this is that it measures total CBF in milliliters per minute without regard for the unknown myocardial mass.

Methods of measuring *regional* CBF are rapidly being developed and offer an exciting new look at coronary artery disease.[222]

CORONARY ARTERY DISEASE

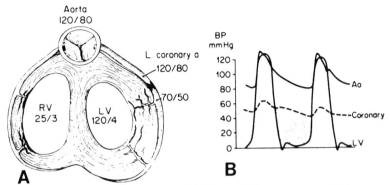

Fig. 6-32. Diagrammatic cross-section of the heart to indicate coronary arterial pressure beyond a severe obstructive arterial lesion. (A) The aortic, distal coronary, and left ventricular pressures. (B) The stippled area indicates the diastolic pressure-time area for the region of the heart supplied by the partially obstructed coronary artery. (From Hoffman JIE, Buckberg GD: Regional myocardial ischemia—causes, prediction and prevention. Vasc Surg 8:115, 1974, with permission.)

1. Steady imaging: This approach is used when the myocardial distribution of the indicator is assumed to be constant. The distribution of the indicator is proportional to the distribution of the CBF. Particulate indicators are most often used, consisting of microspheres of human albumin labeled with isotopes of iodine (^{131}I) or technetium (^{99m}Tc) and ranging in size from 10 to 30 μ. The indicators are detected by scanners or scinticameras and tell the location of poorly perfused areas or changes in the distribution of the CBF.

2. Dynamic imaging: Xenon 133 or thallium 205 is used and is detected by computer analysis of scinticamera pictures. This dynamic study allows regional flow measurement during exercise or drug intervention and permits the evaluation of the site and degree of ischemia as well as response to therapy.

3. Measurement of flow through coronary bypass grafts: This has been measured primarily with electromagnetic flowmeters in the operating room. A number of groups have correlated intraoperative flow measurements with graft patency. Flows of less than 40 ml/min have been associated with increased graft closure. Other groups have found these measurements to be very unreliable, however, and have abandoned the routine intraoperative use of them. In making measurements of flow after CABG, the effects of hemodynamic and anesthetic agents must be considered, since isoflurane has been shown to decrease graft flow.[223]

The coronary perfusion pressure (CPP) is usually defined as the aortic diastolic blood pressure (DBP) minus the left ventricular end-diastolic pressure (LVEDP):

$$CPP = DBP - LVEDP$$

Elevation of the LVEDP will decrease the gradient of blood flow to the vulnerable subendocardial tissue during diastole as will a decrease in the diastolic blood pressure.[224] If coronary artery disease is present (Fig. 6-32), significant stenosis will decrease the coronary artery diastolic pressure well below the aortic diastolic pressure, and elevation of LVEDP can seriously jeopardize the subendocardium as seen in Table 6-6.[225]

An increase in the LVEDP is detrimental in two ways: (1) decreased CBF and (2) increased MVO_2, which explain the severe ischemia seen with overdistention of the left ventricle. Tachycardia is also extremely detrimental because it (1) decreases coronary filling time and thus diastolic pressure–time index (DPTI) and (2) increases oxygen demand. Subendocardial ischemia is commonly produced by a combination of tachycardia and elevated LVEDP.

Table 6-6
Coronary Perfusion Pressure Gradient

Aortic Diastolic BP	Distal Coronary Diastolic BP	–	LVEDP	= CPP
80 ——→	50	–	4	= 46
80 ——→	50	–	30	= 20

Hoffman and Buckberg have described a relationship called the endocardial viability ratio (EVR), or diastolic pressure–time index (DPTI) over tension–time index (TTI), which describes the ratio of myocardial oxygen supply to the myocardial oxygen demand.[226,227] This ratio is used to estimate subendocardial blood flow. To assess the oxygen supply, the DPTI is used, and for the oxygen demand the TTI is used. The formula described by the authors is

$$EVR = \frac{DPTI}{TTP} = \frac{(DBP - LAP) \times d_t}{SP \times S_t}$$

$$= \frac{\text{oxygen supply}}{\text{oxygen demand}}$$

where DBP is the mean aortic diastolic pressure; LAP is the mean left atrial pressure or LVEDP; SP is the mean systemic arterial pressure; d_t is the diastolic time; and s_t is the systolic time.

A normal EVR is 1.0 or above when the DPTI equals or exceeds the TTI. When the EVR is less than 0.7, Hoffman and Buckberg found that the left ventricular endocardial blood flow fell in proportion to the epicardial flow (decreased endocardial-to-epicardial ratio), which indicates subendocardial ischemia. The endocardial to epicardial ratio fell whether the decreased EVR was secondary to decreased aortic diastolic pressure, increased left atrial pressure, or increased heart rate.

REFERENCES

1. Berne RM, Levy MN: Cardiovascular Physiology. St. Louis, CV Mosby, 1977, pp 99–114
2. Van Bergen FH, Weatherhead DS, Treloar AE, et al: Comparison of indirect and direct methods of measuring arterial blood pressure. Circulation 10:481–490, 1954
3. Whitcher C: Blood pressure measurement. In Belvill JW, Weaver CS (eds): Clinical Physiology. London, McMillan, 1969, pp 85–124
4. Reitan JA, Barash PG: Noninvasive monitoring. In Saidman LJ, Smith NT (eds): Monitoring in Anesthesia (ed 2). New York, Butterworth, 1984, pp 117–191
5. Waltemath CL, Preuss ED: Determination of blood pressure in low flow states by the Doppler technique. Anesthesiology 34:77–79, 1971
6. Harken AH, Smith RM: Aortic pressure versus Doppler-measured peripheral arterial pressure. Anesthesiology 38:184–186, 1973
7. Finnie KJ, Watts DG, Armstrong PW: Biases in the measurement of arterial pressure. Crit Care Med 12:965–968, 1984
8. Braissoulis G: Arterial pressure measurement in preterm infants. Crit Care Med 14:735–738, 1986
9. Johnson CJ, Kerr JH: Automatic blood pressure monitors: A clinical evaluation of 5 models in adults. Anaesthesia 40:471, 1985
10. Allen EV: Thromboangitis obliterans: Methods of diagnosis of chronic occlusive arterial lesions distal to the wrist with illustrated cases. Am J Med Sci 178:237–244, 1929
11. Palm T: Evaluation of peripheral arterial pressure in the thumb following radial artery cannulation. Br J Anaesth 49:819–824, 1977
12. Greenhow DE: Incorrect performance of Allen's test—Ulnar artery flow erroneously presumed inadequate. Anesthesiology 37:356–357, 1972
13. Brodsky J: A simple method to determine patency of the ulnar artery intraoperatively prior to radial artery cannulation. Anesthesiology 42:626–627, 1975
14. Ryan JF, Raines J, Dalton BC, et al: Arterial dynamics of radial artery cannulation. Anesth Analg 52:1017–1025, 1973
15. Kaplan JA, Miller ED: Radial artery catheterization. Anesthesiol Rev January: 21–23, 1976
16. Gardner RM, Hollingsworth KW: Optimizing the electrocardiogram and pressure monitoring. Crit Care Med 14:651–658, 1986
17. Gardner RM: Direct blood pressure measurement—Dynamic response requirements. Anesthesiology 54:227–236, 1981
18. Downs JB, Chapman RL, Hawkins IF, et al: Prolonged radial artery catheterization. Arch Surg 108:671–673, 1974
19. Gardner RM, Bond EL, Clark JS: Safety and efficacy of continuous flush systems for arterial and pulmonary catheters. Ann Thorac Surg 23:534–538, 1977
20. Lowenstein E, Little JW, Lo HH: Prevention of cerebral embolization from flushing radial artery cannulae. N Engl J Med 285:1414–1415, 1971
21. Bedford RF, Wollman H: Complications of radial artery cannulation. Anesthesiology 38:228–236, 1973
22. Kin JM, Arakawa K, Bliss J: Arterial cannulation: Factors in the development of occlusion. Anesth Analg 54:836–840, 1975
23. Bedford RF: Radial artery function following percutaneous cannulation with 18-gauge and 20-gauge catheters. Anesthesiology 47:37–39, 1977
24. Downs JB, Rackstein AD, Klein EF, et al: Hazards of radial artery catheterization. Anesthesiology 38:283–286, 1973
25. Bedford RF: Percutaneous radial artery cannulation,

increased safety using Teflon catheters. Anesthesiology 42:219–222, 1975

26. Bedford RF: Wrist circumference predicts the risk of radial arterial occlusion after cannulation. Anesthesiology 48:377–378, 1978

27. Slogoff S, Keats AS, Arlund C: On the safety of radial artery cannulation. Anesthesiology 59:42–47, 1983

28. Bedford RF: Removal of radial artery thrombi following percutaneous cannulation for monitoring. Anesthesiology 46:430–432, 1977

29. Feeley TN: Reestablishment of radial artery patency for arterial monitoring. Anesthesiology 46:73–75, 1975

30. Wyatt R, Glover I, Cooper EJ: Proximal skin necrosis after radial artery cannulation. Lancet 1:1135–1138, 1974

31. Johnson RW: A complication of radial artery cannulation. Anesthesiology 40:598–600, 1974

32. Stamm WE, Colella JJ, Anderson RL, et al: Indwelling arterial catheters as a source of nosocomial bacteremia. N Engl J Med 292:1099–1102, 1975

33. Gardner RM, Schwartz R, Wong HC, et al: Percutaneous in-dwelling radial artery catheters for monitoring cardiovascular function. N Engl J Med 290:1227–1231, 1974

34. Stern DH, Gerson JI, Allen FB, et al: Can we trust the direct radial artery pressure immediately after cardiopulmonary bypass? Anesthesiology 62:557–561, 1985

35. Barnes RW, Petersen JL, Krugmire BB, et al: Complications of brachial artery catheterization: Prospective evaluation with the Doppler ultrasonic detector. Chest 66:363–367, 1974

36. Barnes RW, Foster EJ, Jansen GA, et al: Safety of brachial artery catheters as monitors in the intensive care unit—Prospective evaluation with the Doppler ultrasonic velocity detector. Anesthesiology 44:260–264, 1976

37. Gurman GM, Kriemerman S: Cannulation of big arteries in critically ill patients. Crit Care Med 13:217–220, 1985

38. Seldinger SI: Catheter replacement of the needle in percutaneous arteriography: New technique. Acta Radiol 39:368–376, 1953

39. Ersoz CJ, Hedden M, Lain L: Prolonged femoral artery catheterization for intensive care. Anesth Analg 49:160–164, 1973

40. Kopman EA, Ferguson TB: Intraoperative monitoring of femoral artery pressure during replacement of aneurysms of the descending thoracic aorta. Anesth Analg 56:603–605, 1977

41. Barnhorst BA, Boener HB: Prevalence of generally absent pedal pulses. N Engl J Med 278:264–265, 1968

42. Youngberg JA, Miller ED: Evaluation of percutaneous cannulation of the dorsalis pedis artery. Anesthesiology 44:80–83, 1976

43. Remington JW: Contour changes of the aortic pulse during propagation. Am J Physiol 199:331–334, 1960

44. Johnstone RE, Greenhow DE: Catheterization of the dorsalis pedis artery. Anesthesiology 39:654–655, 1973

45. Verweij J, Kester A, Stroes W, et al: Comparison of 3 methods for measuring central venous pressure. Crit Care Med 14:288–290, 1986

46. Hurst JW, Schlant RC: Examination of veins. In Hurst JW, Logue RB (eds): The Heart (ed 4). New York, McGraw-Hill, 1978, pp 193–201

47. Mangano DT: Monitoring pulmonary arterial pressure in coronary artery disease. Anesthesiology 53:364–370, 1980

48. English IC, Frew RM, Pigott JF, et al: Percutaneous catheterization of the internal jugular vein. Anaesthesia 24:521–531, 1969

49. Defalque RJ: Percutaneous catheterization of the internal jugular vein. Anesth Analg 53:116–121, 1974

50. Kaplan JA, Miller ED: Internal jugular vein catheterization. Anesthesiol Rev May: 21–23, 1976

51. Jernigan WR, Gardner WC, Mahr MM, et al: Use of the internal jugular vein for placement of central venous catheters. Surg Gynecol Obstet 130:520–524, 1973

52. Mosteret JW, Kenny GM, Murphy GP: Safe placement of cardiovascular catheters into the internal jugular vein. Arch Surg 101:431–432, 1970

53. Boulanger M, Delva E, Paiement JM: Une nouvelle voie D'Abord de la veine jugularie interne. Can Anaesth Soc J 23:609–615, 1976

54. Civetta JM, Gabel JC, Gemer M: Internal jugular vein puncture with a margin of safety. Anesthesiology 36:622–623, 1972

55. Petty C: Alternate methods of internal jugular venapuncture for monitoring central venous pressure. Anesth Analg 54:157, 1975

56. Jobes DR, Schwartz AJ, Greenhow DE, et al: Safer jugular vein cannulation: Recognition of arterial puncture. Anesthesiology 59:353–355, 1983

57. Vaughan RW, Weyjandt GR: Reliable percutaneous central venous pressure measurement. Anesth Analg 52:709–716, 1973

58. Kuramoto T, Sakav T: Comparison of success in jugular versus basilic vein techniques for central venous pressure catheter positioning. Anesth Analg 54:696–697, 1975

59. Prince SR, Sullivan RL, Hackel A: Percutaneous catheterization of the internal jugular vein of infants and children. Anesthesiology 44:170–174, 1976

60. Blitt CD, Wright WA, Petty WC, et al: Cardiovascular catheterization via the external jugular vein: A technique employing the J-wire. JAMA 229:817–818, 1974

61. Baum S, Abrams HL: A J-shaped catheter for retro-

grade catheterization of tortuous vessels. Radiology 83:436–437, 1964

62. Kellner GA, Smart JF: Percutaneous placement of catheters to monitor "central venous pressure." Anesthesiology 36:515–516, 1972

63. Webre DR, Arens JF: Use of cephalic and basilic veins for introduction of cardiovascular catheters. Anesthesiology 38:389–392, 1973

64. Johnston AOB, Clark RG: Malpositioning of cardiovascular catheters. Lancet 2:1395–1397, 1972

65. Burgess GE, Marino RJ, Peuler MJ: Effect of head position on the location of venous catheters inserted via the basilic vein. Anesthesiology 46:212–213, 1977

66. Defalque RJ: Subclavian venapuncture: A review. Anesth Analg 47:677–682, 1968

67. Sznajder JI, Zveibil FR, Bitterman H, et al: Central vein catheterization: Failure and complication rates by 3 percutaneous approaches. Arch Intern Med 146:259–261, 1986

68. Ortiz J, Dean WF, Zumbro GL, et al: Arteriovenous fistula as a complication of percutaneous internal jugular vein catheterization. Milit Med 141:171, 1976

69. Brown CS, Wallace CT: Chronic hematoma—A complication of percutaneous catheterization of the internal jugular vein. Anesthesiology 45:368–369, 1976

70. Cook TL, Deuker CW: Tension pneumothorax following internal jugular cannulation and general anesthesia. Anesthesiology 45:554–555, 1976

71. Parikh RK: Horner's syndrome: A complication of percutaneous catheterization of the internal jugular vein. Anaesthesia 27:327–329, 1972

72. Khalil KG, Parker FB, Mukherjee M, et al: Thoracic duct injury: A complication of jugular vein catheterization. JAMA 221:908–909, 1972

73. Bell H, Stubbs D, Pugh D: Reliability of central venous pressure as an indicator of left atrial pressure. Chest 59:169–173, 1971

74. Sarnoff SJ, Berglund E: Ventricular function. I. Starling's law of the heart studied by means of simultaneous right and left ventricular function curves in the dog. Circulation 9:706–718, 1954

75. Forrester JS, Diamond G, McHugh TJ, et al: Filling pressures in the right and left sides of the heart in acute myocardial infarction. N Engl J Med 285:190–193, 1971

76. Civetta JM, Gabel JC, Laver MB: Disparate ventricular function in surgical patients. Surg Forum 22:136–139, 1971

77. Toussaint GPM, Burges JS, Hampson LG: Central venous pressure and pulmonary capillary wedge pressure in critical surgical illness. Arch Surg 109:265–269, 1974

78. Altschule M: Reflections on Starling's laws of the heart. Chest 89:444–445, 1986

79. Goldenheim PD, Kazemi H: Cardiopulmonary mon-

itoring of critically ill patients. N Engl J Med 311:776–780, 1984

80. Swan HJC, Ganz W, Forrester JS, et al: Catheterization of the heart in man with the use of a flow-directed balloon-tipped catheter. N Engl J Med 283:447–451, 1970

81. Humphrey CB, Oury JH, Virgilo RW, et al: An analysis of direct and indirect measurement of left atrial filling pressures. J Thorac Cardiovasc Surg 41:643–647, 1976

82. Lappas D, Lell WA, Gabel JC, et al: Indirect measurement of left atrial pressure in surgical patients—Pulmonary capillary wedge pressure and pulmonary artery diastolic pressure compared with left atrial pressure. Anesthesiology 38:394–397, 1973

83. Walston A, Kendall ME: Comparison of pulmonary wedge and left atrial pressure in man. Am Heart J 86:159–164, 1973

84. Lorzman J, Powers SR, Older T, et al: Correlation of pulmonary wedge and left atrial pressure: A study in the patient receiving positive end-expiratory pressure ventilation. Arch Surg 109:270–277, 1974

85. Heinonen J, Salmenpera M, Takkunen O: Increased pulmonary artery diastolic-pulmonary wedge pressure gradient after cardiopulmonary bypass. Can Anaesth Soc J 32:165–170, 1985

86. Connors AF, McCaffree DR, Gray BA: Evaluation of right heart catheterization in the critically ill patient. N Engl J Med 308:263–267, 1983

87. Waller JL, Johnson SP, Kaplan JA: Usefulness of pulmonary artery catheters during aortocoronary bypass surgery. Anesth Analg 61:221–222, 1982

88. Iberti T, Fisher CJ: A prospective study on the use of the pulmonary artery catheter in a medical intensive care unit—Its effect on diagnosis and therapy. Crit Care Med 11:238, 1983

89. Nichols AB, Owen J, Grossman BA, et al: Effect of heparin bonding on catheter-induced fibrin formation and platelet activation. Circulation 70:843–850, 1984

90. Mantle JA, Massing GK, James TN, et al: A multipurpose catheter for electrophysiologic and hemodynamic monitoring plus atrial pacing. Chest 72:285–290, 1977

91. Waller JL, Kaplan JA, Bauman DI, et al: Clinical evaluation of a new fiberoptic catheter oximeter during cardiac surgery. Anesth Analg 61:676–679, 1982

92. Kelman GR: Applied Cardiovascular Physiology. London, Appleton-Century-Crofts, 1971, p 53

93. Waller JL, Zaidan JR, Kaplan JA, et al: Hemodynamic response to preoperative vascular cannulation in patients with coronary artery disease. Anesthesiology 56:219–221, 1982

94. Quintin L, Whalley DG, Wynands JE, et al: The effects of vascular catheterization upon heart rate and blood pressure before aortocoronary bypass surgery. Can Anaesth Soc J 28:244–247, 1981

95. Nicolson SC, Sweeney MF, Moore RA, et al: Com-

parison of internal and external jugular cannulation of the central circulation in the pediatric patient. Crit Care Med 13:747–749, 1985

96. Kaplan JA, Miller ED: Insertion of the Swan-Ganz catheter. Anesthesiol Rev November: 22–25, 1974

97. Benumof JL, Saidman LJ, Arkin DB, et al: Where pulmonary artery catheters go: Intrathoracic distribution. Anesthesiology 46:336–338, 1977

98. Johnston WE, Royster RL, Choplin RH, et al: Pulmonary artery migration during cardiac surgery. Anesthesiology 64:258–262, 1986

99. Murray MJ, Wignes M, McMichan JC: Assessment of sterility of pulmonary artery catheter sheaths. Anesth Analg 65:1218–1221, 1986

100. Pace NL: A critique of flow-directed pulmonary artery catheterization. Anesthesiology 47:455–465, 1977

101. Shah KB, Rao TK, Laughlin S, et al: A review of pulmonary artery catheterization in 6245 patients. Anesthesiology 61:271–275, 1984

102. McGrath R: Invasive bedside hemodynamic monitoring. Prog Cardiovasc Dis 29:129–144, 1986

103. Patel C, Laboy V, Venus B, et al: Acute complications of pulmonary artery catheter insertion in critically ill patients. Crit Care Med 14:195–197, 1986

104. Grum CM, Reynolds AC: Perils and pitfalls of pulmonary artery catheters. Anesth Rev 12:46–53, 1985

105. Katz JD, Cronau LH, Barash PG, et al: Pulmonary artery flow-guided catheters in the perioperative period: Indications and complications. JAMA 237:2832–2834, 1977

106. Geha DG, David NJ, Lappas DG: Persistent atrial arrhythmias associated with placement of a Swan-Ganz catheter. Anesthesiology 39:651–653, 1973

107. Abernathy WS: Complete heart block caused by a Swan-Ganz catheter. Chest 65:349, 1974

108. Thomson IR, Dalton BC, Lappas DG, et al: Right bundle branch block and complete heart block caused by the Swan-Ganz catheter. Anesthesiology 51:359–362, 1979

109. Nikolic G, French P: Alternate-beat Wenckebach block caused by pulmonary artery catheterization. Crit Care Med 14:646–648, 1986

110. Foote GA, Schabel SI, Hodges M: Pulmonary complications of the flow-directed balloon-tipped catheter. N Engl J Med 290:927–931, 1974

111. Lapin ES, Muriaz JA: Hemoptysis with flow-directed cardiac catheterization. JAMA 220:1246, 1972

112. Buckbinder N, Ganz W: Hemodynamic monitoring: Invasive techniques. Anesthesiology 45:146–155, 1976

113. Lipp H, O'Donoghue K, Resenekov L: Intracardiac knotting of a flow-directed balloon catheter. N Engl J Med 284:220, 1971

114. Ducatman BS, McMichan JC, Edwards WD: Catheter-induced lesions of the right side of the heart. JAMA 253:791–795, 1985

115. Pace NL, Horton W: In-dwelling pulmonary artery catheters: Relationship to aseptic thrombotic endocardial vegetations. JAMA 233:893–894, 1975

116. Greene JF, Fitzwater JE, Colemmer TP: Septic endocarditis in in-dwelling pulmonary artery catheters. JAMA 233:891–892, 1975

117. Cooper GL, Hopkins CC: Rapid diagnosis of intravascular catheter-associated infection by direct gram staining of catheter segments. N Engl J Med 312:1142–1147, 1985

118. Macander PJ, Kuhnlein JL, Buiteweg J, et al: Electrode detachment: A complication of the in-dwelling pacing Swan-Ganz catheter. N Engl J Med 314:1711, 1986

119. Heiselman DE, Maxwell JS, Petro V: Electrode displacement from a multipurpose Swan-Ganz catheter. PACE 9:134–135, 1986

120. Willis C, Wight D, Zidulka A: Hypotension secondary to balloon inflation of a pulmonary artery catheter. Crit Care Med 12:915–917, 1984

121. Kozlowski JH: Inadvertent coronary sinus occlusion by a pulmonary artery catheter. Crit Care Med 14:649, 1986

122. Shin B, McAslan TC, Ayella RJ: Problems with measurements using the Swan-Ganz catheter. Anesthesiology 43:474–476, 1975

123. Suter PM, Lindauer JM, Fairley HB, et al: Errors in data derived from pulmonary artery blood gas values. Crit Care Med 3:175–181, 1975

124. Raper R, Sibbald WJ: Misled by the wedge? Chest 89:427–434, 1986

125. Nadeau S, Noble WH: Misinterpretation of pressure measurements from the pulmonary artery catheter. Can Anaesth Soc J 33:352–363, 1986

126. Schmitt EA, Brantigan CO: Common artifacts of pulmonary artery pressures: Recognition and interpretation. J Clin Mon 2:44–53, 1986

127. Boutros AT, Lee C: Value of continuous monitoring of mixed venous blood oxygen saturation in the management of critically ill patients. Crit Care Med 14:132–134, 1986

128. Guffin A, Girard D, Kaplan JA: Shivering following cardiac surgery: Hemodynamic changes and reversal. J Cardiothorac Anesth 1:24–28, 1987

129. Zaidan JR, Freniere S: Use of a pacing pulmonary artery catheter during cardiac surgery. Ann Thorac Surg 35:633–636, 1983

130. Vincent JL, Thiron M, Brinioulle S, et al: Measurement of right ventricular ejection fraction with a modified pulmonary artery catheter. Intensive Care Med 12:33–38, 1986

131. Hines R, Barash PG: Intraoperative right ventricular dysfunction detected with a right ventricular ejection fraction catheter. J Clin Mon 2:206–208, 1986

132. Guyton AC, Jones EC, Holman TG: Circulatory Physiology: Cardiac Output and Its Regulation (ed 2). Philadelphia, WB Saunders, 1973, pp 9–11

133. Ganz W, Donoso R, Marcus HS, et al: A new tech-

nique for measurement of cardiac output by thermo-dilution in man. Am J Cardiol 27:392–396, 1971

134. Forrester JS, Ganz W, Diamond G, et al: Thermodilution cardiac output determination with a single flow-directed catheter. Am Heart J 83:306–311, 1972

135. Weisel RD, Berger RL, Hectman HB: Measurement of cardiac output by thermodilution. N Engl J Med 292:682–684, 1975

136. Kohanna FH, Cunningham JN: Monitoring of cardiac output by thermodilution after open heart surgery. J Thorac Cardiovasc Surg 73:451–457, 1977

137. Hillis LD, Firth BG, Winniford MD: Comparison of thermodilution and indocyanine green dye in low cardiac output or left-sided regurgitation. Am J Cardiol 57:1201–1202, 1986

138. Noback C: Intraoperative monitoring. In Kaplan JA (ed): Thoracic Anesthesia. New York, Churchill-Livingstone, 1983, pp 197–249

139. Nelson LD, Anderson HB: Patient selection for iced versus room temperature injectate for thermodilution cardiac output determination. Crit Care Med 13:182–184, 1986

140. Nishikawa T, Dohi S: Slowing of the heart rate during cardiac output measurement by thermodilution. Anesthesiology 57:538, 1982

141. Stevens JH, Raffin TA, Mihm FG, et al: Thermodilution cardiac output measurement: Effects of the respiratory cycle. JAMA 253:2240–2242, 1985

142. Ganz W, Swan HJC: Measurement of blood flow by thermodilution. Am J Cardiol 29:241–246, 1972

143. Colgan FJ, Stewart S: An assessment of cardiac output by thermodilution in infants and children following cardiac surgery. Crit Care Med 5:220–225, 1977

144. Bradley EC, Barr JW: Fore-n-aft triangle formula for rapid estimation of curves. Am Heart J 78:643–648, 1969

145. Carey JS, Williamson H, Scott CR: Accuracy of cardiac output computers. Ann Surg 174:762–768, 1971

146. English JB, Hodges MR, Sentker C, et al: Comparison of aortic pulse-wave contour analysis and thermodilution methods of measuring cardiac output during anesthesia in the dog. Anesthesiology 52:56–61, 1980

147. Sahn DJ, Valdes-Cruz LM: New advances in 2-D Doppler echocardiography. Prog Cardiovasc Dis 28:367–382, 1986

148. Labovitz AJ, Buckingham TA, Hebermehl K, et al: The effects of sampling site on the 2-D echo-Doppler determination of cardiac output. Am Heart J 109:327–331, 1985

149. Wyse RK, Robinson PJ: Transcutaneous monitoring of cardiac output during intensive care. Intensive Crit Care Dig 5:12–15, 1986

150. Rose JS, Nanna M, Rahimtoola SH, et al: Accuracy of determination of changes in cardiac output by transcutaneous continuous-wave Doppler computer. Am J Cardiol 54:1099–1101, 1984

151. Vandenbogaerde JF, Scheldewaert RG, Rijckaert DL, et al: Comparison between ultrasonic and thermodilution cardiac output measurements in intensive care patients. Crit Care Med 14:294–297, 1986

152. Rein AJ, Hsieh KS, Elixson M, et al: Cardiac output estimates in the pediatric intensive care unit using a continuous-wave Doppler computer. Am Heart J 112:97–103, 1986

153. Mark JB, Steinrook RA, Gugino LD, et al: Continuous noninvasive monitoring of cardiac output with esophageal Doppler ultrasound during cardiac surgery. Anesth Analg 65:1013–1020, 1986

154. Braunwald E, Ross J, Sonnenblick EH: Mechanisms of Contraction of the Normal and Failing Heart (ed 2). Boston, Little, Brown, 1976

155. Sonnenblick EH, Strobeck JE: Derived indices of ventricular and myocardial function. N Engl J Med 296:978–982, 1977

156. Kaplan JA, Wells PH: Early diagnosis of myocardial ischemia using the pulmonary arterial catheters. Anesth Analg 60:789, 1981

157. Ross J, Sobel BE: Regulation of cardiac contraction. Ann Rev Physiol 34:47, 1972

158. Ross J, Braunwald E: The study of left ventricular function in man by increasing resistance to ventricular ejection with angiotensin. Circulation 29:739, 1964

159. McGregor M, Sniderman A: On pulmonary vascular resistance: The need for more precise definition. Am J Cardiol 55:217–220, 1985

160. Langer GA: The intrinsic control of myocardial contraction—Ionic factors. N Engl J Med 285:1065, 1971

161. Brutsaert DL, Rademaker FE, Sys SU, et al: Analysis of relaxation in the evaluation of ventricular function of the heart. Prog Cardiovasc Dis 28:143–163, 1985

162. Lewis BS, Gotsman MS: Current concepts of left ventricular relaxation and compliance. Am Heart J 99:101, 1980

163. Sarnoff SJ: Myocardial contractility as described by ventricular function curves: Observations on Starling's law of the heart. Physiol Rev 35:107–122, 1955

164. Crexells C, Chatterjee K, Forrester JS, et al: Optimal level of filling pressure on the left side of the heart in acute myocardial infarction. N Engl J Med 289:1263–1266, 1973

165. Forrester JS, Diamond G, Chatterjee K, et al: Medical therapy of acute myocardial infarction by application of hemodynamic subsets. N Engl J Med 295:1356–1362, 1404–1413, 1976

166. Gudwin AL, Goldstein CR, Cohn JD, et al: Estimation of ventricular mixing volume for prediction of operative mortality in the elderly. Ann Surg 168:183–192, 1968

167. Cohn JN, Franciosa JA: Vasodilator therapy of heart failure. N Engl J Med 297:27–31, 254–258, 1977

168. Dilley RB, Ross J, Bernstein EF: Serial hemodynamics during intraaortic balloon counterpulsation for cardiogenic shock. Circulation 47,48(suppl 3):99–104, 1973

169. Braunwald E: On the difference between the heart's output and its contractile state. Circulation 43:171–174, 1971

170. Sonnenblick EH, Parmley WE, Urshel CW: The contractile state of the heart as expressed by force/velocity relationships. Am J Cardiol 23:488–503, 1969

171. Pollack GH: Maximum velocity as an index of contractility in cardiac muscle: A critical evaluation. Circ Res 26:111–127, 1970

172. Morrow DH, Morrow AG: The effects of halothane on myocardial contractile force and vascular resistance: Direct observations made in patients during cardiopulmonary bypass. Anesthesiology 22:537–541, 1961

173. Gleason WL, Braunwald E: Studies on the first derivative of the ventricular pressure pulse in man. J Clin Invest 41:80–90, 1962

174. Wallace AG, Skinner NS, Mitchell JH: Hemodynamic determinants of the maximal rate of rise of left ventricular pressure. Am J Physiol 205:30–36, 1963

175. Braunwald E, Ross J, Gault JH, et al: Assessment of cardiac function. Ann Intern Med 70:369–399, 1969

176. Tomlin PJ, Duck F, McNulty M, et al: A comparison of methods of evaluating myocardial contractility. Can Anaesth Soc J 22:436–448, 1975

177. Nobel M, Trenchard D, Gus A: Left ventricular ejection in conscious dogs: I. Measurement and significance of the maximum acceleration of blood from the left ventricle. Circ Res 19:139–147, 1966

178. Alderman EL: Angiographic indicators of left ventricular function. JAMA 236:1055–1058, 1976

179. Weissler AM: Systolic time intervals. N Engl J Med 296:321–324, 1977

180. Weissler AM, Harris WS, Schoenfeld CD: Systolic time intervals in heart failure in man. Circulation 37:149–159, 1968

181. Tonnesen AS, Gabel JC, Cooper JR, et al: Intraesophageal microphone for phonocardiographic recording. Anesthesiology 46:70–71, 1977

182. Martin CE, Shaver JS, Thompson ME: Direct correlation of external systolic time intervals with internal indices of left ventricular function in man. Circulation 44:419–431, 1971

183. Talley RL, Meyer JF, McNay JL: Evaluation of the pre-ejection period as an estimate of myocardial contractility in dogs. Am J Cardiol 27:384–391, 1971

184. Garrard CL, Weissler AM, Dodge HT: The relationship of alterations in systolic time intervals to ejection fraction in patients with cardiac disease. Circulation 42:455–462, 1970

185. Diamond G, Forrester JS, Chatterjee K, et al: Mean electromechanical $\Delta P/\Delta T$. Am J Cardiol 30:338–341, 1972

186. Reitan JA, Smith NT, Barrison VS, et al: The cardiac preejection period. Anesthesiology 36:76–80, 1972

187. Lewis RP, Rittgess SE, Forrester WF, et al: A critical review of the systolic time intervals. Circulation 56:146–158, 1977

188. Dauchot PJ, Rasmussen JP, Nicholson DH, et al: On-line systolic time intervals during anesthesia in patients with and without heart disease. Anesthesiology 44:472–480, 1976

189. Harrison WK, Friessenger GC, Johnson SL, et al: Relation of the ballistocardiogram to left ventricular pressure measurements in man. Am J Cardiol 23:673–678, 1969

190. Eddleman EE, Harrison WK, Jackson WDH, et al: A critical appraisal of ballistocardiography. Am J Cardiol 29:120–122, 1972

191. Stevens WC, Cromwell TH, Halsey MJ, et al: The cardiovascular effects of a new inhalation anesthetic, Forane, in human volunteers at constant arterial carbon dioxide tension. Anesthesiology 35:8–16, 1971

192. Mann DL, Gillam LD, Weyman AE: Cross-sectional echocardiographic assessment of regional left ventricular performance and myocardial perfusion. Prog Cardiovasc Dis 29:1–52, 1986

193. Belkin RN, Kisslo J: Clinical applications of echocardiography in myocardial and valvular heart disease. Prog Cardiovasc Dis 29:81–106, 1986

194. Smith MD, Kwan OL, Demaria AN: Value and limitations of continuous-wave Doppler echocardiography in estimating severity of valvular stenosis. JAMA 255:3145–3151, 1986

195. Dubroff JM, Clark MB, Wong CYH, et al: Left ventricular ejection fraction during cardiac surgery: A 2D echocardiographic study. Circulation 68:95, 1983

196. Schluter M, Langenstein GA, Polster J, et al: Transesophageal cross-sectional echocardiography with a phased-array transducer system. Br Heart J 48:67, 1982

197. Konstadt SN, Thys D, Mindich BP, et al: Validation of quantitative intraoperative transesophageal echocardiography. Anesthesiology 65:418–421, 1986

198. Rathod R, Jacobs HK, Kramer NE, et al: Echocardiographic assessment of ventricular performance following induction of two anesthetics. Anesthesiology 49:86, 1978

199. Kremer P, Schwartz L, Cahalan MK, et al: Intraoperative monitoring of left ventricular performance by 2D transesophageal echocardiography. Am J Cardiol 49:956, 1982

200. Sagawa K: The end-systolic pressure-volume relation of the ventricle: Definition, modifications, and clinical use. Circulation 63:1223, 1981

201. Kono A, Maughan WL, Sunagawa K, et al: The use of left ventricular end-ejection pressure and peak pressure in the estimation of the end-systolic pres-

sure-volume relationship. Circulation 70:1057–1065, 1984

202. Thys DM: Pulmonary artery catheterization: past, present, and future. Mt Sinai J Med 51:578, 1984

203. Sagawa K: End-systolic pressure-volume relationship in retrospect and prospect. Fed Proc 43:2399, 1984

204. Suga H, Sagawa K: Control of ventricular contractility assessed by pressure-volume ratio. Cardiovasc Res 10:582, 1976

205. Suga H, Sagawa K: Load independence of the instantaneous pressure-volume ratio of the canine left ventricle and effects of epinephrine and heart rate on the ratio. Circ Res 32:314, 1973

206. Sagawa K: The ventricular pressure-volume diagram revisited. Circ Res 43:677, 1978

207. Alderman EL, Glantz SA: Acute hemodynamic interventions shift the diastolic pressure-volume curve in man. Circulation 54:662, 1976

208. Iskandrian AS, Heo J: Left ventricular pressure/volume relationship in coronary artery disease. Am Heart J 112:375–381, 1986

209. Poliner CR, Farber SH, Glasser DH, et al: Alteration of diastolic filling rate during exercise radionuclide angiography: A highly sensitive technique for detection of coronary artery disease. Circulation 70:942–950, 1984

210. Coriat P, Mundler O, Bousseau D, et al: Response of left ventricular ejection fraction to recovery from general anesthesia. Anesth Analg 65:593–600, 1986

211. Iskadrian AS, Hakki AH: Thallium-201 myocardial scintigraphy. Am Heart J 109:113–129, 1985

212. Reeves RC, Evanochko WT, Pohost GA: Potential approaches to evaluating the cardiovascular system using NMR. Prog Cardiovasc Dis 29:53–64, 1986

213. Higgins CV, Kaufman L, Crooks LE: Magnetic resonance imaging of the cardiovascular system. Am Heart J 109:136–152, 1985

214. Braunwald E: Control of myocardial oxygen consumption: Physiologic and clinical considerations. Am J Cardiol 27:416–432, 1971

215. Hoffman JIE, Buckberg GD: The myocardial supply:demand ratio. A critical review. Am J Cardiol 41:327–332, 1978

216. Klocke FJ, Mates RE, Copely DP, et al: Physiology

217. Klocke FJ: Clinical measurements of coronary blood flow. In Yu PN, Goodwin JF (eds): Progress in Cardiology. Philadelphia, Lea & Febiger, 1976, pp 91–130

218. Rowe GG, Thomsen JH, Stenlund RR: A study of hemodynamics and coronary blood flow in man with coronary artery disease. Circulation 39:139–148, 1969

219. Rowe GG, Castillo CA, Afonso S: Coronary flow measured by nitrous oxide method. Am Heart J 67:457–468, 1964

220. Ganz W, Tamura K, Marcus HS: Measurements of coronary sinus blood flow by continuous thermodilution in man. Circulation 44:181–195, 1971

221. Moffitt EA, Barker RA, Glenn JJ, et al: Myocardial metabolism and hemodynamic responses with isoflurane anesthesia for coronary artery surgery. Anesth Analg 65:53–62, 1986

222. Maseri A: Radioactive tracer techniques for evaluating coronary blood flow. In Yu PN, Goodwin JF (eds): Progress in Cardiology. Philadelphia, Lea & Febiger, 1976, pp 141–168

223. Ohquist G, Settergren G, Ekestrom S, et al: The influence of isoflurane on blood flow in coronary bypass grafts. Acta Anaesthesiol Scand 29:758–763, 1985

224. Gamble WJ, LaFarge CG, Fyler DC, et al: Regional coronary venous oxygen saturation and myocardial oxygen tension following abrupt changes in ventricular pressure in the isolated dog heart. Circ Res 34:672, 1974

225. Hoffman JIE, Buckberg GD: Regional myocardial ischemia—Causes, prediction and prevention. Vasc Surg 8:115–130, 1974

226. Hoffman JIE, Buckberg GD: Transmural variations in myocardial perfusion. In Yu PN, Goodwin JF (eds): Progress in Cardiology. Philadelphia, Lea & Febiger, 1976, p 37

227. Hoffman JIE, Buckberg GD: Pathophysiology of subendocardial ischemia. Br Med J 1:76–79, 1975

of the coronary circulation in health and coronary artery disease. In Yu PN, Goodwin JF (eds): Progress in Cardiology. Philadelphia, Lea & Febiger, 1976, pp 1–17

Daniel M. Thys, M.D.
Joel A. Kaplan, M.D.

7

Recent Advances in Electrocardiographic Techniques

It has become standard practice to monitor the electrocardiogram (ECG) in all patients undergoing anesthesia and surgery.[1] One of the earliest indications for the use of ECG monitoring in the operating room was for the diagnosis of dysrhythmias.[2] In recent years, considerable advances have been made in the design of the lead systems that facilitate the recognition of abnormal rhythms. Other advances in the field of dysrhythmia detection have occurred in the automated systems used for rhythm analysis. Another major indication for intraoperative monitoring of the ECG is the diagnosis of myocardial ischemia. Significant advances have been made in the ability to detect and analyze ischemic ECG changes and a number of computerized systems are currently available. This chapter reviews the use of these new techniques in the operating room.

INDICATIONS FOR ECG MONITORING

Intraoperative Dysrhythmias

Interest in the intraoperative detection of cardiac dysrhythmias has grown since 1847, when the first cardiac arrest during surgery was reported.[3] Earlier in this century occasional dysrhythmias were de-scribed in anesthetized patients, and the first large series with ECG studies during anesthesia was published by Kurtz et al in 1936.[4] They observed dysrhythmias in 79 percent of 109 patients receiving cyclopropane, ether, procaine, ethylene, nitrous oxide, vinyl ether, chloroform, or tribromethanol anesthesia. Other studies documenting the incidence of intraoperative dysrhythmias associated with contemporary agents and techniques were reviewed by Katz et al[5] and are summarized in Table 7-1.[5-10]

Dysrhythmias are most common during endotracheal intubation and extubation. Patients with preexisting cardiac disease have a higher incidence of ventricular dysrhythmias than patients without known heart disease (60 percent versus 37 percent). In a study of patients undergoing cardiac surgery, Angelini et al reported that 29 of 50 patients (58 percent) having valve surgery and 35 of 78 patients (45 percent) having coronary revascularization developed significant postoperative dysrhythmias.[11] These dysrhythmias tended to correlate with the severity of the heart disease, led to a prolonged hospital stay, and were responsible for up to 80 percent of the surgical mortality in their series. The following features have been shown to be possible contributors to the etiology of dysrhythmias in the perioperative period.

CARDIAC ANESTHESIA, SECOND EDITION
ISBN 0-8089-1848-6

Table 7-1
Incidences of Intraoperative Dysrhythmias

Study	Year	Total Patients	Dysrhythmias	% Patients with Dysrhythmias
Dodd et al[6]	1962	569	170	29.9
Kuner et al[7]	1967	154	95	61.7
Vanik et al[8]	1968	5013	901	17.9
Russell et al[9]	1969	3177	494	15.5
Bertrand et al[10]	1971	100	84	84.0
Total		9013	1744	19.3

1. Anesthetic agents. Halogenated hydrocarbons, such as halothane or enflurane, have been shown to produce dysrhythmias, probably by a reentrant mechanism.[12] In addition, halothane has been shown to sensitize the myocardium to both endogenous and exogenous catecholamines. Drugs that block the reuptake of norepinephrine, such as cocaine and ketamine, can facilitate the development of epinephrine-induced dysrhythmias.[13]

2. Abnormal arterial blood gases or electrolytes. Edwards et al showed that hyperventilation to a $PaCO_2$ of 30 or 20 mm Hg lowered a normal serum potassium to 3.64 or 3.12 mEq/liter, respectively.[14] If serum and total body potassium start at low levels, it is possible to decrease the serum potassium into the 2 mEq/liter range by hyperventilation, and thus precipitate severe cardiac dysrhythmias. Alterations of blood gases or electrolytes may lead to dysrhythmias either by producing reentrant mechanisms or by altering phase 4 depolarization of conduction fibers.

3. Endotracheal intubation. This may be the most common cause of dysrhythmias during surgery. These dysrhythmias can occasionally be associated with severe hypertension.[15] Several authors have emphasized the hemodynamic alterations that may occur during endotracheal intubation.[15,16]

4. Reflexes. Vagal stimulation may produce sinus bradycardias and allow ventricular escape mechanisms to occur. In addition, specific reflexes such as the occulocardiac reflex can produce severe rhythm disturbances during surgery.[17]

5. Central nervous system (CNS) stimulation.[18] Many ECG abnormalities have been reported with intracranial pathology, especially subarachnoid hemorrhage, including changes in QT intervals, development of Q waves, ST-segment changes, and the occurrence of U waves. The mechanism of these dysrhythmias appears to be due to changes in the autonomic nervous system.

6. Location of surgery. Dental surgery is often associated with dysrhythmias, since profound stimulation of both the sympathetic and parasympathetic nervous systems often occurs.[19] Junctional rhythms commonly occur and may be due to stimulation of the autonomic nervous system via the fifth cranial nerve.

7. Preexisting cardiac disease. Studies by Angelini et al have shown that patients with known cardiac disease have a much higher incidence of dysrhythmias during anesthesia than patients without known cardiac disease.[11]

8. Insertions. The insertion of catheters or wires in the heart may lead to dysrhythmias. This is seen with the placement of pulmonary artery catheters (PACs) and often leads to premature ventricular contractions.

Dysrhythmias may also be attenuated or eliminated by general anesthesia.[20] This could be due to relief of anxiety and loss of sympathetic stimulation, an antiarrhythmic property of the anesthetic agent itself, or the correction of abnormalities of respiration, blood gases, and electrolytes.

Myocardial Ischemia

THE INCIDENCE OF PERIOPERATIVE
MYOCARDIAL ISCHEMIA AND INFARCTION

Many studies have investigated the incidence of myocardial infarction or reinfarction following surgery. In the "normal" surgical population, the incidence of postoperative myocardial infarction is on the order of 0.13 to 0.66 percent.[21-24]

Preoperative myocardial infarction significantly increases the risk for the development of subsequent postoperative reinfarction. Topkins and Artusio found that 43 of 658 patients (6.5 percent) reinfarcted;[24] while Knapp et al reported that 26 of 427 patients (6 percent) developed an infarction postoperatively.[23] Arkins et al, in a series of 240 patients with severe coronary artery disease (CAD), found that 54 patients (22.6 percent) died in the 2 months following surgery.[25] Tarhan et al investigated 422 patients with previous myocardial infarctions and found that 28 of them (6.6 percent) experienced another infarction during the first postoperative week.[22] Steen et al, from the same institution 6 years later, still found that 6.1 percent of patients developed a reinfarction within 1 week of surgery.[26] The time interval between the first infarction and surgery influenced the subsequent risk of reinfarction.[22,24,26] If the first infarction occurred within 3 months prior to surgery, the incidence of reinfarction was 27 to 37 percent. Between 3 and 6 months, this fell to 11 to 16 percent, and, thereafter, stabilized at 4 to 5 percent. Recently, these results have been markedly improved by Rao et al who used aggressive invasive hemodynamic monitoring and prompt treatment of hemodynamic aberrations to produce reinfarction rates of 5.8 percent and 2.3 percent for previous infarctions less than 3 months and 4 to 6 months old, respectively.[21] Thereafter, the reinfarction rate dropped to 1 to 1.7 percent. In this study, the mortality after reinfarction was 36 percent, which is also significantly lower than that reported in previous studies (over 50 percent).

Other studies have attempted to define the incidence of ECG changes occurring in the perioperative period in selected groups of patients who may be at an increased risk for the development of myocardial ischemia. Chamberlain and Edmonds-Seal performed preoperative and postoperative 12-lead ECGs in 217 patients with ischemic heart disease or hypertension.[27] Twenty-two percent developed significant ECG deterioration (2.3 percent sustained frank myocardial infarction), and 33 percent had minor ECG changes of which 68 percent became worse with a subsequent ECG on the fourth postoperative day. They postulated that persistence of ECG changes indicated that severe myocardial muscle injury may have occurred. Driscoll et al studied 145 patients with documented arteriosclerosis with pre- and postoperative ECGs and found that 23 percent developed fresh ischemic changes.[28] The problem with these early studies from the 1960s using serial ECGs to detect ischemic changes is that monitoring was not continuous, and, therefore, the onset of ischemia was not known and transient episodes of ischemia were probably missed.

FACTORS PREDISPOSING TO THE DEVELOPMENT OF ISCHEMIA

It is important to identify the factors that may cause perioperative ischemia and myocardial infarction in order to define appropriate measures for their prevention and treatment. The presence of preexisting CAD is a major risk factor for the subsequent development of perioperative ischemia.[29-31] Coriat et al found that patients with disabling angina (Class III and IV) had the highest incidence of intraoperative myocardial ischemia.[32] Many groups have studied the incidence of perioperative myocardial infarction in patients with CAD with or without previous coronary artery bypass grafting (CABG).[33-37] Patients without prior CABG who developed a perioperative infarction usually had three-vessel CAD. The infarction rate in the CABG group was very low, supporting the "protective" effect of prior CABG before noncardiac surgery.[33-37]

Anesthesia, especially during induction, periods of surgical stress, and emergency procedures, may produce adverse hemodynamic changes which affect the myocardial oxygen balance. Hypertension and tachycardia during intubation may produce myocardial ischemia in healthy patients[38] and in those with CAD.[29,30]

Intraoperative hypotension in patients with ischemic heart disease has been associated with the development of postoperative ECG changes[27] and postoperative reinfarction in patients with preoperative myocardial reinfarction.[21,26,34,36] Rao et al found a higher incidence of reinfarction in patients who developed episodes of intraoperative hypotension or hypertension (with or without tachycardia).[21] Slogoff and Keats found that tachycardia (heart rate > 100), but not hypotension or hypertension, correlated best with myocardial ischemia and infarction.[29]

Although it is attractive to think that a particular anesthetic technique may affect the incidence of perioperative myocardial ischemia and infarction, numerous studies have failed to demonstrate any benefits of different anesthetic regimes.[22-24,26,39,40] In the prospective study of Rao et al, patients receiving nitrous oxide, oxygen, a muscle relaxant, and a narcotic had a higher incidence of reinfarction compared with other anesthetic drugs, but for no apparent reason.[21] The pitfalls of subjecting such data to multiple retrospective analysis, however, have thrown some doubt on these findings.[41] The retrospective study by Steen et al included two groups of patients who had transurethral resections of the prostate under either general (50 patients) or spinal (44 patients) anesthesia.[26] The incidence of perioperative myocardial infarction was similar in both groups, and it appears that regional or general anesthesia is equally safe if properly conducted with maintenance of normal hemodynamic parameters.

The effect of the type and duration of surgery on the development of perioperative infarction and ischemia has also been extensively studied. Several studies have demonstrated an increased risk of reinfarction following intrathoracic or abdominal surgery.[21,22,26,40] However, the data on duration of surgery are not clear. Topkins and Artusio found no correlation between the length of surgery and the occurrence of perioperative myocardial infarction in patients with or without prior infarctions,[24] whereas the studies from the Mayo Clinic were positive regarding the incidence of reinfarction and duration of surgery.[22,26] Similarly, in the study of Rao et al, surgery lasting longer than 4 hours increased the incidence of reinfarction in the retrospective group, but had no influence on the prospective group of patients.[21] This may reflect the advantages of intensive hemodynamic monitoring with prompt treatment of hemodynamic aberrations during prolonged surgery, which may be associated with major physiological and hemodynamic changes (see Chapter 10).

ADVANCES IN ECG DATA ACQUISITION

Lead Systems

STANDARD AND PRECORDIAL LEAD SYSTEMS

The small electric currents produced by the activity of the heart spread throughout the whole body, which behaves like a volume conductor, enabling the surface ECG to be recorded at any site on the body. Electrodes were first placed on the limbs in order to standardize the format of the ECG, and the potential differences between pairs of these electrodes became known as the *standard leads*. Knowledge of these basic leads and their polarity is helpful in understanding the further modifications made in these leads for use in the operating room and intensive care unit.

Einthoven's triangle is a hypothetical, equilateral triangle centered on the heart and formed by connecting the right arm, left arm, and left leg electrodes, such that each lead is equal to the algebraic sum of the other two leads (Fig. 7-1).[42] The three standard limb leads are the most useful leads, with many dys-

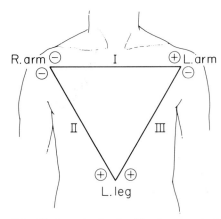

Fig. 7-1. Einthoven's triangle. The three standard leads and their electrical polarity are shown.

rhythmias, heart blocks, and episodes of ischemia being easily identified. Lead I connects the right arm and left arm electrodes; lead II, the right arm and left leg; and lead III, the left arm and left leg. The right leg electrode usually serves only as a ground. The electrodes can be placed anywhere on the extremities. The polarity of the standard leads is also shown in Figure 7-1.

The standard leads are *bipolar leads* since they record the potential difference between two electrodes. Additional information can be obtained by placing electrodes closer to the heart or around the thorax. If the three standard leads are connected through resistances of 5000 ohms each, a *common central terminal* with zero potential is obtained (Fig. 7-2). When this common electrode is used with

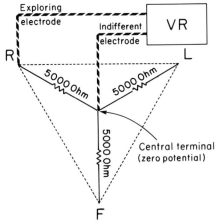

Fig. 7-2. Unipolar lead system. Wilson's unipolar VR lead.

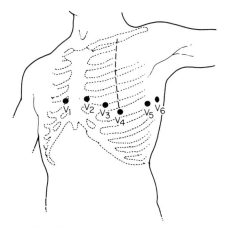

Fig. 7-3. Precordial lead placement.

another active electrode, the potential difference between them represents the actual potential. This is the basis of *unipolar* lead systems, which use a neutral electrode formed by the standard leads and an additional electrode called the *exploring* electrode. The exploring electrode theoretically gives an accurate representation of electrical activity, since it is referred to a zero potential. Unipolar leads that have proven most useful are the *precordial leads* designated by a letter V and a numeral that corresponds to the location of the electrode on the chest wall (Fig. 7-3) as follows:

V_1 just to the right of the sternum in the fourth intercostal space

V_2 just to the left of the sternum in the fourth intercostal space

V_3 midway between V_2 and V_4

V_4 in the midclavicular line in the fifth intercostal space

V_5 in the anterior axillary line in the fifth intercostal space

V_6 in the midaxillary line lateral to V_5

These leads are most useful in diagnosing rotational changes in position of the heart, ventricular hypertrophy, bundle branch blocks, and ischemia of the anterior, anteroseptal, or lateral areas of the ventricles. For detailed analysis of myocardial ischemia, complex precordial lead systems with 35 leads consisting of 5 vertical rows with 7 leads on each row have been used.[42]

Precordial leads are more sensitive than the standard leads in detecting myocardial ischemia. Blackburn has clearly shown that the most sensitive exploring electrode is at the V_5 chest position, where 89 percent of the ST-segment information contained

in a standard 12-lead ECG is found.[43] Mason et al showed that leads V_4, V_5, and V_6 were the most valuable and lead I was the least informative for diagnosing ischemia.[44] There is also good correlation between the site of coronary artery obstruction and the lead in which ischemia is detected.[45] ST-segment changes in leads II, III, and aVF correspond to disease of the right coronary artery, and changes in leads V_4, V_5, and V_6 indicate ischemia from the left anterior descending or circumflex coronary arterial trees. In 1976, based on the above information, Kaplan and King recommended that all patients with CAD should be monitored intraoperatively with a multiple-lead ECG system capable of recording at least leads V_5 and II.[46]

The multiple-lead ECG system recommended by Kaplan and King consisted of four electrodes on the extremities and a fifth electrode in the V_5 position, which allows for selection of any of seven different ECG leads (I, II, III, aVR, aVL, aVF, or V_5).[46] Leads II and V_5 are usually displayed simultaneously, allowing for observation of both inferior wall and anterolateral myocardial ischemia. Over the past decade this system has become the standard way of monitoring patients with significant CAD. The use of the unipolar precordial exploring lead (true V_5) requires a five-electrode system in order to produce the common central terminal. However, many operating room ECG monitors still have only a three-electrode system. These three-electrode systems can be adapted so that similar ECG information can be obtained by using "modified" bipolar standard limb leads.

THE MODIFIED BIPOLAR STANDARD LIMB LEADS

In order to look at one particular area of the heart more closely, several modifications of the basic three-electrode bipolar chest leads have been devised (Fig. 7-4). The nomenclature and classification of these lead systems have evolved over time and can be confusing. Table 7-2 gives the principal bipolar leads that are useful in the operating room and intensive care setting. The nomenclature of these lead systems is based on that used for the precordial leads. In the precordial lead system, the indifferent electrode is placed on the central terminal and the chest electrode is the positive exploring electrode (eg, V_5). In the modified bipolar lead system, the negative electrode is still designated as central (C) followed by its position (eg, CL for left arm). A number (suffix) indicates the position of the exploring electrode on the chest (according to the usual precordial lead posi-

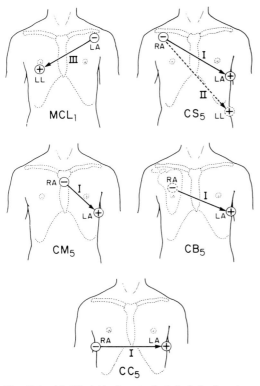

Fig. 7-4. Modified bipolar standard limb lead systems including MCL$_1$, CS$_5$, CM$_5$, CB$_5$, and CC$_5$. See text for details.

tions). The letter "M" before a given lead refers to "modified" (eg, in lead MCL$_1$ the central lead has been modified by moving it down from the left arm to beneath the left clavicle).

MCL$_1$ Lead (Modified Central Lead). This lead is obtained by placing the left arm (negative) electrode under the outer third of the left clavicle, the left leg (positive) electrode in the V$_1$ position (ie, in the fourth intercostal space to the right of the sternum), and the right arm (ground) electrode in its usual position (Fig. 7-4). Lead III is selected so that the left leg lead becomes the exploring lead. This lead gives a good P-wave deflection and QRS complex that enable rapid and accurate diagnosis of atrial dysrhythmias, conduction defects, and bundle branch blocks. Consequently, it is the lead most commonly employed in coronary care units after acute myocardial infarctions. Since dysrhythmias and conduction abnormalities may occur during anesthesia, the MCL$_1$ lead would also appear to be a useful lead to monitor in the operating room.

CS$_5$ (Central Subclavicular). This lead may be more correctly called the MCR$_5$ lead according to the classification previously described. The right arm (negative) electrode is placed under the right clavicle, the left arm (positive) electrode in the V$_5$ position, and the left leg electrode remains in the usual position to serve as the ground (Fig. 7-4). Lead I is then selected. One particular advantage of the CS$_5$ lead is that lead II can also be monitored using the

Table 7-2
Bipolar Leads for Use with Three Electrodes

Lead System	MCL$_1$	CS$_5$	CM$_5$	CB$_5$	CC$_5$
RA electrode	Ground	Under right clavicle (−) (subclavicular)	Manubrium sternum (−)	Center of right scapula (−)	Right anterior axillary line (V$_5$R) (−)
LA electrode	Under left clavicle	V$_5$ (+)	V$_5$ (+)	V$_5$ (+)	V$_5$ (+)
LL electrode	V$_1$ (+)	Ground	Ground	Ground	Ground
Lead selected	III	I	I	I	I
Advantages and indications	Good P wave and QRS complex. Useful for diagnosis of dysrhythmias.	Monitoring for anterior ischemia.	Monitoring for anterior ischemia.	Monitoring for anterior ischemia. Good P wave for diagnosis of dysrhythmias.	Monitoring for ischemia.

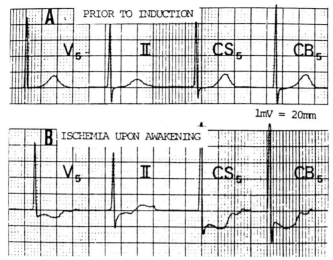

Fig. 7-5. (A) ECG prior to induction. Anterolateral myocardial ischemia upon awakening from anesthesia is shown in (B). Leads CS$_5$ and CB$_5$ show larger ventricular deflections and ST-segment depression than the true V$_5$. (From Griffin RM, Kaplan JA: Comparison of ECG leads V$_5$, CS$_5$, CB$_5$, and II by computerized ST-segment analysis. Anesth Analg 65:S65, 1986, with permission.)

same configuration of electrodes since the left leg electrode is in its usual position. This allows the inferior wall of the heart to be periodically monitored for the development of ischemia, as well as using lead II for dysrhythmia detection.

CM$_5$ (Central Manubrium Lead). This lead is obtained by placing the negative right arm electrode on the manubrium of the sternum, the positive left arm lead in the V$_5$ position, and the ground (left leg) electrode in the left leg position. This lead essentially looks at the same vector as the CS$_5$ lead and provides similar information on ischemia.

CB$_5$ (Central Back Lead). The right arm (negative) electrode is placed over the center of the right scapula and the left arm (positive) electrode is placed in the V$_5$ position. The vector monitored by this lead is in the same direction as that monitored by a true V$_5$ lead (ie, downward, leftward, and anterior). The P wave may not be seen on the true V$_5$ lead, since a certain proportion of the atria may lie to the right or posterior of the origin of the V$_5$ vector. However, the CB$_5$ lead, since it originates to the right and back of the atrium, produces a good P-wave deflection in addition to providing a similar QRS complex to the V$_5$ lead for detection of ischemia. A recent study comparing CB$_5$ and V$_5$ leads in patients with closed and open chests demonstrated a good correlation

between ventricular deflections in both leads.[47] The ventricular deflection was 20 percent larger in the CB$_5$ lead, and, more significantly, the P wave was 90 percent larger. Therefore, with this one lead, monitoring for supraventricular dysrhythmias and ischemia can be obtained. This may be useful in certain patients with ischemic heart disease who may be especially prone to develop dysrhythmias in the perioperative period (Fig. 7-5).[31]

CC$_5$ Lead. The right arm (negative) electrode is placed in the right anterior axillary line over the fifth interspace, and the left arm (positive) electrode in the usual V$_5$ position. Lead I is selected.

INVASIVE ELECTROCARDIOGRAPHIC
MONITORING

In addition to recording the electrical potentials of the heart from the surface of the body, they may also be obtained from body cavities adjacent to the heart (ie, the esophagus and trachea) or from within the heart itself. This type of ECG monitoring is useful in the anesthetized patient, and each particular type of monitoring produces an ECG complex with certain advantages for the diagnosis of dysrhythmias or ischemia. Furthermore, these ECG leads are less prone to signal distortion by patient movement, baseline drift, and the electrocautery; however, inevitably, invasive monitoring is associated with some morbidity.

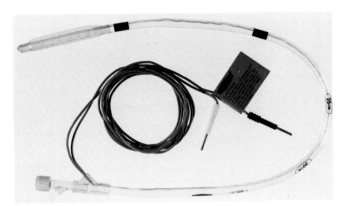

Fig. 7-6. The Portex Cardioesophagoscope® (Wilmington, MA) is shown. The esophageal leads are made of plastic. The ECG wires are attached to the right and left arm electrode sites of the ECG monitor (lead I).

The Esophageal ECG

The concept of placing an electrode in the esophagus, adjacent to the heart, in order to monitor the ECG is certainly not new. Cremer, in 1906, passed a 10 × 15 cm electrode into the esophagus of a professional sword swallower. Since then, numerous studies have confirmed the value of the esophageal lead in nonsurgical patients to facilitate the diagnosis of complex dysrhythmias.[48-50] The principal advantage of the esophageal ECG (EsECG) compared to the surface leads is the ability to record a prominent P wave, and, therefore, identify the presence of atrial depolarization and its temporal relationship to ventricular activity. In addition, the EsECG has been shown to be a useful monitor of posterior ischemia due to its close anatomical location to the posterior aspect of the left ventricle.

The EsECG may be monitored either as a unipolar or bipolar lead. The bipolar lead is more commonly employed since the P:QRS ratio is greater (ie, there is greater augmentation of the P wave).[50] Interpretation of the EsECG in isolation from other surface leads may be difficult, since the P wave may be larger, equal to, or smaller than the QRS complex, and is sometimes difficult to distinguish from the QRS complex.[49]

A disposable EsECG electrode has recently become available that is suitable for use during anesthesia, in the recovery room, or in the intensive care unit. This EsECG monitor consists of an 18-Fr esophageal stethoscope with two external electrodes 7 and 20 cm from the distal end. The wires from the electrodes are extruded through the wall of the stethoscope and welded to conventional ECG lead wires at the proximal ends (Fig. 7-6). To observe a bipolar EsECG, the leads are connected to the right and left arm terminals and lead I is selected on the monitor. A typical EsECG tracing is shown in Figure 7-7; lead V_5 is shown for comparison. To minimize the risk of electrocution or esophageal burn injury, strict electrical safety precautions must be followed. All ECG monitoring equipment should be incapable of delivering more than 10 μamps of leakage current to the patient. In addition, when electrocautery is used, a properly applied groundplate of sufficient surface area should be used; and, as an extra precaution, an electrocautery protection filter capable of filtering

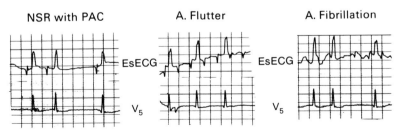

Fig. 7-7. Progression from a normal sinus rhythm (NSR) to atrial flutter and atrial fibrillation is easily observed on the EsECG but not on lead V_5.

Table 7-3

Comparison of Esophageal ECG and Standard ECG for Correct Diagnosis
of Dysrhythmias

Dysrhythmia	Correct Diagnosis			
	No.	*V₅*	*II*	*Esophageal*
Sinus bradycardia	4	4	4	4
Sinus tachycardia	1	1	1	1
1° heart block	1	0	0	1
2° heart block	2	0	0	2
3° heart block	4	0	1	4
Frequent premature ventricular contractions	2	2	2	2
Frequent premature atrial contractions	5	2	3	5
Atrial flutter	2	0	0	2
Atrial fibrillation	3	2	2	3
Paroxysmal atrial tachycardia	1	0	0	1
Nodal rhythm	1	0	0	1
% correct	—	42.3	53.8	100

Source: Kates RA, Zaidan JR, Kaplan JA: Esophageal lead for intraoperative electrocardiographic monitoring. Anesth Analg 61:781, 1982, with permission.

radio frequencies greater than 20 kHz can be inserted between the ECG cable and the esophageal lead.

Kates et al, in a study of 20 patients undergoing CABG, compared the EsECG with standard lead II, precordial lead V₅, and an intra-atrial electrogram obtained with a multipurpose PAC that served as the gold standard for the definite diagnosis of dysrhythmias.[51] The correct diagnosis was made from leads II and V₅ in 53.8 percent and 42.3 percent of cases, respectively; whereas the esophageal lead correctly diagnosed 100 percent of the dysrhythmias that occurred (Table 7-3). The study clearly demonstrated that dysrhythmias may be missed or incorrectly diagnosed if only surface leads II or V₅ are employed (Fig. 7-8). Since leads MCL₁ and CB₅ give a more prominent P wave than leads II and V₅, comparative

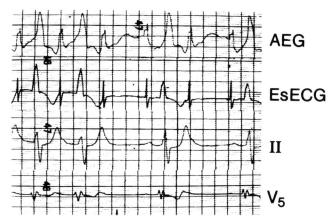

Fig. 7-8. Four ECG leads are demonstrated in a patient after CPB. AEG = atrial electrogram. The patient progressed from a normal sinus rhythm with a first-degree heart block to a Mobitz type II block. The type of bradycardia was misdiagnosed from leads II and V₅ as a sinus bradycardia, while the AEG and EsECG show the heart block. (From Kates RA, Zaidan JR, Kaplan JA: Esophageal lead for intraoperative electrocardiographic monitoring. Anesth Analg 61:781, 1982, with permission.)

studies of these leads with the esophageal lead are needed to confirm the value of EsECG monitoring over all of the conventional surface leads for diagnosing dysrhythmias.

There have been only a relatively small number of patients monitored with an EsECG, but so far there are no reports of postoperative symptoms related to the use of this monitor. In sum, the esophageal ECG appears to be a simple, safe method of monitoring the anesthetized patient, and should be used in more cases, especially when there is a high risk of developing dysrhythmias.

Intracardiac Electrograms

Recording of electrical potentials from within the heart itself produces prominent atrial (P wave) and ventricular (QRS complex) signals that allow for interpretation of complex dysrhythmias. Although more invasive than the EsECG, there is less baseline wandering with the intracardiac electrogram. The techniques available for recording the intra-atrial and intraventricular ECG are discussed below.

SALINE-FILLED CARDIAC CATHETER

In 1949, Hellerstein et al described a method of obtaining intracavitary potentials with a single-lumen catheter.[52] The catheter was passed into the heart while connected to a heparinized saline drip, and a simple electrode was then passed 2 to 4 cm into the proximal end of the catheter and connected to the exploring lead of the ECG. The saline acted as a conductor to transmit the electrical potentials to the ECG electrode. The potentials obtained from the "saline electrode" were identical in form to those obtained simultaneously from a wire electrode inserted into the right ventricle. However, the amplitude of the complexes obtained with the wire electrode was greater than those with saline due to the greater resistance of saline or blood, and alternating current interference was a frequent problem that could not be completely overcome. Use of hypertonic saline has been shown to provide a better electrode and may be used to locate the distal end of a ventricular-atrial shunt for hydrocephalus.[53]

The saline-filled electrode has also been used to locate a catheter in the right atrium or superior vena cava to facilitate aspiration of air during procedures where there is a high risk of air embolism.[54] Thus, the principal uses of the saline-filled electrode have been to locate probes in the heart on a short- or long-term basis for diagnostic or therapeutic purposes.

Use of the electrode as an ECG monitor is limited by susceptibility to artifact and electrical interference.

INTRAVASCULAR WIRE ELECTRODE

Indications for use of an intravascular wire electrode are essentially similar to those for the saline-filled catheter electrode. The wire electrode may be inserted percutaneously via any of the usual venipuncture sites. Richards and Freeman first described the use of a metal stylette inserted into the intracardiac tubing of a Holter valve shunt to form a rigid probe and locate the tip in the atrium.[55] A bipolar lead II was recorded from the intracardiac electrode by connecting the proximal end of the metal stylette to the right arm terminal via an alligator clip and a length of sterile wire. More recently, a J-tipped wire guide has been used as the intravascular ECG lead to position a catheter tip in the right atrium.[56] The increased rigidity of the wire/catheter combination, compared with the saline-filled electrode, results in less artifact caused by "catheter whipping" during insertion. Moreover, the wire guide has a lower electrical resistance and is, therefore, less sensitive to AC interference.

MULTIPURPOSE PAC

Chatterjee et al first described the use of a modified balloon-tipped flotation catheter for recording intracavitary electrograms.[57] They used a standard 7F PAC with two pairs of electrodes situated 17 to 18 cm and 28 to 29 cm from the catheter tip for the ventricular and atrial electrodes, respectively. The wires from the electrodes were insulated and conveyed via a third lumen of the catheter to its proximal end. The atrial and ventricular electrograms were recorded as bipolar leads by attaching the electrode wires to the arm leads and selecting lead I. With the catheter tip properly located in the pulmonary artery, the proximal and distal pairs of electrodes should come to lie in the upper atrium and right ventricle, respectively. In a series of 43 patients with various cardiac diagnoses, stable tracings were obtained that greatly facilitated the diagnosis of complex dysrhythmias. When necessary, atrial, ventricular, or A-V sequential pacing was promptly initiated.[57] Mantle et al modified the thermistor-tipped PAC to incorporate two electrodes at 25 and 26 cm from the tip of the catheter to record the intra-atrial electrogram.[58] The catheter was found to be useful for the diagnosis and treatment of dysrhythmias in 30 patients with serious cardiac disease. On the average, the catheter was left in place for 3 days without the development of serious complications.

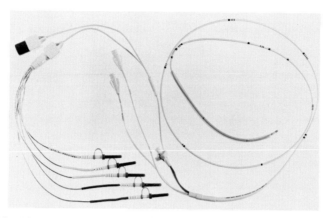

Fig. 7-9. The multipurpose pacing PAC. Three atrial and two ventricular electrodes can be seen.

The multipurpose PAC that is presently available has five electrodes: two intraventricular electrodes situated 18.5 and 19.5 cm from the distal end, and three intra-atrial electrodes situated 28.5, 31.0, and 33.5 cm from the distal end (Fig. 7-9). Incorporation of a third intra-atrial electrode has enabled the electrodes to be properly positioned in heart chambers and great vessels of varying sizes. The multipurpose PAC provides comprehensive hemodynamic monitoring (pulmonary artery pressure, wedge pressure, central venous pressure, and cardiac output); stable intra-atrial (Fig. 7-8) and intraventricular electrogram monitoring; and the capability of atrial, A-V sequential, or ventricular pacing, if necessary.

The ease of insertion and pacing capabilities of the catheter were evaluated in a series of 30 patients undergoing cardiac surgery.[59] The catheter was easily inserted and A-V sequential pacing was successful in approximately 70 percent of the patients. The high-fidelity tracings obtained from intracardiac electrodes are particularly suitable for computer analysis and reliable, consistent operation of any device requiring QRS triggering mechanisms (eg, the intraventricular electrogram provides a large voltage spike which can be used for triggering an intra-aortic balloon pump).[60] The application of the multipurpose pacing catheter, however, should not be limited to cardiac surgical patients, and should be considered whenever critically ill patients with serious cardiac disease present for noncardiac surgery.

The Endotracheal ECG

The endotracheal ECG provides a route for monitoring the ECG in situations in which it is difficult or impossible to use surface ECG leads. The esophageal ECG can play a similar role, but may not be acceptable in small infants. The endotracheal ECG comprises a standard endotracheal tube with distal (1.2 cm long) and proximal (6 cm long) electrodes shrunk onto the exterior of the tube (Fig. 7-10).[61] The electrodes are connected in a teflon-coated wire, through 47,000 ohms resistance, to a battery-powered ECG with an isolated preamplifier that is shown to conform to the current recommended electrical safety standards. Endotracheal ECG tracings were obtained from three pediatric patients and compared to lead II tracings (Fig. 7-11). An inverted QRS complex was obtained with a low-amplitude P wave compared to

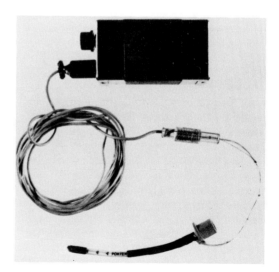

Fig. 7-10. Endotracheal ECG system using a 3.5-mm endotracheal tube. (From Mylrea KC, Calkins JM, Carlson J, et al: ECG lead with the endotracheal tube. Crit Care Med 11:199, 1983, with permission.)

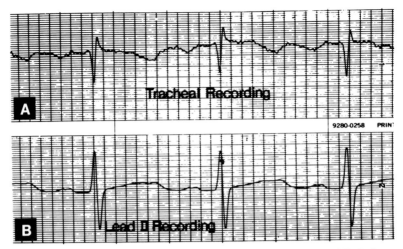

Fig. 7-11. Endotracheal ECG recording (A) compared to a standard lead II (B) in an infant. (From Mylrea KC, Calkins JM, Carlson J, et al: ECG lead with the endotracheal tube. Crit Care Med 11:199, 1983, with permission.)

lead II. Alternating current interference was a major problem that could be improved by use of a reference electrode (a two-electrode system was used for simplicity), improved common mode rejection in the amplifier, and better matching of input impedances. Position and movement of the tube also were critical factors in the quality of the signal.

The endotracheal ECG offers advantages for monitoring small infants where surface electrodes cannot be used (eg, with certain surgical sites, following extensive trauma or burns, and in long-term critical care where surface electrodes may cause skin irritation or hamper temperature maintenance).

ELECTROCARDIOGRAPHIC LEAD SYSTEMS FOR THE DETECTION OF ISCHEMIA

It has long been known that the precordial leads are superior to the standard leads for the detection of myocardial ischemia.[62,63] With the development of the exercise ECG test for the detection of latent coronary insufficiency, many lead systems were introduced for simplicity and good performance during muscular effort. Blackburn et al, in a comparative study of different chest lead configurations, found that for the detection of ischemia the most sensitive exploring electrode position was at the V_5 position.[64] Furthermore, of all the lead configurations tested, the CM_5 lead was superior for the detection of significant ischemia and least affected by variations in body build, electrical frontal plane position, and noise. However, these results were not confirmed in another study of postexercise ECG testing utilizing visual

and computerized techniques.[65] ST-segment depression and slope were compared using standard lead V_5 and the bipolar leads CM_5 and CC_5 in two groups of subjects, one with known CAD and one without. Lead CM_5 was found to be less sensitive than V_5 for the detection of ischemia, and lead CC_5 was more comparable to V_5. Both bipolar leads were less affected by noise than standard lead V_5 (see Chapter 10).

Dalton reported use of lead V_5 monitoring during cardiac surgery by attaching the exploring precordial lead to a sterile spinal needle inserted subcutaneously following skin preparation.[66] Kaplan and King first demonstrated the value of monitoring lead V_5 with a modern multilead system during both cardiac and noncardiac surgery.[46] They were able to monitor leads I, II, III, aVR, aVL, aVF, and V_5 using a five-wire system, and demonstrated that significant ST-segment depression in V_5 could occur in the absence of any changes in the standard leads.

In 1979, Kaplan recommended that a five-electrode ECG system should be used during all cardiac surgery.[42] In this system, four disposable ECG pads are placed on the extremities, with a fifth placed in the V_5 position covered with Steri-drape (3M, St. Paul, MN). The electrodes are positioned before the induction of anesthesia, and the V_5 electrode is included in the skin preparation without detrimental effect on the ECG tracing. Standard and augmented limb leads can be displayed in addition to lead V_5 using an ECG monitor with a lead selector switch. Prior to surgery, all seven leads are displayed and

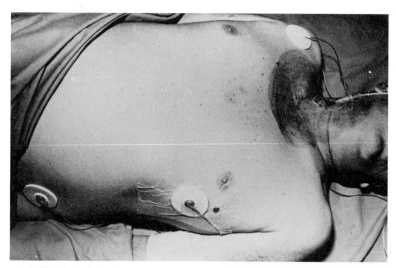

Fig. 7-12. The CS_5 lead arrangement is demonstrated. Standard lead I should be selected to monitor a modified V_5 lead.

recorded to serve as a baseline reference. During induction of anesthesia and surgery, leads II and V_5 can be displayed simultaneously in order to monitor anterior and inferior ischemic changes, respectively.

Many operating room ECG monitors are equipped with a three-electrode system, and, therefore, are unable to monitor a true lead V_5. Modified bipolar leads CM_5 or CS_5 can be employed in this case (Fig. 7-12). Although the comparability of ST-segment changes obtained with various bipolar leads and those recorded with a true V_5 lead during stress testing is disputed, any of these leads is satisfactory during anesthesia (Fig. 7-5).[31,64,65]

Blackburn showed that 89 percent of significant ST-segment depression following exercise was found in precordial lead V_5 of a 12-lead ECG.[64,67] Furthermore, he and his colleagues showed that 100 percent of the ST-segment changes could be detected by recording leads II, aVF, and anterior precordial leads V_3 to V_6. Mason et al demonstrated the value of multiple-lead ECG recording during and after exercise.[68] Nineteen of 67 patients with angina showed a positive test in only one lead. Overall, 30 patients showed anterior ischemia (leads I and V_3 to V_6) and 8 showed inferior ischemia (leads II, III, and aVF). Multiple-lead ECGs are usually not used during anesthesia for routine monitoring since the anesthesiologist may not be able to assimilate the amount of information provided by the continuous simultaneous display of 12 ECG leads. Nonetheless, especially in high-risk cases, the anterior, inferior, and posterior surfaces of the heart should be monitored for the

development of ischemia. The inferior surface of the heart overlies the diaphragm and ischemia is seen in leads II, III, and aVF. Lead II is most often used to detect inferior ischemia, which may remain undetected if only anterior leads are employed,[68,69] since it is also helpful in detecting rhythm problems.

True posterior ischemia may not be detected by leads looking at the inferior or the anterolateral surfaces of the heart. Anatomically, the posterior wall of the left ventricle lies adjacent to the esophagus. An esophageal ECG inserted 40 to 50 cm into the esophagus will reflect the electrical potential of the posterior surface of the heart, and, therefore, may be used for the detection of posterior myocardial ischemia and infarction.[70] The esophageal ECG lead is suitable for use in the anesthetized patient, and Kates et al demonstrated its value in patients undergoing CABG.[51] In their study, a patient with posterior ischemia developed significant ST-segment elevation on the esophageal ECG, but not in leads II and V_5 (Fig. 7-13).

Acute myocardial ischemia and infarction are not confined to the left ventricle. Right ventricular infarction may occur in isolation, or, more frequently, along with inferoposterior infarction of the left ventricle (see Chapter 27). Cohn et al described the hemodynamic consequences of right ventricular infarction along with acute left ventricular inferior wall infarction.[71] Six patients developed hypotension, engorged neck veins, and heart block; and hemodynamic measurements disclosed that right ventricular filling pressure equalled or exceeded left

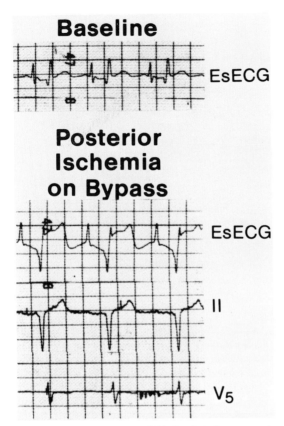

Fig. 7-13. Posterior myocardial ischemia is demonstrated on the EsECG lead during CPB. This occurred after rewarming to normothermia, but prior to complete revascularization of the posterior wall of the heart. (From Kates RA, Zaidan JR, Kaplan JA: Esophageal lead for intraoperative electrocardiographic monitoring. Anesth Analg 61:781, 1982, with permission.)

ventricular end-diastolic pressure (LVEDP). However, these clinical and hemodynamic findings are variable and their time of onset unpredictable. The diagnosis can be confirmed by techniques to detect right ventricular dilatation, dysfunction, and necrosis. These diagnostic criteria are time-consuming, however, and right ventricular infarction may rapidly lead to serious hemodynamic dysfunction. Erhardt et al, having previously found a 43 percent incidence of right ventricular infarction in an autopsy study, first proposed the use of a right-sided precordial lead for early diagnosis.[72] Subsequently, Klein et al used lead V_4R in conjunction with clinical and laboratory criteria to diagnose right ventricular infarctions in a series of 110 patients presenting with acute inferior myocardial infarctions.[73] Right ventricular infarctions were detected in 58 patients (52.7 percent), of

whom 82.7 percent developed ST-segment elevation. The V_4R lead (the unipolar precordial exploring electrode is placed in the *right* midclavicular line in the fifth intercostal space and the V lead is selected) had a reasonably high sensitivity, specificity, and predictive value for right ventricular infarction and ischemia. Although its use has not been reported during anesthesia, the V_4R lead may prove beneficial for monitoring those patients with previous inferior infarction or with right-sided occlusive disease on coronary arteriography.

During anesthesia, Trager et al demonstrated the value of the EsECG in diagnosing right ventricular ischemia.[74] ST-segment depression in the EsECG lead was found in conjunction with the development of V waves in the right atrial pressure tracing, while no changes occurred in lead II or the wedge pressure (Fig. 7-14), in a patient with severe right coronary artery obstruction. It has been previously noted that in some patients there is a marked similarity between the EsECG and right ventricular cavitary recordings. The proposed mechanisms are (1) the proximity of the right ventricle to the esophagus, or (2) the conduction of right ventricular electrical potentials through the inferior vena cava or right atrium to the esophagus.[70]

Monitoring and Recording the ECG

The function of the ECG monitor is to detect, amplify, display, and record the ECG signal. The changes of potential produced by the heart between two electrodes is on the order of 1 mV and has a rapid time course (normal QRS complex is less than 0.12 seconds). Moreover, the skin has a potential of 20 mV with a slow time base and must be separated from the ECG signal. The ECG monitor is essentially an amplifier capable of separating these signals and then amplifying the power of the ECG signal, thereby enabling an output signal to drive a recording or display system. The ECG is usually displayed on an oscilloscope, and several monitors now offer nonfade storage oscilloscopes. These offer no advantages over the use of direct-writing recorders which enable accurate interpretation of difficult ECGs and provide a written record for the patient's chart. The capability of recording the ECG on paper should be available in every cardiac surgical operating room. Different recording methods, however, have to be considered if an attempt is made to collect information on cardiac electrical activity over prolonged periods of time.

Holter monitoring has been utilized by a number

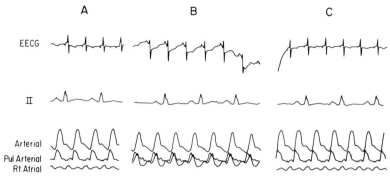

Fig. 7-14. Baseline tracings (A). The ischemic event is shown in (B) with marked J-point depression, 2 mm ST-segment depression, and loss of R-wave amplitude in the EsECG lead. This was associated with a drop in systemic and pulmonary artery pressures, and an increase in the right atrial pressure with the appearance of V waves. Resolution of the ischemia occurred when the blood pressure was increased (C). (From Trager M, Feinberg BI, Kaplan JA: Right ventricular ischemia diagnosed by an esophageal electrocardiogram and right atrial pressure tracing. J Cardiothorac Anesth, in press, with permission.)

of investigators to document the perioperative incidence of dysrhythmias and ischemia. In Holter monitoring, ECG information from one or two bipolar leads is recorded by a miniature magnetic tape recorder (Fig. 7-15). Up to 48 hours of ECG signals can be collected. Subsequently, the tape is processed by a playback system and the ECG signals are analyzed. On most modern systems the playback unit includes a dedicated computer for rapid analysis of the data and automatic recognition of dysrhythmias.

Michelson et al, studying 70 patients undergoing cardiac surgery, obtained 24-hour continuous ECG recordings on the day before surgery and on the first and fifth days after discharge from the surgical intensive care unit.[75] New dysrhythmias were recognized in 52 percent of the patients undergoing CABG, and in 40 percent of those undergoing valve replacement. While ventricular dysrhythmias were uncommon preoperatively in both groups, they occurred frequently after CABG (36 percent). In a similar study, de Soyza et al examined 57 patients with Holter monitors on the day before CABG and 3 months after the surgery.[76] They could not establish a significant difference in the number of patients who had dysrhythmias before or after surgery.

More recently, Dewar et al studied 52 patients undergoing cardiac surgery with a Holter monitor adapted for intraoperative use.[77] Their results show a high incidence of various dysrhythmias during induction of anesthesia and thoracotomy for cardiac surgery. They further demonstrated a high incidence of continued atrial activity during cardioplegia and a lack of correlation between peak serum CPK-MB levels and dysrhythmias. Valve replacement patients tended to have a higher overall incidence of dysrhythmias.

Although one of Holter's initial publications described the recording of ST-T changes during an anginal attack, the use of this method for the recording of ischemic changes has not been widely applied.[78] Particularly in the early days of Holter monitoring, a number of authors voiced their concern about the reliability of this technique for the recognition of ST-segment changes.[79,80] One of the reasons was that on early instruments narrow band-width recordings were utilized to eliminate artifacts and to provide a stable baseline. As ST-segment changes often have a low frequency, the narrow band-width that stabilized the baseline produced considerable ST-segment distortion. The introduction of frequency modulated (FM) recording systems partially solved this problem. Balasubramanian et al, comparing various recording systems, demonstrated that FM recorders were able to accurately detect ST-segment changes at rest and during exercise.[81]

Bragg-Remschel et al studied the frequency response characteristics of ambulatory ECG recording equipment from eight manufacturers.[82] They established that none of the systems fully met the American Heart Association low-frequency and high-frequency response values, and that only three systems were able to accurately reproduce the actual degree of ST depression, as well as provide flat ST-segment depression. Even FM systems did not

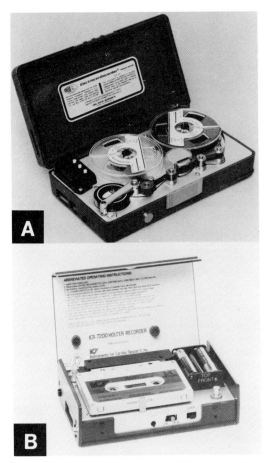

Fig. 7-15. Modern Holter recorders. (A) Reel-to-reel type with rechargeable battery. (B) Cassette type with alkaline disposable battery. (From HL Kennedy: Ambulatory Electrocardiography Including Holter Recording Technology. Philadelphia, Lea-Febiger, 1981, with permission.)

always faithfully reproduce the ST segment. Tzivoni et al have recently compared ECG findings recorded simultaneously by two-lead Holter and 12-lead ECGs in 144 patients undergoing a Bruce protocol treadmill exercise test.[83] The two exploring electrodes of the Holter system were attached to the V_3 and V_5 positions, while the two negative electrodes were placed at the right side of the upper sternum. They found that in 96 percent of the patients the results of the two recording techniques were concordant and concluded that V_3, V_4, and V_5 Holter recordings were as accurate as 12-lead ECG systems for the detection of ischemic changes during exercise.

Intraoperatively, Coleman and Jordan obtained continuous ECG recordings from 36 healthy patients undergoing elective general surgical procedures.[38]

They observed ST-segment changes around the time of induction and intubation in six of these patients, while two others exhibited ST-segment changes at the end of surgery. Coriat et al, studying 51 patients with ischemic heart disease undergoing vascular surgery, recorded ST-segment changes in 20 of these patients.[32] The Holter recording was started 30 minutes before induction of anesthesia and lasted 24 hours. In 11 of the cases, the ischemic changes occurred during induction; while in two cases they first appeared 2 hours after extubation.

In a different study, but with a similar group of patients, Coriat et al further observed that continuous administration of nitroglycerin (NTG) did not prevent a high incidence of myocardial ischemia.[84] They continuously monitored lead CM_5 for 24 hours and defined as an ischemic episode ST-segment depression greater than 1 mm lasting for more than 10 beats. Ischemic changes occurred in 18 of the 45 patients, but in only 8 of these episodes were the changes detected by the anesthesiologist. Thomson et al used Holter monitoring of leads II and CS_5 to study ischemic changes in 20 patients undergoing CABG.[85] They also observed a high incidence of myocardial ischemia and were unable to demonstrate a reduction in ischemic episodes with the prophylactic administration of NTG.

Artifacts Affecting the ECG in the Operating Room

Electrocardiographic monitoring in the operating room is subject to many types of interference that may prevent reliable interpretation. Artifacts simulating dysrhythmias may occur and even lead to inappropriate therapeutic intervention. Some of the artifacts produced are common to ECG monitoring outside of the operating room, whereas others are problems unique to the operating room environment.

1. Artifacts related to the patient:
   a. Muscle tremor produces a characteristic fine fibrillatory pattern on the ECG. It may be evident in anxious patients prior to induction of anesthesia, and also in the awake, shivering patient on emergence from anesthesia.
   b. Movement of the patient may cause sudden changes in potential differences between the electrodes or disturb the electrode contacts.
   c. Hiccoughing and movements of the diaphragm.
   d. Respiratory-induced variations in the electrical axis may be produced during spontaneous or controlled ventilation.

e. Assumption of the lateral or Trendelenburg position may cause axis deviations.

2. Artifacts related to the lead systems and ECG monitoring equipment:

a. Loose electrodes and broken leads may produce a variety of artifacts that may simulate dysrhythmias, Q waves, or inverted T waves.[86] Pregelled, disposable silver/silver chloride electrodes are usually used in the operating room. It is important that all the electrodes be moist, uniform, and not out of date. To ensure good contact between the electrode and the skin, the electrical resistance of the skin should be minimized (ie, rubbed with alcohol) and excess body hair removed. Some ECG monitors have built-in cable testers that enable a lead to be tested by plugging in the distal end. A high resistance causes a large voltage drop indicating that the lead is faulty.

b. Abnormal waveforms may be produced due to incorrect placement of the leads. If the right and left arm leads are reversed, a mirror image of the normal lead I will be produced and leads II and III will be reversed.

c. A simple fault in the ECG monitor, such as weak batteries, may simulate a dysrhythmia.[87]

3. Artifacts produced by external sources of interference:

a. During CPB the roller pumps can produce an artifactual trace resembling atrial flutter. Automatic infusion pumps may cause similar problems.

b. Direct contact with the patient by other operating room personnel.

4. Electrical interference:

a. Electrocautery is the most important source of interference on the ECG in the operating room, since usually the electrocautery completely obliterates the ECG tracing. Analysis of the electrocautery has identified three component frequencies.[88] The *radiofrequency* between 800 kHz and 2000 kHz comprises most of the interference, coupled with 60 Hz *AC frequency* and 0.1 to 10 Hz *low frequency* noise from intermittent contact of the electrosurgical unit with the patient's tissue. Preamplifiers may be modified to suppress radiofrequency interference, but these filter circuits are still not widely available in the operating room.

b. All equipment in the operating room should be properly grounded, otherwise 60 Hz alternating current can produce gross interference.

ADVANCES IN ECG ANALYSIS

Automatic Dysrhythmia Detection

There is little doubt that during prolonged visual observation of the ECG on an oscilloscope, certain dysrhythmias will go undetected. This was clearly demonstrated by Romhilt et al who showed that coronary care unit nurses failed to detect serious ventricular dysrhythmias in 84 percent of their patients.[89] In a similar study, Holmberg et al found that in their coronary care unit the detection rate for ventricular tachycardia was as low as 42 percent.[90]

Various computers have been designed for the automatic detection of dysrhythmias to increase the detection of abnormal rhythms. An early method to sample the ECG in a form suitable for continuous real-time analysis was a preprocessing algorithm called AZTEC.[91] The system utilized measurements of QRS width, offset, amplitude, and area to classify complexes in morphologic families. In one study the computer accurately detected 78 percent of ventricular ectopic beats.[92] Utilizing a slightly modified version of the AZTEC system, Yanowitz et al increased the accuracy for the detection of PVCs to 90 percent.[93]

Other systems have depended on QRS recognition and cross-correlation with stored QRS complexes.[94,95] In cross-correlation, each detected QRS complex is compared with a list of previously detected complexes. If a complex does not correlate better than 0.9 with a previously stored complex it is considered to have a new configuration and is added to the list. A number of points of the complex, such as the PR interval and ST segment, are stored as a template for future comparison (Fig. 7-16).[96] Whenever a new complex matches an existing template, it is averaged into that template so that each template represents a running average of all complexes of a particular configuration. Each template is defined as normal, abnormal, or questionable according to previously defined criteria. In a prospective evaluation of such a system, Shah et al found that the computer accurately detected 95.4 percent of ventricular premature beats, but only 82.4 percent of supraventricular premature beats.[95]

In the analysis of Holter recordings, similar templates are utilized to differentiate among various

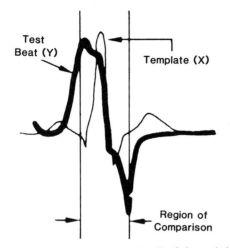

Fig. 7-16. Computerized "template" of the underlying normal QRS complex (X) and an ectopic complex termed a "test beat" (Y). Beat Y is matched to beat X by the computer during the region of comparison by cross-correlation algorithms. (From Morganroth J: Ambulatory Holter electrocardiography. Ann Int Med 102:73, 1985, with permission.)

types of QRS complexes. More recently, cross-correlation has also been applied to P-wave patterns, so that not only abnormal QRS shapes, but also abnormal P-wave shapes, can be recognized. The P-wave recognition allows accurate definition of the RR, PP, and PR intervals and enables reliable detection of a wide variety of dysrhythmias.[97]

Analysis of the ST Segment

The patterns of ST-segment change that fulfill the criteria of myocardial ischemia have been extensively studied in subjects with and without CAD undergoing exercise stress testing in the laboratory. Since anesthesia and surgery may be regarded as a potentially stressful situation, these criteria may be applied to anesthetized patients.

For the accurate diagnosis of ischemia, a knowledge of the normal morphology of the ST segment and the response to exercise is essential. A normal, resting ECG complex is shown in Figure 7-17A. The J point is the junction between the S wave and the ST segment. Exercise causes a downward displacement of the J point, such that the baseline is depressed below the isoelectric line in the resting tracing (Fig. 7-17B). The ST segment normally becomes up-sloping, slightly concave, and returns to the baseline (PR junction) within 0.04 to 0.06 seconds after the J point. J-point depression with an up-sloping ST segment may also be the earliest indication of myocardial ischemia. This is differentiated from the normal J-point depression produced with exercise by the degree of upsloping of the ST segment (Fig. 7-18). Salzman et al attempted to quantify J-point slope and suggested that a J-point slope of 30° above horizontal was probably not indicative of ischemia.[98] Stuart and Ellestad concluded that an up-sloping ST segment was indicative of ischemia if the ST segment was depressed at least 2.0 mm below the baseline of the PR segment at 0.08 seconds from the J point (Fig. 7-19).[99] With ongoing ischemia, the J-point depression evolves into progressive horizontal depression

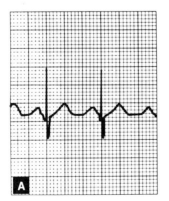
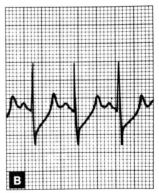

Fig. 7-17. Normal resting ECG complex (A), and an exercise ECG tracing showing depression of the J point and an up-sloping ST segment (B). (From Ellestad MH: Stress Testing: Principles and Practice. Philadelphia, F.A. Davis, 1975, with permission.)

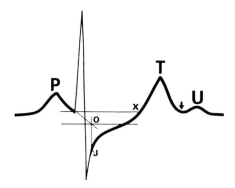

Fig. 7-18. Methods of measuring true and false ST-segment depression and the degree of horizontality of the ST segment. The line of the sloping PR segment is continued until it meets, at point O, a vertical line drawn from the junction of the QRS complex and ST segment (J point). The distance O-J indicates the true amount of ST-segment depression. (From Schamroth L: The ECG of Coronary Artery Disease. Oxford, Blackwell, 1984, with permission.)

of the ST segment (Fig. 7-20). Significant myocardial ischemia is present when there is greater than 1 mm of ST-segment depression measured 0.06 seconds from the J point.[100] The ST-segment depression may be convex in form or down-sloping. The magnitude of ST-segment depression correlates with the amount of myocardium involved and the extent to which it is made ischemic.[100,101]

There is also a relationship between the severity of CAD and the ST-segment configuration induced by exercise. Robb and Marks were able to demonstrate an increased mortality and worse prognosis for patients with downsloping ST-segment depression as compared with horizontal depression.[102] Goldshlager et al compared ST-segment depression with extent of disease as demonstrated by coronary angiography and found a correlation between downsloping ST-segment depression and increasing number of diseased vessels.[103] Down-sloping ST-segment depression represents profound myocardial ischemia and possibly even transmural ischemia. ST-segment elevation greater than 1 mm is also indicative of severe, transmural ischemia.

ST-segment changes have been reported in normal subjects. Armstrong et al, using ambulatory ECG monitoring in 50 normal males, demonstrated a 30 percent incidence of transient ST-segment depression.[104] Posture and positional changes can also affect the ST segment.[105] Patients with nonspecific T-wave abnormalities in their resting ECG may develop ST-segment depression while standing or with hyperventilation.[106] Intermittent ST-segment depression associated with respiration has been observed during stress testing in apparently normal subjects, and may be a preliminary finding to the subsequent development of classical ischemia. Elles-

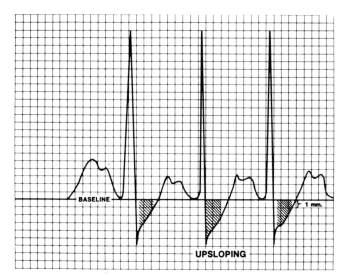

Fig. 7-19. Up-sloping ST-segment depression showing early ischemia. (From Ellestad MH: Diagnostic and prognostic information derived from exercise testing. *In* Wenger NK (ed): Exercise and the Heart. Philadelphia, F.A. Davis, 1978, with permission.)

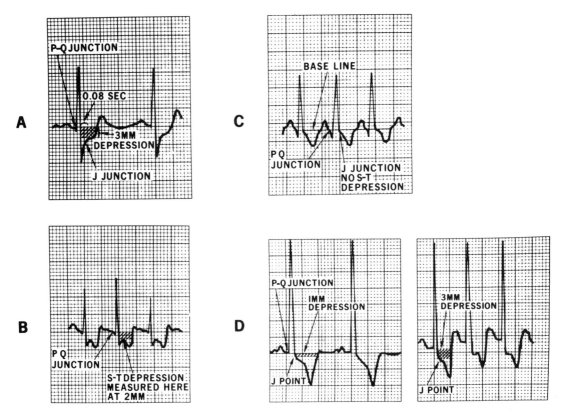

Fig. 7-20. Tracings showing ST-segment depression. (A) Horizontal ST depression is measured from a point 0.06 seconds after the J point. (B) Convex ST-segment depression is measured from the top of the curve to the PQ junction. (C & D) With down-sloping ST segments, the depression is measured at the point where the ST segment changes slope. (From Ellestad MH: Stress Testing: Principles and Practice. Philadelphia, F.A. Davis, 1975, with permission.)

tad et al postulated that, in a left ventricle with slightly decreased compliance, different rates of filling during inspiration and expiration could produce an increased end-diastolic pressure, and, therefore, ST-segment depression for a few beats.[100] Drugs, such as digitalis and diuretics, by depletion of potassium or hypokalemia per se, disturbances of conduction such as left bundle branch block or Wolff-Parkinson-White syndrome, and left ventricular hypertrophy with strain, can all affect the ST segment.

When ST-segment elevation occurs in the absence of any obvious hemodynamic or rhythm disturbances, coronary artery spasm (Prinzmetal's angina) should be suspected as the cause of the myocardial ischemia. Coronary artery spasm has been reported during anesthesia[107] when the diagnosis is especially important, since appropriate treatment with verapamil, nifedipine, or NTG is effective.

THE INTRAOPERATIVE ANALYSIS OF THE ST SEGMENT

For the accurate evaluation of ST-segment changes, it is essential that the ECG monitor is properly calibrated before use so that a signal of 1 mV will produce a vertical deflection of 10 mm. It is also important that the ECG signal displayed on the oscilloscope is an accurate representation of the true signal. This becomes a major consideration when the ST segment is subject to computer analysis. Many of the oscilloscopes currently used in the operating room can distort the ST segment and T wave of the ECG. This is largely the result of electronic filtering circuits that are used to remove artifacts from the ECG, such as baseline wandering and 60-cycle interference. The lower end of the normal frequency response of the ECG is 0.14 cycles per second, below which electrical signals are attenuated by low-frequency filters. On some monitors this filter may

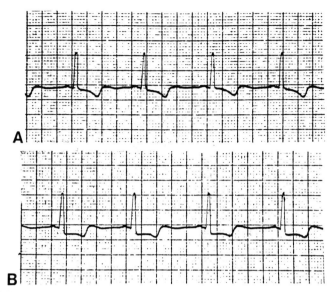

Fig. 7-21. Tracing A shows the proper ECG using the diagnostic filter mode. In tracing B, the ECG has been switched to the monitoring filter mode and the ST segments are depressed due to artifact. (From Kaplan JA: The ECG and anesthesia. *In* Miller RD (ed): Anesthesia (ed 1). New York, Churchill-Livingstone, 1981, p 228, with permission.)

be selected as the "diagnostic mode" and should be used to evaluate ST-segment changes. However, in this mode, the ECG is very susceptible to baseline wandering caused by respiration, movement, or electrode artifact. The baseline may be stabilized by further filtering low frequency signals up to 4 cycles per second in the "monitor mode." Unfortunately, the addition of more filtration may cause spurious shifts in the ST segment due to the absence of the usual low-frequency components.[108,109] An isoelectric ST segment may become elevated or depressed, resembling ischemia (Fig. 7-21). Moreover, elevated or depressed ST segments may be shifted towards the isoelectric line, effectively masking ongoing ischemia.

Changes in the ST segment indicative of ischemia may be evaluated visually or subjected to analysis by computer. Computer analysis was first applied to stress testing as an alternative to close scrutiny of tracings that may inevitably introduce an element of

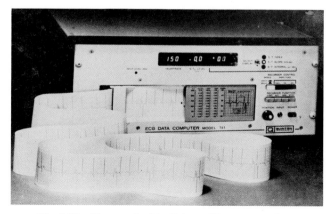

Fig. 7-22. Photograph of the Quinton ST-segment analyzer.

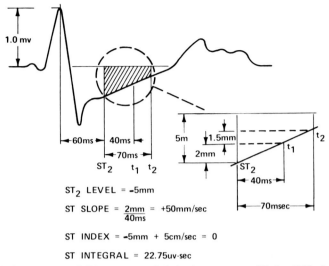

ST$_2$ LEVEL = -5mm

ST SLOPE = $\frac{2mm}{40ms}$ = +50mm/sec

ST INDEX = -5mm + 5cm/sec = 0

ST INTEGRAL = 22.75uv-sec

Fig. 7-23. Diagram of ST segment and derived parameters: ST$_2$ level/ST slope/ST index/ST integral. The ST$_2$ level is the change in the ST segment in millimeters. ST slope is measured between ST$_2$ and t$_1$ as mm/sec. The ST index is the sum of the ST$_2$ level and ST slope without a unit value. The ST integral is the area of ST depression measured as an integrated voltage between ST$_2$ and t$_2$.

human error.[110] Accurate computer analysis of changes in ST-segment configuration depends upon selection of ECG complexes that are unaffected by artifact. In 1967, Rosner et al described one of the first digital computer systems for analyzing the exercise ECG.[111] The subsequent development of computer averaging techniques over several beats with the rejection of ectopic beats has reduced the amount of random noise and enabled studies of the ECG during and after graded exercise.[112] Computer analysis of the ECG has also established precise numerical measurements for the objective ECG diagnosis of ischemia.[113] However, the usefulness of derived

parameters and the criteria for defining ischemia when computerized techniques are employed are still controversial.[64,65]

The technology of computerized ST-segment monitoring is equally applicable to the conscious and the anesthetized patient. Roy et al first described the use of a computerized exercise testing system to detect ischemia during anesthesia.[30] During induction, leads V$_4$, V$_5$, and V$_6$ were continuously recorded on paper. For the remainder of the procedure, leads V$_5$ and II were continuously displayed, and leads II, aVF, V$_3$, V$_4$, V$_5$, and V$_6$ were recorded on paper every 3 minutes. The diagnosis of ischemia

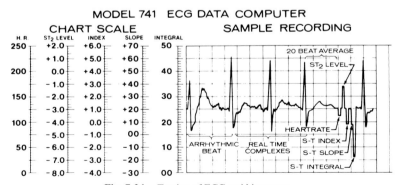

Fig. 7-24. Tracing of ECG and histogram.

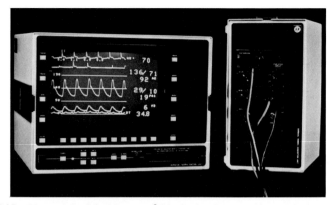

Fig. 7-25. Photograph of the Marquette® Monitoring System with the ST-segment analyzer.

was aided by a continuous digital readout of the magnitude of ST-segment depression and an averaged picture of the last 16 QRST complexes in lead V_5. Every 20 minutes a written histogram retrospectively demonstrated the amount of ST-segment displacement over 1 minute intervals.

Recently, Griffin and Kaplan evaluated the use of a simple ST-segment computer during anesthesia.[31] The device received a signal from an ECG preamplifier and displayed in digital form the ST_2 level, ST index, ST slope, and ST integral (Figs. 7-22 and 7-23). The computations were performed on an ECG complex produced from the average of the previous 20 beats. The averaged beat was recorded on paper followed by a histogram of all the derived ST-segment information (Fig. 7-24). Although the averaging process of the computer greatly reduced the amount of random noise, interference from electrocautery was a major problem since the ECG trace was completely lost and a further 20 beats had to elapse before another useful analysis

could be obtained. Although the written record was unaffected in the exercise monitor used by Roy et al, the computer also would not accept any data for processing during electrocautery.[30]

Kotrly et al reported the use of a modified microcomputer-based ECG which displayed, as a trend line, the summed ST-segment deviations from the isoelectric line in leads V_5, aVF, and $-V_1$.[114] The trend line was continuously displayed for 20 minutes, and thereafter was retained in hard copy form. In addition, the three ECG complexes were electronically stored every 10 minutes (Figs. 7-25 and 7-26). This ST-segment analyzer has been recently updated and presently can analyze leads I, II, and V_5.

The value of computer monitoring of the ST segment is still being evaluated. The visual quantification of ST-segment shifts in absolute terms as a digital display or trend line may provide the anesthesiologist with a simple, almost instantaneous means for the early and accurate ECG diagnosis of ischemia.

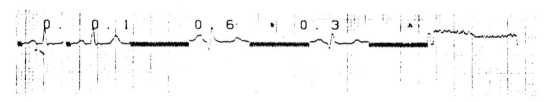

Fig. 7-26. The Marquette® ST-segment analysis is shown. From left to right are leads I, II, and V_5. The ST-segment trend line (28 minutes) is shown at the far right. It can be seen that the ST-segment trend line has returned back toward the baseline in the past 15 minutes. The change in ST-segment from baseline in millimeters is shown above each of the leads.

REFERENCES

1. Thys D, Kaplan JA (eds): The ECG in anesthesia and critical care. New York, Churchill-Livingstone, 1987

2. Cannard TH, Dripps RD, Helwig J, et al: The ECG during anesthesia and surgery. Anesthesiology 21:194, 1960

3. Beecher HK: First anesthesia death with some remarks suggested by it on the fields of the laboratory and the clinic in the appraisal of new anesthetic agents. Anesthesiology 2:443, 1941

4. Kurtz CM, Bennet JH, Shapiro H: Electrocardiographic studies during surgical anesthesia. JAMA 106:434, 1936

5. Katz RL, Bigger JT: Cardiac arrhythmias during anesthesia and operation. Anesthesiology 33:193, 1970

6. Dodd RB, Sims WA, Bone DJ: Cardiac arrhythmias observed during anesthesia. Surgery 51:440, 1962

7. Kuner J, Enescu V, Utsu F, et al: Cardiac arrhythmias during anesthesia. Dis Chest 52:580, 1967

8. Vanik PE, Davis HS: Cardiac arrhythmias during halothane anesthesia. Anesth Analg 47:299, 1968

9. Russell PH, Coakley CS: Electrocardiographic observation in the operating room. Anesth Analg 48:784, 1969

10. Bertrand CA, Steiner NV, Jameson AG, et al: Disturbances of cardiac rhythm during anesthesia and surgery. JAMA 216:1615, 1971

11. Angelini L, Feldman MI, Lufschonowski R, et al: Cardiac arrhythmias during and after heart surgery: Diagnosis and management. Prog Cardiovasc Dis 16:469, 1974

12. Atlee JL, Rusy BF: Ventricular conduction times and AV nodal conductivity during enflurane anesthesia in dogs. Anesthesiology 47:498, 1977

13. Koehntop DE, Liao JC, Van Bergen FH: Effects of pharmacologic alterations of adrenergic mechanisms by cocaine, tropolone, aminophylline, and ketamine on epinephrine-induced arrhythmias during halothane-nitrous oxide anesthesia. Anesthesiology 46:83, 1977

14. Edwards R, Winnie AL, Ramamurthy S: Acute hypocapnic hypokalemia: An iatrogenic anesthetic complication. Anesth Analg 56:786, 1977

15. Fox EJ, Sklar GS, Hill CH, et al: Complications related to the pressor response to endotracheal intubation. Anesthesiology 47:524, 1977

16. Stoelting RK: Circulatory changes during direct laryngoscopy and tracheal intubation: Influence of duration of laryngoscopy with and without prior lidocaine. Anesthesiology 47:381, 1977

17. Pratila MG, Pratilas V: Anesthetic agents and cardiac electromechanical activity. Anesthesiology 49:338, 1978

18. Smith M, Ray CT: Cardiac arrhythmias, increased intracranial pressure, and the autonomic nervous system. Chest 61:125, 1972

19. Alexander JP: Dysrhythmia and oral surgery. Br J Anaesth 43:773, 1971

20. Borg DE: Paradox of cardiac arrhythmias in anaesthesia. Br J Anaesth 41:709, 1969

21. Rao TLK, Jacobs KH, El-Etr AA: Reinfarction following anesthesia in patients with myocardial infarction. Anesthesiology 59:499, 1983

22. Tarhan S, Moffitt EA, Taylor WF, et al: Myocardial infarction after general anesthesia. JAMA 220:1451, 1972

23. Knapp RB, Topkins MJ, Artusio JF: The cerebrovascular accident and coronary occlusion in anesthesia. JAMA 182:332, 1962

24. Topkins MJ, Artusio JF: Myocardial infarction and surgery: A five-year study. Anesth Analg 43:716, 1964

25. Arkins R, Smessaert AA, Hicks RG: Mortality and morbidity in surgical patients with coronary artery disease. JAMA 190:485, 1964

26. Steen PA, Tinker JH, Tarhan S: Myocardial reinfarction after anesthesia and surgery. JAMA 239:2566, 1978

27. Chamberlain DA, Edmonds-Seal J: Effects of surgery under general anesthesia on the electrocardiogram in ischemic heart disease and hypertension. Br J Med 2:784, 1964

28. Driscoll AC, Hobika JH, Etstein BE, et al: Clinically unrecognized infarction following surgery. N Engl J Med 264:633, 1961

29. Slogoff S, Keats AS: Does perioperative myocardial ischemia lead to postoperative myocardial infarction? Anesthesiology 62:107, 1985

30. Roy WL, Edelist G, Gilbert B: Myocardial ischemia during non-cardiac surgical procedures in patients with coronary artery disease. Anesthesiology 51:393, 1979

31. Griffin RM, Kaplan JA: Comparison of ECG leads V_5, CS_5, CB_5, and II by computerized ST segment analysis. Anesth Analg 65:S65, 1986

32. Coriat P, Harari A, Daloz M, et al: Clinical predictors of intraoperative myocardial ischemia in patients with coronary artery disease undergoing non-cardiac surgery. Acta Anaesthesiol Scand 26:287, 1982

33. Mahar LJ, Steen PA, Tinker JH, et al: Perioperative myocardial infarction in patients with coronary artery disease with and without aorta-coronary artery bypass grafts. J Thorac Cardiovasc Surg 76:533, 1978

34. Scher KS, Tice DA: Operative risks in patients with previous coronary artery bypass. Arch Surg 111:807, 1976

35. McCollum CH, Garcia-Rinaldi R, Graham JM, et al: Myocardial revascularization prior to subsequent

major surgery in patients with coronary artery disease. Surgery 81:302, 1977

36. Bernhard VM, Johnson SD, Peterson JJ: Carotid artery stenosis: Association with surgery for coronary artery disease. Arch Surg 105:837, 1972

37. Crutchley P, Kaplan JA, Hug CC, et al: Non-cardiac surgery in patients with prior myocardial revascularization. Can Anaesth Soc J 30:629, 1983

38. Coleman AJ, Jordan C: Cardiovascular responses to anaesthesia. Influence of beta-adrenoreceptor blockade with metoprolol. Anaesthesia 35:972, 1980

39. Stein I, Caginalp N: The postoperative electrocardiogram. Angiology 17:323, 1966

40. Eerola M, Eerola R, Kaukinen S, et al: Risk factors in surgical patients with verified preoperative myocardial infarction. Acta Anaesthesiol Scand 24:219, 1980

41. Lowenstein E, Yusef S, Teplick R: Perioperative myocardial reinfarction: A glimmer of hope—a note of caution. Anesthesiology 59:493, 1983

42. Kaplan JA: Electrocardiographic monitoring. *In* Kaplan JA (ed): Cardiac Anesthesia. New York, Grune & Stratton, 1979, p 117

43. Blackburn H: The exercise electrocardiogram: Technological, procedural, and conceptual development. *In* Measurements in Exercise Electrocardiography. Springfield, IL, Charles C. Thomas, 1967

44. Mason RE, Likar I, Biern RO, et al: Multiple-lead exercise electrocardiography. Circulation 36:517, 1967

45. Robertson D, Kostok WJ, Ahuja SP: The localization of coronary artery stenosis by 12-lead ECG response to graded exercise test. Am Heart J 91:437, 1976

46. Kaplan JA, King SB: The precordial electrocardiographic lead (V_5) in patients who have coronary artery disease. Anesthesiology 45:570, 1976

47. Bazaral MG, Norfleet EA: Comparison of CB_5 and V_5 leads for intraoperative electrocardiographic monitoring. Anesth Analg 60:849, 1981

48. Brown WH: A study of the esophageal lead in clinical electrocardiography, Part I. Am Heart J 121:306, 1936

49. Kistin AD, Bruce JC: Simultaneous esophageal and standard electrocardiographic leads for the study of cardiac arrhythmias. Am Heart J 53:65, 1957

50. Copeland GD, Tullis IF, Brody DA: Clinical evaluation of a new esophageal electrode, with particular reference to the bipolar esophageal electrocardiogram. Am Heart J 53:863, 1959

51. Kates RA, Zaidan JR, Kaplan JA: Esophageal lead for intraoperative electrocardiographic monitoring. Anesth Analg 61:781, 1982

52. Hellerstein HK, Pritchard WH, Lewis RL: Recording of intracavitary potentials through a single lumen, saline filled cardiac catheter. Proc Soc Exp Biol Med 71:58, 1949

53. Robertson JT, Schick RW, Morgan F, et al: Accurate placement of ventriculo-atrial shunt for hydrocephalus under electrocardiographic control. J Neurosurg 18:255, 1961

54. Michenfelder JD, Terry HR Jr, Daw EF, et al: Air embolism during neurosurgery: A new method of treatment. Anesth Analg 45:390, 1966

55. Richards CC, Freeman A: Intra-atrial catheter placement under electrocardiographic guidance. Anesthesiology 25:388, 1964

56. Westheimer DN: Right atrial catheter placement: Use of a wire guide as the intravascular ECG lead. Anesthesiology 56:478, 1982

57. Chatterjee K, Swan HJC, Ganz W, et al: Use of a balloon-tipped flotation electrode catheter for cardiac monitoring. Am J Cardiol 36:56, 1975

58. Mantle JA, Massing GK, James TN, et al: A multipurpose catheter for electrophysiologic and hemodynamic monitoring plus atrial pacing. Chest 72:285, 1977

59. Zaidan ZR: Experience with the pacing pulmonary artery catheter. Anesthesiology 53:S118, 1980

60. Lichtenthal PR: Multipurpose pulmonary artery catheter. Ann Thorac Surg 36:493, 1983

61. Mylrea KC, Calkins JM, Carlson J, et al: ECG lead with the endotracheal tube. Crit Care Med 11:199, 1983

62. Russell PH, Coakley CS: Electrocardiographic observation in the operating room. Anesth Analg 48:784, 1969

63. Wood FC, Wolferth CC: Angina pectoris. The clinical and electrocardiographic phenomenon of the attack and their comparison with the effects of experimental temporary occlusion. Arch Intern Med 47:339, 1931

64. Blackburn H, Taylor HL, Okamoto N, et al: Standardization of the exercise electrocardiogram. A systematic comparison of chest lead configurations employed for monitoring during exercise. *In* Karoonen MJ, Barry AJ (eds): Physical Activity and the Heart. Springield, IL, Charles C. Thomas, 1967, p 101

65. Froelicher VF Jr, Wolthius R, Keiser N, et al: A comparison of two bipolar exercise electrocardiographic leads to lead V_5. Chest 70:611, 1976

66. Dalton B: A precordial ECG lead for chest operations. Anesth Analg 55:740, 1976

67. Blackburn H, Katigbak R: What electrocardiographic leads to take after exercise? Am Heart J 67:184, 1964

68. Mason RE, Likar I, Biern RO, et al: Multiple-lead exercise electrocardiography. Experience in 107 normal subjects and 67 patients with angina pectoris and comparison with coronary cinearteriography in 84 patients. Circulation 36:517, 1967

69. Kirstner JR, Miller ED, Epstein RM: More than V_5 needed. Anesthesiology 47:75, 1977

70. Scherlis L, Wener J, Grishman A, et al: The ventricular complex in esophageal electrocardiography. Am Heart J 41:246, 1951

71. Cohn TN, Guilia NH, Broder MI, et al: Right ventricular infarction: Clinical and hemodynamic features. Am J Cardiol 33:209, 1974

72. Erhardt LR, Sjogren A, Wahlberg I: Single right-sided precordial lead in the diagnosis of right ventricular involvement in inferior myocardial infarction. Am Heart J 91:571, 1976

73. Klein HO, Turdjman T, Nino R, et al: The early recognition of right ventricular infarction: Diagnostic accuracy of the electrocardiographic V₄R lead. Circulation 67:558, 1983

74. Trager MA, Feinberg BI, Kaplan JA: Right ventricular ischemia diagnosed by an esophageal electrocardiogram and right atrial pressure tracing. J Cardiothorac Anesth (in press)

75. Michelson E, Morganroth J, MacVough H: Postoperative arrhythmias after coronary artery and cardiac valvular surgery detected by long-term electrocardiographic monitoring. Am Heart J 97:442, 1979

76. de Soyza N, Thenabadu P, Murphy M, et al: Ventricular arrhythmia before and after aortocoronary bypass surgery. Int J Cardiol 1:123, 1981

77. Dewar M, Rosengarten M, Blundell P, et al: Perioperative Holter monitoring and computer analysis of dysrhythmias in cardiac surgery. Chest 87:593, 1985

78. Holter NJ: New method for heart studies. Continuous electrocardiography of active subjects over long periods is now practical. Science 134:1214, 1961

79. Crawford MJ, Mendoza CA, O'Rourke RA, et al: Limitations of continuous ambulatory electrocardiogram monitoring for detecting coronary artery disease. Ann Intern Med 89:1, 1978

80. Hinkle LE, Meyer J, Stevens M, et al: Tape recording of the ECG of active man: Limitations and advantages of the Holter-Avionics instruments. Circulation 36:752, 1967

81. Balasubramanian V, Lahini A, Green HL, et al: Ambulatory ST segment monitoring problems, pitfalls, solutions and clinical applications. Br Heart J 44:419, 1980

82. Bragg-Remschel DA, Anderson CM, Winkle RA: Frequency response characteristics of ambulatory ECG monitoring systems and their implications for ST segment analysis. Am Heart J 103:20, 1982

83. Tzivoni D, Benhorin J, Gavish A, et al: Holter recording during treadmill testing in assessing myocardial ischemic changes. Am J Cardiol 55:1200, 1985

84. Coriat P, Daloz M, Bousseau D, et al: Prevention of intraoperative myocardial ischemia during noncardiac surgery with intravenous nitroglycerin. Anesthesiology 61:193, 1984

85. Thomson IR, Mutch WAC, Culligan JD: Failure of intravenous nitroglycerin to prevent intraoperative myocardial ischemia during fentanyl-pancuronium anesthesia. Anesthesiology 61:385, 1984

86. Borello G: ECG artifacts simulating atrial flutter. JAMA 223:439, 1973

87. Shapiro LA, Jejeikin R, Hoffman S: Misdiagnosis due to ECG failure. Anesthesiology 60:166, 1984

88. Doss JD, McCabe CW, Weiss GK: Noise-free data during electrosurgical procedures. Anesth Analg 52:156, 1973

89. Romhilt DW, Bloomfield SS, Chai TC, et al: Unreliability of conventional electrocardiographic monitoring of arrhythmia detection in coronary care units. Am J Cardiol 31:457, 1973

90. Holmberg S, Ryder L, Waldenstrom A: Efficiency of arrhythmia detection by nurses in a coronary care unit using a decentralized monitoring system. Br Heart J 39:1019; 1977

91. Cox JR, Nolle FM, Fozzard MA, et al: AZTEC, a preprocessing program for the real-time ECG analysis. IEEE Trans Biomed Eng 15:128, 1968

92. Oliver GE, Nolle FM, Wolff GA, et al: Detection of premature ventricular contractions with a clinical system for monitoring electrocardiographic rhythms. Comput Biomed Res 4:523, 1971

93. Yanowitz F, Kinias P, Rawling D, et al: Accuracy of continuous real-time ECG dysrhythmic monitoring system. Circulation 50:65, 1974

94. Feldman CL, Amazeen PG, Klein MD, et al: Computer detection of ventricular ectopic beats. Comput Biomed Res 3:666, 1971

95. Shah PM, Arnold JM, Haberen NA, et al: Automatic real-time arrhythmia monitoring in the intensive coronary care unit. Am J Cardiol 39:701, 1977

96. Morganroth J: Ambulatory Holter electrocardiography: Choice of technologies and clinical uses. Ann Intern Med 102:73, 1985

97. Govrin O, Sadeh D, Akselrod S, et al: Cross-correlation technique for arrhythmia detection using PR and PP intervals. Comput Biomed Res 18:37, 1985

98. Salzman SH, Hellerstein HK, Radke JD, et al: Quantitative effects of physical conditioning on the exercise electrocardiogram of middle-aged subjects with arteriosclerotic heart disease. In Blackburn H (ed): Measurements in Exercise Electrocardiography. Springfield, IL, Charles C. Thomas, 1969

99. Stuart RJ, Ellestad MH: Upsloping ST segment in exercise stress testing. Am J Cardiol 37:19, 1976

100. Ellestad MH, Cooke BM Jr, Greenberg PS: Stress Testing: Principles and Practice. Philadelphia, F.A. Davis, 1980, p 85

101. Ellestad MH, Cooke BM Jr, Greenberg PS: Stress Testing: Clinical application and predictive capacity. Prog Cardiovasc Dis 21:431, 1979

102. Robb GP, Marks H: Post-exercise electrocardiogram in arteriosclerotic heart disease. JAMA 200:918, 1967

103. Goldshlager N, Selzer A, Cohn K: Treadmill stress tests as indicators of presence and severity of coronary artery disease. Ann Intern Med 85:277, 1976

104. Armstrong WF, Jordon JW, Morris SN, et al: Prevalence of and magnitude of ST segment and T wave abnormalities in normal men during continuous ambulatory electrocardiography. Am J Cardiol 49:1638, 1981

105. Lachman AB, Semler HJ, Gustafson RH: Postural ST-T wave changes in the radioelectrogram simulating myocardial ischemia. Circulation 31:557, 1965

106. Holmgren A, Strom G: Vasoregulatory asthenia in a female athlete and Da Costa's syndrome in a male athlete successfully treated by physical training. Acta Med Scand 164:113, 1959

107. Briard C, Coriat P, Commin P, et al: Coronary artery spasm during noncardiac surgical procedures. Anaesthesia 38:467, 1983

108. Berson AS, Pipberger HV: The low-frequency response of electrocardiographs, a frequent source of recording errors. Am Heart J 71:779, 1966

109. Arbeit SR, Rubin IL, Gross H: Dangers in interpreting the electrocardiogram from the oscilloscope monitor. JAMA 211:453, 1970

110. Acheson RM: Observer error and variation in interpretation of electrocardiograms in epidemiological study of coronary heart disease. Br J Prev Soc Med 14:99, 1960

111. Rosner SR, Leinbach RC, Presto AJ, et al: Computer analysis of the exercise electrocardiogram. Am J Cardiol 20:356, 1967

112. Davies CT, Kitchin AH, Knibbs AV: Computer quantitations of ST segment response to graded exercise in untrained and trained normal subjects. Cardiovasc Res 5:201, 1971

113. Sheffield LT, Holt HJ, Lester FM, et al: On-line analysis of the exercise electrocardiogram. Circulation 40:935, 1969

114. Kotrly KJ, Kotter GS, Mortara D, et al: Intraoperative detection of myocardial ischemia with an ST segment trend monitoring system. Anesth Analg 63:343, 1984

Daniel M. Thys, M.D., Zaharia Hillel, M.D. Ph.D.
Steven N. Konstadt, M.D., Martin E. Goldman, M.D.

8

Intraoperative Echocardiography

Physicians managing patients with cardiac disease have relied on invasive hemodynamic monitoring to assess ventricular filling, myocardial performance, and the hemodynamic disturbances caused by myocardial ischemia. These assessments are indirect and in some clinical situations have been misleading. With echocardiography, ventricular filling, diastolic compliance, and global or regional ventricular function can be evaluated directly and noninvasively.

Since echocardiographic (echo) information has proven useful in clinical medicine, a rapid expansion of the field has ensued, and it now plays a prominent role in the medical diagnosis of cardiac disorders. The recent introduction of transesophageal echocardiography has given anesthesiologists access to the same valuable technology. Hemodynamic data can be obtained noninvasively in intubated patients, can be used to guide patient management, or can be stored for subsequent review. The possible applications of the technique are unlimited, and the findings could revolutionize hemodynamic monitoring.

In echocardiography, the heart is probed by ultrasound, which is sound above the human audible range. Initial investigations with ultrasound explored its potential for the localization of submerged objects, and the sinking of the Titanic in 1912 gave this research a major impetus. During World War I,

Langevin was already able to detect submarines and large schools of fish with an ultrasound technique later known as *sonar* (*so*und, *na*vigation, and *rang*ing).[1]

In 1937, Dussik first applied ultrasound in humans to visualize the cerebral ventricles by measuring the attenuation of an ultrasound beam through the head.[2] Unfortunately, his measurements were later proven invalid since variations in attenuation caused by the skull were more significant than those caused by the ventricular system.[3]

The second World War brought major advances in radar and sonar technology as well as marked improvements in the performance of ultrasonic instruments. These advances allowed pioneers such as Howry and Wild in the United States and Edler in Sweden to extend medical ultrasound to its full potential.[4,5] In 1953, Edler and Hertz demonstrated that echoes from the moving heart could be received and displayed on an ultrasonic flow detector.[6] This monumental achievement signified the birth of clinical echocardiography. By 1955, Edler had reported the ability to diagnose mitral stenosis, thrombus in the left atrium, and pericardial effusions.[7] These pioneering efforts provided the impetus for other investigators such as Reid, Wild, Feigenbaum, Joyner, and many others to advance echocardiography into a modern, sophisticated diagnostic tool that today is widely utilized in adult and pediatric cardiology.

The aim of this chapter is to provide insight into the basic principles of ultrasound technology and to describe the function of various echocardiographic instruments. Clinical applications are reviewed, with a particular emphasis on the measurement of hemodynamic performance and the diagnosis of myocardial ischemia. For a broader view on echocardiography, the reader is referred to standard texts.[8-10]

PHYSICS AND PRINCIPLES

Properties of Ultrasound

The ultrasound or echo technique provides information on distance, velocity, and density of objects much as a submarine's sonar detection system does.[8] This section describes the application of ultrasound for the imaging of structures. Blood flow velocity measurements are discussed in the section on Doppler echocardiography.

An ultrasound beam is a continuous or intermittent train of waves originating at the transducer or wave generator. It is composed of density or pressure waves and can exist in any medium with the exception of a vacuum (Fig. 8-1). Ultrasound waves are characterized by their wavelength, frequency, and velocity. *Wavelength* is the distance between the two nearest points of equal pressure or density in an ultrasound beam, while *velocity* is the speed at which the waves propagate through a medium. The waves travel by at any fixed point in an ultrasound beam and the pressure cycles regularly and continuously between a high and a low value. The number of cycles per second (Hertz) is called the *frequency* of

the wave. Ultrasound is sound with frequencies above 20,000 cycles each second, which is the upper limit of the human audible range.[11] The relationship among the frequency (f), wavelength (λ) and velocity (v) of a sound wave is defined by the formula

$$v = f \times (\lambda) \qquad (8\text{-}1)$$

Waves interact with the medium in which they travel and with one another. Interaction among waves is called *interference*.[12] The manner in which waves interact with a medium is determined by its density and homogeneity. When a wave is propagating through an inhomogeneous medium, and all living tissue is essentially inhomogeneous, it is partly absorbed, partly reflected, and partly scattered (Fig. 8-2). Reflected echoes, also called *specular echoes,* are usually much stronger than scattered echoes. A grossly inhomogeneous medium, such as a stone in a water bucket or a cardiac valve in a blood-filled heart chamber, produces strong specular reflections at the water–stone or blood–valve interface. Conversely, media that are inhomogeneous at the microscopic level, such as muscle, produce more scatter than specular reflection. Specular reflections are obtained when the width of the reflecting object is larger than one fourth of the wavelength of the ultrasound. It is clear that to visualize smaller objects, ultrasound of shorter wavelength must be used. Since the velocity of sound in soft tissue is approximately constant (1540 m/sec), shorter wavelengths are obtained by increasing the frequency of the ultrasound beam (Equation 8-1). While smaller objects can be visualized with higher frequencies, more scatter is produced by insignificant inhomogeneities in the medium, and confusing signals are generated.

Any ultrasound beam traveling through tissues

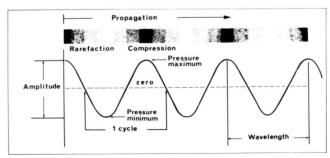

Fig. 8-1. A sound wave is a series of compressions and rarefactions. The combination of one compression and one rarefaction represents one cycle. The distance between the onset (peak compression) of one cycle to the next is the wavelength. (From Feigenbaum H: Echocardiography (ed 4). Philadelphia, Lea & Febiger, 1986, with permission.)

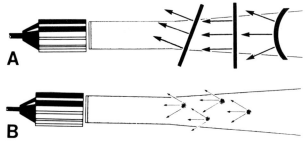

Fig. 8-2. Specular echoes (A) originate from relatively large, strongly reflective, regularly shaped objects with smooth surfaces and are relatively intense and angle dependent. Scattered echoes (B) originate from small, weakly reflective, irregularly shaped objects and are less angle dependent and less intense. (From Feigenbaum H: Echocardiography (ed 4). Philadelphia, Lea & Febiger, 1986, with permission.)

will be weakened or attenuated as it progresses. Table 8-1 gives the distance in various tissues at which the intensity or amplitude of an ultrasound wave of 2 MHz is halved (the half-power distance). Clearly, echo studies across lung or other gas-containing tissues are not feasible. Nor are they feasible across dense structures such as bone or strongly scattering tissues such as thick muscle.

Modern ultrasound transducers employ piezo-electric crystals to transmit ultrasound and receive echoes (Fig. 8-3). A high-frequency electric signal stimulates the crystal, which emits ultrasound. Conversely, reflected ultrasound echoes striking the crystal's surface generate vibrations that are converted to electric impulses, amplified, processed, and then imaged on a television screen (Fig. 8-4). Electronic circuits measure the time delay between the emitted and received echo, and, using the known speed of ultrasound in tissue, convert this time delay into the precise distance between transducer and tissue.

The commonly used transducer spends a small amount of time, typically on the order of 1 μsec (10^{-6} seconds), to emit a pulse of ultrasound waves. It then "listens" for the returning echoes for about 0.25 msec and pauses for 0.75 msec or less before repeating the cycle. Ultrasound takes about one tenth of a millisecond to travel through 10 cm of human tissue and to be reflected or echoed back to the transducer. There is no time loss in the reflection process.

Table 8-1

Half-Power Distances for Tissues and Substances Important in Echocardiography

Material	Half-Power Distance (cm)
Water	380
Blood	15
Soft tissue*	5–1
Muscle	1–0.6
Bone	0.7–0.2
Air	0.08
Lung	0.05

*Except muscle.

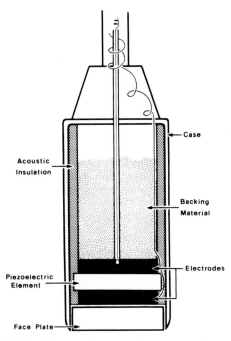

Fig. 8-3. Diagram of a conventional echocardiographic transducer with the principal components labeled. See text for further details. (From Weyman AE: Cross-Sectional Echocardiography. Philadelphia, Lea & Febiger, 1982, with permission.)

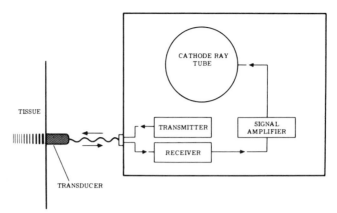

Fig. 8-4. Simplified block diagram of a pulse-echo instrument, omitting scanning electronics. (From Feigenbaum H: Echocardiography (ed 4). Philadelphia, Lea & Febiger, 1986, with permission.)

Techniques and Instrumentation

ULTRASOUND TECHNIQUES

Early methods of ultrasound examination were nonimaging, since they did not produce an image resembling the studied object. These techniques, the A-, B-, and M-mode, required simple instruments but considerable expertise for the interpretation of the results. Of the three, M-mode is the only one still currently used in clinical practice. Two-dimensional or cross-sectional echocardiography, a fourth type of ultrasound examination, produces true images of anatomic structures.

The A-mode display. In the A-mode, the intensity or amplitude (hence *A*-mode) of the reflected echo and the distance between the transducer and the target generating that echo are displayed on a television screen as a line signal or bar (Fig. 8-5 A, B, and D–F). The height of the bar is proportional to the echo signal amplitude, while the distance between the line signal and the edge of the screen is proportional to the distance between the transducer and the target. Motion of the reflecting object will produce motion of the line signal on the screen (Fig. 8-5C,F).

The B-mode display. The B-mode displays a dot whose brightness (hence *B*-mode) is proportional to the strength of the reflected echo. On the display screen, the dot's position, relative to a reference point, is determined by the distance between transducer and object. An example of a B-mode examination is depicted in Figure 8-5G–I, in which a moving object is seen to produce a bright spot moving in a

straight horizontal display line. The advantage of the B-mode over the A-mode is that while the two techniques provide similar information, the B-mode only utilizes one of the two screen dimensions available for imaging.

The M-mode display. The M-mode is based on the same imaging technique as the B-mode. If motion of the study object away or toward the transducer is

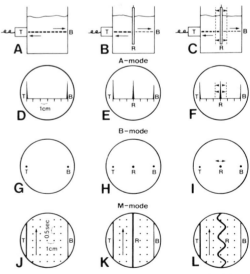

Fig. 8-5. (A–L) These diagrams illustrate the principles of acoustic imaging using pulsed, reflected ultrasound. See text for details. (Abbreviations: T, transducer; B, beaker; R, rod.) (From Feigenbaum H, Zaky A: Use of diagnostic ultrasound in clinical cardiology. J Indiana State Med Assoc 59:140, 1966, with permission.)

displayed by horizontal motion on the screen, time can be displayed as vertical motion (Fig. 8-5J). Sweeping the screen from bottom to top, a display that varies continuously with time is obtained. Current time is at the bottom edge of the screen, and the time history of the motion is displayed for a brief duration, continuously moving toward the top of the screen. The *M* in M-mode stands for *motion.* A stationary object in an ultrasound field will produce a straight vertical line on this type of display (Fig. 8-5K). An object that oscillates back and forth toward the transducer will produce wavy, sinusoidal lines sweeping from top to bottom on the screen (Fig. 8-5L). Most cardiac structures move in a manner that is cyclic or repetitive. An M-mode display of the heart will therefore produce a pattern of wavy lines across the screen (Fig. 8-6). Since an ultrasound beam is narrow and well-focused, much like a pointed ice-pick, a narrow view of the heart is obtained. By convention, the distance away from the transducer is displayed on the vertical axis; thus, the objects closest to the transducer will be displayed near the top of the screen, and objects farther away from the transducer will be visualized lower down on the screen. Timed motion of cardiac structures is

displayed from right to left. Using a strip-chart recorder, this moving display can be inscribed on a permanent record.

The two-dimensional (2D) scan. Information from a B-mode scan is essentially unidimensional. By moving the narrow ultrasound beam across the target field (scanning), information can be obtained on position and motion in a second dimension perpendicular to the ultrasound beam. The ultrasound beam thus examines an entire plane or cross-section of the target object. The actual image consists of a series of adjacent B-mode line displays in which the bright dots and lines are fused by the observer's eye to form an integrated picture (Fig. 8-7). Since emitted and reflected echoes take little time to cross distances of clinical interest, the beam scans the field so rapidly that very few changes can occur in the field during a single scan period. This scanning technique is called real-time B-mode cross-sectional scanning of the heart, or, more commonly, two-dimensional (2D) echocardiography. Once a cross-sectional view of the heart has been obtained, changes within the cross-section can be followed by repeating the scan, often as frequently as every 17 msec. For more

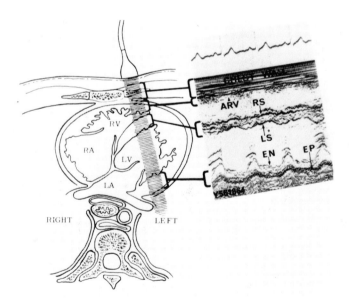

Fig. 8-6. Transverse section of the heart with corresponding echocardiogram showing the path of the ultrasonic beam during an M-mode examination of the left ventricle. (Abbreviations: ARV, anterior right ventricular wall; RS, right septum; LS, left septum; EN, left ventricular posterior endocardium; EP, left ventricular posterior epicardium.) (From Feigenbaum H, Popp RL, Wolfe SB, et al: Ultrasound measurement of the left ventricle: A correlative study with echocardiography. Arch Intern Med 129:461, 1972, with permission.)

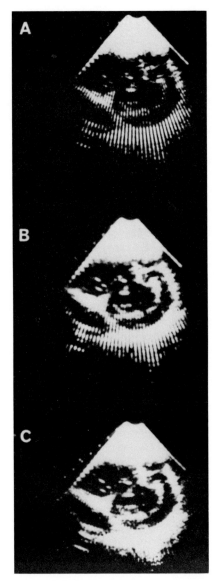

Fig. 8-7. This illustrates two methods of increasing the apparent line density. (A) A single field of data is displayed. At the line density of this image, there is a clear separation between the individual data lines producing a "spoking" effect. (B) The system gain has been increased, causing the individual data points to bloom. The data lines widen, and the separation between lines decreases. (C) The technique of interlacing has been used. In this example, a second field has been laid down so that the data lines are placed between the lines of the field illustrated in A. Interlacing further smooths the image; however, some blurring results because the data in the second field are recorded slightly later. (From Weyman AE: Cross-Sectional Echocardiography. Philadelphia, Lea & Febinger, 1982, with permission.)

details on 2D imaging technology, see the technical section at the end of this chapter.

TRANSDUCERS

In echocardiography, the goal is to aim ultrasound waves at a given tissue section and subsequently to receive undistorted echoes from that tissue section alone. Different transducers accomplish this task with varying efficiency. The simplest uses a single, small piezoelectric element, which produces a very widely dispersed beam of circular concentric ultrasound waves (Fig. 8-8A). The problem with this simple system is that it generates echoes indiscriminately from tissues in all directions around it; hence, it has poor resolution and locates objects poorly.

A more advanced transducer consists of a linear array of crystals emitting synchronously (Fig. 8-8B). Each individual crystal produces its own circular ultrasound waves. The end result is a planar (flat) beam moving in a direction perpendicular to the array. For some distance away from the transducer, the width of this beam is approximately the same as the width of the array, allowing the beam to interrogate tissues selectively. A single large-element transducer produces the same effect (Fig. 8-8C).

Even the straightest parallel beam eventually diverges after it has traveled a certain distance from the transducer, however. This distance (L), or depth of field, at which the beam is no longer parallel is estimated as

$$L = D^2/\lambda \qquad (8\text{-}2)$$

in which D represents the size of the transducer surface.[13] The depth of field sets the limit for the practical depth of the ultrasound examination. From Equation 8-2, it appears that the larger the transducer, or the smaller the ultrasound wavelength, the greater the depth of field.

SCANNERS

In order to generate 2D echo images, the transducer must be able to scan the target field with a linear arc or sector scanner (Fig. 8-9). In clinical echocardiography, either mechanical or electronic 2D sector scanners are most commonly utilized. The former employs oscillating or rotating transducer heads, while in the latter the beam is steered or aimed electronically (Fig. 8-9). Electronic scanners use linear phased-array transducers, which can contain as many as 48 piezoelectric elements. Electronic beam steering is achieved by multiple circuits, each of

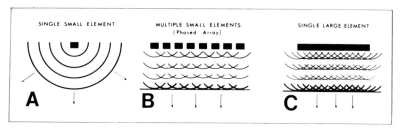

Fig. 8-8. This diagram demonstrates how longtitudinal ultrasonic wavefronts are produced. (A) The ultrasonic wavelets travel in a circular fashion from a single, small element. With either (B) multiple-element or (C) single large-element transducers, the circular wavelets combine to produce a longitudinal wavefront directed away from the face of the transducer. (From Feigenbaum H: Echocardiography (ed 4). Philadelphia, Lea & Febiger, 1986, with permission.)

which provides a properly delayed electric impulse to their dedicated array element. Wave summation produces a planar or flat wave front at any desired angle within a theoretical 180° sector (Fig. 8-10). In practice, however, scanning transducers are limited to sectors of approximately 90°. A significant advantage of the electronic phased-array scanner is that it can simultaneously display a 2D as well as an M-mode image on two separate television screens. More advanced phased-array scanners even have

dual M-mode displays on the same screen, allowing the simultaneous study of the motion of two cardiac valves. The mechanical 2D scanners can also perform M-mode and 2D examinations but only in a sequential manner. In a phased-array scanner, the returning echoes are also received selectively. By a mechanism of time delays similar to the one used in emission, a phased array can "focus" on signals from designated regions.

A comparison between the mechanical and the

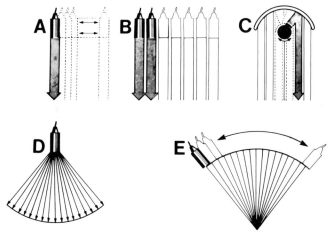

Fig. 8-9. This series of diagrams illustrates the different scan formats that have been used to produce cross-sectional images. (A–C) These indicate the various methods used to generate linear scans. (A) A single transducer is rapidly moved from one point to another while maintaining a constant orientation relative to the heart. (B) A series of transducers is aligned in a row and activated in sequence to produce a series of parallel pulses. (C) A rotating transducer is used to reflect pulses off a parabolic mirror so that they enter the tissue in a parallel orientation. (D) In this sector scan format, the transducer is held in a fixed location while the sound beam is gradually swept through an arc of varying width. (E) In an arc scanner, the transducer is moved along an arcuate path while the beam is directed at a fixed point in space. (From Weyman AE: Cross-Sectional Echocardiography. Philadelphia, Lea & Febiger, 1982, with permission.)

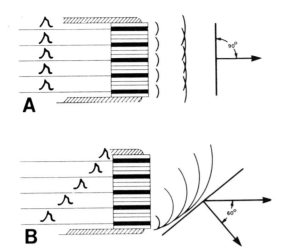

Fig. 8-10. These diagrams illustrate the method of beam transmission and steering in the phased-array format. (A) A series of electrical pulses is depicted moving from left to right toward the transducer elements in the array. The pulses activate the elements, simultaneously producing a series of small wavelets. As these wavelets move from the transducer face, they summate to form a beam that propagates away from the transducer. (B) The transducer elements are activated slightly out of phase. In this example, the upper transducer is activated first, producing an acoustic wavelet that propagates to the right and away from the array. Rapidly thereafter, the second element is excited, producing a second wavelet slightly behind the first. The sequence continues until the bottom element in the array is activated. In tissue, these five individual wavefronts summate to produce an acoustic beam that approximates in shape and direction the beam that would be produced by a transducer aimed in that direction. (From Weyman AE: Cross-Sectional Echocardiography. Philadelphia, Lea & Febiger, 1982, with permission.)

electronic phased-array 2D scanners is provided in Table 8-2. Image quality is about the same with either technique. The phased-array scanner is driven by large electronic equipment but offers a smaller, lighter transducer, hence a better "window." In addition, it is more flexible in its Doppler or combined 2D-Doppler capabilities. The mechanical scanner requires a smaller electronic enclosure but has a bulkier transducer. The use of a cathode ray tube display (transient image) rather than a video monitor (persistent image) has allowed production of a 2D echo scanner that is about the same size as a portable ECG monitor. Unfortunately, it is a mechanical system, and it cannot be used with an esophageal probe, since most esophageal probes are of the phased-array type.

ESOPHAGEAL ECHOCARDIOGRAPHY

Because fat, bone, and air-containing lung interfere with sound wave penetration, clear transthoracic echocardiographic views are particularly difficult to obtain in patients with obesity, emphysema, or abnormal chest wall anatomy. To avoid these problems, esophageal echo transducers have been developed. Sound waves emitted from an esophageal transducer only have to pass through the esophageal wall and the pericardium before reaching the heart; thus, there is less likelihood of image distortion. Other advantages of transesophageal echocardiography (TEE) include the stability of the transducer position and the possibility of obtaining continuous recordings of cardiac activity for extended periods of time. Because of these advantages, the potential for continuous intraoperative echocardiographic examinations has been recognized and has led to the evaluation of TEE as a monitoring tool. While initially only M-mode instruments were available for esophageal echocardiography, current equipment provides a combination of M-mode and 2D capabilities.

M-mode echocardiograms are obtainable using a Picker Echocardiogram Model 80CI or a Hoffrel Ultrasonoscope Model 101C with a 3.5-mHz nonfocused esophageal transducer.[14] The transducer is 10 mm in diameter and has a pulse-repetition frequency of 1000 Hz.

Two-dimensional TEE was first performed with a mechanical system.[15] The system was composed of two mechanical scanners (one horizontal and one vertical) that were each connected to a 3.5-mHz ultrasonic transducer contained in a $12 \times 20 \times 6$ mm oil bag. The transducers were rotated by a single-phase commutator motor via flexible shafts.

Currently, only one 2D-TEE transducer is widely available in the United States. This system, manufactured by Diasonics, consists of a specially designed phased-array probe that can be connected to a number of standard echo instruments (Diasonics Cardiovue 3400 and 6400). The transducer is 17 mm long, 15 mm wide, and 16 mm thick[16] (Fig. 8-11A). To avoid esophageal injury, it is embedded in soft plastic with rounded edges. The transducer is attached to a standard gastroscope, consisting of a 110-cm flexible shaft and a 7-cm deflection section (Fig. 8-11B). Deflection controls permit 180° angulation of the probe in two planes. The use of the controls and rotation of the entire unit make it possible to obtain many echocardiographic views. Internally, the probe consists of 32 linearly arranged elements with a center frequency of 3.5 mHz, corres-

Table 8-2

Comparison of Mechanical and Phased-Array Real-Time Sector Scanners

Features	Mechanical	Phased Array
Simultaneous M-mode and 2D echo	No	Yes
Sequential M-mode and 2D echo	Yes	Yes
Dual M-mode echo	No	Yes
Simultaneous 2D and Doppler	No	Yes
Sequential 2D and Doppler	Yes	Yes
Small acoustic window for wide-angle scan	No	Yes*
Can be electronically focused in lateral (y) axis	No	Yes
Compatible with ring or annular phased-array transducer technology	Yes	No
Minimal side lobe artifacts	Yes	No
Easily compatible with transducers 7.5-MHz or above	Yes	No
Portable	Yes	±
Relatively inexpensive	Yes	No

*Size of phased-array transducer depends on whether it is dynamically focused and on the frequency used.

ponding to a wavelength of 0.43 mm. The array has a 9-mm total aperture, and, with the appropriate phasing of the single elements, an 84° sector angle is obtained for real-time imaging. The spherical acoustic lens gives an anatomically appropriate depth of field of 2–10 cm in front of the array.

The 6400 Cardiovue Ultrasonograph is a sophisticated system that utilizes three microprocessors and software control for the emission and detection of ultrasound pulses, the processing of echo signals, and the reconstruction and display of the resultant images (Fig. 8-12). In addition to 2D imaging, it also permits M-mode and Doppler examination. Various software packages are available for on-line data analysis.

Although passage of the TEE probe in awake

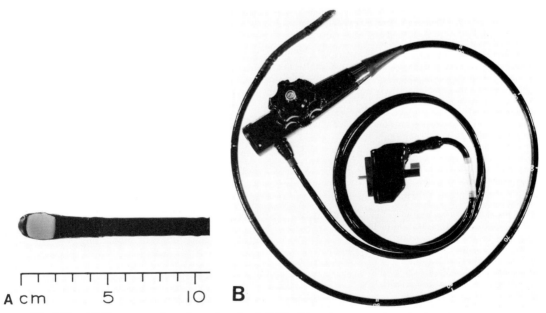

Fig. 8-11. (A) The transesophageal transducer head. (B)The Diasonics transesophageal echoprobe mounted on a standard gastroscope.

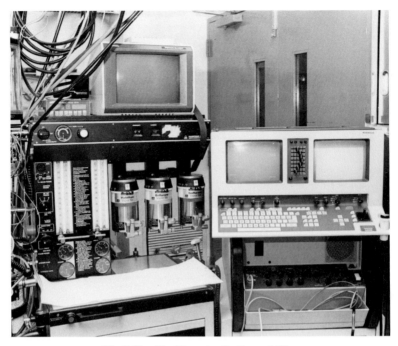

Fig. 8-12. The Diasonics Cardiovue 6400.

patients and volunteers has been described, the size of the device makes it more suitable for use in intubated anesthetized patients. In the awake subject, passage of the probe is preceded by intravenous sedation and topical anesthesia of the oropharynx with viscous lidocaine. With the controls of the gastroscope in the neutral, unlocked position, the transducer is inserted to the level of the cricopharyngeal sphincter. The patient is then asked to swallow; this helps guide the transducer into the esophagus. Schluter et al reported that in 84 of 103 patients the probe was successfully passed.[16] For all patients in whom the probe was successfully introduced, clear echocardiograms were obtained.

In anesthetized patients, also with the controls in the neutral, unlocked position, the transducer is introduced into the esophagus after tracheal intubation, either blindly or with the aid of a laryngoscope. Once in the esophagus, manipulation of the scope with simultaneous observation of the image is necessary.

To facilitate structure identification and interpretation of anatomic relations, Schluter et al have compared 2D-TEE recordings with the corresponding anatomic sections.[17a] They described six transesophageal transducer positions of diagnostic value: aortic valve, mitral valve, short-axis left ventricle, apical,

pulmonary, and biatrial. Of these six views, four are similar to views described by the Committee on Nomenclature and Standards of the American Society of Echocardiography (ASE).[17b] The aortic valve view is similar to the suprasternal long-axis view, and the mitral valve view approximates the apical long-axis view (Fig. 8-13). The left ventricular view is equivalent to the parasternal short-axis view at the mid-papillary muscle level, and the apical view is similar to a parasternal short-axis view of the apical region (Fig. 8-14). In addition to the six views described by Schluter et al, a four-chamber view equivalent to the ASE's apical four-chamber view and a short-axis view at the level of the aortic root are also obtainable by TEE (Fig. 8-15). It should be noted that because the transducer in TEE is posterior to the heart while it is anterior with transthoracic echocardiography (TTE), the TEE images are inverted when compared with TTE images.

Intraoperatively, TEE can be used as a diagnostic tool or for continuous monitoring. The two most commonly used views are the short-axis view at mid-papillary level (Fig. 8-14B) and the four-chamber view (Fig. 8-15B). The four-chamber view is used to assess atrial size, mitral and tricuspid valve function, septal thickness, regional wall motion, and the presence of air emboli. The short-axis left ventricular

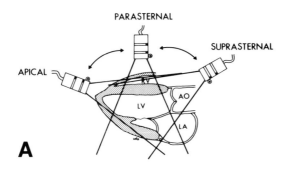

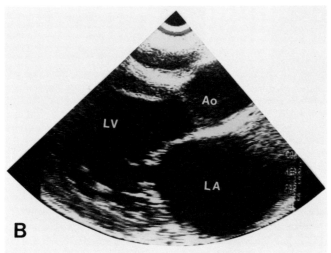

Fig. 8-13. Long-axis view. (A) Diagrammatic representation of the possible transducer orientations. (Abbreviations: LV, left ventricle; LA, left atrium; AO, aortic root.) (From Henry WL, DeMaria A, Gramiak R, et al: Report of the American Society of Echocardiography Committee on Nomenclature and Standards in Two-dimensional Echocardiography. Circulation 62:212, 1980, with permission.) (B) Representative long-axis echocardiographic image.

(LV) view is used to determine global ventricular function. Since myocardium perfused by the three major coronary arteries is represented at this level, this view is also useful to monitor changes in regional wall function due to myocardial ischemia. Insertion of the esophageal transducer is contraindicated in patients with esophageal pathology, descending thoracic aneurysms, left atrial myxomas, or coagulopathies (Table 8-3).

Although no complications related to the use of TEE have thus far been reported in supine patients, a number of potential problems related to the passage of the probe and operation of the ultrasonograph must be kept in mind. Potential complications include esophageal bleeding, burning, tearing, and dyspha-

gia and laryngeal discomfort or dysfunction. During ultrasound transmission, the transducer generates heat, and in vitro temperatures up to 42°C at the transducer tip have been observed when maximal transmission power was utilized.

Though TEE provides clearer images than TTE, it has potential limitations. It is possible that since TEE examines the heart from a retrocardiac position with a different orientation and somewhat more oblique angulation than routine echocardiography, the images and the measurements derived by TEE may be relatively inaccurate. However, Matsumoto et al compared standard parasternal M-mode echocardiography prior to induction of anesthesia with transesophageal M-mode after induction with

PARASTERNAL

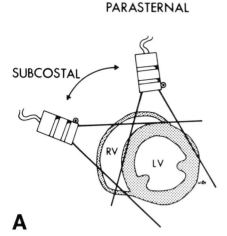

SUBCOSTAL

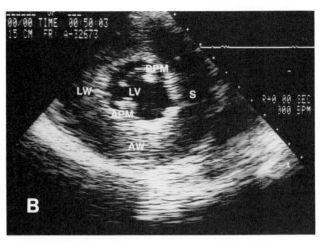

Fig. 8-14. Short-axis view. (A) Diagrammatic representation of the possible transducer orientations. (Abbreviations: RV, right ventricle; LV, left ventricle.) (From Henry WL, DeMaria A, Gramiak R, et al: Report of the American Society of Echocardiography Committee on Nomenclature and Standards in Two-dimensional Echocardiography. Circulation 62:212, 1980, with permission.) (B) Representative short-axis echocardiographic image. Abbreviations: LW, lateral wall; AW, anterior wall; S, septum; LV, left ventricle; APM, anterior papillary muscle; PPM, posterior papillary muscle.

enflurane.[14] They observed a close correlation for the end-diastolic dimensions ($r = 0.96$) and end-systolic dimensions ($r = 0.93$). Matsuzaki et al validated transesophageal M-mode echocardiography for the evaluation of left ventricular anterior wall (LVAW) motion by comparing TTE and TEE recordings to left ventriculographic findings.[18] TEE not only

obtained adequate images in more patients, but it had a higher correlation with measured left ventricular anterior wall motion than TTE.

Left ventricular diameters can also be accurately measured by TEE. Kremer et al demonstrated a good correlation ($r = 0.84$) between preinduction transthoracic 2D left ventricular diameter measure-

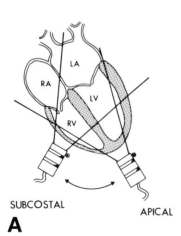

SUBCOSTAL   APICAL

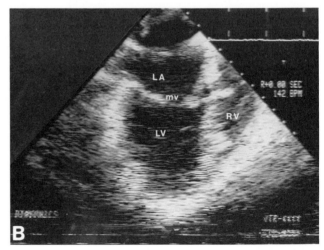

Fig. 8-15. Four-chamber view. (A) Diagrammatic representation of the possible transducer orientations. (Abbreviations: RV, right ventricle; RA, right atrium; LV, left ventricle; LA, left atrium.) (From Henry WL, DeMaria A, Gramiak R, et al: Report of the American Society of Echocardiography Committee on Nomenclature and Standards in Two-dimensional Echocardiography. Circulation 62:212, 1980, with permission.) (B) Representative four-chamber echocardiographic image. (Abbreviations: LA, left atrium; LV, left ventricle; mv, mitral valve; RV, right ventricle.)

Table 8-3
Transesophageal Echocardiography

Indications	Contraindications
Assessment	Absolute
Chamber size	Esophageal pathology:
Valvular function	stricture, varices,
Septal thickness	scleroderma, esophagitis,
Intracardiac shunts	or a history of esophageal
Monitoring	surgery
Global ventricular function	Relative
Regional ventricular function	Coagulopathy or
Intracardiac contrast	heparinization
	Large descending thoracic
	aneurysm
	Left atrial myxoma

ments and postinduction 2D-TEE-derived measurements.[19] Studies comparing measurements obtained at two distinct intervals separated by the induction of anesthesia may be invalid, however, since the induction of anesthesia can alter ventricular filling, contractility, and systemic vascular resistance.

Konstadt et al therefore compared measurements of end-diastolic area, end-systolic area, and ejection fraction area obtained by TEE with those obtained by almost simultaneous on-heart echocardiography (OHE) under identical hemodynamic conditions.[20] They found a close correlation between the two techniques for each of the three measurements (end-systolic area, $r = 0.94$; end diastolic area, $r = 0.88$; and ejection fraction area, $r = 0.92$) (Fig. 8-16). Furthermore, they found minimal interobserver variability ($r = 0.91$) (Fig. 8-17). TEE is therefore an accurate tool with which to measure ventricular dimensions in anesthetized patients.

DOPPLER ECHOCARDIOGRAPHY

General Principles

In the ultrasonic examination of the heart and great vessels, 2D and Doppler echocardiography are complementary techniques. Whereas the cardiac structures and their motion are visualized with 2D echocardiography, Doppler echocardiography studies the flow of blood within these structures. The physical principles on which the flow measurements are based were first described in 1842 by the Austrian physicist, Christian Doppler.[21]

At the time it was already known that the color perceived by the eye varies with the light wave fre-

quency. Doppler postulated that the observed color and, thus, the frequency changed with the relative motion between the source of the light and the observer. Unfortunately, he tried to prove his hypothesis by erroneously claiming that blue stars were moving toward the earth while red ones were moving away. As a result of this false explanation, he suffered severe criticism and his theories were rejected.

A few years later, however, Buys Ballot was able to apply the frequency-shift principle to the study of sound waves using three stationary trumpet players and one on a moving train.[22] While the four players were playing the same note, it appeared to the stationary observer that, as the train approached, the moving trumpet player's sound was of a higher pitch than the sound of the three stationary trumpeters. As soon as the train passed the observer, the tone shifted to a lower pitch. After these demonstrations, the Doppler principle became universally recognized, and it is now widely applied in science and engineering.

In the clinical applications of the Doppler principle, ultrasound is reflected from a moving target while the transmitter and receiver are stationary. For the study of blood flow velocities, ultrasound is emitted by a transducer, the red blood cells act as the moving reflectors, and the reflected ultrasound is recorded by the same or a different transducer (Fig. 8-18). To understand how the measurement of the frequency shift between the emitted and reflected ultrasonic beam provides information on blood velocity, it is necessary to refer to the Doppler equation:[23]

$$f_d = 2f_o \frac{v \cos \theta}{c} \qquad (8\text{-}3)$$

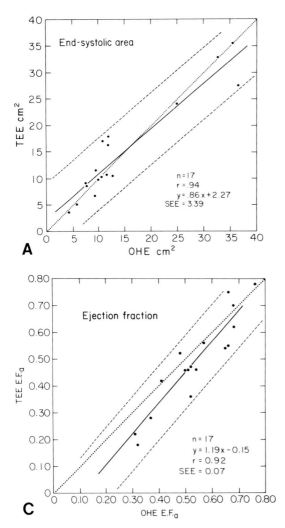

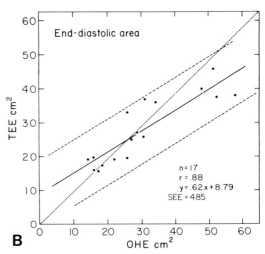

Fig. 8-16. Validation of quantitative transesophageal echocardiography. (A) End-systolic area measured by TEE versus values obtained by on-heart echocardiography (OHE). In these graphs, the solid line represents the slope derived by linear regression analysis; the two dashed lines represent two standard errors of the estimate above and below the slope, and the dotted line represents the line of identity. (B) End-diastolic area measured by TEE plotted versus end-diastolic area by OHE (see above). (C) Ejection fraction area calculated by TEE versus ejection fraction area calculated by OHE (see above). (From Konstadt S, Thys D, Mindich B, et al: Validation of quantitative intraoperative transesophageal echocardiography. Anesthesiology 65:418–421, 1986, with permission.)

where f_d represents the observed frequency shift between the emitted and reflected signals, f_o equals the frequency of the emitted ultrasound signal, v stands for the velocity of the blood flow, c equals the velocity of sound in tissues (1540 m/sec), and θ represents the angle of incidence between the direction of the blood flow and the direction of the ultrasonic signal.

Blood flow velocity is obtained by rearranging Equation 8-3 to

$$v = \frac{c}{2f_o} \times \frac{f_d}{\cos \theta} \qquad (8\text{-}4)$$

The only ambiguity in Equation 8-4 is that, theoretically, the direction of the ultrasonic signal could either refer to the transmitted or the received beam.[24] By convention, however, Doppler displays are made with reference to the received beam, and thus if the blood flow and the reflected beam travel in the same direction, the incidence angle is 0° and the cosine is +1. As a result, the frequency of the reflected signal will be higher than the frequency of the emitted signal.

Equipment currently utilized in clinical practice displays blood flow velocities as waveforms. The waveforms consist of a spectral analysis of velocities on the ordinate (Fig. 8-19) over time on the abscissa.[23] On such a display, blood flow toward the transducer is by convention represented above the baseline. If the blood flows away from the transducer, the incidence angle will be 180°, the cosine

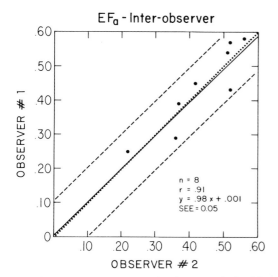

Fig. 8-17. A plot of ejection fraction area obtained by observer #1 versus observer #2 (see Fig. 8-16). (From Konstadt S, Thys D, Mindich B, et al: Validation of quantitative intraoperative transesophageal echocardiography. Anesthesiology 65:418–421, 1986, with permission.)

will equal −1, and the waveform will be displayed below the baseline. When the blood flow is perpendicular to the ultrasonic beam, the incidence angle will be 90° or 270°. The cosine of either angle being zero, no frequency shift will be detected. The inclusion of the cosine of the incidence angle in the Doppler equation results in the observation that blood

flow velocities will be most accurately measured when the ultrasonic beam is, as nearly as possible, parallel (or antiparallel) to the direction of blood flow (Fig. 8-20). In clinical practice, a deviation from parallel of up to 20° can be tolerated, since this only results in an error of 6 percent or less.[25]

Most modern echo scanners combine 2D imaging capabilities with Doppler capabilities. After the desired view of the heart has been obtained by 2D echocardiography, the Doppler beam, represented by a cursor, is superimposed on the 2D image. The operator positions the cursor as parallel as possible to the assumed direction of blood flow and then empirically adjusts the direction of the beam to optimize the audio and visual representations of the reflected Doppler signal.[24] At the present time, Doppler technology can be utilized in at least four different ways to measure blood flow velocities; these are pulsed, high-repetition frequency, continuous wave, and color-flow Doppler. Although each of these methods has specific applications, they are seldom concurrently available and then only on the most sophisticated and expensive echocardiographic devices.

Pulsed-Wave Doppler

In pulsed-wave Doppler, a short burst of ultrasound is transmitted at a given pulse-repetition frequency and sampled at an identical sampling frequency (fs). The depth at which the velocities are measured is called the sampling volume and is deter-

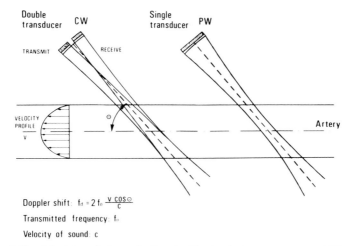

Doppler shift: $f_d = 2 f_0 \dfrac{V \cos \Theta}{c}$

Transmitted frequency: f_0

Velocity of sound: c

Fig. 8-18. Principles of ultrasonic Doppler blood velocity measurement. (Abbreviations: CW, continuous-wave; PW, pulsed-wave.) (From Blood velocity using the Doppler effect of backscattered ultrasound. *In* Hatle L, Angelsen B (eds): Doppler Ultrasound in Cardiology. Philadelphia, Lea & Febiger, 1985, with permission.)

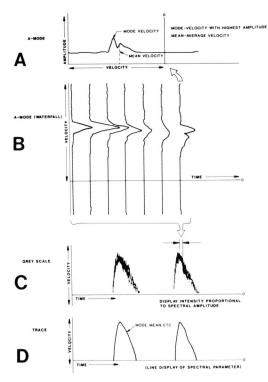

Fig. 8-19. A variety of Doppler displays are illustrated. (A) An amplitude velocity mode shows the cross-section of the spectrum at any one point in time and designates the fact that the most frequently found velocity is the "modal velocity" as opposed to the arithmetic mean velocity. (B) The A-mode waterfall display shows individual amplitude versus velocity cross-sections of the spectrum, with the A-mode waterfall shown above, having been selected from it. (C,D) Derived arithmetical estimates of the gray scale spectral velocity versus time display are the mode, mean, etc., which may be calculated and shown in addition to the spectral display. (From Recommendations for Terminology and Display for Doppler Echocardiography. Raleigh, NC, American Society of Echocardiography, 1984, with permission.)

mined by the time delay between the emission of the ultrasound signal burst and the sampling of the reflected signal. To sample at a given depth (D), sufficient time must be allowed for the signal to travel a distance of 2 × D (from the transducer to the sample volume and back).[23] The time delay, Td, between the emission of the signal and the reception of the reflected signal is related to D and to the speed of sound in tissues (c) by the following formula:

$$D = \frac{cTd}{2} \qquad (8\text{-}5)$$

The operator varies the depth of sampling by varying the time delay between the emission of the ultrasonic signal and the sampling of the reflected wave. In practice, the sample volume is represented by a small marker, which can be positioned at any point along the Doppler beam by moving it up or down the Doppler cursor. On some devices, it is also possible to vary the width and height of the sample volume.

The major advantage of the pulsed-wave Doppler is its range resolution or its ability to measure velocities at very specific locations within the circulation. It also has a major disadvantage, however, since it is limited in its ability to measure moderate-to-high velocities.

A simple reference to Western movies will clearly illustrate this point. When a stagecoach gets underway, its wheel spokes are observed as rotating in the correct direction. As soon as a certain speed is attained, however, rotation in the reverse direction is noted. This reversal is due to the fact that the camera frame rate is too slow to correctly observe the motion of the wheel spokes. In pulsed-wave Doppler, the ambiguity exists because the measured Doppler frequencies (fd) and the sampling frequency (fs) are in the same frequency (kiloHertz) range.

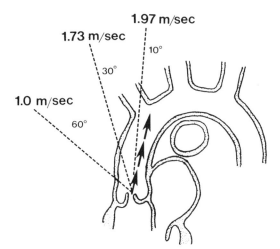

Fig. 8-20. Schematic diagram showing the importance of being parallel to flow. The solid arrows represent the direction of a systolic jet of 2 m/sec. If the interrogating beam is only 10° from parallel, the maximum velocity that can be recorded is 1.97 m/sec. Moving 60° from parallel only allows a peak velocity of 1.0 m/sec to be recorded. (From Kisslo J, Adams D, Mark DB (eds): Basic Doppler Echocardiography. New York, Churchill Livingstone, 1986, with permission.)

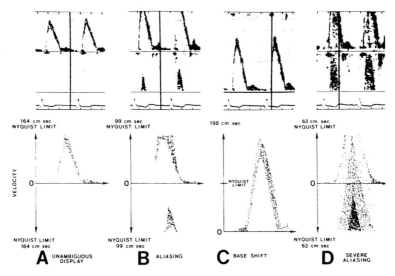

Fig. 8-21. Diagrammatic and spectral illustration of normal (A) and aliased Doppler (B) displays. (C) A baseline shift allows flow to be shown above the Nyquist limit; (D) severe aliasing with more than one wraparound is seen. (From Recommendations for Terminology and Display for Doppler Echocardiography. Raleigh, NC, American Society of Echocardiography, 1984, with permission.)

Ambiguity will only be avoided if the Doppler frequency is less than half the sampling frequency:

$$fd < \frac{fs}{2} \qquad (8\text{-}6)$$

The expression, fs/2, is also known as the Nyquist limit.

Doppler shifts above the Nyquist limit will create artifacts described as "aliasing" or "wraparound," and blood flow velocities will appear in a direction opposite to the conventional one (Fig. 8-21). Blood flowing with high velocity toward the transducer will result in a display of velocities above and below the baseline. This artifact can be avoided by increasing the sampling frequency (fs), but this then limits the time available for a pulse to travel to the sample volume and back, thus limiting the range. The relationship between the maximal detectable velocity and the range at which it can be detected is known as the range velocity product or $v_m R$:

$$v_m R = \frac{c^2}{8fo} \qquad (8\text{-}7)$$

where v_m is the maximal velocity that can be unambiguously measured and R is the range or distance from the transducer at which the measurement is to be made (Fig. 8-22).

High-Pulse-Repetition Frequency Doppler

To allow the measurement of high velocities with a single transducer, the pulsed-wave Doppler method can be modified to a high-pulse-repetition (high-PRF) method. While in pulsed-wave Doppler only a single burst of ultrasound is considered to be in the body at any given time, in high-PRF Doppler two to five sample volumes are simultaneously present in the tissues (Fig. 8-23). Information coming back to the transducer may be coming back from depths of either two, three, or four times the initial sample volume depth. The returning signals can be a mix of signals that have previously been emitted and have traveled to distant gates and other signals that were just sent and returned from the first range gate.

This method allows implementation of rapid–pulse-repetition frequency since the device does not wait for the return of the information from distant gates. It nonetheless receives that information back within the specified time gate period. Higher velocities can be measured with this method than with pulsed-wave Doppler; however, the depth from

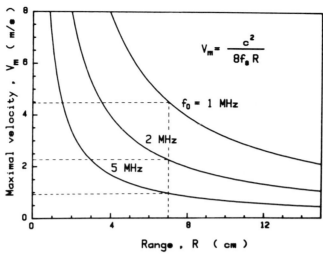

Fig. 8-22. The range–velocity product. (From Blood velocity measurements using the Doppler effect of backscattered ultrasound. *In* Hatle L, Angelsen B (eds): Doppler Ultrasound in Cardiology. Philadelphia, Lea & Febiger, 1985, with permission.)

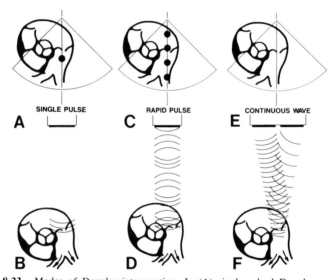

Fig. 8-23. Modes of Doppler interrogation. In (A) single-pulsed Doppler, a single range, or time gate, is established distal to the pulmonary valve, as shown here, and ultrasound information from that gate, shown as the wavelets in the diagram below (B), is processed for the Doppler shift. In continuous Doppler, one transducer (E) is sending and the other (F) is receiving ultrasound from all along the line of site. Therefore, velocities from along the complete line of the right ventricular outflow tract are summed into the resultant display (F). (C) A rapid-pulse, or high–pulse-repetition frequency Doppler has been implemented. Individual sample volumes are shown with Doppler information being processed from gates with depths that are multiples of the depth of the first gate. This is illustrated by the position of four sample volumes in C and by the fact that ultrasound information is coming and going at the same time from within the tissue (D). The multiple sampling depths (D) are also illustrated by the individual wavelet packets. Information may be coming back to the transducer from depths of either two, three, or four times the initial sample volume depth, returning from previous pulse bursts and having traveled and arrived back at the transducer at the same instant in time as the information from the first range gate from the pulse just sent. (From Recommendations for Terminology and Display for Doppler Echocardiography. Raleigh, NC, American Society of Echocardiography, 1984, with permission.)

which the velocity signal was reflected is unknown (range ambiguity).

Continuous-Wave Doppler

In continuous-wave (CW) Doppler, separate crystals are used to transmit and receive the ultrasound. The transmitting element continuously sends ultrasound while the other element continuously receives it. As a result of the continuous sampling technique, depth determination or range gating is not available; however, analysis of high velocities is possible (Fig. 8-23). This ability is of particular importance in the evaluation of patients with valvular and congenital heart disease, since high velocities are frequently detected in these disorders. CW Doppler is also the preferred method for the measurement of continuous flows.

Real-Time Doppler Color-Flow Mapping

To obtain better spatial orientation of flow within the cardiovascular system, real-time Doppler color-flow mapping has recently been introduced.[26] In Doppler flow mapping, a number of individual gates (± 8) are established along a line of sight within a 2D sector image. Along each line of sight, echo information is first obtained, followed by flow information at each of the gates. After these measurements are performed, the next line of sight is interrogated. Flow information from the various lines of sight within the sector is then assembled and superimposed on the 2D sector image. To quantitate the velocities measured at each of the gates, the signals are processed by an autocorrelator, which estimates velocities. These are then passed on to a digital scan converter and color converter for display. Because there are limitations to the speed at which these computations can be performed and to the speed at which ultrasound travels through tissue, the highest pulse-repetition frequency available in this system is 8 kHz. In several systems,

flows toward the transducer have been coded in increasing brightness of red to yellow, while flows away from the transducer are represented in increasing brightness of blue to magenta (Fig. 8-24).

Abnormal or turbulent flows are represented by a multicolored mosaic pattern. Currently, limitations of the real-time Doppler color-flow mapping are the low pulse-repetition frequency leading to aliasing even at physiologic velocities, the low sector-scanning frequency due to the complexity of the computations, and high signal-to-noise problems for signals from deep structures.

CLINICAL APPLICATIONS

Global Hemodynamic Performance

In clinical cardiology, echocardiography plays a major role in the hemodynamic evaluation of patients with heart disease. Valuable information concerning ventricular function can be gathered from either M-mode, 2D, or Doppler echocardiography. The data are obtained with minimal discomfort to the patient, and the examination can be repeated over time. Although similar techniques could be applied in the evaluation of the cardiac performance of anesthetized patients, they have not yet gained wide acceptance in clinical anesthesiology.

M-MODE ECHOCARDIOGRAPHY

For the diagnosis of cardiac lesions, M-mode echocardiography has to a great extent been surpassed by 2D echocardiography. By virtue of its simplicity and high image quality, however, it retains a certain advantage over 2D for the determination of hemodynamic performance. Indeed, M-mode measurements can easily be quantitated with calipers, pencil, and a ruler, while the 2D measurements often require sophisticated computer analysis. Since most modern echo scanners combine 2D and M-mode

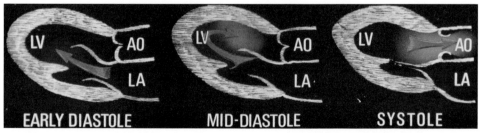

Fig. 8-24. Normal Doppler color-flow pattern with transducer at the apex of the heart. (From Omoto R (ed): Color Atlas of Real-Time 2-Dimensional Doppler Echocardiography. Tokyo, Shindas, 1984, with permission.)

capabilities, M-mode measurements are best obtained under 2D guidance. After a selected tomographic plane has been displayed on a 2D screen, the M-mode cursor is directed toward the desired ventricular axis.

The major disadvantage of the M-mode measurements is their unidimensional nature. Single dimensions are not always representative of the global ventricle, particularly in the presence of ischemic regional dysfunction or atypical geometry in dilated hearts.[27]

Left ventricular dimensions. The evaluation of hemodynamic function by M-mode echocardiography begins with the recording of left ventricular dimensions. This can be done across the chest wall with a transthoracic echotransducer or from the esophagus with the use of an esophageal transducer. In cardiac surgery, epicardial placement of the transducer has also been utilized. To obtain accurate measurements of the left ventricular cavity, the M-mode beam is directed at the cavity between the mitral valve and the papillary muscles. An M-mode recording at this level displays a clear view of the interventricular septum, the left ventricular cavity dimensions, and the posterior left ventricular wall. Occasionally, some elements of the mitral valve apparatus such as chordae tendineae are also visible

on the recording (Fig. 8-25). The ASE has published a number of guidelines concerning the measurement of left ventricular dimensions at this level.[28] The ASE recommends that the measurements be made from leading edge to leading edge and that the end-diastolic dimension (LVIDd) coincide with the Q wave on the ECG. The end-systolic dimension (LVIDs) is best measured at the time of peak downward motion of the interventricular septum. If abnormal septal motion is observed, the measurement should be obtained at the time of peak upward motion of the posterior endocardium. As considerable beat-to-beat variation is known to occur, it is recommended that measurements be made for several consecutive beats and that the results be averaged.[29]

Spotnitz et al have combined the intraoperative measurement of end-diastolic internal diameters with end-diastolic pressure determinations to assess the effects of open-heart surgery on left ventricular compliance in humans.[30] They obtained the M-mode recordings by retrocardiac placement of a 3.5-MHz low-profile M-mode echo transducer, which was embedded in a silicone disc for stability. In 7 of 15 patients, they observed a decrease in left ventricular compliance after ischemic cardiac arrest; they attributed these changes to ischemia. Utilizing the same technique, Wong and Spotnitz studied the effects of sodium nitroprusside on left ventricular

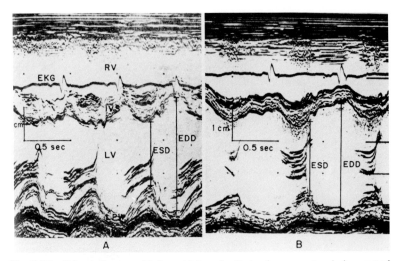

Fig. 8-25. Echocardiogram of left ventricle and mitral valve apparatus during control period (A) and halothane (B) administration. Note increase in end-systolic dimension (ESD) at halothane, 2 percent, with end-diastolic dimension (EDD) remaining virtually unchanged. This is consistent with a decrease in stroke volume. (Abbreviations: RV, right ventricle; LV, left ventricle; EKG, electrocardiogram.) (From Barash P, Glanz S, Katz J, et al: Ventricular function in children during halothane anesthesia: An echocardiographic evaluation. Anesthesiology 49:79–85, 1978, with permission.)

compliance.[31] They concluded that nitroprusside had no significant direct effect on the diastolic properties of the human myocardium.

Ejection phase indices. After the systolic and diastolic internal diameters have been measured, it becomes possible to calculate a variety of ejection phase indices. These indices were initially described for the angiographic evaluation of ventricular function and were later adapted for use in echocardiography. In numerous studies, the values of ejection phase indices obtained by echocardiography have been compared with the angiographic values. Some of the studies showed a good correlation between echo and angiographic results; in others, the correlation was poor.[32-34]

Fractional shortening (FS) is the simplest of the ejection phase indices since in its calculation no assumptions are made about the shape or the volume of the left ventricle.[35] FS is often expressed as a percentage, and it is obtained by the formula

$$FS(\%) = \frac{LVIDd - LVIDs}{LVIDd} \times 100 \qquad (8\text{-}8)$$

A very similar ejection phase index is called circumferential fiber shortening. In its measurement, it is assumed that the ventricle is composed of a series of concentric circles and that the M-mode dimensions are the diameters of these circles. The circumferential fiber shortening is then calculated as the difference between the diastolic and systolic circumferences over the diastolic circumference.[36]

$$\frac{\text{Circumferential}}{\text{fiber shortening}} = \frac{\pi LVIDd - \pi LVIDs}{\pi LVIDd} \qquad (8\text{-}9)$$

If the circumference of the ventricle and its contractility are symmetrical, the values for fractional shortening and circumferential fiber shortening are identical because the M-mode slices are representative of the entire ventricle.

When the left ventricular ejection time (LVET) is known, another ejection phase index, the mean rate of circumferential fiber shortening (Vcf), can be computed by the formula

$$\text{Mean Vcf} = \frac{LVIDd - LVIDs}{LVIDd \times LVET} \qquad (8\text{-}10)$$

In a number of studies, the addition of the time element was found to enhance the ability of M-mode echocardiography to separate normal from abnormal subjects.[37,38]

The M-mode–derived ejection phase index most closely related to the angiographic indices is the ejection fraction. The computation of ejection fraction (EF) requires the conversion from a linear dimension to a volume dimension. Although numerous formulas have been suggested for this conversion, the results have often been found to be erroneous and unreliable.[39] It is generally accepted that the best equation for these conversions was described by Teichholz et al:[27]

$$V = \frac{7 \cdot D^3}{2.4 + D} \qquad (8\text{-}11)$$

where V stands for volume and D stands for internal diameter.

After the left ventricular end-diastolic volume (LVEDV) and end-systolic volume (LVESV) have been calculated, the EF is obtained with the following formula:

$$\frac{LVEDV - LVESV}{LVEDV} \times 100 = EF(\%) \qquad (8\text{-}12)$$

A number of these ejection phase indices have been utilized intraoperatively to assess the effects of cardiac valve replacement or the administration of anesthetic agents on ventricular function.[40] Wong and Spotnitz demonstrated that in patients with chronic mitral regurgitation, valve replacement resulted in a marked decrease in FS.[41] Barash et al studied the effects of halothane on ventricular function in healthy children.[42] Data were obtained prior to the induction of anesthesia and at halothane concentrations ranging from 0.5 to 2.0 percent. At 2.0 percent halothane, Barash et al noted a 26 percent reduction in EF and a 36 percent decrease in the mean Vcf. No significant change in LVEDV was noted. Gerson and Gianaris performed a comparable study on healthy adult patients and observed similar results regarding the depressant effects of halothane on left ventricular performance.[43]

Rathod et al studied 20 healthy patients scheduled for minor surgical procedures.[44] They compared the effects of halothane and enflurane on ventricular performance and found that 0.93 percent end-tidal concentration of halothane caused a significant decrease in LVIDd and a significant increase in LVIDs. The calculation of FS showed a highly significant decrease. Vcf and percentage of systolic thickening of the left ventricular posterior wall also decreased significantly. Enflurane in a 2.4 percent end-tidal concentration caused a significant reduction in both end-systolic and end-diastolic dimensions; however, enflurane did not produce significant changes in FS, Vcf, or percentage of systolic thickening of the left ventricular posterior wall.

In addition to these early studies of anesthetic effects on myocardial performance, M-mode echocardiography has been utilized in recent investigations of the effects of narcotics on ventricular function. Schieber et al used M-mode echocardiography and invasive hemodynamic monitoring to assess the cardiovascular effects of high-dose fentanyl in newborn piglets. No significant change in FS was observed.[45] Moore et al, studying the cardiovascular effects of sufentanil as the sole anesthetic for pediatric cardiac surgery, reported no significant change in EF after induction with 5, 10, or 20 μg/kg of sufentanil.[46]

Cardiac output. After calculation of the LVEDV and LVESV, it is also possible to derive stroke volume and cardiac output, since the difference between LVEDV and LVESV is equal to the stroke volume. If the heart rate is known, the cardiac output can be calculated as the product of stroke volume and heart rate.

Matsumoto et al utilized transesophageal M-mode echocardiography to continuously monitor the left ventricular dimensions in 21 patients undergoing open heart surgery.[14] They observed only a modest correlation between cardiac output measurements by dye dilution and the echocardiographic technique ($r = 0.72$). In contrast, Terai et al, studying the effects of positive end-expiratory pressure on cardiac function using M-mode transesophageal echocardiography, found an excellent correlation ($r = 0.97$) between M-mode and thermodilution cardiac outputs.[47]

Systolic time intervals. Another measure of hemodynamic performance that can be obtained using M-mode echo measurements is systolic time intervals. When the M-mode beam is directed across the aortic orifice, opening and closing of the aortic valve leaflets can be easily detected. The time between the opening and the closing of the aortic valve represents the LVET while the time between the beginning of the Q wave on ECG and the opening of the valve represents the preejection period (PEP) (Fig. 8-26).[48] The usefulness and limitations of the systolic time intervals for the assessment of left ven-

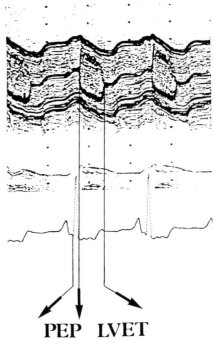

PEP LVET

Fig. 8-26. Systolic time intervals. The preejection period (PEP) is defined from the Q wave on the ECG to the opening of the aortic valve, while the left ventricular ejection time (LVET) represents the time between opening and closing of the aortic valve.

tricular function have been extensively reviewed elsewhere[49,50] (see Chapter 6).

Right ventricular ejection time (RVET) and PEP can also be measured by simultaneous recording of an M-mode echocardiogram at the pulmonary valve and an electrocardiogram.[51] In a number of reports, the PEP/RVET ratio has been utilized as a measure of pulmonary artery pressure.[52-54] In children with congenital heart disease, this measurement was shown to be useful in assessing the adequacy of surgical banding of the pulmonary artery.[55]

Wall thickness and wall stress. M-mode echocardiography is uniquely suited for the determination of wall thickness. It is well established that the thickness of the left ventricular wall varies from systole to diastole and that with decreased ventricular function the rate of thickening is reduced.[56]

During ischemia, occasional systolic thinning of the wall rather than thickening can be observed.[57] The ASE recommends that to assess wall thickness, measurements should be made from leading edge to leading edge.[28] The combination of thickness and cavity dimensions into a thickness/volume ratio provides an estimate of the relationship between left ventricular hypertrophy and dilatation.[58] This ratio has also been utilized to predict systolic left ventricular pressure.[59] If systolic arterial pressure is combined with wall thickness and cavity dimension, meridional end-systolic wall stress can be obtained, which is a quantitative index of left ventricular afterload.[60,61]

The formula utilized to calculate wall stress was derived by Sandler and Dodge from the basic Laplace equation:[62]

$$\text{Wall stress} = \frac{1.33 \times P \times LVID}{4\ WT\ (1 + WT/LVID)} \qquad (8\text{-}13)$$

where P equals the systolic blood pressure, WT represents wall thickness, LVID represents cavity dimension, and 1.33 converts mm Hg to dynes/cm^2. For peak systolic wall stress, the LVID is measured in diastole, and the wall thickness is equal to half the sum of the diastolic interventricular and posterior wall thicknesses. The diastolic dimensions are selected on the assumption that no significant changes occur in these dimensions between end-diastole and the time at which peak systolic wall stress is developed. In clinical practice Equation 8-13 is often simplified to the equation

$$\text{Wall stress} = \frac{\text{radius}}{\text{wall thickness}} \qquad (8\text{-}14)$$

Elevated wall stress has been reported in patients with aortic stenosis, aortic regurgitation, and systemic hypertension. In untreated hypertension, even at the early stages, Hartford et al have demonstrated elevated wall stress, usually combined with supranormal myocardial contractility.[63] Recent evidence suggests that wall stress is a better indicator of left ventricular afterload than systemic vascular resistance and that changes in these two variables do not necessarily correlate.[64,65]

Contractility. In a number of studies, ventricular dimensions derived by M-mode echocardiography have been combined with end-systolic pressures to determine contractility. Marsh et al studied 13 normal subjects during methoxamine infusion and established the linearity between the end-systolic pressure and the end-systolic diameter.[66] In asymptomatic or mildly symptomatic patients with chronic aortic regurgitation, Branzi et al demonstrated that the end-systolic pressure–volume relation was the most sensitive index of myocardial depression (see Chapters 6 and 16).[67] Utilizing the same index of contractility in humans after cardiac transplantation, Borow et al have shown that left ventricular contractility in transplanted patients was not significantly different from normal.[68]

Other M-mode measurements. The motion of the mitral valve, as recognized on M-mode, has long been utilized to provide information on left ventricular function.[69] The motion of the anterior mitral valve leaflet describes a specific and easily recognizable pattern resembling the letter *M* (Fig. 8-27). The various peaks and troughs of the anterior mitral leaflet have been labeled on Figure 8-27. D represents the end of systole and is located immediately before the opening of the valve. The first peak is labeled E and occurs during rapid ventricular filling. The nadir of the early diastolic closing is labeled F. The second peak follows atrial contraction and is represented by the letter A, while complete closure occurs at C, following the onset of the ventricular systole. A decrease in the E to F slope was recognized many years ago in patients with mitral stenosis (MS) and was suggested as a diagnostic sign for MS.[70] Since then, however, it has also been observed in patients with normal mitral valve function but reduced left ventricular compliance.[71] More recently, it has become evident that a reduction in the EF slope is a nonspecific sign that can occur in patients with reduced ventricular compliance but also in patients with pulmonary hypertension in whom no evidence of reduced left ventricular compliance can be detected.[72] The D to E slope has been studied as an indicator of blood velocity across the mitral valve and has been shown to be decreased in patients with severe low-output states.[73]

When the mitral valve echocardiogram is recorded simultaneously with the ECG, the valve stroke volume can be calculated (Fig. 8-28). In 80 patients, simultaneous mitral valve echograms and either thermodilution or Fick cardiac outputs were measured.[74] In 73 patients without mitral valve regurgitation, the correlation between the echocardiographic determinations of stroke volume and the stroke volume determined by other methods was good ($r = 0.90$).

Mitral valve echograms have also been combined with phonocardiograms and electrocardiograms to determine pulmonary capillary wedge pressure noninvasively.[75,76] Pulmonary capillary wedge pressure (PCWP) was predicted from the ratio of the interval between the Q wave of the ECG and

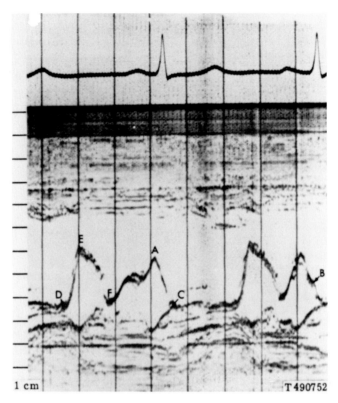

Fig. 8-27. M-mode echocardiogram of a normal mitral valve (see text). (From Feigenbaum H: Echocardiography (ed 4). Philadelphia, Lea & Febiger, 1986, with permission.)

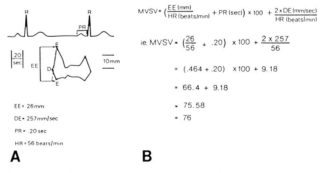

$$MVSV = \left(\frac{EE \ (mm)}{HR \ (beats/min)} + PR \ (sec) \right) \times 100 \ + \frac{2 \times DE \ (mm/sec)}{HR \ (beats/min)}$$

$$ie. \ MVSV = \left(\frac{26}{56} + .20 \right) \times 100 + \frac{2 \times 257}{56}$$

$$= (.464 + .20) \times 100 + 9.18$$

$$= 66.4 + 9.18$$

$$= 75.58$$

$$= 76$$

EE = 26mm
DE = 257mm/sec
PR = .20 sec
HR = 56 beats/min

A   **B**

Fig. 8-28. (A) This diagram illustrates variables used in one technique to calculate stroke volume from the mitral valve echogram and the electrocardiogram. EE is measured from the outermost echoes. DE represents the most rapid slope from the D to E points. Heart rate (HR) is calculated by dividing 60 by the R-to-R interval in seconds. (B) Formula for calculating mitral valve stroke volume (MVSV). (From Rasmussen S, Conya BC, Feigenbaum H, et al: Stroke volume calculated from the mitral valve echogram in patients with and without ventricular dyssynergy. Circulation 58:125, 1978, by permission of the American Heart Association, Inc.)

278

the closure of the mitral valve (Q-C) and from the interval between the closure of the aortic valve and the E point on the mitral echogram (A_2–E). These measurements have been obtained in patients with mitral stenosis and mitral regurgitation and have been found useful for the longitudinal follow-up of these patients.[77,78]

TWO-DIMENSIONAL ECHOCARDIOGRAPHY

Because anatomic structures are easily recognized on a 2D image, qualitative assessment of cardiac function can often be performed by simple visual analysis of the echo images either on-line or from video recordings. By the continuous monitoring of a left-ventricular short-axis view, information on myocardial contractility, systolic wall motion, and wall thickening can be obtained.

Contractility is determined by the observation of left ventricular emptying. In systole, all segments of the normal left ventricular myocardium move, by the same degree, toward the geometric center of the cavity. In a ventricle with generalized depression of contractility, this motion can be equally reduced for all segments of the ventricular wall. In ischemia, only a localized segment of the wall may contract poorly—ie, less than the rest of the wall (hypokinesis) or not at all (akinesis). A third index of ventricular function is systolic wall thickening, which relates myocardial thickness at end-systole to the thickness at end-diastole. Normal myocardium shows significant thickening (30–50 percent) at end-systole in roughly homogeneous fashion around the entire left-ventricular perimeter. Poorly functioning or infarcted myocardium shows little or no thickening. All of the methods of estimating ventricular function rely on the detection of endocardial and epicardial ventricular borders and their motion. Once the borders have been defined, a variety of performance indices can also be derived quantitatively.

Since 2D echocardiography provides tomographic cuts of the heart, the major questions concerning the determination of global ventricular function evolve around the choice and number of cuts required to accurately characterize the whole ventricle. Folland et al have compared left ventricular EF and volumes calculated with five different algorithms with standard cineangiographic and radionuclide values.[79] They established that for the determination of EF, the modified Simpson's rule was the algorithm that gave the best correlation with the non-echo techniques. In the Simpson's rule method, the ventricle is divided into a number of slices of known thickness (Fig. 8-29).[80] The volume of each of the slices is

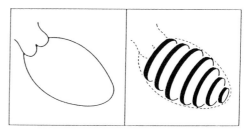

Fig. 8-29. These diagrams demonstrate Simpson's rule; the left ventricle is expressed as a series of circular slices. (From Rogers EW, Feigenbaum H, Weyman AE: Echocardiography for quantitation of cardiac chambers. *In* Yu PN, Goodwin JF (eds): Progress in Cardiology, vol 8. Philadelphia, Lea & Febiger, 1979, with permission.)

derived by multiplying the surface areas of the slices by their thickness. The volume of the ventricle is equal to the sum of the volumes of the slices. The number of slices required to define the volume of the ventricle accurately depends on the shape of the ventricle. The more irregular the shape, the more slices are required.

Dubroff et al, studying left ventricular EF during cardiac surgery, utilized up to four different short-axis views for each left ventricular volume determination.[81] They observed a decrease in EF after correction of mitral or aortic regurgitation and an increase in EF after relief of aortic and mitral stenosis.

Since in adults it is often difficult to obtain a sufficient number of slices, it is common in clinical practice to utilize modifications of the Simpson's rule. One such modification utilizes two perpendicular tomographic views of the ventricle to calculate the volume.[82] An apical two-chamber view and a short-axis view at the level of the papillary muscles are traced at the endocardial border, while a computer utilizes a modification of the Simpson's rule to calculate the left ventricular volume. This technique was recently utilized by Ren et al to assess the effects of myocardial revascularization or valve replacement on left ventricular function.[83] In 27 patients undergoing cardiac catheterization and intraoperative 2D echo within 1 week, a good correlation was found between 2D and angiographic left ventricular EF and left ventricular end-systolic volumes. Like Dubroff et al,[81] Ren et al found that patients undergoing valve replacements for regurgitant lesions had a postoperative decrease in left ventricular function. In 7 coronary artery bypass patients with evidence of perioperative ischemia, a significant reduction from 52 ± 10 percent to 43 ± 12 percent in left ventricular EF was observed.

The advantage of 2D measurements over M-mode measurements for the calculation of EF was clearly demonstrated in the study of Folland et al.[79] When compared with angiography, the 2D-derived EF yielded a higher correlation coefficient ($r = 0.78$) than the unidimensional M-mode measurement ($r = 0.55$); however, 2D did not offer a clear advantage for the calculation of ventricular volumes in this study.

Most of the currently utilized algorithms for the calculation of the left ventricular volumes or EF include a measurement of the long axis of the left ventricular cavity in the two-chamber or four-chamber apical view. A true long-axis view cannot always be obtained, however, and therefore the length of the ventricle is often underestimated.[84] This is particularly true with TEE and has led to the use of short-axis area measurements, rather than volume measurements, for the determination of left ventricular performance.

Left ventricular end-diastolic area (EDA) represents a better index of left ventricular preload than PCWP. In one report, the measurement of end-diastolic area by TEE allowed Cahalan et al to establish that the etiology of a hypotensive episode was hypovolemia although the PCWP was normal.[85]

The ejection fraction area (EFA), a measure of left ventricular performance, is obtained by the formula

$$\frac{EDA - ESA}{EDA} \times 100 = EFA(\%) \qquad (8\text{-}15)$$

where ESA represents end-systolic area.

Roizen et al were able to demonstrate that EFA was a more sensitive indicator of left ventricular performance than cardiac output alone.[86] Indeed, in some patients undergoing abdominal aortic cross-clamping, they observed marked reductions in EFA while changes in cardiac output were minimal.

As with M-mode echocardiography, wall stress can be calculated when 2D echo information is combined with the systolic blood pressure. In 15 normal subjects and in 15 patients with severe chronic aortic regurgitation, St. John Sutton et al obtained 2D short-axis views at the level of the tips of the papillary muscles and apical four-chamber views for long-axis determination.[87] After digitizing the echo images, they calculated left ventricular end-systolic meridional and circumferential wall stress and demonstrated that these variables were increased in patients with aortic regurgitation when compared with normal patients. The meridional stress values

obtained from 2D echo correlated closely ($r = .89$) with values obtained from simultaneously recorded M-mode echocardiograms.

Information on left ventricular contractility can also be derived from the combined analysis of 2D short-axis echocardiograms and peak systolic arterial pressure. In recent experiments, Hillel et al demonstrated that, during preload manipulations, the correlation between the end-systolic volume, derived from a 2D short-axis area, and the systolic arterial pressure was linear.[88] In patients undergoing coronary artery bypass surgery, they further showed that the method was sufficiently sensitive to detect changes in contractility after administration of dopamine or halothane.[89,90] Left ventricular volume calculations in these experiments were based on a modified elipsoid model for single-plane data using the following equation:

$$V = SA^{3/2} \frac{SA + 36}{SA + 12} \qquad (8\text{-}16)$$

where V stands for volume and SA for short-axis area at the papillary muscle level.[91] When this formula was utilized to calculate cardiac output as the difference between end-diastolic and end-systolic volume, multiplied by heart rate, a good correlation was found with thermodilution cardiac output measurements ($r = 0.87$).[65]

DOPPLER ECHOCARDIOGRAPHY

In anesthesia, Doppler echocardiography has particular appeal as a method to determine flow in various vessels. When the flow measurement is applied to the aorta, cardiac output is obtained. A more recent application of intraoperative Doppler echocardiography relates to the esophageal determination of mitral inflow.

Cardiac output. The determination of cardiac output by Doppler echocardiography is based on the measurement of blood flow velocities in the ascending aorta.[92] Doppler sampling in the aorta produces a time-dependent velocity curve. During systole, the blood flow velocities in the aorta describe a bell-shaped curve over time. The area under this curve must be integrated manually or automatically and multiplied with the aortic cross-sectional area to yield stroke volume. Cardiac output is the product of stroke volume and heart rate. As in any Doppler examination, the Doppler beam should be aimed in a direction parallel to the flow for accurate signal collection. In most patients, a parallel alignment can satisfactorily be obtained when the Doppler signal is recorded from the suprasternal notch.[93] The major difficulties in Doppler cardiac output determinations evolve around the measurement of the aortic cross-sectional area, beat-to-beat variations in stroke volume, respiratory disturbances, and changes in probe position (see Chapter 6).

Whereas the aorta is often thought of as a curved tube with unchanging dimensions from inlet to arch, in practice considerable variations in aortic cross-sectional area are observed from the aortic orifice to the arch. The narrowest diameter is at the aortic orifice, and because of blood acceleration in the left ventricular outflow tract, the velocity profile is flat. This would therefore be the ideal location to measure aortic flow.[95] In practice, however, the measurements in this area are often disturbed by the movement of the aortic leaflets, and a slightly superior location is preferred. The aortic diameter is best measured on a long-axis view of the left ventricle. Numerous investigators have found a good correlation between the cardiac output measured by combined Doppler echo methods and thermodilution or Fick cardiac outputs.[96-99]

Recently, a dedicated CW Doppler device has been introduced for the intraoperative measurement of cardiac output. The Doppler transducers are mounted on a 24-Fr esophageal stethoscope, which continuously measures blood flow velocities in the descending aorta. A single measurement of ascending aortic flow is obtained by suprasternal sampling, after the aortic diameter has been measured by echo-cardiography or calculated by an algorithm. The relationship between ascending and descending aortic flow is assumed constant. In two recent studies, a fairly good correlation was observed between esophageal Doppler and thermodilution cardiac output determinations.[100,101]

Mitral inflow. Doppler echocardiography is ideally suited to assess flow velocity patterns across the mitral valve. With the pulsed Doppler sample volume located in the left ventricular inlet, a typical flow velocity pattern is observed.[102] In normal sinus rhythm, an initial early velocity peak (E) is followed by a low-velocity pause and a second peak (A) corresponding to the atrial contraction (Fig. 8-30). With increases in heart rate, the duration of the pause is shortened, while in atrial fibrillation the A peak disappears. A number of recent investigations suggest that the E-A peak ratio is related to left ventricular compliance; a reduction in the E-A ratio occurs as compliance decreases, during ischemia, or in association with aortic stenosis or hypertension (Fig. 8-31).[102-104]

Ryan et al have shown that in dogs after coronary artery occlusion, ischemic changes in LV relaxation were associated with a reduction in the E-A ratio;[105] however, a relationship between the extent of filling dysfunction and infarct size could not be clearly established.[106] Using either transthoracic or esophageal Doppler techniques, several investigators have demonstrated changes in the E-A ratio in patients with ischemic heart disease.[102,107]

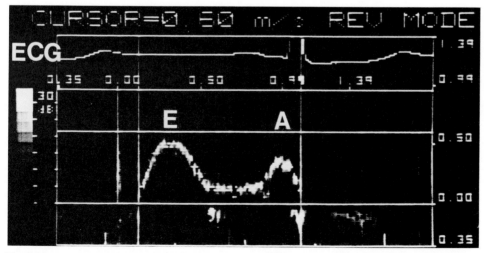

Fig. 8-30. Normal mitral inflow velocity profile. Time is represented on the horizontal axis while a spectral display of the velocities is shown on the vertical axis. The early left ventricular phase (E) is followed by a period of low-velocity flow and the contribution of atrial contraction (A).

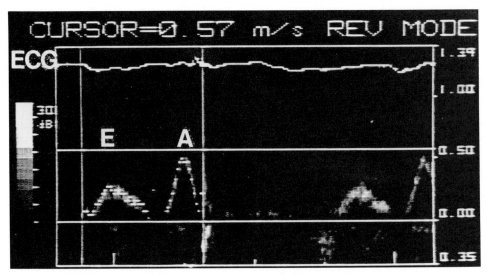

Fig. 8-31.   Reversal of the E-A velocity ratio in a patient with ischemic heart disease.

The Doppler-derived E-A ratio has also been found useful as a predictor of outcome in patients with acute myocardial infarction (MI). In 60 patients with acute MI, Visser et al observed a significant trend toward a lower E-A ratio in patients with a higher Killip class.[108] They also found that a low E-A ratio obtained on admission to the hospital helped to identify the patients at risk of subsequent death from cardiogenic shock.

Regional Performance

INDEX OF MYOCARDIAL PERFUSION

In 1935, Tennant and Wiggers first demonstrated that left ventricular contractile function was impaired shortly after coronary artery ligation.[109] Subsequently, Herman et al described four patterns of abnormal regional ventricular wall motion: (1) asynchrony, or disturbed temporal sequence of contraction; (2) asyneresis, or local hypokinesis; (3) akinesis; and (4) dyskinesis, or paradoxical systolic expansion (Fig. 8-32).[110] Though the areas of these localized disturbances of wall motion were in close anatomic relation to regions of known areas of ischemic heart disease, no specific causal relationship between the ischemic heart disease and the contractile abnormalities was established.

Recently, the correlation between myocardial blood flow and ventricular function has become clearer. Forrester et al have demonstrated that stepwise reductions in perfusion pressure produce a predictable progression of segmental contractile abnormalities from dysynchrony to hypokinesis to akinesis and finally to dyskinesis.[111] Similarly, coronary blood flow correlates closely with ventricular function.[112] Importantly, wall motion abnormalities may be more sensitive indicators of ischemia than ECG changes. Lowenstein et al have documented regional wall motion abnormalities (RWMA) in myocardial regions perfused by narrowed coronary arteries while the epicardial ECG did not change.[113] Therefore, regional wall motion, which is readily evaluated by echo, is now considered a reliable indicator of myocardial blood flow. Since RWMAs do not always correlate with ventricular contractility, however, investigators have examined regional wall thickening as an index of myocardial perfusion.[114,115] Gallagher et al have demonstrated that the degree of systolic wall thickening (%WT) is proportional to the myocardial blood flow.[116] They measured systolic wall thickening with sonomicrometry and regional blood flow by tracer microspheres in 15 open-chest anesthetized dogs at progressive degrees of coronary artery stenosis (Fig. 8-33).[114-116] When perfusion to the subendocardium was decreased, a 75 percent reduction in %WT was observed. When myocardial flow was reduced to the point that only subepicardial zones were perfused, akinesis was observed. Wall thinning also occurred with transmural reductions in blood flow. Similar results have been obtained by other investigators.[117]

The above studies have failed to distinguish between the effects of ischemia and the effects of

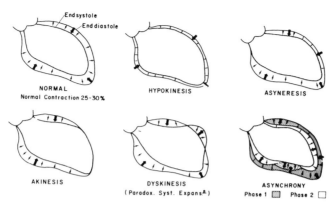

Fig. 8-32. Localized and generalized abnormalities in cardiac contraction. This schematic representation shows various localized and generalized abnormalities in cardiac contraction. Motion from end-diastole to end-systole is illustrated by arrows. Hypokinesis is a generalized reduction in the normal degree of contraction. See text for definitions and descriptions. (From Herman M, Heinle R, Klien M, et al: Localized disorders in myocardial contraction. Asynergy and its role in congestive heart failure. N Engl J Med 277:222–232, 1967, with permission.)

changing loading conditions on regional myocardial function. For example, an area of myocardium may be able to contract against a low afterload, but in the face of an acute increase in resistance, it may no longer contract normally. Therefore, Osakada et al defined an index of regional wall function that is independent of ventricular loading conditions.[118] They developed the end-systolic pressure–wall thick-

ness relationship, which is analogous to the load-independent end-systolic pressure–volume relationship used to assess global contractility. The end-systolic pressure–wall thickness relationship was displaced to the left by progressive coronary stenosis, but it remained unaffected by changes in ventricular loading. Though Osakada et al used microcrystals for the determination of ventricular dimensions, these measurements can also be obtained by echocardiography.

ECHOCARDIOGRAPHY IN THE DIAGNOSIS OF REGIONAL DYSFUNCTION

Echocardiography is an ideal method with which to detect RWMAs in clinical practice. Comparing echocardiography to left ventriculography in patients with ventricular aneurysms and localized ventricular dysfunction, Weyman et al observed an excellent correlation in location, contour, and wall-motion pattern.[119] In a more quantitative fashion, Kislo et al compared 2D echocardiography and cineangiography for the detection of RWMA.[120] In 82 percent of the analyzed segments (430 of 525), the echocardiographic images of the examined regions were adequate. In a double-blind analysis of the two techniques, there was agreement in 365 of 430 segments examined. Retrospective analysis of the 55 discrepancies revealed that 34 were due to echocardiographic error, 6 were indeterminant, and 15 were due to angiographic error. Kislo et al concluded that echocardiography was useful in the assessment of left ventricular asynergy.

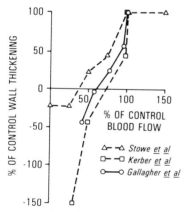

Fig. 8-33. Comparison of data on the relationship of mean transmural blood flow to systolic wall thickening. Data are presented as percentages of control blood flow and control systolic thickening. The data from Kerber et al[114] were normalized to conform with data of Stowe et al[115] and Gallagher et al.[116] (From Kerber RE, Marcus ML, Ehrhardt J, et al: Correlation between echocardiographically demonstrated segmental dyskinesis and regional myocardial perfusion. Circulation 52:1097–1104, 1975, with permission.)

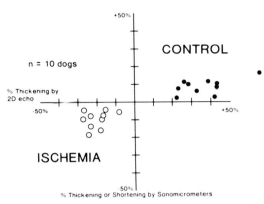

Fig. 8-34. Comparison of two-dimensional echocardiograms and sonomicrometers in detecting transient ischemia. In dogs with severe coronary stenosis but no resting ischemia, both techniques showed systolic thickening during control conditions (solid circles). When isoproterenol and acute aortic constriction were superimposed on coronary stenosis, both techniques demonstrated regional systolic thinning (negative thickening), which indicates ischemia (open circles). (From Pandian N, Kerber R: Two-dimensional echocardiography in experimental coronary stenosis. I. Sensitivity and specificity in detecting transient myocardial dyskinesis: Comparison with sonomicrometers. Circulation 66:597–602, 1982, with permission.)

Two-dimensional echocardiography has been shown to be sensitive and specific in detecting the precise location of transient ischemia. When a 90 percent reduction in circumflex artery diameter was created, there was complete agreement between sonomicrometric and 2D echocardiographic diagnosis of systolic wall thinning (Fig. 8-34).[121]

The diagnosis of acute myocardial ischemia can be made by evaluating endocardial motion or systolic wall thickening. To measure endocardial motion or thickening, it is necessary first to identify the epicardial and endocardial borders of a diastolic frame. An approximate center of the cavity is then assigned, and an end-systolic frame is superimposed. In a system with a fixed reference system, the center of the cavity is assumed unchanged between diastole and systole. In a floating axis system, a small correction is applied to correct for the rotational and translational motion of the heart during systole. In nonsurgical patients, the fixed reference system is used because systolic translation is minimal; however, in patients with open chests undergoing cardiac surgical procedures, there is enhanced systolic translation, and the fixed reference system may be inaccurate. With the use of the fixed reference system, the enhanced translation gives the impression of septal hypokinesis in patients without other evidence of ischemia.[122]

In 13 patients with ventriculographic confirmation of anterior wall motion hypokinesis, Ren et al have shown that %WT was abnormal in 92 percent (12 of 13) of patients, while endocardial motion abnormalities were only observed in 46 percent (6 of 13) of patients.[123] Dyskinesis was detected by %WT in 100 percent of the patients and by endocardial wall motion in only 60 percent. Therefore, wall thickening as measured by 2D echocardiography is an accurate means to detect dysfunctional segments, and %WT is a more sensitive indicator of ischemia than endocardial motion.

Though it is clear that 2D echocardiography is able to detect RWMAs, and that ischemia will cause RWMAs, not every RWMA is due to ischemia. Several investigators have studied wall thickening and motion by 2D echocardiography in normal subjects and have found that both technologic and physiologic factors contribute to significant heterogeneity in regional wall motion.[124,125] The septal area at the base is the least contractile, but contractility increases greatly from base to apex and is the greatest in the posterior region of the left ventricle. Since ventricular contractility is not uniform, it should not be assumed that all hypokinetic segments represent ischemic areas. Though this may affect baseline studies, changes in regional contractility induced by drugs or stress should still be significant signs of newly developed ischemia.

Another potential problem is that the extent of RWMA may exceed the actual area of ischemia. It has been shown that myocardial segments with normal myocardial blood flow, adjacent to an ischemic area, may have significantly depressed function (Fig. 8-35).[126] Lima et al have demonstrated by echocardiography that transmural ischemia results in profound dysfunction of the normally perfused zones immediately adjacent to the ischemic area.[127] Some dysfunction relatively distant to the ischemia zone was also observed. During subendocardial ischemia, there was minor functional impairment of the lateral border immediately adjacent to the ischemic zone. These observations may represent a mechanical tethering of non-ischemic myocardium.

Despite the above-mentioned problems, echocardiography is extremely valuable and sensitive in the diagnosis of intraoperative ischemia. Using transthoracic M-mode echocardiography, Elliott et al detected significant changes in wall motion in 10 of 24 patients studied with M-mode echocardiography during the induction of anesthesia for coronary artery bypass surgery, while only one patient developed corresponding ECG changes.[128] 2D-TEE can also

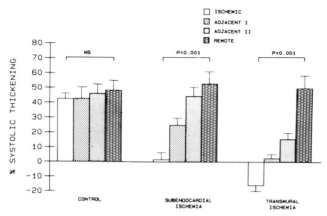

Fig. 8-35. Percentage of systolic thickening of the four anatomic regions at control and during subendocardial and transmural ischemia. In the ischemic region, systolic thickening was abolished during subendocardial ischemia and was replaced by thinning during transmural ischemia. In adjacent zone I, function was depressed during subendocardial ischemia and practically abolished during transmural ischemia, while in adjacent zone II, function was impaired only during transmural ischemia. In the remote region, there were no changes in regional myocardial function at any time. (From Homans D, Asinger R, Elsperger J, et al: Regional function and perfusion at the lateral border of ischemic myocardium. Circulation 71:1038–1047, 1985, with permission.)

detect myocardial ischemia prior to ECG changes. Beaupre et al reported two cases in which 2D-TEE revealed important clinical information.[129] In one case, only 1 mm of ST-segment depression was evident in leads I, aVL, and V_5 at the time of diagnosis despite "pronounced anteroseptal akinesis." The patient later developed ECG changes consistent with a transmural anteroseptal myocardial infarction, and creatine phosphokinase (CPK) was noted to be greater than 3000 IU/l postoperatively. In the second case, improved segmental wall motion was documented after cardiopulmonary bypass and aortocoronary grafting without any improvement in the ECG signs of ischemia. Konstadt et al reported another case in which TEE aided in the diagnosis of myocardial ischemia in the absence of ST-segment changes.[130] They showed a good correlation between the appearance of RWMAs and the presence of pathologic V waves on the PCWP waveform tracing. In addition, nitroglycerin resulted in normalization of the RWMA and a reduction in the PCWP and V waves. These clinical observations have recently been confirmed by a prospective study reported by Smith et al.[131] Using TEE to detect altered endocardial motion and myocardial thickening, they found that 24 of 50 patients developed RWMAs consistent with intraoperative myocardial ischemia. During this period ECG monitoring detected only six episodes of myocardial ischemia, and no patient had ST-segment

changes without corresponding RWMAs. In addition to being more sensitive than ECG monitoring in detecting myocardial ischemia, echocardiographic monitoring was able to diagnose an ischemic episode earlier and to predict the likelihood of progression to a myocardial infarction better than the ECG.

Numerous studies have previously shown that, in response to decreased myocardial blood flow, changes in regional wall motion consistently occur prior to ECG changes. In anesthetized dogs with the left anterior descending coronary artery constricted, changes in segmental shortening of the myocardium were demonstrated by ultrasound prior to changes in the ECG.[132] Similar results were obtained by other investigators (Fig. 8-36).[133,134] Upton et al studied ventricular function by radionuclide angiocardiography during exercise in 25 patients.[135] At a low level of exercise, no patients developed angina or ST-segment depression, but 14 of the 25 patients had segmental contractile abnormalities. Sugishita et al, also using radionuclide scanning, found that RWMAs occurred on the average 30 seconds after the onset of exercise, whereas ECG changes took 90 seconds to occur in patients with coronary artery disease.[136] Thus, RWMAs often appear prior to ECG changes in response to ischemia.

Intraoperative echocardiography can also be used to identify myocardium at risk of ischemia. In patients with multivessel coronary artery disease, the

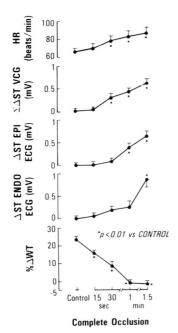

Complete Occlusion

Fig. 8-36. Effects of complete coronary occlusion on the percentage of systolic wall thickening (%WT), elevation from control of endocardial ST segments (ΔST ENDO ECG), epicardial ST segments (ΔST EPI ECG), the sum of ST-segment displacements from control in the vectorcardiographic leads X, Y, and Z (E ST VCG) and heart rate (HR). Negative values for %WT represent regional dyskinesis. (From Battler A, Froelicher VF, Gallagher KP, et al: Dissociation between regional myocardial dysfunction and ECG changes during ischemia in the conscious dog. Circulation 62:735–744, 1980, with permission.)

lesion with the greatest severity does not necessarily supply the area of myocardium that is most compromised. After identification of the areas of greatest risk, selective cardioplegic infusion and preferential coronary artery bypass grafting may be performed. When Goldman et al used rapid atrial pacing to stress the myocardium, new contractile abnormalities occurred in 18 of 60 segments analyzed by 2D echo.[137] Though the region that developed hypocontractility could not always be predicted by coronary angiography, the regions did correlate with cardioplegic perfusion defects also detected by 2D echocardiography.

Another application of echocardiography is to evaluate the efficacy of interventions, both surgical and pharmacologic, on ischemic myocardium. Using TEE, Topol et al studied the effect of coronary revascularization on dysfunctional myocardial segments in 20 patients before and after coronary artery bypass

surgery and showed that systolic wall thickening increased significantly after revascularization (Fig. 8-37).[138] Furthermore, the segments with the worst preoperative function showed the most improvement after surgery.

Most pharmacologic studies use hemodynamic parameters to assess the effects of a drug. These hemodynamic parameters reflect global rather than regional changes. Since echocardiography can be used to assess regional function, it is particularly valuable in investigating the effects of vasodilators on ischemic myocardium.[139-142] Komer et al studied the effects of nitroglycerin (NTG) on left ventricular wall thickness during coronary occlusion and found that although NTG infusion reduced left ventricular end-diastolic pressure, it did not alter the abnormal wall thickening in the area of ischemia.[139] Kerber et al performed a similar study comparing the effects of NTG and sodium nitroprusside (SNP) on systolic wall thinning, wall stress, and myocardial perfusion.[140] They found that myocardial perfusion and systolic wall thinning were unaffected, but due to the drop in left ventricular end-diastolic pressure, the wall stress was decreased by 50 percent (Fig. 8-38). Since wall stress is a major determinant of myocar-

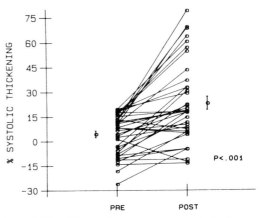

Fig. 8-37. Effect of coronary revascularization on severely dysfunctional segments. Percentage of systolic wall thickening before (PRE) and immediately after (POST) coronary revascularization as assessed by transesophageal echocardiography is shown. Values are mean ± standard error of the mean. Despite overall significant improvement, two apparent subgroups are identified; those segments that improved and those that did not. (From Topol EL, Weiss J, Guzman P, et al: Immediate improvement of dysfunctional myocardial segments after coronary revascularization: Detection by intraoperative transesophageal echocardiography. J Am Coll Cardiol 4:1123–1134, 1984, with permission.)

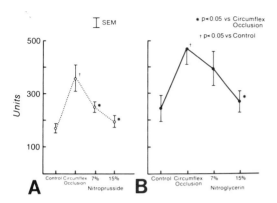

Fig. 8-38. Effect of circumflex occlusion and (A) nitroprusside and (B) nitroglycerin on the end-systolic posterior wall stress index. After occlusion, the stress index doubled; it fell to control levels in response to both nitroglycerin and nitroprusside. (From Kerber R, Martins J, Marcus M: Effect of acute ischemia, nitroglycerin, and nitroprusside on regional myocardial thickening, stress, and perfusion. Experimental echocardiographic studies. Circulation 60: 121–129, 1979, with permission.)

dial oxygen consumption, they postulated that it was this reduction in wall stress that was responsible for the beneficial effect of NTG and SNP during acute ischemia.

Other Intraoperative Applications

In addition to the assessment of global and regional ventricular function, there are a number of other important intraoperative applications of 2D echocardiography. In particular, ultrasound can be utilized for the evaluation of valvular function, coronary perfusion, and the presence of intracardiac shunts. Intraoperative echocardiography can be performed with a transthoracic, esophageal, or epicardial transducer.[143] For epicardial intraoperative echocardiography, the transducers are either gas sterilized or wrapped in sterile drapes. After sternotomy and pericardiotomy, the surgeon can obtain a long-axis view and a series of short-axis views by rotating the transducer on the right ventricular epicardium. Four-chamber or two-chamber views can be obtained by apical placement of customized phased-array transducers. This apical window is not obtainable with larger mechanical transducers.

VALVULAR FUNCTION

The use of prosthetic heart valves can lead to many problems, including valve dysfunction, endocarditis, emboli, and the sequelae of anticoagula-

tion.[144,145] Additionally, in younger patients tissue heterografts are prone to premature calcification.[146] Preservation of native valves by reconstructive techniques is therefore a valuable alternative to valve replacement. Unfortunately, the routine methods for intraoperative evaluation of valve competency following repair are inaccurate.[147] Echocardiography with contrast injection has been found to be very useful during surgery. It can evaluate the presence and amount of baseline regurgitation and can help determine the amount of residual regurgitation following valve annuloplasty, commissurotomy, or replacement.

Mitral valve disease. Goldman et al first applied intraoperative contrast echocardiography to the assessment of mitral valve surgery.[148] Imaging of the valvular and subvalvular apparatus allows the surgeon to assess the extent of fibrous or calcific involvement and to determine whether a conservative repair is feasible.

The presence and severity of both left- and right-sided valvular regurgitation can be determined from the "contrast" pattern generated by the injection of 5 ml of agitated saline solution or 5 percent dextrose in water through a long needle placed into the left or right ventricle. The needle and syringe generate microbubbles by creating surface agitation and microcavitation within the fluid even after all visible air bubbles have been removed.[149,150] These injections appear safe; in a collective registry report, over 40,000 contrast studies have been performed without any permanent deleterious effect.[151] Normally, when agitated fluid is injected into the left ventricle, contrast fills the left ventricular cavity and completely exits into the aorta during systole (Fig. 8-39). Depending on the severity of mitral regurgitation, the left atrium fills with variable amounts of contrast during ventricular systole (Fig. 8-40). By evaluating contrast density and clearing from the left atrium, valvular regurgitation can be graded in a manner similar to that for the standard angiographic and echocardiographic techniques.[147,152,153] Contrast injection and imaging in the short-axis view allows precise localization of the regurgitant flow along the free atrial wall or interatrial septum. Precise localization is extremely useful in detecting regurgitation after prosthetic valve replacement or repair procedures. Importantly, intraoperative contrast quantification of mitral valve insufficiency has an excellent correlation with preoperative left ventriculography ($r = 0.93$).

After the baseline contrast echocardiogram is completed, the operative procedure on the mitral

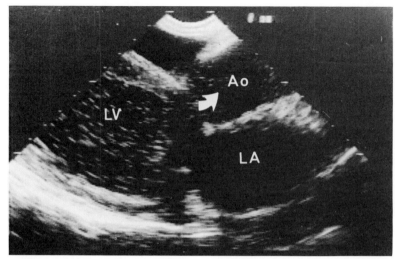

Fig. 8-39. Normal contrast echocardiogram. The left ventricle fills with microbubbles, which all exit out the aorta. (Abbreviations: Ao, aorta; LA, left atrium; LV, left ventricle.)

valve is performed. Once the patient has been weaned from cardiopulmonary bypass and has a stable, spontaneous, or paced rhythm, a repeat left ventricular contrast echocardiogram is performed. If the repair is adequate, no microbubbles should be seen in the left atrium. If more than one quarter of the left atrium is filled by contrast in either the long- or the short-axis view, there is more than a minimal degree of regurgitation. Cardiopulmonary bypass can be reinstituted and additional valve repair or correction of the prosthesis performed.

Goldman et al reported more than 175 echocardiographic contrast left ventriculograms successfully performed for the evaluation of mitral regurgitation in native and prosthetic valves. During surgery, the ultrasound method of mitral valve evaluation proved

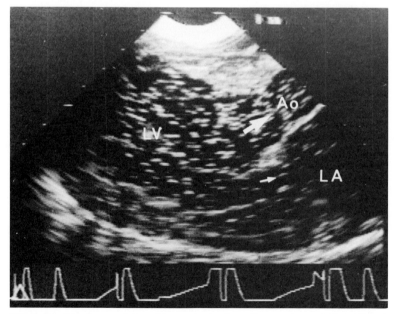

Fig. 8-40. Mitral regurgitation. The contrast echocardiogram demonstrates antegrade exit of microbubbles out the aorta as well as reflux into the left atrium.

superior to the standard methods, such as digital palpation and hemodynamic measurement of V wave size.[148] Recently, Equaras et al reported similar success using intraoperative contrast echocardiography to evaluate 15 patients with mitral regurgitation.[154]

Experience with both the technical performance and interpretation of the contrast echocardiogram is required for a successful study. Spontaneous bubbles are frequently generated in the left atrium after open heart surgery and should not be confused with truly regurgitant bubbles.[155] Careful frame-by-frame review of the echocardiogram in the operating room may be necessary to determine whether the contrast seen in the left atrium is due to true mitral regurgitation, to an injection in diastole, or to a dysrhythmia (Fig. 8-41). With use of intraoperative contrast echocardiography, potential valve problems can be detected before chest closure.

Intraoperative echocardiography is particularly valuable in patients with combined aortic stenosis and mitral regurgitation. In some of these patients, the mitral regurgitation may regress spontaneously after aortic valve replacement, thereby eliminating the need for mitral valve surgery. Intraoperative contrast echocardiography can assess mitral valve competency immediately after aortic valve surgery.

A few investigations have also evaluated the usefulness of esophageal pulsed Doppler echocardiography in the assessment of mitral regurgitation.[156,157] Schluter et al were able to detect mitral regurgitation in all patients by the transesophageal technique but in only 58 percent by the precordial approach.[158] Shively et al found the two techniques comparable.[159] 2D color-flow Doppler echocardiography can also be used for intraoperative determination of residual mitral regurgitation.

Tricuspid valve disease. Functional tricuspid regurgitation secondary to mitral regurgitation or stenosis is difficult to quantify adequately because current methods (physical examination, Doppler ultrasound, and cardiac catheterization) are inaccurate.[157] Failure to appreciate the severity of tricuspid regurgitation increases the postoperative morbidity and mortality after mitral valve operations.[160-162] Intraoperatively, a right ventricular contrast injection, generating microbubbles, can be used to determine the presence and degree of tricuspid regurgitation by semiquantifying the concentration and time for clearing of contrast from the right atrium during ventricular systole (Fig. 8-42). Goldman et al have applied intraoperative contrast echocardiography, in a manner similar to that developed for mitral regurgitation, to determine the baseline severity of tricuspid regurgitation in 85 patients.[163] Though tricuspid regurgitation may diminish spontaneously

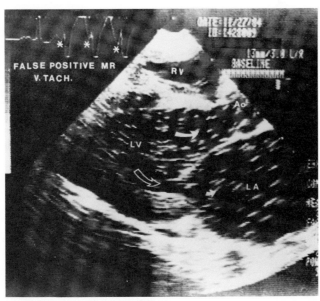

Fig. 8-41. False-positive mitral regurgitation (MR). The intraoperative echocardiogram in the long-axis view demonstrates systolic contrast in the left atrium (LA) after a left ventricular injection. The ECG shows ventricular tachycardia (V. TACH; starred) (RV, right ventricle).

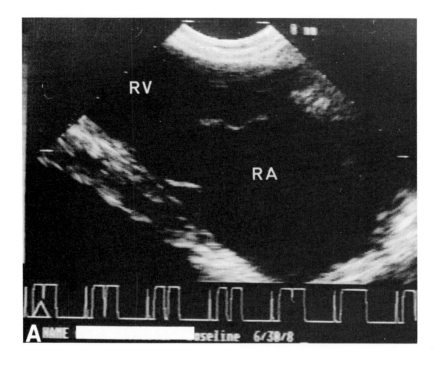

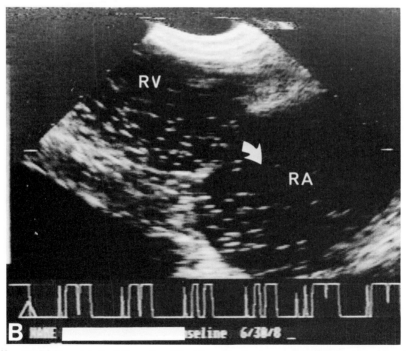

Fig. 8-42. (A) Right ventricular inflow view. The tricuspid valve is seen between the right atrium (RA) and right ventricle (RV). (B) Tricuspid regurgitation. Following contrast injection into the right ventricle, the reflux of microbubbles into the right atrium is seen.

after repair of the mitral lesion, in some patients persistent severe regurgitation will lead to increased morbidity and mortality. The results of intraoperative contrast echocardiography of tricuspid regurgitation correlate well with those of preoperative pulsed-wave Doppler studies.[163] The advantage of the intraoperative 2D echo technique, however, is that it allows the surgeon to evaluate the degree of tricuspid regurgitation immediately after the mitral valve procedure to determine whether tricuspid valve repair is still necessary. If the tricuspid valve is repaired, it can be evaluated before the patient leaves the operating suite.

Aortic valve disease. Occasionally, the presence of aortic valve stenosis or regurgitation is inadequately assessed preoperatively, especially when aortic valve disease is not clinically suspected or the patient is too critically ill to undergo catheterization. Intraoperative echocardiography can adequately visualize all three cusps of the aortic valve (in the short-axis view) and valve mobility (in the long-axis view). Aortic regurgitation can be demonstrated by injecting saline solution or dextrose in water into the proximal aortic root and visualizing diastolic reflux of microbubbles into the left ventricle. The degree of aortic regurgitation is assessed in a manner similar to that used to assess mitral regurgitation, from the degree of filling of the left ventricle during diastole and the time for clearing of the contrast. After aortic valve repair or prosthesis insertion, a postoperative contrast injection can determine the possible presence or severity of regurgitation. This is extremely valuable in congenital aortic valve anomalies when surgical treatment is reparative and residual or new aortic regurgitation may be present. In 75 aortic root echocardiographic contrast injections performed, there was excellent correlation with catheterization-determined severity of aortic regurgitation.[143] Equaras et al reported similar results in 14 patients.[154]

CORONARY PERFUSION

An exciting application of intraoperative echocardiography is the evaluation of myocardial perfusion. Studies have shown that different agents can be injected into the aortic root or directly into the coronary arteries to demonstrate myocardial perfusion. Normal perfusion is confirmed by the "whiting out" of myocardial segments as the fluid reaches the capillary level. Since cold potassium cardioplegia solution is routinely infused into the aortic root, it appears to be an ideal agent with which to study myocardial perfusion. Goldman and Mindich reported the ability

to image cardioplegic flow as it perfused the myocardium in a manner similar to a thallium perfusion scan.[164] As cardioplegia solution entered the heart, the myocardial region appeared whiter. Areas not perfused and, therefore, unprotected did not lighten, continued to finely fibrillate, and could be easily detected by on-heart echocardiography. In 42 patients studied, the overall sensitivity and specificity values for predicting significant (greater than 70 percent stenosis) coronary artery lesions based on preoperative angiographic determination were 82 and 92 percent, respectively. The method was most beneficial in detecting septal perfusion, which is difficult to assess by visualization or epicardial temperature probes. Based on the identification of underperfused regions, the surgeon can provide selective cardioplegia distal to a stenosis and perform the distal coronary bypass anastomosis to the ischemic region first.

Several studies have demonstrated the ability to visualize human coronary arteries and intracoronary plaques by epicardial application of high-frequency transducers.[165-167] At present, problems of resolution, cardiac motion, and ultrasound beam distortion due to calcified plaques present major obstacles in the practical application of this technique. Additionally, there is not always a direct correlation between anatomic obstruction and physiologic significance of the obstruction. However, the visualization and precise definition of intracoronary luminal abnormalities might become possible with the design of better transducers and with the use of higher frequency ultrasound, which would allow more precise insertion of coronary grafts and a more aggressive attitude toward intraoperative coronary endarterectomy and angioplasty.[168] Intraoperative echocardiography combined with intracoronary Doppler flow studies should significantly enhance the ability to assess the patency rate of bypassed vessels intraoperatively.

INTRACARDIAC CONTRAST

Because air has a different density than blood and is easily visualized by echocardiography, it has been suggested that TEE may be useful in the detection of venous or arterial air embolism.

Using M-mode TEE, Oka et al studied patients undergoing cardiac surgical procedures requiring cardiopulmonary bypass.[169] Evidence of air emboli was detected in 79 percent of the patients who underwent open cardiotomy and in only 11 percent of the patients who did not. They concluded that open cardiotomy significantly increased the risk of air embolism and that M-mode TEE was useful to detect the presence of air.

Two-dimensional echocardiography, because of its broader view, may be better suited for the monitoring of air embolism. Topol et al, using 2D echocardiography, observed microbubbles in 74 percent of patients undergoing intracardiac operations.[170] Postoperative neurologic examination, however, failed to reveal new neurologic focal deficits in any of the study patients. While in 7 patients generalized encephalopathy or confusion was noted postoperatively, only in 3 of these was any air detected at the end of the bypass period.

Furuya et al studied the sensitivity of 2D echocardiography to detect air when injected either as a bolus or an infusion.[171] The first part of the experiment was performed in dogs. After positioning the TEE probe to visualize the right and left ventricular outflow tracts by contrast echocardiography (iced saline injection), they determined the detection threshold for air injected by bolus to be 0.02 ml/kg for TEE and 0.5 ml/kg for transthoracic Doppler. At these levels of air injection, there were no changes in pulmonary artery pressure or end-tidal CO_2. In a similar study, Glenski et al also demonstrated that TEE was more sensitive than Doppler ultrasound for the detection of venous air embolism in dogs.[172]

Furuya et al also compared TEE to Doppler, pulmonary artery pressure, and end-tidal CO_2 analysis in patients undergoing craniotomy in the sitting position.[171] Though they were unable to quantify the amount of air that had been entrained, they noticed that TEE detected venous air embolism in 5 out of 6 patients. Similar results, however, were obtained by pulmonary artery pressure, Doppler, and end-tidal CO_2 monitoring. These authors further noted that in the event of a "paradoxical air embolism" (right-sided to left-sided via a patent foramen ovale or other intracardiac intrapulmonary shunt), TEE is the only monitoring technique that would potentially detect this event.

Cucchiara et al compared precordial Doppler to TEE monitoring for venous air embolism detection.[173] Transthoracic Doppler definitely detected air in 7 of the 15 patients and questionably detected air in 2 of 15 patients, whereas TEE consistently verified venous air embolism in the same 9 of 15 patients. Additionally, one episode of paradoxical air embolism was detected. From these studies, it is clear that TEE may be useful in the detection of venous air embolism or at the termination of cardiopulmonary bypass to determine whether or not air is still present in the left atrium or left ventricle.

As in the assessment of valvular lesions, intraoperative contrast echocardiography can also be utilized to evaluate the presence and severity of intracardiac shunts.[174,175] Saline solution injected on the right side of the heart can detect right-to-left shunts, and injections on the left side of the heart can assess left-to-right shunts. A minimal residual shunt may persist postoperatively along the patch material used for repair of interventricular and interatrial shunts.[174,175] Therefore, possible significant residual shunt after an operative procedure can be evaluated by intraoperative contrast echocardiography to detect potential suture dehiscence or inadequate repair. Possibly, in the future, color-flow Doppler will be preferred for this application.

Diagnosis of Cardiac Lesions

MITRAL VALVE

The mitral valve with its anterior and posterior leaflets, chordae tendineae, and papillary muscles is easily visualized from several different planes. The valve leaflet mobility can be examined and the valvular orifice can be planimetered on-line. The orifice is normally greater than 4 cm^2. In mitral stenosis, the thickened leaflets, commissural fusion, and fibrotic subvalvular apparatus decrease the valve orifice to varying degrees. M-mode measurement of the E-F slope can only roughly approximate the degree of stenosis. With 2D echo, however, not only can the actual valve orifice be measured in the short-axis view, but the size of the left atrium and right heart chambers, as well as the presence of possible atrial thrombi, can also be visualized (Fig. 8-43).[176] In one study of 24 patients, 2D echocardiographic planimetry of the mitral valve correlated well ($r = 0.93$) with hemodynamically calculated mitral valve area.[177] However, potential overestimation of the severity of stenosis can occur in low cardiac output states; in the presence of heavily calcified valve orifices, which do not allow accurate visualization of the actual mitral orifice; or following mitral commissurotomy with subsequent distortion of the orifice. Underestimation of the degree of stenosis can occur if there is excessive echo dropout on a single still-frame picture or if the narrowest orifice is not measured due to technical difficulties. Therefore, corroboration of mitral valve area should be made by Doppler techniques. By measuring the velocity of blood flow in the area of the left ventricular inflow in the apical four-chamber view (thereby being parallel to blood flow), the gradient across the mitral valve can be calculated ($p_1 - p_2 = 4 v^2$, where $p_1 - p_2$ is the pressure gradient

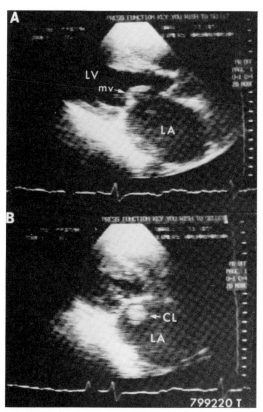

Fig. 8-43. 2D echo demonstrating a clot (CL) in the left atrium (LA) in a patient with a stenotic mitral valve (MV) (LV, left ventricle). (A) Long-axis view of stenotic MV. (B) View of CL. (From Feigenbaum H: Echocardiography (ed 4). Philadelphia, Lea & Febiger, 1986, with permission.)

across the valve, and v is the maximum velocity measured by Doppler.[178] The pressure half-time is another Doppler technique that utilizes the relationship between delayed diastolic left ventricular filling and the severity of mitral stenosis. One study showed a correlation of 0.91 between Doppler pressure half-time and hemodynamically derived valve areas.[179]

Mitral valve prolapse, one of the most common cardiac abnormalities, can be confirmed by echocardiography. M-mode echo may reveal either late or holosystolic posterior displacement of the mitral valve corresponding to the auscultation of a systolic click and murmur. Because the M-mode transducer beam may not always be perpendicular to the mitral valve, however, the 2D echo can better demonstrate actual prolapse of either leaflet into the left atrium (Fig. 8-44).[180]

Frequently, the etiology of mitral regurgitation can be determined rapidly with echocardiography. Flailing of either leaflet of the mitral valve, ruptured single or multiple chordae tendineae, or inferior wall hypocontractility with subsequent papillary muscle dysfunction is easily visualized. Additionally, 2D echo can confirm the diagnosis of endocarditis by the presence of white, fluffy densities of varying size attached to either leaflet (Fig. 8-45). Pulsed-wave Doppler echocardiography is the noninvasive method of choice to detect mitral regurgitation. Real-time Doppler color-flow mapping can be utilized to semiquantify the severity of valvular regurgitation by measurement of both the depth and area of reflux of color-coded flow into the left atrium. In a study of

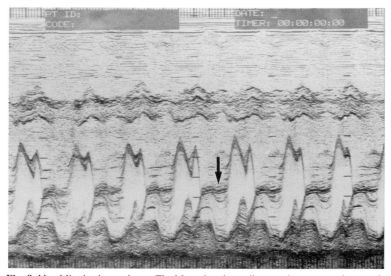

Fig. 8-44. Mitral valve prolapse. The M-mode echocardiogram demonstrates hammocking of the mitral valve during systole (arrow).

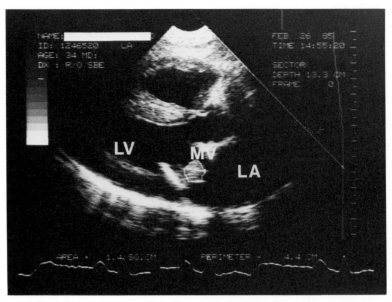

Fig. 8-45. Mitral valve endocarditis. The two-dimensional echocardiogram, parasternal long-axis view, demonstrates a fluffy density on the anterior leaflet of the mitral valve consistent with a vegetation.

109 patients, a significant correlation ($r = 0.87$) was found between color-flow Doppler and left ventriculographic estimation of mitral regurgitation.[181]

AORTIC VALVE

Aortic stenosis may present as heart failure, angina, or syncope, and may be difficult to assess by auscultation alone. Therefore, direct echocardiographic visualization of systolic doming of a calcified valve and a limited maximum aortic cusp separation in the parasternal long-axis view are invaluable in confirming the diagnosis of aortic stenosis. Usually the valve area cannot be measured as in mitral stenosis due to dense calcifications and irregular orifices.[182] However, CW Doppler can accurately calculate the transvalvular gradient using the apical, suprasternal, or right parasternal view.[183] The pressure drop across the valve ($p_1 - p_2$) is equal to four times the square of the blood velocity ($4v^2$) measured in the ascending aorta.

Aortic regurgitation can have various etiologies: primary valve pathology (endocarditis or prolapse) or root abnormalities (aneurysms, dissection, or inflammation). The classic M-mode finding in aortic regurgitation is diastolic fluttering of the anterior leaflet of the mitral valve when the regurgitant jet is directed toward the mitral valve. Color-flow Doppler allows semiquantification of the degree of insufficiency seen in diastole in the apical or long-axis views. Not only can echocardiography accurately diagnose the precipitating cause, but it can also evaluate how the aortic regurgitation has influenced ventricular dimensions and function. In an early study, echo criteria for the timing of surgery in asymptomatic patients with aortic regurgitation were proposed; they were an end-systolic dimension of greater than 55 mm and a fractional shortening less than 25 percent.[184] In recent studies, however, the use of rigid echocardiographic measurements has been avoided and symptomatology or noninvasively measured ventricular performance has been suggested as a more sensitive predictor of postoperative ventricular function in aortic regurgitation.[185-187]

MASSES

Prior to the introduction of echocardiography, the diagnosis of intraventricular or atrial masses (tumors and thrombi) was very difficult to confirm; however, with echo their precise location, size, shape, and mobility can be visualized in real time.

The most common intracardiac malignancies, myxomas, usually occur more frequently in the left than in the right atrium (3:1 ratio) and are usually attached to the interatrial septum. Frequently, because of the risk of dislodgement or fragmentation of the mass during cardiac catheterization, patients proceed to surgical excision of the tumors with the echocardiogram as the only preoperative examination.[188]

Ventricular thrombi occur in approximately 30 percent of large anterior wall myocardial infarctions, with reduced ejection fraction and apical wall motion abnormalities, and are easily visualized by echocardiography. Thrombi that are mobile and protrude into the ventricular chamber, rather than being laminar, have greater embolic potential.[189] Although atrial thrombi can sometimes be seen in dilated left atria (Fig. 8-43), particularly in mitral disease or atrial fibrillation, they can also be located in the atrial appendage, which cannot be routinely imaged. Therefore, failure to visualize an atrial thrombus when its presence is clinically suspected should not alter the decision to anticoagulate the patient.

MYOCARDIAL ISCHEMIA

In addition to its use in the diagnosis of myocardial ischemia by assessment of regional function, echocardiography can identify complications of acute infarction, such as aneurysms, thrombi, ventricular septal defects, and pseudoaneurysms.[190,191] Routine echocardiography can visualize the proximal coronary anatomy, particularly in the parasternal short-axis view, at the base of the heart.[192] Recently, exercise echocardiography, imaging either during or immediately following a stress intervention, has been utilized to detect underlying coronary artery disease.[193] Since echocardiography is the only routine imaging technique that can directly assess myocardial contractility, studies obtained during or immediately following exercise may be a valuable method with which to identify stress-induced RWMAs. Studies have shown that echocardiography is superior to routine electrocardiography in the detection of exercise-induced ischemic abnormalities.[194]

PERICARDIAL EFFUSION

Ordinarily, there is 15–30 ml of fluid in the pericardial space for lubrication; however, under diverse pathological circumstances—such as heart failure, renal failure, hypothyroidism, metastatic infiltrations, radiation, vasculitis, trauma, or following operations—pericardial effusions can be observed. If the fluid accumulates rapidly and is of sufficient volume, hemodynamic compromise may ensue, leading eventually to pericardial tamponade. Echocardiogra-

phy cannot only assess the extent of the effusion but may also be used to help guide the needle during therapeutic or diagnostic pericardiocentesis.

MYOCARDIAL DISEASE

Primary cardiomyopathies can be divided into three pathologic categories: hypertrophic, idiopathic dilated (congestive), and restrictive. Echocardiography can identify each distinctive subtype.

Hypertrophic cardiomyopathy (HCM) connotes a primary, nonphysiologic hypertrophy of the myocardium, involving the septum (asymmetric septal hypertrophy), particularly the basal septum (idiopathic hypertrophic subaortic stenosis [IHSS]), but occasionally the apical septum or the entire ventricle. Since M-mode echocardiography may show a falsely thick septum if the heart is vertically oriented, a 2D echo study can be performed to accurately localize and measure the site of hypertrophy in several views. However, the hallmark indices of resting outflow obstruction are derived from the M-mode, guided by the 2D echo study. These indices include a very thick septum, a mid-systolic notching of the aortic valve, and a sustained apposition of the mitral valve (either anterior or posterior leaflet) against the septum.[195] Two-dimensional echocardiography can reveal cavity obliteration and a ground-glass myocardial texture of the hypertrophic segment characteristic of HCM.

Dilated, congestive cardiomyopathy is characterized by a dilated left ventricle with severe, diffuse hypocontractility. Usually, there is biatrial and biventricular dilatation, with dysfunction of the right ventricle as well. An M-mode echocardiogram taken distal to the mitral valve is representative of the entire ventricle, but a 2D study allows a more qualitative evaluation of all four chambers, as well as detection of thrombi. Importantly, even without underlying coronary artery disease, there may be some variation in regional wall contractility. Usually the lateral wall is less severely involved; however, in contrast to ischemic heart disease following myocardial infarctions with visible scarring and thinning of the involved myocardial segments, in a dilated cardiomyopathy the ventricular walls are uniform in thickness.

Restrictive cardiomyopathy is the result of various infiltrative diseases, including amyloidosis, hemachromatosis, sarcoidosis, and endomyocardial fibrosis. The ventricular cavity is normal or small, and, though the walls are diffusely and markedly thickened, they are hypocontractile. Early in the dis-

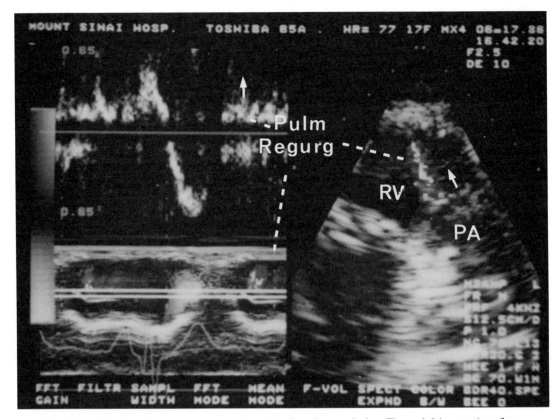

Fig. 8-46. Color-flow Doppler study of a patient with pulmonic regurgitation. The top left is regurgitant flow shown by pulsed Doppler; the bottom left is M-mode echo with color-flow Doppler; and the right is a 2D echo study with color-flow Doppler.

ease process, however, systolic function may be normal and only diastolic function is impaired, leading to pulmonary congestion despite a normal ejection fraction. Digitized M-mode echocardiograms or Doppler studies may be beneficial in the detection of early diastolic dysfunction.[196]

CONGENITAL HEART DISEASE

Echocardiography and Doppler studies have virtually revolutionized the approach to congenital heart disease. Even prenatal diagnosis of cardiac pathology is now possible with fetal echocardiography. The etiology of cyanotic conditions can be determined immediately after birth, avoiding cardiac catheterization.[197]

The orientation of the great vessels, intactness of the atrial and ventricular septum, valvular anatomy, and ventricular function can be assessed. Doppler blood flow velocities can localize intracardiac shunts that are too small to be visualized by 2D echo. Color-

flow Doppler has the potential to semiquantify shunt flow or regurgitant volumes (Fig. 8-46).

TWO-DIMENSIONAL IMAGING: TECHNICAL DETAILS

Image Generation

The conversion of reflected ultrasound echoes into 2D video images is a complicated process involving numerous electronic and digital manipulations. These manipulations are so complex that one echoscanner, currently utilized for intraoperative TEE (Diasonics Cardiorevue 6400), employs three interconnected microprocessors (computers) to control the process of image generation.[198]

BASIC PRINCIPLES

A 2D echo image is generated by scanning the heart every 17 msec or 60 times each second. The image generated from a single 1/60th of a second scan is called a "field" (Fig. 8-7A). A process called interlacing combines two scans or fields into a frame of 1/30th of a second. Since the eye cannot capture an image lasting 1/30th of a second, microprocessors further process the frame electronically in real time. The intrinsic persistence of the television screen enhances image quality, and the end result is a fairly smooth picture (Fig. 8-7B).

RESOLUTION

Resolution is the ability of ultrasound to distinguish fine detail. The resolution of an echo system is the minimum distance that must separate two distinct reflectors so that they can be imaged as separate entities. Image resolution is markedly dependent on transducer characteristics and is different along the two major image axes. Along the direction of the beam, the axial resolution of a pulsed instrument is approximately equal to

0.77 × number of cycles in one pulse per frequency (8-17)

Typically, for a 2.5-MHz transducer with a narrow, three-cycle pulse duration, the acoustic transducer resolution is calculated at

$$\frac{0.77 \times 3}{2.5} \approx 1 \text{ mm} \qquad (8\text{-}18)$$

Lateral resolution is the minimum distance perpendicular to the ultrasound beam at which two objects can be imaged as distinct. It is determined almost entirely by the beam diameter; the narrower the beam, the better the lateral resolution. Typical values for lateral resolution are 2–3 mm. Axial resolution is better than lateral resolution, because along the axis of the beam, image data are used as detected; in the lateral direction, the image is formed by the juxtaposition of many line scans.

PREPROCESSING

Ultrasound echoes are received and converted to electric signals by the transducer. On most modern echo scanners, the analog electronic signals undergo several modifications before being digitized, further manipulated, and eventually displayed as an image. Preprocessing describes the modifications performed on the analog and digital signal prior to storage in the computer memory.

Dynamic range manipulation. The intensity of echo signals spans a wide range from very weak to very strong. Very strong signals falling beyond the saturation level of the electronic circuitry and very weak signals below the sensitivity of the instrument are automatically eliminated. The dynamic range (DR) of the instrument is defined by the limits at which extremely strong or weak signals are eliminated; DR is under operator control (Fig. 8-47). In this manner, signals of low intensity that contain little useful information, but mostly noise, can be selectively rejected.

A wide DR is needed for high resolution, while a narrow range facilitates the discrimination between true image signals and noise. In clinical echocardiography, strong signals that arise from dense tissues, such as cardiac valves, and weaker signals arising from soft tissues, such as myocardium, are of interest.

To give the weaker signals a greater representation in the dynamic range, an amplifier converts the linear signal-intensity scale into a logarithmic scale. While this increases the number of weaker signals detected, it also unfortunately tends to amplify noise.

Gain attenuation and damping. The gain and attenuation controls of a scanner increase and decrease the intensity of all signals in a proportional manner. As a result, they change the number of detected echo signals by bringing them above or below the rejection threshold of the dynamic range. To deal with the potential loss of image quality caused by the display of the larger number of insignificant echoes obtained at high gain settings, a "damping" adjustment exists. Damping does not modify the received signal directly, but it decreases the strength of the emitted ultrasound beam by limiting the duration of the pulses that form the beam. Since less power is sent toward the target, fewer noise signals are generated. Damping also enhances the image since it improves resolution by decreasing the number of cycles in each ultrasound pulse (see Equation 8-17).[199]

Time-gain compensation. Since any wave traveling through tissues is attenuated to a degree proportional to the traveled distance, it is necessary to compensate for the fact that echoes returning from more distant objects will be weaker than those from equally dense objects closer to the transducer. A mechanism called depth compensation, or time-gain compensation (TGC), is used to achieve this. The

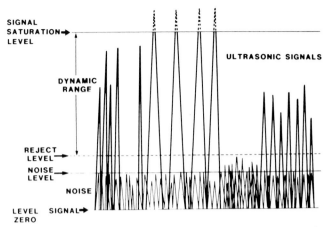

Fig. 8-47. This diagram depicts the dynamic range of a representative echocardiographic display system. As indicated, all ultrasonic signals begin at a zero signal level and
can increase in amplitude until they reach the system "signal saturation" level. Many of
the low-intensity signals fall within the range of the background noise and are therefore
obscured. All systems have a built-in system reject, which eliminates both the system
noise and the low-intensity echoes that lie just above the noise level. The dynamic range
of the system, therefore, is between the system reject level and the signal saturation level
and represents the echoes that actually appear on the display scope. (From Weyman AE:
Cross-Sectional Echocardiography. Philadelphia, Lea & Febiger, 1982, with permission.)

manner in which TGC is obtained is illustrated in
Figure 8-48. TGC can be controlled manually or
automatically.

Leading-edge enhancement. Leading-edge enhancement, or differentiation, is another type of preprocessing used to sharpen the video image.[200] The
reflected echo signal undergoes half-wave rectifica-
tion and is smoothed into a signal envelope (Fig. 8-
49A and B). An amplifier then differentiates the
leading edge of the smoothed signal envelope to its
first mathematical derivative (Fig. 8-49C), and a narrower and brighter image spot is formed (Fig.
8-49D). Since a 2D echo image is composed of multiple radially juxtaposed B-mode lines, excessive
edge enhancement narrows bright spots in the direction of the travel of the echo beam, ie, axially but not
laterally. For this reason, leading-edge enhancement
is primarily performed on M-mode scans, while
instruments with 2D capability use little or no edge
enhancement in the 2D mode. Therefore, M-mode
images often have better resolution than 2D images
and are better suited for quantitative measurements.

DIGITAL SIGNAL PROCESSING

Digital scan conversion. After completing analog preprocessing, ultrasound devices digitize the

image data with an analog-to-digital (A-D) converter
(Fig. 8-50). Further processing is done while data are
stored in the digital memory (input processing) or as
they are retrieved from the memory (output processing).[201] An early step in digital processing uses a scan
converter to transform the information obtained as
radial sector scan lines into a rectangular (cartesian)
format for television screen display.

The memory stores the information of two adjacent scan fields consisting of a total of 128 scan lines.
Each scan line is assigned to one column of memory.
There is also one row of memory for each of the 512
horizontal television image lines (raster lines).
Therefore, a typical television display of an echo
image consists of 128 columns by 512 rows for a
total of 65,536 picture elements or pixels. While the
monitor only displays 64 shades of gray for each
pixel, the memory unit assigned to each pixel has the
capacity to store 1024 degrees of brightness. Each
pixel is assigned 10 binary bits of memory for a total
of 2^{10} (1024) possible storage combinations.

Temporal processing. As digital data are
entered into memory, they can undergo temporal
averaging in one of two modes. In the variable persistence mode, information from previous images is
combined with current image data. A weighted average of the old and new data is then entered in mem-

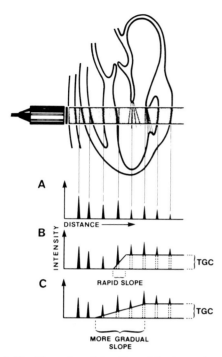

Fig. 8-48. Illustration of the effect of the time-gain compensation (TGC) on the echoes from more distant structures. (A) The normal loss in echo strength is due to the decreasing intensity of the beam as it propagates through the heart. (B) The effect of the TGC in boosting the intensity of far-field signals is shown. Intensity is selectively increased to display far-field signals at an appropriate height relative to the near-field echoes. (C) The position of this gain function and its rate of employment can be individualized to suit the needs of the operator. (From Weyman AE: Cross-Sectional Echocardiography. Philadelphia, Lea & Febiger, 1982, with permission.)

ory as the new current data. A mechanism is built in to allow variable representation of old data into the new image. A different input-processing option calculates the arithmetic mean of the new data and up to nine frames of existing data.

Input processing is mainly utilized to improve the signal-to-noise ratio. In a 2D echo image, a lower signal-to-noise ratio means a less granular appearance (the result of microscopic scatter) and less echo dropout (the result of very weak signals that are difficult to detect on the screen). Time averaging is most useful for enhancing slowly varying images.

Histogram equalization. The video image is generated from data retrieved from memory via the scan converter. During retrieval, data can be subjected to histogram equalization. This process redis-

tributes the gray level assignment of each pixel according to the relative frequency of occurrence of the gray level in the entire image in an equalitarian manner. All levels of gray receive some representation even though the original image may have been formed from only a limited range of grays (Fig. 8-51).

Gray-scale processing. Each unit of memory assigned to a pixel can store 1024 values of echo intensity, while the pixel itself can only display 64 shades of gray; thus, each gray level must represent multiple echo intensities. The gray level reassignment is done by transfer functions of variable shapes, slopes, and end points. An inverting transfer function allows the M-mode display to exist as a dark background with white lines or as a light background with dark lines. Gray-scale processing greatly affects image quality (Fig. 8-52).

Spatial processing or convolution operations. Spatial processing is a very sophisticated type of averaging, which involves modifications in the content of a pixel based on the content of its neighbors. In Figure 8-53A, the gray level at pixel A_{11} is replaced by the average gray level of all pixels within the "kernel" $W_1 \ldots W_9$ or, simply stated, by

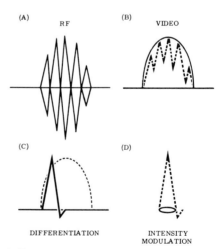

Fig. 8-49. Ways of processing the returning ultrasonic echo. (A) RF or radiofrequency type of echo display. (B) This video display represents the average height of the upper half of the RF signal. (C) Differentiation is obtained by taking the first derivative of the video display. (D) Intensity modulation represents the conversion of signal amplitude to intensity, changing the signal from a spike to a dot. (From Feigenbaum H: Echocardiography (ed 4). Philadelphia, Lea & Febiger, 1986, with permission.)

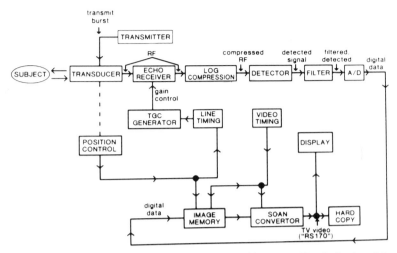

Fig. 8-50. Block diagram of a modern echocardiographic system. Note indication of the various forms that the received echocardiographic data take during the signal processing steps (see also Fig. 8-4). (From Skorton DG, Collins SM, Garcia E, et al: Digital signal and image processing in echocardiography. The American Society of Echocardiography Subcommittee on Digital Imaging Processing. Am Heart J 110:1268–1283, 1985, with permission.)

the average of itself and the eight surrounding gray levels [$A_{11} = 1/9 (A_2 + A_3 + A_4 + A_{10} + A_{11} + A_{12} + A_{18} + A_{19} + A_{20})$]. This operation is done for all pixels, and the new pixels are stored in a new image memory area. This produces spatial smoothing of the image and is particularly useful for parts of the image in which no abrupt changes in the echo density occur. It also eliminates "noise." When the detection of subtle changes in density is desired, such as in endocardial border detection, an edge-enhanc-

ing, convolution process is used. Applying the kernels shown in Figure 8-53B, the new A_{11} value would be $A_{11} = 1/9 (A_2 + A_3 + A_4 - A_{18} - A_{19} - A_{20})$. To enhance vertical edges, a similar transformation can be used with the values of the kernel mask rotated 90°. Edge enhancement has limited success because most ultrasound image edges are relatively smooth and the enhancement operator works best with images in which light and dark regions change abruptly.

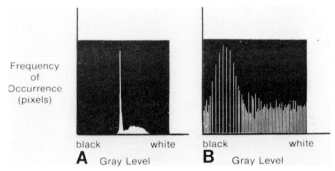

Fig. 8-51. Histogram equalization. (A) Gray level histogram of an image, showing the relative frequency of occurrence of all gray levels within the image. (B) After the image has undergone histogram equalization, the histogram demonstrates greater relative uniformity among all gray levels in the image, with utilization of the entire range of possible gray levels. (From Skorton DG, Collins SM, Garcia E, et al: Digital signal and image processing in echocardiography. The American Society of Echocardiography Subcommittee on Digital Image Processing. Am Heart J 110:1268–1283, 1985, with permission.)

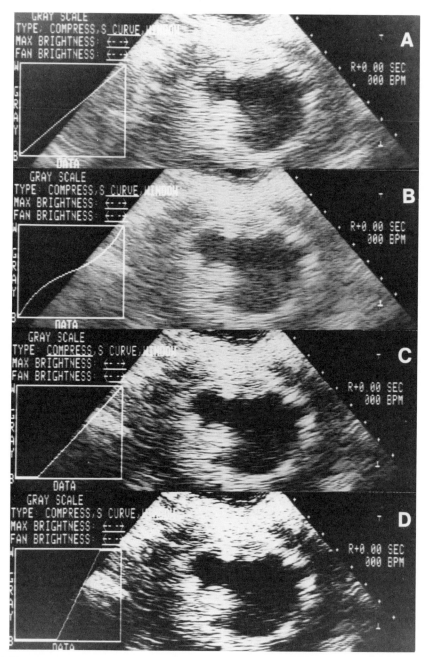

Fig. 8-52. Gray scale manipulation of a two-dimensional echocardiogram. The gray scale curves and the resultant images with a variety of postprocessing possibilities are presented. (A) 1:1 relationship for gray scale and echo amplitude. (B) The echoes with low gray scale are enhanced. (C) Suppression of the low gray level echoes slight enhancement of the high-level signals. (D) The low gray level echoes are suppressed even more, while high-level echoes are enhanced.

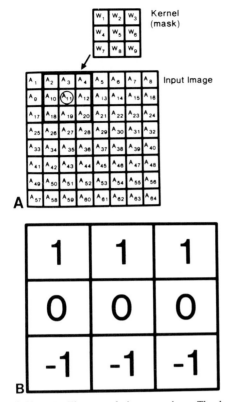

Fig. 8-53. (A) The convolution procedure. The lower panel shows an input image matrix, with A being the value of pixel 11. A 3 × 3 pixel convolution kernel or mask is shown at the top. Convolution is performed by passing the mask "over" the image, multiplying the image pixels "underneath" the mask by the corresponding mask weights, summing the individual terms, and assigning the result to the "center" pixel. (From Skorton DJ, Collins SM, Garcia E, et al: Digital signal and image processing in echocardiography. The American Society of Echocardiography Subcommittee on Digital Image Processing. Am Heart J 110:1268–1283, 1985, with permission.) (B) Digital edge enhancement operator. Application of the 3 x 3 convolution kernel shown here will result in "zero" values for pixels in uniform regions of the image and in large values (positive or negative) for pixels on a horizontal edge. (From Skorton DJ, Collins SM, Garcia E, et al: Digital signal and image processing in echocardiography. The American Society of Echocardiography Subcommittee on Digital Image Processing. Am Heart J 110:1268–1283, 1985, with permission.)

Digital data storage and retrieval. Off-line analysis and processing of the digital echo data have recently become very popular with the advent of microprocessors, minicomputers, and inexpensive data-handling hardware. Dedicated work stations are being marketed (Microsonics, Franklin) for the pur-

pose of image analysis with or without digital signal processing. In nondigital video-based systems, the analog signal is digitized by a computer interface, and the digital images must then be stored in real time. Since multiple images, each with large data content, need to be stored in short periods of time, special disk storage mechanisms, different from the ordinary disk storage devices, are necessary. Both floppy disks (with the capacity of 1024 kilobytes of data) and hard disks (with the capacity of up to 100 megabytes of data) have been used for storage. However, a single floppy disk can only store a few images while a complete ultrasound study may generate data on the order of 100 megabytes. To deal with this limitation, only edited data are currently stored on digital medium. Due to the band-width limitations of the initial video recording, image quality is significantly degraded in the storage process.

Image Artifacts

Image artifacts fall into three broad categories: failure to image objects (echo dropout), production of totally spurious images (display of nonexistent objects), and imaging of objects in a distorted fashion (either at the improper location or as having improper shape, size, or brightness).

ECHO DROPOUT

Failure to image an object can be due to shadowing by adjacent structures or to the poor intrinsic reflecting properties of the target itself. Shadowing can be caused by dense structures, such as prosthetic valves, which reflect most of the beam; by very light structures, such as gas bubbles, which do not transmit ultrasound; or by thick muscle layers, which scatter most of the beam away.

Properties of the target tissue that affect ultrasound reflection are their orientation in the scan plane, their surface characteristics, and differences in acoustic impedance between the target structures and the surrounding medium. For surfaces that are perpendicular to the beam, imaging is most influenced by the difference in density between the studied object and the medium. The larger this difference, the better the imaging. For objects with surfaces parallel or oblique to the beam, the incidence angle between the object and the beam and the texture of the surface are the major factors that affect imaging. Imaging is better if the incidence angle approaches 90° or if the reflecting surface is irregular.

Because the geometry of the endocardium and epicardium varies throughout the cardiac cycle,

examin___ ___age frames may
show___ ___s, ie, "echo dropout"___ ___articular problem in
M-___ ___ history of the struc-
t___ ___en, making it easier to
___ ___uous 2D imaging, it is
___se the observer's eyes can
___ting to quantitate informa-
___nes, however, this compen-
___ne either manually by the
___cally. Averaging of frames
___time in the cardiac cycle allevi-
___a certain extent.
___s, 2D view of the heart, the poste-
___vill image better than any other con-
___is contrasted against the lungs, which
___ly lower acoustic density. Since blood
___ardium have similar densities, the endo-
___es not image as well. In systole, however,
___larities of the endocardium become more

pronounced; hence, a sharper endocardial echo
image is produced.[202]

SPURIOUS IMAGES

The processes responsible for the appearance of
totally spurious images are reverberation (multiple
reflection), multipath propagation, and video persistence. Echoes reflected from dense objects are strong
and can be partly reflected by the transducer surface.
They are sent in the same direction as the main beam
and will duplicate the original echo of the dense
object. Since the duplicate echo has traveled twice
the distance to the object (true distance × 2), however, it produces a second image of the object at
twice the distance from the transducer—hence, an
echo of an echo, or a reverberation.

An example of such an artifact associated with a
catheter is shown in Figure 8-55. Additional reverberation artifacts may be caused by the plastic material used to house some transducers. They can be

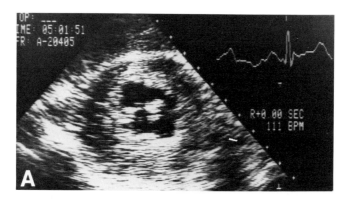

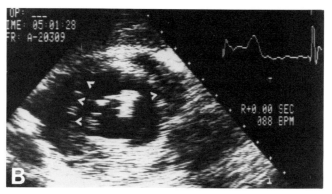

Fig. 8-54. Short-axis images demonstrating echo dropout of endocardial borders during
the cardiac cycle in two nearly consecutive heart beats: (A) end-systole; (B) end-diastole;
arrows identify missing border regions.

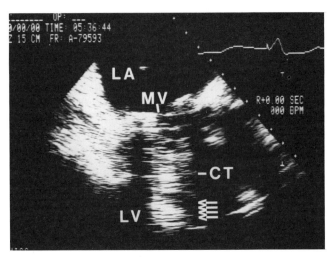

Fig. 8-55. Echocardiogram demonstrating reverberations (arrows) from a catheter in the left ventricle.

eliminated by adjusting the angle between the transducer and the target.

Unlike normal ultrasound transmission where the paths of the emitted and reflected beams are the same, in multipath propagation part of the reflected beam bounces off a second reflector before it is detected by the transducer. The reflected beam thus takes a longer path and time to be received and creates a second image of the target at a location farther from the transducer than the true image. The orientation and intrinsic properties of both reflectors determine the relative intensities of the true and virtual images. In standard television broadcasting, multipath propagation is responsible for the occasionally observed image "ghosts."

Screen persistence causes spurious images of objects undergoing rapid changes in shape, location, or density. The television screen continues to display the image of a very bright structure at the screen location where it was originally displayed, although that particular structure is not currently in the path of the beam.

Display of a structure at an improper location can be caused by off-axis ultrasound emission, mirror image formation, and wave refraction.[203] In off-axis emission, secondary beams or side lobes, generated at the edges of the transducer, give the transducer the undesirable ability to "see sideways." As a result, objects outside the main beam are imaged at the correct distance from the transducer and displayed as though they were in the main beam.

When side lobes scan objects of densities much higher than those studied by the main beam—for example, foreign objects such as catheters or prosthetic valves—the side lobes produce strong confusing echoes (Fig. 8-56). Even dense tissues, like the fibrous portions of the heart found in the atrioventricular grooves, can produce noticeable side lobe echoes.

In the mirror image artifact, a single object is displayed at two different locations in the image. The first reflection is generated when the ultrasound beam comes across the intended object. The second reflection occurs when, during the scan, the beam comes across a strong reflector with a favorable orientation toward the target object. This strong reflector will also reflect ultrasound signals to and from the object, causing the object to be imaged at a second position.

Ultrasound beam refraction, which is due to changes in acoustic impedance of the medium between the transducer and the target, causes bending of both emitted and reflected beams. This results in misplacement of structures on the display screen.

DISTORTION

Occasionally, cardiac structures can appear distorted in size or shape on echo images. Factors that contribute to these distortions are the directionality and gain dependence of image resolution, as well as the operator's inability to access all planes of the heart.

The higher the instrument gain, the larger an imaged object appears on display, particularly if the object is small in reality. Furthermore, axial and lateral gain controls differ so that lateral dimensions are more gain dependent than the axial ones. In quantita-

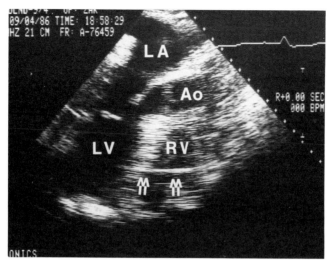

Fig. 8-56. Echocardiogram demonstrating a side lobe artifact (arrow heads) traversing from the right ventricle (RV) into the left ventricle (LV). This artifact is due to a pulmonary artery catheter in the RV.

tive assessment, it is very important to minimize gain settings. A dramatic example of how gain affects measurement of a stenotic valve area is shown in Figure 8-57.

The inability to freely view a specific anatomic plane results in the simplest and occasionally most annoying artifact of image generation. What appears to be the correct plane can in reality be a distorted representation of the wrong plane. For example, a short-axis mid-ventricular view may not really be halfway down the ventricle. It may also be in a slightly oblique plane rather than truly perpendicular to the long axis of the heart. In a different example, a long-axis view of the ventricle may not include an image of the true apex but may display a false one.

These artifacts are major sources of errors in the quantitative assessment of echo images.

Image Analysis

It is much easier for the eye to trace the myocardial border from a continuously moving display than from a single still frame, because the image composed by the brain represents the integration of multiple frames. Thus, although qualitative 2D echo assessment may not be very precise or accurate, it is based on more data, which are often of better quality than in quantitative single-frame off-line measurements.

Quantitative analysis is usually performed off-

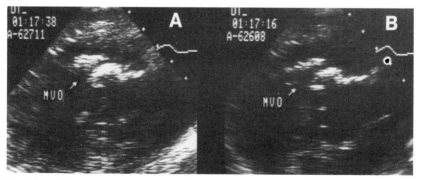

Fig. 8-57. Echocardiograms demonstrating how the mitral valve orifice (MVO) can be significantly influenced by gain. The orifice (A) is virtually eliminated with a high gain setting. (B) shows the MVO with a normal gain setting.

line from a videotape recording or occasionally from a digital recording. Video has the disadvantage of reproducing images of low quality because of the limited recording band width of the original recording. As a result, myocardial echo dropout is often significant. On the other hand, video allows easy access to data, since it can be played forward or backward over a large range of speeds. Another advantage of the videotape recordings is the ability to capture sound as well as images, which allows the examiner to place sound cues on the video tape.

After data are stored in digital format, myocardial borders can be enhanced by time averaging over several cardiac cycles; however, during averaging, image resolution is degraded because of transducer movement, respiratory motion, and variability in cycle length. On-line image averaging significantly increases the cost of the processing hardware, and most manufacturers of echo equipment do not provide this feature.

Based on the complexity of the analysis, three types of quantitative image measurements can be distinguished:[204]

1. Length or area measurements, which can be performed manually or with the aid of simple automated equipment
2. More complex measurements, such as regional myocardial wall measurements, for which computer-assisted analysis is usually preferred

3. Extremely complex measurements, such as three-dimensional ventricular chamber reconstruction, which can only be performed by computers[204]

For length or area measurements, the interpreter uses a pointing device (magnetic pen, light pen, or joystick-controlled screen cursor) to identify image points, which are electronically converted into digital x and y coordinates. The image can be either in video or hard-copy format. Such digitizing systems have a better than 0.1-mm resolution.

The digitized data can then be entered into a computer system where simple contour length or closed loop areas are calculated (Fig. 8-58). Ventricular or atrial chamber diameters, perimeters, or areas can thus be computed; however, any echo-generated image line or contour has a finite thickness related to the gain setting. Also, any image line or contour possesses a leading edge (LE), which is closest to the transducer, and a trailing edge (TE), which is farthest away from the transducer. When performing endocardial wall measurements, intuitively (though not logically), the proximal wall TE, the distal wall LE, and the inner aspects of the lateral and medial walls would be traced. A moment's reflection shows this to be wrong because the thickness of the endocardial line is artificially determined by the gain setting. TE–TE or LE–LE measurements of endocardial borders are more accurate. Figure 8-59 demonstrates the

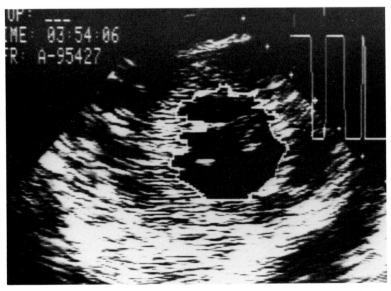

Fig. 8-58. Two-dimensional echocardiogram demonstrating how area measurements can be obtained from two-dimensional examinations. The measurements are usually obtained from the trailing edge of the anterior echoes, the leading edge of the posterior echoes, and the inner aspects of the lateral and medial echoes.

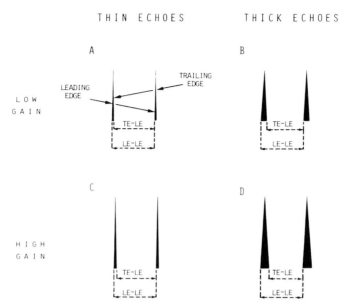

Fig. 8-59. This series of diagrams demonstrates how echocardiographic measurements can differ according to whether leading edge (LE) or trailing edge (TE) measurements are used. Echocardiographic measurements are commonly from leading edge to leading edge (LE–LE) or from trailing edge to leading edge (TE–LE). If the echocardiographic system has thin echoes (A and C), the gain makes little difference in either measurement. However, if the echocardiograph displays relatively thick echoes (B and D), then the TE–LE measurement is significantly reduced with an increase in gain (D). The LE–LE measurement is uninfluenced by gain. (From Feigenbaum H: Echocardiography (ed 4). Philadelphia, Lea & Febiger, 1986, with permission.)

principle of linear LE–TE measurements and also shows that as the gain setting increases, the potential for introducing errors in quantitative measurements becomes greater. The difference between measurements obtained by TE–LE and LE–LE techniques is the greatest when studying strong echoes, which produce thick contours. In automated computer border detection, the LE–LE principle of endocardial border measurement is often ignored.

FUTURE DEVELOPMENTS

Tissue Diagnosis of Ischemia

Recently, contrast echocardiography has been shown to aid in the diagnosis of myocardial ischemia. Sakanaki et al injected agitated saline–renografin, an echocardiographic contrast agent, into the left main coronary artery of dogs before and after left anterior descending artery occlusion (Fig. 8-60).[205] After 45 minutes or 5 hours of occlusion, the size of the area free of echo contrast correlated well with the

area delineated as ischemic at necropsy. Another use of contrast echocardiography to define ischemic zones consists of the measurement of the washout rate of contrast from areas supplied by normal or diseased coronary arteries.[206] The washout time increases as the degree of coronary stenosis becomes more severe. These studies were performed by injection of contrast directly into the coronary arteries, which appears impractical in clinical practice. Ten Cate et al have attempted to opacify the left ventricular chamber by right-sided injections of contrast, but they were only able to obtain myocardial enhancement in 16 percent of injections.[207] If the opacification rate can be improved, this technique could provide a safe method with which to study the effects of various manipulations on myocardial perfusion.

Another new application of echocardiography is the analysis of ultrasonic backscatter to assess tissue characteristics. The amplitude and frequency of an ultrasonic signal are altered as the signal traverses tissue. Abnormal tissue will alter the signal in a different fashion than normal tissue. For example, fibrotic or scarred tissue increases the magnitude of

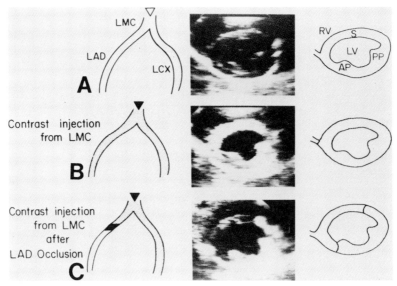

Fig. 8-60. This illustration indicates the quality of myocardial contrast echocardiographic opacification in two-dimensional echocardiographic cross-sections after injection of saline–renografin echo contrast agent in the left main coronary artery. (A) Shown is a mid-papillary level short-axis view of the left ventricle before coronary artery occlusion and before contrast injection. Note the epicardial and endocardial outlines, with relatively echolucent intervening myocardium. (B) The same cross-section is shown in the preocclusion control state, after contrast agent injection from the left main coronary artery. The entire circumference of the left ventricular myocardium is opacified. (C) This shows the effect of a left main coronary artery contrast agent injection after left anterior descending coronary artery occlusion. Note that a substantial portion of the interventricular septum and a part of the left ventricular anterior wall are devoid of contrast echo. This negative echo contrast area represents the underperfused myocardium during the coronary artery occlusion. (Abbreviations: AP, anterior papillary muscle; LAD, left anterior descending coronary artery; LCx, left circumflex coronary artery; LMC, left main coronary artery; LV, left ventricle; PP, posterior papillary muscle; RV, right ventricle; S,interventricular septum.) (From Sakanaki T, Tei C, Meerbaum S, et al: Verification of myocardial contrast two-dimensional echocardiographic assessment of perfusion defects in ischemic myocardium. J Am Coll Cardiol 3:34–38, 1984, with permission.)

integrated ultrasonic backscatter. Hoyt et al, studying the relationship between ultrasonic backscatter and collagen deposition in 10 excised human hearts with old myocardial infarctions, found a linear correlation ($r = 0.78$) between the magnitude of integrated backscatter and the collagen content of the myocardium (Fig. 8-61).[208]

Ischemic tissue becomes edematous, and it will also reflect ultrasound in a different fashion than normal tissue. Schnittger et al, studying the effects of acute myocardial ischemia on the ultrasonic signal, found that the baseline mean amplitude over the standard deviation of the amplitude (MSR) was significantly elevated after 30 minutes of acute ischemia (Fig. 8-62).[209] Thus, statistical analysis of the ultrasonic signal may help in the recognition of ischemic and infarcted areas of myocardium.

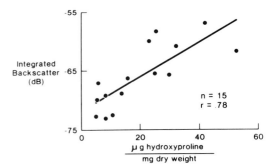

Fig. 8-61. Correlation between the magnitude of the integrated ultrasonic backscatter (average of five measurements for each specimen) and the collagen content of the myocardium as estimated by hydroxyproline assay. (From Hoyt R, Collins S, Skorton D, et al: Assessment of fibrosis in infarcted human hearts by analysis of ultrasonic backscatter. Circulation 71:740–744, 1985, with permission.)

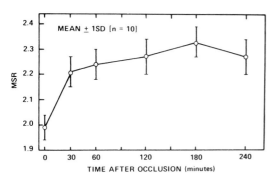

Fig. 8-62. MSR as a function of time after occlusion of the left anterior descending coronary artery (LAD) in 10 dogs. All error bars are expressed as mean ± S.D. (From Schnittger I, Vieli A, Heiserman J, et al: Ultrasonic tissue characterization: Detection of acute myocardial ischemia in dogs. Circulation 72:193–199, 1985, with permission.)

Three-Dimensional Echocardiography

By reconstructing planar projections of the heart, a computer linked to an echo scanner can generate what is termed *3D imaging*.[204] In fact, since only planar or 2D imaging modalities exist today, no real 3D image can be generated. The computer merely aquires a sufficient number of 2D views from the ultrasound scanner to be able to mathematically generate any desired projection. "Wire frame" representation of such superimposed 2D projections (Fig. 8-63) gives the impression of three-dimensionality. Data required for 3D reconstructions are synchronous 2D views of the epicardium and/or endocardium at different levels through the heart. They must be obtained at exactly the same time point in consecutive cardiac cycles. As few as five to ten of these

views may be sufficient. The relative location of these images in real space needs to be known, and the more images used, the more accurate the 3D reconstruction. There are three different ways to track the position and orientation of the transducer in space in order to orient the 2D image data sets. The first method uses electronic potentiometers at the elbows of an articulated mechanical arm and is accurate to several millimeters. The second method uses an ultrasonic signal emitted by the transducer and received by three remote receivers. This method is accurate to 2–3 mm and allows unrestricted motion of the transducer, but it limits the number of accessible transducer orientations. The last method uses optical laser light reflected by reflectors mounted on the transducer. It has an accuracy of about 3 mm, but like the second method, it limits the number of possible transducer orientations.

Three-dimensional echo reconstructions yield more precise cardiac chamber volumes than 2D echocardiography since data from multiple different views are used, and fewer geometric assumptions are made. Practical applications of the method are limited by the long time required for data collection during which breathing, motion of the heart, and beat-by-beat variations in hemodynamics can cause artifacts. Thus, real-time 3D echocardiography is presently only a research tool with exciting potential for the future.

AUTOMATED OR COMPUTER-ASSISTED BORDER DETECTION

For numerous reasons, automatic or semiautomatic endocardial border identification would be desirable. It reduces the time spent on manual analy-

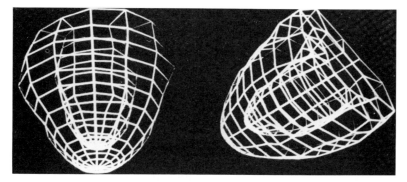

Fig. 8-63. 3D "wire frame" representations of a human left ventricle at end-systole. Data from individual echocardiographic views were placed in proper 3D orientation with the use of information from a mechanical transducer position registration system. (From Skorton DJ, Collins SM, Garcia E, et al: Digital signal and image processing in echocardiography. The American Society of Echocardiography Subcommittee on Digital Image Processing. Am Heart J 110:1268–1283, 1985, with permission.)

sis, while increasing objectivity and accuracy. The tracing of an echo image border is divided into the following tasks: (1) selection of a good quality image; (2) selection of a frame at the correct time in the cardiac cycle; (3) identification of the border of interest; and (4) tracing of the border contour. In the semiautomated border detection systems, the operator chooses a starting frame and roughly defines the border of interest. The computer refines the border outline and tracks it on subsequent frames. More sophisticated fully automatic border detection systems exist; however, echo dropout and spurious echo content limit their applicability. As mentioned earlier, various digital processing steps, such as space or time averaging and histogram equalization, can improve image quality. Borders can be further sharpened by using "differential" or gradient operations on the image data. After all border-enhancing operations have been completed, the key border identification step can be performed in three ways: (1) an operator can assign a starting border and the computer delineates subsequent borders using defined "prior constraints"; (2) a radial search algorithm can be applied; or (3) a binary image can be formed. The first method is semiautomated since it requires a subjective interpreter's initial tracing. Additional constraints, such as temporal rate of motion of the border and its general shape, guide the computer in the assignment of new borders in subsequent echo frames. This method is limited by the subjectivity in the initial tracing and also partly by the imposed constraints. In the radial search method, the computer searches for borders in a circular fashion starting in the center of the cavity. A border is reached when predetermined thresholds of change in echo amplitude in one or several neighboring pixels are observed. The rate of these changes in a spatial dimension increases the sensitivity of the method. Using equally spaced radial search lines, a complete border is generated when all locations identified as "border" are connected by some mathematical fitting formula.

In the binary method of border generation, all image information is transformed into either a single white or a single black intensity level (the image data content of each pixel is assigned either a 1 or a 0 binary value). All pixels that fulfill the amplitude threshold criteria for representing echoes and those satisfying the edge criteria (spatial rate of change in amplitude) are imaged in white while the intensity of all other pixels is set to black (Fig. 8-64). This procedure produces an image with sharp border outlines. The border outline is subsequently tracked at the

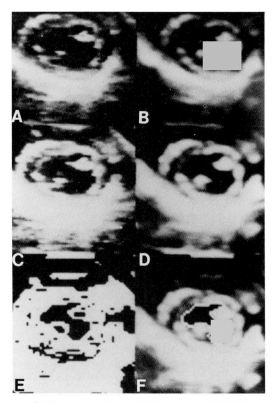

Fig. 8-64. Edge detection algorithm implementation in echocardiographic images. (A) Selected digitized frame of a short-axis cross-section at the level of the papillary muscles. (B) Corresponding frame following space-time smoothing. (C and D) Images corresponding to those in A and B after histogram equalization are shown. Note the decreased dropout in the equalized images. (E and F) Shown are binary image (E) and tracked endocardial outlines (F). (From Skorton DJ, Collins SM, Garcia E, et al: Digital signal and image processing in echocardiography. The American Society of Echocardiography Subcommittee on Digital Image Processing. Am Heart J 110:1268–1283, 1985, with permission.)

boundary between black and white pixels. This method is superior to the radial search algorithm in that all pixels containing border information are used rather than a sample of selected border points connected by a mathematical curve-fitting approximation. A limitation of this method is that it tends to underestimate areas enclosed within the borders. Manually tracing the endocardial border of an enhanced image using the LE–LE principle or simply using the center of the border line would yield an area significantly larger than the one identified by automatic border detection. This is particularly important when high gain settings or other types of processing produce thick border images. When automated border analysis is attempted, automated rather than manual time gain compensation should be utilized.

Although automatic edge detection has not yet reached sufficient sophistication to be useful in clinical practice, there is little doubt that in the near future it will become available for patient care. When that milestone is reached, intraoperative echocardiography will become a powerful and versatile monitoring tool, and it may surpass all currently available hemodynamic monitoring modalities.

REFERENCES

1. Langevin MP: Les ondes ultrasonores. Rev Gen Elect 23:626–634, 1928
2. Dussik TK: Uber die moglichkeit hochfrequente mechanische schwingungen als diagnostisches hilfmittel zu verwerten. Z Neurol Psychiatr 174:153–168, 1942
3. Guttner Von W, Fiedler G, Patzold: Uber Ultrashall abbildungen am Menschlichen Schadel. Acustica 2:148–156, 1952
4. Brown RE: History of diagnostic ultrasound. In Brown RE (ed): Ultrasonography. St. Louis, Warren H. Green, 1975
5. Holmes JP: Diagnostic ultrasound: Historical perspective. In King DL (ed): Diagnostic Ultrasound. St. Louis, CV Mosby, 1974
6. Edler I, Hertz CH: The use of the ultrasonic reflectoscope for the continuous recording of movements from the heart walls. Kungl Fysiog Sallsk Lund Fork 24:1–19, 1954
7. Edler I: Ultrasound cardiography. Acta Med Scand [Suppl] 170:1–124, 1961
8. Feigenbaum H: Echocardiography (ed 4). Philadelphia, Lea & Febiger, 1986
9. Hagan AD, DiSessa TG, Bloor CM, et al: Two-dimensional echocardiography. Boston, Little, Brown, 1983
10. Arvan S: Echocardiography. New York, Churchill Livingstone, 1984
11. Joyner CR: Ultrasound in the Diagnosis of Cardiovascular-Pulmonary Disease. Chicago, Year Book Medical, 1974
12. Gramiak R, Waag RC (eds): Cardiac Ultrasound. St. Louis, CV Mosby, 1975
13. Hagen-Ansert SL: Textbook of Diagnostic Ultrasonography (ed 2). St. Louis, CV Mosby, 1983
14. Matsumoto M, Oka Y, Strom J, et al: Application of transesophageal echocardiography to continuous intraoperative monitoring of left ventricular performance. Am J Cardiol 46:95–105, 1980
15. Hisanaga K, Hisanaga A, Nagata K, et al: Transesophageal cross-sectional echocardiography. Am Heart J 100:605–609, 1980
16. Schluter M, Langenstein B, Polster J, et al: Transesophageal cross-sectional echocardiography with a phased array transducer system. Technique and initial clinical results. Br Heart J 48:68–72, 1982

17a. Schluter M, Hinricks A, Thier W, et al: Transesophageal two-dimensional echocardiography: Comparison of ultrasonic and anatomic sections. Am J Cardiol 53:1173–1178, 1984
17b. Henry WL, DeMaria A, Gramiak R, et al: Report of the American Society of Echocardiography Committee on nomenclature and standards in two-dimensional echocardiography. Circulation 62:212, 1980
18. Matsuzaki M, Matsuda Y, Ikee Y, et al: Esophageal echocardiographic left ventricular anterolateral wall motion in normal subjects and patients with coronary artery disease. Circulation 63:1085–1092, 1981
19. Kremer P, Schwartz L, Cahalan M, et al: Intraoperative monitoring of left ventricular performance by transesophageal M-mode and 2-D echocardiography. Am J Cardiol 49:976, 1982
20. Konstadt S, Thys D, Mindich B, et al: Validation of quantitative intraoperative transesophageal echocardiography. Anesthesiology 65:418–421, 1986
21. Doppler CJ: Uber das farbige Licht der Doppelsterne. Abhandlungen der Koniglishen Bohmischen Gesellschaft der Wissenschaften 2:465, 1842
22. White DN: Johann Christian Doppler and his effect: A brief history. Ultrasound Med Biol 8:583, 1982
23. Hatle L, Angelsen B: Blood velocity measurements using the Doppler effect of backscattered ultrasound. In Hatle L, Angelsen B (eds): Doppler Ultrasound in Cardiology. Philadelphia, Lea & Febiger, 1985
24. Schuster AH, Nanda NC: Doppler examination of the heart, great vessels and coronary arteries. In Nanda N (ed): Doppler Echocardiography. New York, Igaku-Shoin, 1985
25. Goldberg SJ, Allen HD, Marx GR, et al: Doppler physics. In Doppler Echocardiography. Philadelphia, Lea & Febiger, 1985
26. Sahn DJ: Real-time two-dimensional Doppler echocardiographic flow mapping. Circulation 71:849–853, 1985
27. Teichholz LE, Kreulen T, Herman MV, et al: Problems in echocardiographic volume determinations: Echocardiographic-angiographic correlations in the presence or absence of asynergy. Am J Cardiol 37:7, 1976
28. Sahn DJ, DeMaria A, Kisslo J, et al: Recommendations regarding quantitation in M-mode echocardiog-

raphy: Results of a survey of echocardiographic measurements. Circulation 58:1072, 1978

29. Bett JHN, Dryburgh LG: Beat-to-beat variation in echocardiographic measurements of left ventricular dimensions and function. JCU 9:119, 1981

30. Spotnitz HM, Bregman D, Bowman FO, et al: Effects of open-heart surgery on end-diastolic pressure-diameter relations of the human left ventricle. Circulation 59:662–670, 1979

31. Wong YH, Spotnitz HM: Effects of nitroprusside on end-diastolic pressure-diameter relations of the human left ventricle after pericardiotomy. J Thorac Cardiovasc Surg 82:350–357, 1981

32. Quinones MA, Gaasch WH, Alexander JK: Echocardiographic assessment of left ventricular function with special reference to normalized velocities. Circulation 50:42, 1974

33. Fortuin NJ, Hood WP Jr, Craige E: Evaluation of left ventricular function by echocardiography. Circulation 46:26, 1972

34. Rosenblatt A, Clark R, Burgess J, et al: Echocardiographic assessment of the level of cardiac compensation in valvular heart disease. Circulation 54:509, 1976

35. Quinones MA, Pickering E, Alexander JK: Percentage of shortening of the echocardiographic left ventricular dimension: Its use in determining ejection fraction and stroke volume. Chest 74:59, 1978

36. Benzing G, Stockert J, Nave E, et al: Evaluation of left ventricular performance: Circumferential fiber shortening and tension. Circulation 49:925, 1974

37. Cooper R, Karliner JS, O'Rourke RA, et al: Ultrasound determinations of mean fiber-shortening rate in man. Am J Cardiol 29:257, 1972

38. Cooper RH, O'Rourke RA, Karliner JS, et al: Comparison of ultrasound and cineangiographic measurements of the mean rate of circumferential shortening in man. Circulation 46:914, 1972

39. Feigenbaum H: Echocardiographic examination of the left ventricle. Circulation 51:1, 1975

40. Kronik G, Slany J, Mosslacher H: Comparative value of eight M-mode echocardiographic formulas for determining left ventricular stroke volume. A correlative study with thermodilution and left ventricular single-plane cineangiography. Circulation 60:1308, 1979

41. Wong CYH, Spotnitz HM: Effect of nitroprusside on end-diastolic pressure-diameter relations of the human left ventricle after pericardiotomy. J Thorac Cardiovasc Surg 82:350–357, 1981

42. Barash P, Glanz S, Katz J, et al: Ventricular function in children during halothane anesthesia: An echocardiographic evaluation. Anesthesiology 49:79–85, 1978

43. Gerson J, Gianaris C: Echocardiographic analysis of human left ventricular diastolic volume and cardiac performance during halothane anesthesia. Anesth Analg 58:23–29, 1979

44. Rathod R, Jacobs H, Kramer N, et al: Echocardiographic assessment of ventricular performance following induction with two anesthetics. Anesthesiology 49:86–90, 1978

45. Schieber M, Stiller R, Cook R: Cardiovascular and pharmacodynamic effects of high-dose fentanyl in newborn piglets. Anesthesiology 63:166–171, 1985

46. Moore R, Yang S, McNicholas K, et al: Hemodynamic and anesthetic effects of sufentanil as the sole anesthetic for pediatric cardiovascular surgery. Anesthesiology 62:725–731, 1985

47. Terai C, Venishi M, Sugimoto H, et al: Transesophageal echocardiographic dimensional analysis of four cardiac chambers during positive end-expiratory pressure. Anesthesiology 63:640–646, 1985

48. Hirschfeld S, Meyer R, Schwartz DC, et al: Measurement of right and left ventricular systolic time intervals by echocardiography. Circulation 51:304, 1975

49. Weissler AM: Systolic time intervals. N Engl J Med 296:321–324, 1977

50. Lewis RP, Rittgers SE, Forester WF, et al: A critical review of the systolic time intervals. Circulation 56:146, 1977

51. Riggs T, Hirschfeld S, Borkat G, et al: Assessment of the pulmonary vascular bed by echocardiographic right ventricular systolic time intervals. Circulation 57:939, 1978

52. Spooner EW, Perry BL, Stern AM, et al: Estimation of pulmonary/systemic resistance ratios from echocardiographic systolic time intervals in young patients with congenital or acquired heart disease. Am J Cardiol 42:810, 1978

53. Johnson GL, Meyer RA, Korfhagen J, et al: Echocardiographic assessment of pulmonary arterial pressure in children with complete right bundle branch block. Am J Cardiol 41:1264, 1978

54. Gutgesell HP, Pinsky WW, Duff DF, et al: Left and right ventricular systolic time intervals in the newborn: Usefulness and limitation in distinguishing respiratory disease from transposition of the great arteries. Br Heart J 42:27, 1979

55. Garcia EJ, Riggs T, Hirschfeld S, et al: Echocardiographic assessment of the adequacy of pulmonary arterial banding. Am J Cardiol 44:487, 1979

56. Corya BC, Rasmussen S, Feigenbaum H, et al: Systolic thickening and thinning of the septum and posterior wall in patients with coronary artery disease, congestive cardiomyopathy, and atrial septal defect. Circulation 55:109, 1977

57. Feneley MP, Hickie JB: Validity of echocardiographic determination of left ventricular systolic wall thickening. Circulation 70:226, 1984

58. Aziz KU, vanGrondelle A, Paul MH, et al: Echocardiographic assessment of the relation between left ventricular wall and cavity dimensions and peak systolic pressure in children with aortic stenosis. Am J Cardiol 40:775, 1977

59. Schwartz A, Vignola PA, Walker HJ, et al: Echocar-

diographic estimation of aortic valve gradient in aortic stenosis. Ann Intern Med 89:329, 1978

60. Reichek N, Wilson J, St. John Sutton M, et al: Noninvasive determination of left ventricular end-systolic stress: Validation of the method and initial application. Circulation 65:99, 1982

61. Quinones MA, Moketaff DM, Nouri S, et al: Noninvasive quantification of left ventricular wall stress. Am J Cardiol 45:782, 1980

62. Sandler H, Dodge HT: Left ventricular tension and stress in man. Circ Res 13:91, 1963

63. Hartford M, Wikstand JCM, Wallentin I, et al: Left ventricular wall stress and systolic function in untreated primary hypertension. Hypertension 7:97–104, 1985

64. Brown KM, Lang R, Neuman A, et al: Systemic vascular resistance: An unreliable index of left ventricular afterload. J Am Coll Cardiol 7:35A, 1986

65. Thys DM, Hillel Z, Goldman M, et al: A comparison of hemodynamic indices derived by invasive monitoring and by two-dimensional echocardiography. Anesthesiology 65:A143, 1986

66. Marsh JD, Creen LH, Wynne J, et al: Left ventricular end-systolic pressure-dimension and stress-length relations in normal human subjects. Am J Cardiol 44:1311–1317, 1979

67. Branzi A, Lolli C, Piovaccari G, et al: Echocardiographic evaluation of the response to afterload stress test in young asymptomatic patients with chronic severe aortic regurgitation: Sensitivity of the left ventricular end-systolic pressure-volume relationship. Circulation 70:561–569, 1984

68. Borow KM, Neumann A, Arensman FW: Left ventricular contractility and contractile reserve in humans after cardiac transplantation. Circulation 71:866–872, 1985

69. Feigenbaum H: Hemodynamic information derived from echocardiography. In Feigenbaum H (ed): Echocardiography (ed 4). Philadelphia, Lea & Febiger, 1985, p 200

70. Duchak JM Jr, Chang S, Feigenbaum H: The posterior mitral valve echo and the echocardiographic diagnosis of mitral stenosis. Am J Cardiol 29:628, 1972

71. Goodman DJ, Harrison DC, Popp RL: Echocardiographic features of primary pulmonary hypertension. Am Heart J 86:847, 1973

72. McLaurin LP, Gibson TC, Waider W, et al: An appraisal of mitral valve echocardiograms mimicking mitral stenosis in conditions with right ventricular pressure overload. Circulation 48:801, 1973

73. Pennock R, Kingsley B, Kawai N, et al: Stroke volume and cardiac output measured by echocardiography. Am J Cardiol 25:121, 1970

74. Rasmussen S, Corya BC, Feigenbaum H, et al: Stroke volume calculated from the mitral valve echogram in patients with and without ventricular dyssynergy. Circulation 58:125, 1978

75. Askenazi J, Koenigsberg DI, Ziegler JH, et al: Echo-

cardiographic estimates of pulmonary artery wedge pressure. N Engl J Med 305:1566, 1981

76. Askenazi J, Koenigsberg DI, Ribner HS, et al: Prospective study comparing different echocardiographic measurements of pulmonary capillary wedge pressure in patients with organic heart disease other than mitral stenosis. J Am Coll Cardiol 2:919, 1983

77. Rahko PS, Shaver JA, Salerni R, et al: A critical review of echophonocardiographic estimates of pulmonary artery wedge pressure in patients with mitral stenosis. Am J Cardiol 55:462–569, 1985

78. Gamble WH, Salerni R, Shaver JA: The noninvasive assessment of pulmonary capillary wedge pressure in mitral regurgitation. Am Heart J 107:950–958, 1984

79. Folland ED, Parisi AF, Moynihan PF, et al: Assessment of left ventricular ejection fraction and volumes by real-time, two-dimensional echocardiography. Circulation 60:760, 1979

80. Rogers EW, Feigenbaum H, Weyman AE: Echocardiography for quantitation of cardiac chambers. In Yu PN, Goodwin JF (eds): Progress in Cardiology, vol 8. Philadelphia, Lea & Febiger, 1979

81. Dubroff JM, Clark MB, Wong CYH, et al: Left ventricular ejection fraction during cardiac surgery: A two-dimensional echocardiographic study. Circulation 68:95–103, 1983

82. Schiller NB, Acquatella H, Ports TA, et al: Left ventricular volume from paired biplane two-dimensional echocardiography. Circulation 60:547, 1979

83. Ren JF, Panidis IP, Kotler MN, et al: Effect of coronary bypass surgery and valve replacement on left ventricular function: Assessment by intraoperative two-dimensional echocardiography. Am Heart J 109:281–289, 1985

84. Gordon EP, Schnittger I, Fitzgerald PJ, et al: Reproducibility of left ventricular volumes by two-dimensional echocardiography. J Am Coll Cardiol 2:506, 1983

85. Cahalan M, Kremer P, Schiller N, et al: Intraoperative monitoring with two-dimensional transesophageal echocardiography. Anesthesiology 57:A153, 1982

86. Roizen M, Beaupre P, Alpert R, et al: Monitoring with two-dimensional transesophageal echocardiography. Comparison of myocardial function in patients undergoing supraceliac, suprarenal-infraceliac, or infrarenal aortic occlusion. J Vasc Surg 1:300–305, 1984

87. St. John Sutton M, Plappert TA, Hirshfeld JW, et al: Assessment of left ventricular mechanics in patients with asymptomatic aortic regurgitation: A two-dimensional echocardiographic study. Circulation 69:259–268, 1984

88. Hillel Z, Thys DM, Mindich BP, et al: A new method for the intraoperative determination of contractility. Anesth Analg 65:S72, 1986

89. Hillel Z, Thys DM, Mindich BP, et al: Intraoperative measurement of the effects of dopamine on LV contractility. Anesthesiology 63:A25, 1985

90. Thys DM, Hillel Z, Mindich BP, et al: Halothane is a potent myocardial depressant during fentanyl anesthesia. Anesth Analg 65:S159, 1986

91. Parisi AF, Moynihan PF, Feldman CL, et al: Approaches to determination of left ventricular volume and ejection fraction by real-time two-dimensional echocardiography. Clin Cardiol 2:257–263, 1979

92. Skjaerpe T, Hegrenaes L, Ihlen H: Cardiac output. In Hatle L, Angelsen B (eds): Doppler Ultrasound in Cardiology (ed 2). Philadelphia, Lea & Febiger, 1985

93. Angelsen BAJ, Brubakk AO: Transcutaneous measurement of blood flow velocity in the human aorta. Cardiovasc Res 10:368–379, 1976

94. Gisvold SE, Brubakk AO: Measurements of instantaneous blood-flow velocity in the human aorta using pulsed ultrasound. Cardiovasc Res 16:26–33, 1982

95. Ihlen H, Amlie JP, Dale J, et al: Determination of cardiac output by Doppler echocardiography. Br Heart J 51:54–60, 1984

96. Leoppky JA, Greene ER, Hoekenga DE, et al: Beat-by-beat stroke volume assessment by pulsed Doppler in upright and supine exercise. J Appl Physiol 50:1173–1182, 1981

97. Goldberg SJ, Sahn DJ, Allen HD, et al: Evaluation of pulmonary and systemic blood flow by 2-dimensional Doppler echocardiography using fast Fourier transform spectral analysis. Am J Cardiol 50:1394–1400, 1982

98. Fisher DC, Sahn DJ, Friedman MJ, et al: The effect of variations of pulsed Doppler sampling site on calculation of cardiac output: An experimental study in open-chest dogs. Circulation 67:370–376, 1983

99. Magnin PA, Stewart JA, Myers S, et al: Combined Doppler and phased-array echocardiographic estimation of cardiac output. Circulation 63:388–392, 1981

100. Kumar A, Minagoe S, Thangaturai D, et al: Non-invasive measurement of cardiac output during general anesthesia by continuous wave Doppler esophageal probe: Comparison with simultaneous thermodilution cardiac output. Anesthesiology 63:A68, 1985

101. Freund PR, Padovich CA: A comparison of cardiac output techniques: Transesophageal Doppler versus thermodilution cardiac output during general anesthesia in man. Anesthesiology 63:A191, 1985

102. Spirito P, Maron BJ, Borow RO: Non-invasive assessment of left ventricular diastolic function: Comparative analysis of Doppler echocardiographic and radionuclide angiographic techniques. J Am Coll Cardiol 7:518–526, 1986

103. Fujii J, Yazaki Y, Sawada H, et al: Noninvasive assessment of left and right ventricular filling in myocardial infarction with a two-dimensional Doppler echocardiographic method. J Am Coll Cardiol 5:1155–1160, 1985

104. Snider AR, Gidding SS, Rocchini AP, et al: Doppler evaluation of left ventricular diastolic filling in children with systemic hypertension. Am J Cardiol 56:921–926, 1985

105. Ryan T, Armstrong WF, Feigenbaum H: Doppler assessment of left ventricular filling during experimental myocardial ischemia. Circulation 72:III59, 1985

106. Rosoff M, Funai J, Wang SS, et al: Left ventricular filling dynamics in acute myocardial infarction: Immediate effects of ischemia, time course in first 6 hours and relation to infarct size. J Am Coll Cardiol 7:227A, 1986

107. Thys DM, Hillel Z, Konstadt S, et al: Esophageal Doppler echocardiography for the intraoperative evaluation of transmitral flow velocity. Montreal, Abstract, Annual Meeting of the Society of Cardiovascular Anesthesiologists, 1986

108. Visser CA, deKonig H, Delemarre B, et al: Pulsed, Doppler-derived mitral inflow velocity in acute myocardial infarction: An early prognostic indicator. J Am Coll Cardiol 7:136A, 1986

109. Tennant R, Wiggers CJ: Effects of coronary occlusion on myocardial contraction. Am J Physiol 112:351–361, 1935

110. Herman M, Heinle R, Klien M, et al: Localized disorders in myocardial contraction. Asynergy and its role in congestive heart failure. N Engl J Med 277:222–232, 1967

111. Forrester JS, Wyatt HL, Paluz PL, et al: Functional significance of regional ischemic contraction abnormalities. Circulation 54:64–70, 1976

112. Vatner SF: Correlation between acute reductions in myocardial blood flow and function in conscious dogs. Circ Res 47:201–207, 1980

113. Lowenstein E, Foex P, Phil D, et al: Regional ischemic ventricular dysfunction in myocardium supplied by a narrowed coronary artery with increasing halothane concentration in the dog. Anesthesiology 55:349–359, 1981

114. Kerber RE, Marcus ML, Ehrhardt J, et al: Correlation between echocardiographically demonstrated segmental dyskinesis and regional myocardial perfusion. Circulation 52:1097–1104, 1975

115. Stowe DF, Mathey DG, Moores WY, et al: Segmental stroke work and metabolism depend on coronary blood flow in the pig. Am J Physiol 234:H597–H607, 1978

116. Gallagher K, Kumada T, Koziol J, et al: Significance of regional wall thickening abnormalities relative to transmural myocardial perfusion in anesthetized dogs. Circulation 62:1266–1274, 1980

117. Pandian N, Kieso R, Kerber R: Two-dimensional echocardiography in experimental coronary stenosis, II. Relationship between systolic wall thinning and regional myocardial perfusion in severe coronary stenosis. Circulation 66:603–611, 1982

118. Osakada G, Hess O, Gallagher K, et al: End-systolic dimension-wall thickness relations during myocar-

dial ischemia in conscious dogs. Am J Cardiol 61:1750–1758, 1983

119. Weyman A, Peskoe S, Williams E, et al: Detection of left ventricular aneurysms by cross-sectional echocardiography. Circulation 54:936–944, 1976

120. Kislo J, Robertson D, Gilbert B, et al: A comparison of real-time two-dimensional echocardiography and cineangiography in detecting left ventricular asynergy. Circulation 55:134–141, 1977

121. Pandian N, Kerber R: Two-dimensional echocardiography in experimental coronary stenosis. I. Sensitivity and specificity in detecting transient myocardial dyskinesis: Comparison with sonomicrometers. Circulation 66:597–602, 1982

122. Force T, Bloomfield P, O'Boyle JE, et al: Quantitative two-dimensional echocardiographic analysis of regional wall motion in patients with perioperative myocardial infarction. Circulation 70:233–241, 1984

123. Ren J, Kotler M, Hakki A, et al: Quantitation of regional left ventricular function by two-dimensional echocardiography in normals and patients with coronary artery disease. Am Heart J 110:552–560, 1985

124. Pandian N, Skorton D, Collins S, et al: Heterogeneity of left ventricular segmental wall thickening and excursion in two-dimensional echocardiograms of normal human subjects. Am J Cardiol 51:1667–1673, 1983

125. Haendchen R, Wyatt H, Maurer G, et al: Quantitation of regional cardiac function by two-dimensional echocardiography. I. Patterns of contraction in the normal left ventricle. Circulation 67:1234–1245, 1983

126. Homans D, Asinger R, Elsperger J, et al: Regional function and perfusion at the lateral border of ischemic myocardium. Circulation 71:1038–1047, 1985

127. Lima J, Becker L, Melin J, et al: Impaired thickening of nonischemic myocardium during acute regional ischemia in the dog. Circulation 71:1048–1059, 1985

128. Elliott PL, Schauble JF, Weiss J, et al: Echocardiography and LV function during anesthesia. Anesthesiology 53:S105, 1980

129. Beaupre P, Kremer P, Cahalan M, et al: Intraoperative detection of changes in left ventricular segmental wall motion by transesophageal two-dimensional echocardiography. Am Heart J 107:1021–1023, 1984

130. Konstadt S, Goldman M, Thys D, et al: Intraoperative diagnosis of myocardial ischemia. Mt Sinai J Med 52:521–525, 1985

131. Smith J, Cahalan M, Benefield D, et al: Intraoperative detection of myocardial ischemia in high-risk patients: Electrocardiography versus two-dimensional transesophageal echocardiography. Circulation 72:1015–1021, 1985

132. Miller MM, Thorvaldson J, Ilebekk A, et al: Myocardial ischemia. Relationship between local

flow, function and ST segment elevation. Eur J Cardiol 10:7–8, 1979

133. Battler A, Froelicher VF, Gallagher KP, et al: Dissociation between regional myocardial dysfunction and ECG changes during ischemia in the conscious dog. Circulation 62:735–744, 1980

134. Smith HJ, Kent KM, Epstein SE: Relationship between regional contractile function and ST segment elevation after experimental coronary artery occlusion in the dog. Cardiovasc Res 12:444–448, 1978

135. Upton MT, Resych SK, Newman GE, et al: Detecting abnormalities in left ventricular function during exercise before angina and ST segment depression. Circulation 62:341–439, 1980

136. Sugishita Y, Susumu K, Matsuda M, et al: Dissociation between regional myocardial dysfunction and ECG in patients with angina pectoris. Am Heart J 106:1–8, 1983

137. Goldman M, Mindich B, Guarino T, et al: Rapid identification of ischemic myocardium before and after bypass surgery by combined use of intraoperative two-dimensional echocardiography and atrial pacing. J Am Coll Cardiol 7:151A, 1986

138. Topol EL, Weiss J, Guzman P, et al: Immediate improvement of dysfunctional myocardial segments after coronary revascularization: Detection by intraoperative transesophageal echocardiography. J Am Coll Cardiol 4:1123–1134, 1984

139. Komer R, Edalji A, Hood W: Effects of nitroglycerin on echocardiographic measurements of left ventricular wall thickness and regional myocardial performance during acute coronary ischemia. Circulation 59:926–937, 1979

140. Kerber R, Martins J, Marcus M: Effect of acute ischemia, nitroglycerin and nitroprusside on regional myocardial thickening, stress and perfusion. Experimental echocardiographic studies. Circulation 60:121–129, 1979

141. Gueret P, Meerbaum S, Corday E, et al: Differential effects of nitroprusside on ischemic and nonischemic myocardial segments demonstrated by computer-assisted two-dimensional echocardiography. Am J Cardiol 48:59–68, 1981

142. Saurada H, Fujii J, Kuboki M, et al: Evaluation of regional wall motion of the left ventricle before and after nitroglycerin administration in patients with ischemic heart disease: Comparison between two-dimensional echocardiograms and coronary angiograms. J Cardiography 12:904–914, 1982

143. Goldman ME, Mindich BP: Intraoperative two-dimensional echocardiography: New application of an old technique. J Am Coll Cardiol 7:374–382, 1986

144. Fuster V, Pumphrey CW, McGoon MD, et al: Systemic thromboembolism in mitral and aortic Starr-Edwards prostheses: A 10–19 year follow-up. Circulation 66(suppl I):157–161, 1982

145. Starr A, Grunkemeir GL: Selection of a prosthetic heart valve. JAMA 251:1739–1742, 1984

146. Milano A, Bartolotti V, Talente E, et al: Calcific degeneration as the main cause of porcine bioprosthetic valve failure. Am J Cardiol 53:1066–1070, 1984

147. Carpentier A, Chavraud S, Fabiani JN, et al: Reconstructive surgery of mitral valve incompetence: Ten-year appraisal. J Thorac Cardiovasc Surg 79: 338–348, 1980

148. Goldman ME, Mindich BP, Stavile K, et al: Intraoperative contrast two-dimensional echocardiography to assess mitral valve operations. J Am Coll Cardiol 4:1035–1040, 1984

149. Feinstein SB, Folkert JTC, Zwehl W, et al: Two-dimensional contrast echocar diography: Development and quantificative analysis of echocardiographic contrast agents. J Am Coll Cardiol 3:14–20, 1984

150. Austen SG, Houry DH: Ultrasound as a method to detect bubbles of particulate matter in the arterial line during cardiopulmonary bypass. J Surg Res 51:273–284, 1965

151. Bommer WJ, Shah PM, Allen H, et al: The safety of contrast echocardiography. Report of the Committee on Contrast Echocardiography for the American Society of Echocardiography. J Am Coll Cardiol 3:6, 1984

152. Grossman W: Cardiac Catheterization and Angiography. Philadelphia, Lea & Febiger, 1977, p 312

153. Reid CH, Kawanishi DT, McKay CR, et al: Accuracy of evaluation of the presence and severity of aortic and mitral regurgitation by contrast two-dimensional echocardiography. Am J Cardiol 52:519–524, 1983

154. Equaras BG, Pasalodos J, Gonzalez V, et al: Intraoperative contrast two-dimensional echocardiography: Evaluation of the presence and severity of aortic and mitral regurgitation during cardiac operations. J Thorac Cardiovasc Surg 89:573–579, 1985

155. Rodigas PC, Meyer JM, Haasler GB, et al: Intraoperative two-dimensional echocardiography: Ejection of microbubbles from the left ventricle after cardiac surgery. Am J Cardiol 50:1130–1132, 1982

156. David TE, Burns RJ, Bacchus CM, et al: Mitral valve replacement for mitral regurgitation with and without preservation of the chordae tendineae. J Thorac Cardiovasc Surg 88:718–725, 1984

157. David TE, Uden DE, Strauss HD: The importance of the mitral apparatus in left ventricular function after correction of mitral regurgitation. Circulation 68(suppl II):76–82, 1983

158. Schluter M, Langenstein BA, Hamath P, et al: Assessment of transesophageal pulsed Doppler echocardiography in the detection of mitral regurgitation. Circulation 66:784–789, 1982

159. Shively B, Cahalan M, Benefield D, et al: Intraoperative assessment of mitral valve regurgita-

tion by transesophageal Doppler echocardiography. J Am Coll Cardiol 7:228A, 1986

160. Cairns KB, Kloster FE, Bristow FD, et al: Problems in the hemodynamic diagnosis of tricuspid regurgitation. Am Heart J 75:173, 1968

161. King RM, Schaft HV, Danielson GK, et al: Surgery for tricuspid regurgitation late after mitral valve replacement. Circulation 70(suppl I):I193–197, 1984

162. Breyer RH, McClenathan JK, Michaelis LL, et al: Tricuspid regurgitation: A comparison of non-operative management, tricuspid annuloplasty and tricuspid valve replacement. J Thorac Cardiovasc Surg 72:867–872, 1976

163. Goldman ME, Mindich BP, Guarino T, et al: Intraoperative contrast echo: A new method to evaluate tricuspid regurgitation. J Am Coll Cardiol 5:459, 1985

164. Goldman ME, Mindich BP: Intraoperative cardioplegic contrast echocardiography for assessing myocardial perfusion during open heart surgery. J Am Coll Cardiol 4:1021–1027, 1984

165. Sahn DJ, Barratt-Boyes BG, Graham K, et al: Ultrasonic imaging of coronary arteries in open-chested humans: Evaluation of coronary atherosclerotic lesions during cardiac surgery. Circulation 66:1034–1044, 1982

166. Sahn DJ, Copeland JG, Temkin LP, et al: Anatomic-ultrasound correlation for intraoperative open chest imaging of coronary artery atherosclerotic lesions in human beings. J Am Coll Cardiol 3:1169–1177, 1984

167. McPherson D, Armstrong M, Marcus M, et al: Evaluation of the coronary arterial wall and lumen by high-frequency two-dimensional epicardial echocardiography: Comparisons with histologic measurements. J Am Coll Cardiol 3:565, 1984

168. Hiratzka LF, McPherson DD, Lamberth WC, et al: Intraoperative evaluation of CABG anastamoses with high frequency epicardial echocardiography. Circulation 73:1199–1205, 1986

169. Oka Y, Boriwaki K, Hong Y, et al: Detection of air emboli in the left heart by M-mode transesophageal echocardiography following cardiopulmonary bypass. Anesthesiology 63:109–113, 1985

170. Topol EH, Humphrey LS, Bashan M, et al: Value of intraoperative left ventricular microbubbles detected by transesophageal two-dimensional echocardiography in predicting neurologic outcome after cardiac operations. Am J Cardiol 56:773–775, 1985

171. Furuya H, Suzuki T, Okumura F, et al: Detection of air embolism by transesophageal echocardiography. Anesthesiology 58:124–129, 1983

172. Glenski FA, Cucchiara RF, Michenfelder JD: Transesophageal echocardiography and transcutaneous O_2 and CO_2 monitoring for detection of venous air embolism. Anesthesiology 64:541–545, 1986

173. Cucchiara R, Nugent M, Seward J, et al: Air embo-

lism in upright neurosurgical patients: Detection and localization by two-dimensional transesophageal echocardiography. Anesthesiology 60:353–355, 1984

174. Valdes-Cruz L, Pieroni D, Roland J, et al: Recognition of residual postoperative shunts by contrast echocardiographic techniques. Circulation 55:148–152, 1977

175. Fraker T, Harris P, Behar V, et al: Detection and exclusion of interatrial shunts by two-dimensional echocardiography and peripheral venous injection. Circulation 59:379–384, 1979

176. Wann LS, Weyman AE, Feigenbaum H, et al: Determination of mitral valve area by cross-sectional echocardiography. Ann Intern Med 88:337, 1978

177. Martin RP, Rakowski H, Kleiman JH, et al: Reliability and reproducibility of two-dimensional echocardiographic measurement of the stenotic mitral orifice area. Am J Cardiol 43:560, 1979

178. Stamm RB, Martin RP: Quantification of pressure gradients across stenotic valves by Doppler ultrasound. J Am Coll Cardiol 2:707, 1983

179. Hatle L, Angelsen B, Tromsdol A: Noninvasive assessment of atrio-ventricular pressure half-time by Doppler ultrasound. Circulation 60:1096–1104, 1979

180. Morganroth J, Jones RH, Chen CC, et al: Two-dimensional echocardiography in mitral, aortic, and tricuspid valve prolapses. The clinical problem, cardiac problem, cardiac nuclear imaging considerations and a proposed standard for diagnosis. Am J Cardiol 46:1164, 1980

181. Mytake K, Lzumi S, Okamoto K, et al: Semi-quantitative grading of severity of mitral regurgitation by real-time two-dimensional Doppler flow imaging technique. J Am Coll Cardiol 7:82–88, 1986

182. Godley RW, Green D, Dillon JC, et al: Reliability of two-dimensional echocardiography in assessing the severity of valvular aortic stenosis. Chest 79:657–662, 1981

183. Hatle L, Angelsen BA, Tromsdol A: Noninvasive assessment of aortic stenosis by Doppler ultrasound. Br Heart J 43:284–292, 1980

184. Henry WL, Bonow RO, Rosing DR, et al: Observations on optimum time for operative intervention for aortic regurgitation, II. Serial echocardiographic evaluation of asymptomatic patients. Circulation 61:484, 1980

185. Daniels WG: Chronic aortic regurgitation: Reassessment of the prognostic value of preoperative left ventricular end-systolic dimension and fractional shortening. Circulation 71:669, 1985

186. Bonow RO, Picone AL, Mcintosh CL, et al: Survival and function results after valve replacement for aortic regurgitation from 1976 to 1983: Impact of preoperative ventricular function. Circulation 72:1244–1256, 1985

187. Bonow RO, Rosing DR, Mcintosh LL, et al: The natural history of asymptomatic patients' aortic regurgitation and normal left ventricular function. Circulation 58:509, 1983

188. Moses HW, Nanda NC: Real-time two-dimensional echocardiography in the diagnosis of left atrial myxoma. Chest 78:788, 1980

189. Visser CA, Kan G, Lie KI, et al: Left ventricular thrombus following acute myocardial infarction. Eur Heart J 4:333–337, 1983

190. Pichler M: Non-invasive assessment of segmental left ventricular wall motion: Its clinical relevance in detection of ischemia. Clin Cardiol 1:173, 1978

191. Weiss J: Relationship of systolic thickening to transmural extent of myocardial infarction in the dog. Circulation 62(suppl II):328, 1980

192. Romderos R, Salcedo EE, Kramer JR, et al: Value and limitation of two-dimensional echocardiography for the detection of left main coronary artery disease. Cleve Clin Q 51:7, 1984

193. Robertson WS, Feigenbaum H, Armstrong WF, et al: Exercise echocardiography: A clinically practical addition in the evaluation of coronary artery disease. J Am Coll Cardiol 2:1085, 1983

194. Crawford MH, Amon KW, Vance WS: Exercise 2-dimensional echocardiography. Am J Cardiol 51:1, 1983

195. Maron BJ, Epstein SE: Hypertrophic cardiomyopathy. Recent observations regarding the specificity of the three hallmarks of the disease: Asymmetric septal hypertrophy, septal disorganization, and systolic anterior motion of the anterior mitral leaflet. Am J Cardiol 45:141, 1980

196. Miyatake K, Okamoto M, Kinoshita N, et al: Augmentation of atrial contribution to left ventricular inflow with aging as assessed by intracardiac Doppler flowmetry. Am J Cardiol 53:586, 1984

197. Macartney FJ: Cross-sectional echocardiographic diagnosis of congenital heart disease. Br Heart J 50:501, 1983

198. Kremkau FW: Diagnostic Ultrasound: Principles, Instrumentation, and Exercises (ed 2). Orlando, FL, Grune & Stratton, 1984

199. Brown RE: Ultrasonography. St.Louis, WH Green, 1975

200. Kleid JJ: Echocardiography: Interpretation and Diagnosis. New York, Appleton-Century-Crofts, 1978

201. Diasonics Cardiovue 60 Operators Manual. Salt Lake City, Diasonics, 1983

202. Weyman AE: Cross-Sectional Echocardiography. Philadelphia, Lea & Febiger, 1982

203. McDicken WN: Diagnostic Ultrasonics: Principles and Use of Instruments (ed 2). New York, John Wiley & Sons, 1981

204. Skorton DJ, Collins SM, Garcia E, et al: Digital signal and image processing in echocardiography. The American Society of Echocardiography Sub-

committee on Digital Image Processing. Am Heart J 110:1268–1283, 1985

205. Sakanaki T, Tei C, Meerbaum S, et al: Verification of myocardial contrast two-dimensional echocardiographic assessment of perfusion defects in ischemic myocardium. J Am Coll Cardiol 3:34–38, 1984

206. Tei C, Kondo S, Meerbaum S, et al: Correlation of myocardial echo contrast disappearance rate and severity of experimental coronary stenosis. J Am Coll Cardiol 3:39–46, 1984

207. Ten Cate F, Feinstein S, Zwehl W, et al: Two-dimensional contrast echocardiography II: Transpulmonary studies. J Am Coll Cardiol 3:21–27, 1984

208. Hoyt R, Collins S, Skorton D, et al: Assessment of fibrosis in infarcted human hearts by analysis of ultrasonic backscatter. Circulation 71:740–744, 1985

209. Schnittger I, Vieli A, Heiserman J, et al: Ultrasonic tissue characterization: Detection of acute myocardial ischemia in dogs. Circulation 72:193–199, 1985

Warren J. Levy, M.D.

9

Central Nervous System Monitoring

The interest in neurophysiologic monitoring during cardiopulmonary bypass (CPB) is as old as extracorporeal circulation. Concern with the adequacy of cerebral perfusion during this unphysiologic state, as well as a desire to prevent catastrophic neurologic complications during a successful cardiac repair, placed neurologic monitoring in a position of some importance. Such monitoring also provided an assurance of pump function when blood gases were not routine measurements and perfusion systems not mass produced. This latter function is less significant now, but the apparent routine nature of cardiac surgery has also increased the importance of preventing neurologic damage during its performance. Whether neurologic monitoring can directly reduce the incidence of neurologic damage during routine cardiac surgery remains to be demonstrated; however, such monitoring is clearly indicated for specific types of cardiovascular procedures in which therapeutic decisions may be based on the results of this monitoring.

Electroencephalography (EEG) and the analysis of evoked potentials (EP) are the two most common forms of neurophysiologic monitoring used during cardiovascular surgery. Although often lumped together, they are very different forms of monitoring with unique indications, anesthetic effects, equipment requirements, and technical problems. Thus,

they will be discussed as two separate entities. The underlying neurophysiology of each will be discussed, as well as some aspects of recording technology. Since there are a variety of computerized EEG analysis systems commercially available and the analyses are somewhat complex, this technology will be addressed in some detail. Finally, specific indications for the use of EP and EEG monitoring will be discussed.

THE ELECTROENCEPHALOGRAM

Neuronal Origins of the EEG

The EEG is the recording from the scalp of the spontaneous electrical activity of the brain generated in the most superficial layers of the cerebral cortex. These layers contain pyramidal cells that are oriented perpendicular to the cortical surface. It is the generation of electrical gradients within these cells that produces the electrical changes which are ultimately identified as the EEG.[1]

Neuronal electrical activity can be subdivided into two general classes: action potentials and postsynaptic potentials. Action potentials occur during the propagation of an electrical event through a neu-

CARDIAC ANESTHESIA, SECOND EDITION
ISBN 0-8089-1848-6

319

ron. They are relatively large changes in voltage, but last only a very brief period of time. They have been shown to be unrelated to the EEG. On the other hand, postsynaptic potentials have been repeatedly demonstrated to have an appropriate time course and to be correlated with EEG activity. These studies have also confirmed the very superficial position in the cortex of the source of the EEG.[2]

The electrical activity that is recorded at the scalp by the EEG differs from the electrical changes in the superficial cortex due to the transmission of this cortical activity through bone and soft tissue. These tissues are largely passive, and thus the scalp potential is the summation of the activity of the underlying cortex.[3] If the cortex (over an area of several square centimeters) is behaving in a synchronous fashion, the EEG amplitude will be large, approximating that of the cortical recording. However, areas of cortex only millimeters apart may show striking differences in activity, and, under such conditions, the scalp EEG will be markedly reduced in amplitude compared with the cortical recording.[4]

This passive transmission also produces a reduction in EEG amplitude as the recording site moves farther from the source of activity. Studies using EP (whose site of action is known) have demonstrated that the measured surface amplitude of the electrical activity drops by almost 80 percent as the recording electrode is moved 2 cm from the site of maximal activity.[5] Accordingly, the contribution of the adjacent cortex to the recorded EEG far outweighs the contributions from more distant cortical activity. For this reason, changes in distant cortical activity cannot be identified with any reliability, and multiple recording electrodes must be utilized to ensure EEG monitoring of all areas of the cortex.

EEG Rhythms

Although an alpha rhythm is usually considered to be the "normal" EEG, under some conditions it may be quite abnormal, and in other circumstances non-alpha rhythms may be quite normal. Accordingly, it is useful to understand the normal variations that can be seen in the EEG to appreciate the specific conditions under which these patterns may be seen, and to apply the language of the electroencephalographer more critically when discussing the EEG under anesthesia.

The alpha rhythm is defined not only by its frequency (8–13 Hz), but by its amplitude (10–50 microvolts), spacial distribution (posterior), and behavior when the patient is stimulated (it is reduced

in amplitude or disappears, particularly during visual activity). Since there are other types of activity in the same frequency range which do not represent an alpha rhythm (eg, mu rhythm, and some anesthetic-induced rhythms), it is most important to differentiate alpha rhythms from activity in the alpha range of frequencies. Non-alpha EEG activity may also be quite normal. Although 80–90 percent of adults demonstrate predominantly alpha activity posteriorly when the EEG is recorded in an unstimulated state,[6] with age up to 50 percent of adults show slowing (7–8 Hz alpha variant) or acceleration (beta-EEG).[7] The anxiety associated with impending surgery (and the concurrent attention to the stimuli in the operating room and surroundings) may also reduce the incidence of alpha rhythms when the EEG is monitored prior to the induction of anesthesia.

Many electroencephalographic rhythms have focal distributions, the posterior prominence of the alpha rhythm being one previously mentioned example. The mu rhythm is most prominent centrally, while beta activity associated with sedation is more prominent frontally. Episodic rhythmic activity during some stages of sleep (sleep spindles) is most prominent in frontal and central regions, and other characteristic waves associated with sleep (V waves) are most prominent at the vertex of the calvarium. There are many other regional waves observed in the EEG, and focal changes due to local pathology are also well known. This is not an exhaustive list of localized EEG phenomena, but does re-emphasize the importance of the location of the recording electrode when interpreting the EEG.

It is beyond the scope of this chapter to review the specific effects of all anesthetics agents on the EEG. Classic reviews include articles by Clark and Rosner,[8] and Martin et al,[9] and material relevant to some of the more modern agents can be found in the text by Pichlmayr.[10] Anesthetic agents are capable of producing enormous variation in the EEG patterns, including a flat EEG with large doses of barbiturates, seizure activity with enflurane, burst-suppression with isoflurane or barbiturates, and EEG slowing with large doses of narcotics which is quite similar to that seen with ischemia. Furthermore, mixtures of anesthetics may have effects different from what would be predicted based on the known behavior of the EEG when the agents are administered individually. In addition, surgical stimulation can produce changes in the EEG.[11] Thus, the EEG cannot be considered in a vacuum; it must be analyzed in light of the known surgical and anesthetic conditions under which it is recorded. A flat EEG following the induction of anesthesia with barbiturates is likely to be benign, but the same EEG recorded after cross-clamping the carotid artery cannot be ignored. When EEG monitoring is used, surgical and anesthetic conditions should be controlled in order to minimize the possibility for confusion between anesthetic-induced benign changes and surgically-induced pathological ones.

EEG Recording Techniques

When monitoring the EEG, attention to technical details is necessary to ensure the acquisition of a high-quality signal representative of the electrical activity of the underlying cortex. Even under nearly optimal conditions in the neurophysiology laboratory, artifact can distort or obliterate the EEG. In the operating room, an electrically hostile environment, casual or careless recording techniques can eliminate any hope of effectively monitoring cortical activity. Under normal conditions, the amplitude of the EEG is less than 5 percent of the QRS complex on an electrocardiogram (ECG), and the identification of cerebral cortical ischemia demands resolution of changes on the EEG of only a very few microvolts. Movement of the patient or cables, nearby equipment, and even the ECG may produce artifact many times the amplitude of the cortical activity, and once amplified as signal, such artifact may be impossible to eliminate. In addition, rather than eliminating arti-

Table 9-1

Relative Ranking of Electrodes for Various Characteristics*

	Needle	Disk	Stick-on	Cap
Stability	4	1	3	2
Impedance	4	1	3	2
Ease of Placement	2	4	3	1
Trauma	4	2	1	2

*Clearly there is no perfect electrode, and the relative importance of each factor plays a major role in the selection process.

1 = best-type electrode; 4 = worst-type electrode

fact, sophisticated processing techniques may make it more difficult to identify. Fortunately, many of these difficulties may be reduced or eliminated by careful recording techniques.

There are many types of EEG electrodes in use (Fig. 9-1). Needles may be made of platinum or stainless steel; disk electrodes may be made of tin, silver, or gold; prepared stick-on types (similar to miniature ECG electrodes) and even caps covering the entire head are available. There are advantages to each type of electrode (Table 9-1). Speed of placement and the ability to place electrodes within a sterile surgical field are really the only factors favoring the use of needle electrodes. The latter is a relatively unimportant issue for monitoring during cardiac sur-

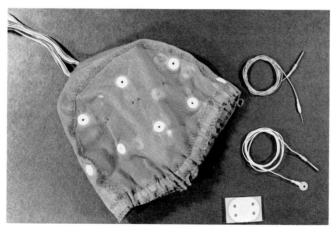

Fig. 9-1. EEG Electrodes. Shown above are four different types of EEG electrodes for intraoperative monitoring. The Ag-AgCl disk (center right) and the needle electrode (upper right) are standard EEG electrodes. The small pad electrode is distributed by Neurometrics Inc. with their monitoring system. The large cap at the upper left is manufactured by Electro-Cap International, Dallas, Texas, and contains a complete montage (or any subset desired).

gery, and the potential for bleeding following heparinization makes needle electrodes relatively contraindicated for use during cardiac surgery.

Stick-on electrodes would be the ideal EEG monitoring system if all patients were bald. Unfortunately, many are not, and these electrodes produce inadequate recordings when placement in hair is attempted. Thus, the routine use of such electrodes tends to result in placement where it is convenient, rather than where it is appropriate for recording cortical activity. The inability to record changes in cortical activity from distant electrodes has already been discussed, and placing the electrodes as dictated by the patient's hair style can only lead to inadequate and unsuccessful attempts at monitoring the EEG.

Electrode caps have much to offer in convenience; however, in practice they may fall short of this potential. The cap may slip during intubation or surgical positioning, causing the loss of recording capabilities from numerous electrodes at once. Such losses can be minimized by using chest or chin straps, but these are unwieldy during anesthesia and may impede access to the surgical site. It may be possible to reduce the incidence of these problems by taping the cap to the head; however, this is still not entirely satisfactory, and pressure sores or hair loss might occur if hypoperfusion occurred for an extended period. Perhaps other improvements in the design of these caps will further their usefulness as intraoperative recording devices.

Finally, there is the "gold standard" for EEG electrodes: Ag-AgCl disk electrodes filled with electrode jelly and secured with collodion and gauze. They are the most difficult to apply. However, this effort is rewarded with high-quality recordings. The time to apply four or even eight channels of EEG electrodes is not excessive, certainly no longer than placing a catheter in the pulmonary artery, and, if ECG monitoring is as important for the patient's care as is the measurement of cardiac output, then the expenditure of an equal amount of time for EEG monitoring is appropriate.

The placement of EEG monitoring electrodes should not be haphazard. Standard techniques for placing the electrodes in relation to the dimensions of the cranium result in reproducible placement of electrodes over identifiable cortical structures. Not only does such careful positioning improve the correlation between EEG events and cortical activity, it also allows intelligent discussion and comparison of EEG recordings. Although a number of systems are available, the International 10-20 system, in which the positions of electrodes are defined as shown in Figure 9-2, is preferred.[12]

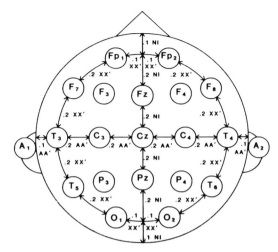

Fig. 9-2. Electrode positions on the scalp. This figure summarizes the position of the electrodes in the International 10-20 system according to scalp measurements. The sagittal hemicircumference is measured from the nasion to the inion, identified on the figure as NI. The coronal hemicircumference (labeled AA') is measured from the root of the one zygoma (just anterior to the ear) to the other, across the vertex. The third measure is the ipsilateral hemicircumference (XX') measured from a point 10 percent of the sagittal hemicircumference above the nasion to 10 percent of this circumference above the inion, running through a point 10 percent of the coronal hemicircumference above the zygoma. Through these intersecting lines, all of the scalp electrodes except for the frontal (F_3 and F_4) and the parietal (P_3 and P_4) may be located. These electrodes are placed along the frontal or parietal coronal line midway between the midline electrode and the electrode marked in the circumferential ring.

The 21 electrodes that comprise the montage could be connected in at least 1330 different ways in order to record the EEG. Clearly, some orderly mechanism must be utilized, and three such systems–bipolar, average reference electrode, and common reference electrode–have evolved. The advantages and disadvantages of each have been reviewed by MacGillivray.[13] The average reference electrode montage is rarely used for intraoperative monitoring because it requires a large number of electrodes and artifact on any electrode will appear on all channels.

In bipolar recordings, adjacent pairs of electrodes are connected and the EEG represents the difference in activity between the two electrodes. This is demonstrated by the right parasagittal electrodes in Figure 9-3. This montage is most useful for identifying foci of unusual activity, since the polarity of the activity changes as the chain of electrode pairs crosses the active focus. The alternative montage,

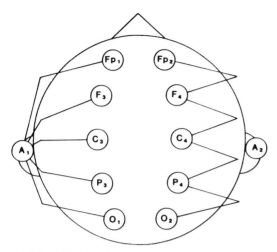

Fig. 9-3. Bipolar and common reference montages. The left parasagittal electrodes are connected in a common reference montage using the left earlobe (A_1) as the common reference electrode. Five channels would be recorded, each of them between the parasagittal electrode and the ear electrode. Differences among these channels would represent the differences in cerebral activity among the various parasagittal electrodes, because each channel is recorded as the difference between the activity at the parasagittal electrode and the activity at the ear electrode. For comparison, the right parasagittal electrodes have been connected in a bipolar chain. In this configuration, only four channels of EEG data are recorded. Each channel of data represents the electrical difference between the two adjacent electrodes.

the common reference electrode montage, is exemplified by the left parasagittal electrodes in Figure 9-3 in which each EEG is recorded with one electrode (usually the ipsilateral earlobe) in common. Thus, differences between channels represent differences in the activity in the adjacent electrodes. The EEG amplitude recorded from such separate electrodes (such as $F_3 - A_1$) is usually higher than that recorded from the adjacent pairs used in a bipolar chain. This is advantageous in the operating room; however, the loss of the single common reference electrode could result in the loss of monitoring from several channels at a single time. For this reason, bipolar chain montages may be more popular for intraoperative monitoring; however, there are no comparative studies indicating which montage is preferable for monitoring during anesthesia.

Although it is an exceedingly rare anesthesiologist who would be called upon to design or build an EEG amplifier, some knowledge of the technical aspects of amplifier design is most valuable for optimizing EEG recordings. The critical portion of the amplifier in this regard is the very first stage, to

which the EEG electrodes are connected. This portion of the amplifier is known as a differential amplifier because it amplifies the difference between the active electrodes. As a result of this design, artifact such as 60 Hz noise will not be amplified as long as it is of equal amplitude on each of the active electrodes. In general, this situation will hold true if the electrodes make good electrical contact (have low impedances). If, however, the electrode impedances are not equal, or vary due to movement of the electrode, the amplitude of the noise is not equal on each active electrode and the noise is not eliminated by differential amplification; it is amplified as signal. Thus, the quality of electrode contact is critical to the proper function of an EEG amplifier. As a result, the anesthesiologist wishing to use EEG monitoring must learn not only to apply electrodes properly, but also to measure the electrode impedances before beginning monitoring and correct those electrodes that have unacceptable impedance levels (usually considered 5 kohms or above).

There are many other types of artifact that occur during intraoperative EEG recording. Muscle artifact, due to the electrical activity in myofibrils, is common in awake, anxious patients awaiting their surgery in cold operating rooms. This muscle artifact usually disappears promptly following the induction of anesthesia; however, the fasciculations associated with depolarizing muscle relaxants may be quite prominent during induction. Artifact may also be produced by movement of the patient's head, the electrode wires, or other cabling. This problem can be lessened by keeping the cables as short as possible, protecting the head from movement with a cage or inverted bowl, and using a small preamplifier adjacent to the head, which minimizes the artifact that might occur during the transmission of very low voltage signals from the patient to the EEG machine.

The ECG can also appear on the EEG, and, when present, usually indicates the presence of problems with one or more EEG electrodes. Electrocardiogram activity may also be recorded when the ground electrode for the EEG is not placed on the head, but is placed on the shoulder or elsewhere on the body. In the unprocessed EEG, ECG artifact is easily identified, particularly if an audible QRS signal is generated by the ECG. After processing, however, it may be much more difficult to recognize ECG artifact. The high-voltage spike produced by a unipolar temporary pacemaker is one particular form of ECG artifact that is difficult to eliminate. Bipolar pacing usually results in less EEG artifact because the current loop is confined to the heart, minimizing the appearance of this electrical activity on the EEG.

Another ubiquitous form of intraoperative artifact is generated by electrosurgery units. Recognizing such artifact is no problem; but, with current technology, recording the EEG during electrocautery is essentially impossible. Finally, and most relevant to monitoring during CPB, roller-pumps can produce artifact of the same amplitude and frequency as the EEG. The problem arises due to the development of static electricity on the tubing of the roller-pump, and its elimination may be very difficult unless a problem can be identified with the electrode impedances or the EEG amplifiers.

It is a common misconception that filtering the EEG is useful as a means of eliminating these and other forms of artifact. In general, EEG activity is recorded between 1 and 70 Hz. Filtering the EEG to eliminate activity above 30 or 35 Hz is sometimes used to reduce muscle artifact; however, this is rarely necessary under anesthesia. The most common forms of intraoperative artifact have frequency distributions from 1 Hz to 3 or 4 Hz, and attempting to eliminate these through the use of filters may result in the loss of considerable amounts of EEG activity. In addition, artifact such as that generated by the roller-pump has a frequency distribution in the mid-range of EEG activity, and, therefore, this artifact cannot be removed with any type of filtering system without severely damaging the EEG. In short, the limitations of filtering make it an unacceptable replacement for careful electrode placement and proper recording technique. Filtering is only a stop-gap measure designed to allow the recording of a distorted EEG under otherwise unacceptable conditions.

Displaying the EEG

Having acquired a satisfactory EEG signal, the problem of intraoperative monitoring shifts to the display of the information contained in this signal. If the EEG were as easily quantified and as closely correlated with neuronal function as the ECG is with cardiac function, the complexities of displaying the information in the EEG would be vastly reduced. Unfortunately, this is not the case, and it is desirable to display the data as completely as possible. In this regard, the unprocessed signal, written as a trace on paper, is the standard. Unfortunately, using this information for intraoperative monitoring is almost impossible since paper is generated at a rate of 6 pages per minute and piles up faster than it can be read while managing the anesthetic. Since a monitor that cannot be read and cannot be interpreted in the available time is not very useful, the goal of auto-

mated EEG processing techniques is to display the relevant information in a form that is more readily interpreted than the raw tracing.

It is important to appreciate the difference between the technique used to analyze the EEG and that used to display the processed data. Although some analyses require specific types of displays, in many cases the same analysis can be displayed in a number of different fashions. Although there may be obvious theoretical advantages to one type of display or another, there are no data to suggest that these theoretical factors are actually practical issues for intraoperative monitoring. Like the vast assortment of laryngoscope blades of which only one or two are adequate for almost all patients, one or two EEG display techniques are likely to satisfy almost all reasonable needs for intraoperative monitoring.

Certainly, the one display modality with which all anesthesiologists must familiarize themselves is the raw EEG, displayed on an oscilloscope or strip chart. This is the best quality-control system existing for EEG recordings, and familiarity with the normal wave patterns will often allow rapid identification of amplifier malfunction, artifact, electrode slippage, and a host of similar problems. Univariant descriptors of the EEG (such as mean frequency or root mean square, [RMS], voltage) vary with time, and are easily interpreted when displayed on a slow-moving strip chart recorder in a trended format.

Many EEG processing techniques provide two-dimensional data that vary with time. These analyses provide information about the amplitude and frequency of component waves in the EEG, and the display must plot both amplitude and frequency in a form that allows their variation over time. Such a three-dimensional display of amplitude, frequency, and time is inherently complex, and no display format is entirely adequate. The true three-dimensional display must obscure some information in order to give perspective. Depending on the perspective taken and the data displayed, the result may be more or less difficult to interpret (Fig. 9-4).

Carrying the rotation of the time axis (z-axis) in Figure 9-4 to the vertical position produces a display of data with time and amplitude on the same axis. This is best known as the compressed spectral array (CSA),[14] although it need not be limited to use with power spectrum analysis of the EEG. In Figure 9-5, it seems that the CSA is more legible than the original three-dimensional display, because the peak hidden on the three-dimensional display is more apparent. Such differences are not always more evident on the CSA, and this particular example is sim-

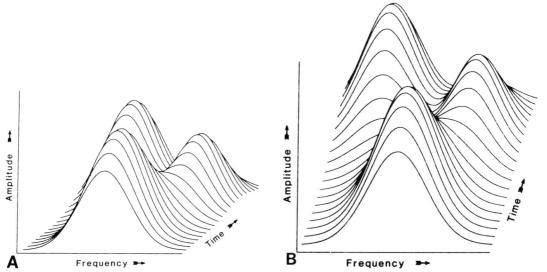

Fig. 9-4. Display of three-dimensional data. Shown above are displays of frequency and amplitude information from a hypothetical EEG recording. In order to give the figure perspective, only the front of the "hills" can be shown. In (A) one "hill" is hidden behind another, and the display is particularly difficult to interpret; however, a small change in perspective (B) greatly improves the readability. This difference is largely coincidence, since with different data, (A) might have been far more readable than (B).

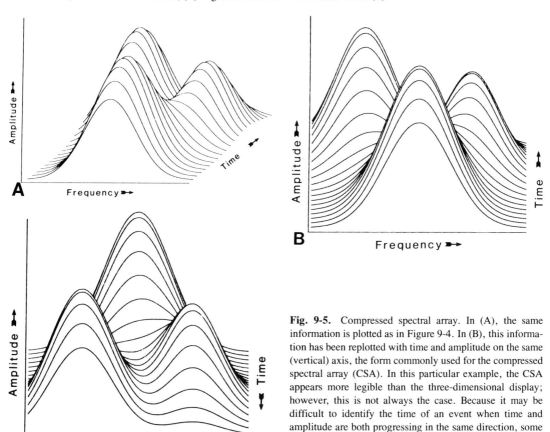

Fig. 9-5. Compressed spectral array. In (A), the same information is plotted as in Figure 9-4. In (B), this information has been replotted with time and amplitude on the same (vertical) axis, the form commonly used for the compressed spectral array (CSA). In this particular example, the CSA appears more legible than the three-dimensional display; however, this is not always the case. Because it may be difficult to identify the time of an event when time and amplitude are both progressing in the same direction, some authors use a display like that shown in (C), in which time advances downward.

325

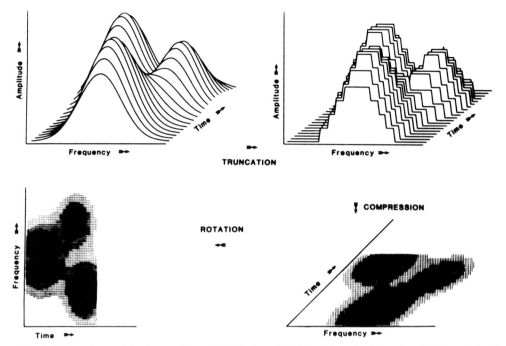

Fig. 9-6. Density-modulated spectral array. The display of the three-dimensional data in a density-modulated display format requires three steps. First, the amplitude information is quantified so that it may be encoded in a gray-scale form. Once encoded, the vertical displacement on the three-dimensional axis is redundant, and the display may be compressed onto a plane surface consisting of time and frequency as shown in the lower right-hand portion of the figure. At this point, the orientation of the time and frequency axes have not been changed. The axes are then rotated, placing time on the horizontal axis and frequency on the vertical axis, resulting in a display which is similar to a strip-chart recording.

ply a function of the perspective used in displaying the three-dimensional data. Figure 9-5 also demonstrates that determining the time of a peak is more difficult when time is shifted to the *y* axis. In an attempt to clarify this display, time is sometimes shown as advancing downward, producing a different, but questionably more readable, display (Fig. 9-5C).

An alternative display technique, called a density-modulated spectral array (DSA), involves topographic compression of the three-dimensional picture (Fig. 9-6).[15] This approach (utilized by cartographers for many years) quantifies the vertical data, codes it in a color or gray scale, and compresses it onto two axes, one of which is time. This display can therefore be rotated so that time is on the horizontal axis (not unlike a strip chart), but both frequency and amplitude data are still legible. Although the quantification of the amplitude data results in some loss of precision, this display provides the clearest recognition of the waveform in the hidden portions of the three-dimensional display. The ability to conveniently dis-

play the EEG with hemodynamic data is another advantage of this format.

Yet another alternative display technique for three-dimensional data is the three-dimensional histogram.[16] Overlapping data are a major problem with this display, and, in Figure 9-7B, only every fourth data point has been plotted. In addition, the perspective has been changed slightly between Figures 9-6 and 9-7 in order to improve the resolution of the histographic display technique. In the commercial unit that displays data in this fashion, color is used to further reduce this problem.

There is yet another way of displaying processed EEG data, one which considers a different aspect of electroencephalography. The display techniques described thus far apply to a single channel of EEG data, but, as has been discussed, more than one channel is necessary to evaluate the physiologic status of the brain. In brain-mapping displays, a univariate descriptor of the EEG such as mean frequency, total power, power in a particular frequency band, or spectral edge is derived from each channel of data and is

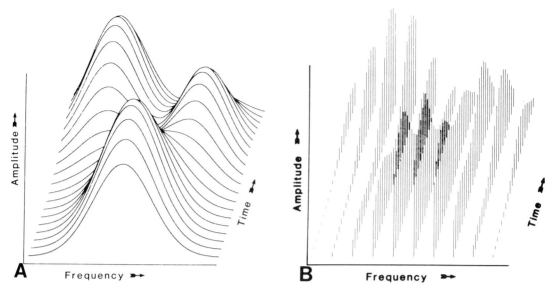

Fig. 9-7. (A) Three-dimensional histogram. The same data which have been used in Figures 9-4 to 9-6 are now plotted as a three-dimensional histogram. (B) Only every fourth data point has been plotted, and the perspective has been shifted slightly in order to improve legibility. For comparison, a three-dimensional display with a similar perspective is also shown.

displayed over a map of the brain. In theory, this type of display simplifies the identification of regional abnormalities, with the disadvantage that the tracking of change is more difficult because there is no simple means of displaying historical information. Whether the added ability to localize activity in this display will offset the theoretical disadvantage of univariate descriptors of the EEG is not known.

EEG Analysis Techniques

The earliest methods of EEG analysis consisted of the identification of specific waves (eg, sleep spindles, V waves), estimates of voltage, and estimates of average frequency from visual inspection of a "typical segment."[17] Such manual analysis is impractical intraoperatively, and need not be considered further, except to note that all quantitative analyses share with the manual techniques a desire to extract frequency and amplitude information from the EEG and to display this information using one of the techniques described previously.

Although there are many variations on each basic type of analysis (and no data to suggest which approach is most desirable), these analysis techniques may be lumped into two categories, analysis

in the frequency domain and analysis in the time domain. The former are best known as variations on power spectrum analysis, while the latter include aperiodic analysis, zero-crossing frequency analysis, and voltage analysis.

The zero-crossing frequency is the automated equivalent of the earliest manual techniques for analyzing the EEG.[18] As shown in Figure 9-8, the average frequency of the EEG is estimated by counting the number of changes in polarity and dividing by two since a sine wave changes polarity twice in each cycle. Although very sensitive to baseline drift and artifact (Fig. 9-9), this form of analysis has an inherent simplicity that is appealing. It has been shown to reflect the gross changes in the EEG produced by hypoxia;[19] however, it may not be sufficiently sensitive to be useful for analyzing the EEG for more subtle changes.

Since zero-crossing analysis of the EEG produces no information about the amplitude of the EEG, analysis in the time domain usually includes a form of amplitude analysis in order to represent this aspect of the EEG waveform. Since the EEG is biphasic, the average voltage is 0, and estimates such as RMS or peak rectified (PR) voltage are usually used as estimates of the EEG amplitude (Fig. 9-10).

Another means of quantifying the EEG is known

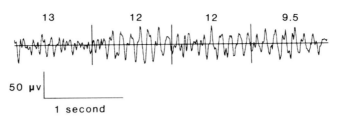

Fig. 9-8. Zero-crossing frequency. This sample of EEG demonstrates the computation of the zero-crossing frequency. The number of times the EEG crosses the isoelectric line is divided by 2 since a sine wave changes polarity twice during a single cycle.

as aperiodic analysis.[16] This technique, utilized in the Lifescan monitor (Neurometrics, Inc., San Diego, CA), displays both frequency and amplitude information about waves identified by a proprietary analysis algorithm. Recent comparison with 16-channel EEG recordings during carotid endarterectomy suggests that this technique may not be as sensitive for the identification of intraoperative ischemia as is the multichannel EEG;[20] however, the use of a limited sample size and the failure to distinguish the effects of lead placement from those of the analysis technique may be misleading.

Power spectrum analysis is the best-known example of EEG analysis in the frequency domain rather than in the time domain. The transformation from time to frequency domain is performed in several steps. First, the data are digitized at specific intervals. A number of these (usually representing 2–30 seconds of EEG) comprise an epoch, which is then subjected to a complex mathematical manipulation known as fast Fourier transformation. The details of this analysis and the underlying assumptions may be found in the engineering literature.[21] For purposes of this discussion, the Fourier transform of an EEG may be considered to be a mathematically equivalent description of the EEG,

composed of regularly spaced frequency components whose amplitude and relationship to each other are defined by the transformation. The size of the frequency steps is defined by the duration of the epoch, while the bandwidth is related to the number of samples in the epoch. The advantage of this transformation is that mathematical manipulations can be performed on the transformed EEG with substantially greater ease than on the original signal. It is the ease in performing these computations that makes the transformation of the raw EEG from the time to the frequency domain so popular.

Although there are many possible analyses that can be performed on the Fourier transform of the EEG, the most common is the computation of the power spectrum (power spectral analysis). This computation provides an estimate of the amplitude of the EEG at each component in the original transformation. This computation is repeated for each epoch transformed, and plotted using one of the three-dimensional techniques described previously.

Because the power spectrum is inherently a complex representation of the EEG, there have been numerous attempts to further simplify this information by computing a one-dimensional (univariate) descriptor of the power spectra. Many such values

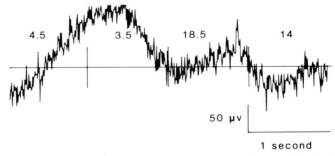

Fig. 9-9. Sensitivity to artifact. This sample of EEG is badly contaminated with drift and artifact, and the zero-crossing frequency reflects this artifact more than it reflects the EEG activity.

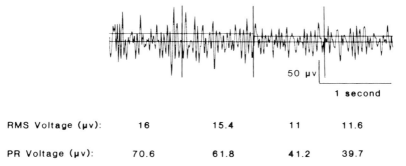

| RMS Voltage (μv): | 16 | 15.4 | 11 | 11.6 |
| PR Voltage (μv): | 70.6 | 61.8 | 41.2 | 39.7 |

Fig. 9-10. Measures of amplitude. This figure demonstrates the formation of the RMS and PR voltages from a segment of EEG. Since the PR voltage is a measure of range rather than central tendency, it is more variable than is the RMS voltage, which is indicated by the horizontal line above the baseline in each 1-second segment.

have been proposed, including median power frequency,[22] peak power frequency,[23] and spectral edge frequency (SEF)[24] (Fig. 9-11). In most cases, such simplified approaches to the power spectrum fail to convey much of the information that is contained in the full spectrum.[25] Whether the information omitted is critical may depend on both the purpose for recording the EEG, and the EEG pattern itself. Rampil et al demonstrated good correlations between outcome and SEF in patients undergoing carotid endarterectomy,[26] and Scott et al found SEF to be valuable for

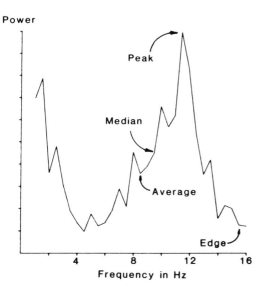

Fig. 9-11. Univariate descriptors. This power spectrum, derived from a patient during isoflurane anesthesia, has been marked to indicate the average, median, peak, and spectral edge frequencies. Because this distribution is not gaussian, the average, median, and peak power frequencies are three different values.

some pharmacodynamic studies.[27] However, Levy was unable to correlate hypothermic EEG changes with the SEF or average frequency, but did demonstrate a relationship using total power and a measure of peak power.[28] Until the behavior of various derivatives of the power spectrum is elucidated, it is preferable to interpret the entire power spectrum, rather than relying on a univariate descriptor.

EEG Changes During Cardiopulmonary Bypass

During extracorporeal circulation, there are several uncommon influences affecting the EEG. Abrupt hemodilution during the initiation of bypass, hypothermia, and changes in perfusion and anesthesia during cardiopulmonary bypass (CPB) are all capable of producing dramatic changes in the EEG. Several effects, such as hemodilution and hypotension may occur simultaneously, making identification of their independent effects more difficult.

During CPB, hypothermia produces characteristic changes in the EEG. During mild hypothermia, slowing of the EEG is observed (Fig. 9-12).[28] Burst suppression (Fig. 9-13) is often seen during deeper hypothermia, even when the patient has not received drugs that typically produce this EEG pattern. Burst suppression due to hypothermia is easily distinguished from the EEG changes produced by hypoxia by the regularity of the pattern of periods of activity and suppression. When hypothermia is being induced slowly, a pattern of waxing and waning EEG activity may be observed before the full burst suppression pattern develops. Finally, at deep hypothermia, an isoelectric EEG may be observed.[29] Under these conditions, the hypothermic EEG may be indis-

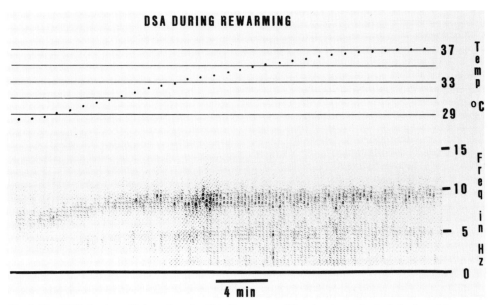

Fig. 9-12. EEG slowing with hypothermia. This figure exemplifies the change in the behavior of the power spectrum during mild hypothermia. The EEG, which has slowed during cooling, gradually accelerates as rewarming takes place. (From Levy WJ: Quantitative analysis of EEG changes during hypothermia. Anesthesiology 60:291–297, 1984, with permission.)

BURST-SUPPRESSION

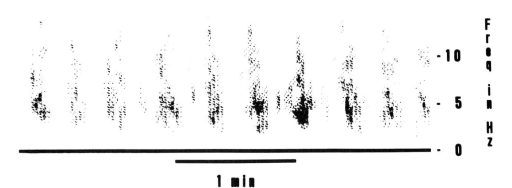

Fig. 9-13. Burst-suppression activity. This figure demonstrates the power spectrum of burst-suppression activity during hypothermia. Periods of little or no power are interspersed between epochs of nominal EEG activity. There is a regular rhythmicity to the periods of activity and quiescence, which allows this pattern to be easily distinguished from slowing or isoelectric EEG due to hypoxia. (From Levy WJ: Quantitative analysis of EEG changes during hypothermia. Anesthesiology 60:291–297, 1984, with permission.)

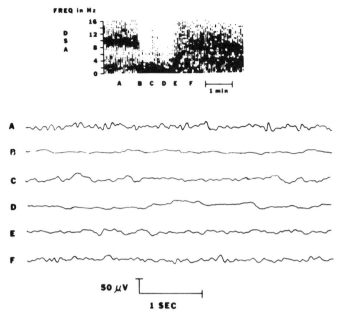

Fig. 9-14. Ischemic EEG on initiating cardiopulmonary bypass. This segment of EEG, recorded during the initiation of cardiopulmonary bypass, exemplifies the changes seen during cerebral hypoxia. Coincident with beginning bypass, there was a fall in blood pressure, the previously stable rhythm (at A) terminated abruptly, and slow activity in the EEG predominated. After several minutes, cerebral perfusion was improved, and the EEG returned to a more normal pattern seen in segments E and F. (From Levy WJ, Shapiro HM, Maruchak G, et al: Automated EEG processing for intraoperative monitoring. Anesthesiology 53:231, 1980, with permission.)

tinguishable from that seen in hypoxia, and it may be impossible to determine when the hypothermic protection of the brain is being exhausted and ischemia is occurring.

The identification of cerebral hypoxia is the primary purpose for EEG monitoring during CPB. In the absence of confounding situations, such as severe hypothermia or a very slow EEG due to anesthetic drugs, the onset of ischemia is associated with an abrupt reduction of the high-frequency activity in the EEG and the development of low-frequency activity in its place (Fig. 9-14). If the ischemia is sufficiently severe, the slow activity may disappear, resulting in an isoelectric EEG; however, a flat EEG is not necessary for ischemia to be present. Like ST-segment depression on the ECG, these changes reflect ischemia at an early stage, well before damage has occurred. This safety zone, between the onset of ischemic changes and the development of permanent damage, makes EEG monitoring valuable; that functional damage does not ensue in every case does not mean that it is safe to ignore ischemic EEG changes

any more than it is safe to ignore ischemic changes on the ECG.

Although EEG monitoring was once considered a means of ensuring adequate oxygenator function when the techniques of extracorporeal circulation were first developed, modern techniques of blood gas monitoring as well as improved oxygenator design have reduced or eliminated its need in this regard. Whether routine EEG monitoring can reduce or eliminate the neurologic complications seen following cardiac surgery largely depends on the source of the central nervous system insults and the potential for prevention or successful treatment of the complication. If most strokes result from small emboli, then routine EEG monitoring is unlikely to identify their occurrence and is equally unlikely to produce a significant improvement in patient care. However, if ischemia is due to unrecognized cerebrovascular stenoses, it is likely that routine EEG monitoring could reduce the incidence of complications. The definitive studies to compare these hypotheses have not been performed since the low incidence of neuro-

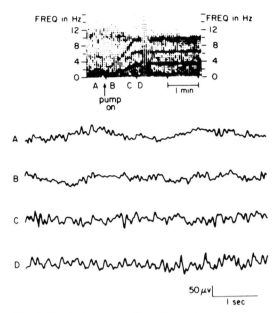

Fig. 9-15. Roller-pump artifact. Shown above is an example of the artifact generated by the roller-pump during the initiation of cardiopulmonary bypass. Beginning when the pump is turned on, two bands of artifact are seen to increase in frequency, becoming stable when full bypass flows have been achieved. This artifact may be identified in the DSA by its unchanging pattern, but it is very difficult to identify in the unprocessed EEG, shown below. Since this activity is in the range of activity expected to be found in the EEG, it is impossible to remove by filtering. (From Levy WJ, Shapiro HM, Meathe E: The identification of rhythmic EEG artifacts by power-spectrum analysis. Anesthesiology 53:505–507, 1980, with permission.)

logic complications (only a few percent in most studies) requires the prospective study of an enormous number of patients.

The identification of EEG changes during CPB may be important, but the artifact produced by perfusion pumps must be ruled out since it may be deceptively similar to the EEG.[30] In particular, roller-pumps often produce an EEG artifact whose fundamental frequency is in the 3 Hz-range and may contain higher frequency harmonics as well (Fig. 9-15). When such artifact is present, the loss of EEG activity due to ischemia *may go unrecognized.* Thus, the recognition and elimination of this artifact is most important. Unfortunately, the origin of this artifact is complex, and the only sure technique for its elimination (grounding the patient) is unsafe. The elimination of roller-pump artifact is dependent on both proper electrode placement technique and a bit of

luck. One easy method of eliminating this artifact is the replacement of the roller-pump with a vortex perfusion pump (Bio Medicus, Inc., Eden Prairie, Minnesota). Unfortunately, this device is substantially more expensive than the conventional roller-pump tubing.

EEG Monitoring During Cerebrovascular Surgery

Although EEG monitoring may not yield sufficient information to warrant its routine use on CPB, during cerebrovascular surgery there can be little doubt of its value.[31] Even when placement of a bypass shunt is routine, EEG monitoring can provide warning of inadequate shunt function and early detection of intravascular dissection or clotting. When shunting is performed electively (on the basis of EEG changes), the surgical complexity is reduced in cases in which a shunt is not required, and the risk of intraoperative stroke may be reduced threefold as shown in Figure 9-16. The estimates used in this figure for both the sensitivity and specificity of the EEG as indications of cerebral ischemia are probably conservative. Multichannel EEG monitoring is the standard against which other techniques are compared, and a sensitivity and specificity in excess of 99 percent is probable. However, the more conservative values used in the figure have been selected in order to demonstrate the value of monitoring even though the use of fewer than 16 channels or the use of automated analysis techniques may result in some reduction of sensitivity and specificity. This figure also demonstrates that over half of the strokes would occur in patients in whom the ischemia went unrecognized. Thus, improving the sensitivity (eg, by increasing the number of channels monitored) would be more important than improving the specificity. Improving the sensitivity alone to 99 percent could reduce the stroke rate by more than half, but a comparable increase in specificity would produce no improvement.

When using two- or four-channel automated monitoring systems, the position in which electrodes are placed may be critical to the identification of ischemia. Theoretical factors suggest that the optimal lead configuration for a two-channel machine would be $F_P - C$ or $F - P$ bilaterally. With four channels, $F - C - P$, or $F - C - T$ bilaterally would seem to be good choices. $F_P - A$, the configuration often used with stick-on electrodes, would not seem to be nearly as good a choice, although there are no defini-

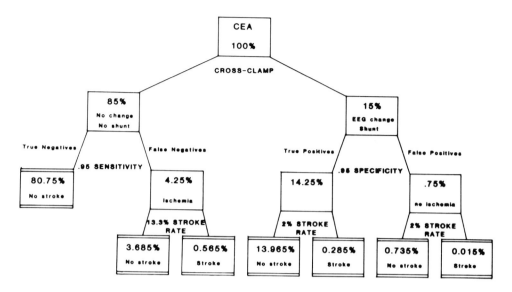

Overall incidence of stroke: 0.865%

Fig. 9-16. Distribution of outcomes with selected shunting during carotid endarterectomy. This figure demonstrates the distribution of outcomes when vascular shunting is performed only on the indication of the EEG. The data are based on the following estimates, which represent reasonable values for the incidence of ischemia and stroke during carotid endarterectomy. (1) It is assumed that 15 percent of patients will demonstrate ischemic changes in the EEG coincident with carotid cross-clamp. (2) The EEG is assumed to be 95 percent sensitive and 95 percent specific for these changes. (3) The incidence of stroke that has been reported by surgeons who do not shunt is approximately 2 percent. Assuming that these patients are comparable to the total population of patients undergoing carotid endarterectomy (15 percent of whom show ischemia), and assuming that only those patients who demonstrate ischemia are at risk for stroke when a shunt is not placed, this yields the 13.3 percent risk of stroke in patients who have demonstrated ischemia, but who are not shunted. (4) Series in which all patients are shunted show an incidence of stroke of approximately 2 percent. Since this, presumably, occurs due to embolic phenomena or damage to the intima of the vessel by the shunt, this 2 percent incidence of stroke applies to all patients in whom a shunt was placed, whether they were truly ischemic or not.

tive studies documenting a reduction in sensitivity with this configuration.

The anesthetic considerations for carotid endarterectomy in conjunction with cardiac surgery extend somewhat beyond "avoiding hypoxia and hypotension." High-dose narcotic anesthesia typically produces EEG slowing during which the identification of ischemia may be more difficult.[32] Because their cardiac condition may be more tenuous, these patients may also show cerebral ischemia due to hemodynamic instability brought on by ischemia, hypovolemia, or dysrhythmias. In patients with severe coronary artery disease, the hemodynamic alternative to shunting (increasing the blood pressure) may be hazardous;[33] thus shunts may be required somewhat more often. Although the use of modest doses of barbiturates for cerebral protection may be possible, this seriously interferes with the use

of EEG monitoring. Added to an isoflurane anesthetic, doses of thiopental as low as 100 mg may produce a period of prolonged EEG suppression easily confused with ischemia. During the redistribution of this drug, the EEG change is easily recognized to have been due to the barbiturate, not ischemia, but this retrospective diagnosis does little to allay the anxiety of the surgeon and anesthesiologist during the period of EEG suppression.

Some surgeons may elect to repair the carotid artery during hypothermic CPB, employing the hypothermia for an added margin of safety during cerebral ischemia. In such cases, EEG monitoring during the initiation of CPB may reveal slowing due to hemodilution or hypotension. Hypothermia produces substantial increases in the ischemic tolerance of the central nervous system, but, unless very deep hypothermia is used, the EEG will still reflect the development of hypoxia in the central nervous system. Unfortunately, the same factors that provide cerebral protection against ischemia increase the likelihood that the ischemia will not be identified by a brief test occlusion, but may still occur later during the endarterectomy. Since no guidelines exist for the allowable duration of ischemia, such an occurrence may necessitate placement of a shunt at an inconvenient stage in the repair.

THE EVOKED POTENTIAL

Generation of the Evoked Potential

Unlike the EEG, which is a recording of the spontaneous electrical activity of the cortex, the EP is a recording of the electrical activity produced by a stimulus. This activity may be recorded from any area of the nervous system which can be stimulated, including spinal cord (for extracranial nerves), thalamus and other subcortical structures, or the cortex. EP monitoring thus is complementary to EEG monitoring and is of particular value when the structures at risk are readily activated by sensory stimulation. For the dorsal column of the spinal cord, stimulation of an appropriate peripheral nerve provides a useful somatosensory evoked potential (SEP). During a craniotomy, auditory or visual evoked potentials may prove of value in assessing the integrity of the subcortical pathways at risk; however, these are of limited clinical interest during CPB.

When recording from the scalp, the electrical activity produced by the stimulation of a peripheral nerve is substantially smaller than the amplitude of the spontaneously occurring EEG. Since it is not possible to silence the EEG in order to record the SEP, another approach must be used to extract the EP signal. This approach, well known to engineers, treats the EEG as random noise in relation to the EP signal. By repeatedly measuring the cortical activity (EEG and EP) following a stimulus, the amplitude of the EEG component decreases relative to the EP component. The magnitude of the decrement is related to the number of repetitions of sampling (Fig. 9-17). For SEP, 100–250 repetitions are usually summated; although for other EPs, as many as 4000 repetitions may be necessary.

The SEP derived from such a process (Fig. 9-18) consists of a series of negative and positive voltage deviations which are described by their amplitude and time of occurrence after the initial stimulation (latency). Neurophysiologists have expended great effort in locating the neural generators responsible

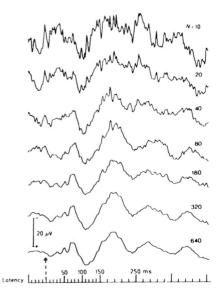

Fig. 9-17. Effect of repetition count on the evoked potential. This figure demonstrates the increased smoothing of the evoked potential (improvement in signal-to-noise ratio), which occurs as the number of repetitions is increased over a ten-fold range. (From Cooper R, Osselton JW, Shaw JC: EEG Technology, Third Ed. Boston, Butterworths, 1980, p 6, with permission.)

for individual peaks and valleys in the EP, since such identification greatly enhances the usefulness of the EP in localizing subcortical lesions. Such localization may be less critical when using SEPs for the evaluation of spinal cord perfusion during aortic surgery; however, differential effects of hypothermia and anesthetics do occur in various sections of the EP. In general, the earlier the wave in the EP (the shorter the latency), the more resistant is that wave to the depressant effects of anesthetics. Thus, the earliest cortical responses in the SEP, occurring at 30–40 milliseconds after stimulation, are influenced by anesthetics and hypothermia to a lesser extent than the later components. In fact, the later components (after 100–150 milliseconds) are so strongly affected by even small changes in anesthetic drugs and surgical conditions that their use for intraoperative monitoring is not recommended.

Since anesthetics do interfere with the measurement of the SEP, it is important to maintain a stable anesthetic state and to utilize controls to determine whether the observed changes are due to anesthetic drugs or other surgical events.[34] In general, narcotics produce less depression of the EP than do halogenated hydrocarbons, making narcotic-based anesthetics preferable when EP monitoring is to be used. Unfor-

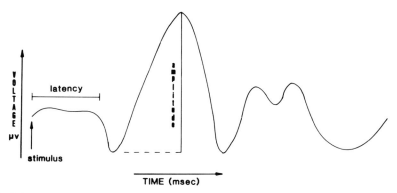

Fig. 9-18. Typical somatosensory evoked potential. Shown above is a typical (stylized) somatosensory evoked potential. The latency of the evoked potential is measured from the time of the stimulus to the beginning of the negative deflection. The amplitude is measured from the maximum negative deflection to the maximum positive deflection. (From Laschinger JC, Cunningham JN, Jr, Cooper MM, et al: Prevention of ischemic spinal cord injury following aortic cross-clamping. Use of corticosteroids. Thoracic Surg 38:501–507, 1984, with permission.)

tunately, this is not always practical, since the surgical procedure or the patient's condition may dictate the use of halogenated agents to control blood pressure or high oxygen concentrations during intrathoracic procedures. The most important baseline for EP measurements is that recorded following the induction of anesthesia, but before the initiation of surgical manipulation, which may threaten the blood supply to the spinal cord. Values that reflect the absolute normalcy or abnormalcy of the EP, particularly as it relates to unanesthetized patients, are of substantially less value in anesthetic monitoring.

EP Recording Techniques

Somatosensory evoked potentials are recorded from cortical electrodes adjacent to the sensory cortex for either the hand or leg. The optimal locations for this recording are slightly (2 cm) posterior to the standard C_3, C_4, and C_z electrode positions and are identified as C_3', C_4', and C_z'. A midline frontal electrode, F_{Pz}, is used as the reference electrode for each of these active electrodes. Alternative sites may also be used for recording SEPs when there is an interest in assessing central conduction time or other aspects of neuronal function; however, these are less important as intraoperative monitors.

The stimulation required for the generation of an SEP is normally 3–20 mA given as a square wave of approximately 0.25-millisecond duration and repeated at 1–2 Hz. Higher stimulus rates may produce artifact because the terminal components of one EP may overlap early components of the next one.

Since up to 250 repetitions may be required for a single SEP, the duration of sampling for a single measurement is several minutes and may be substantially longer if artifact interferes with the acquisition of data. Such artifact, whether from motion, electrocautery, or electrical equipment in immediate proximity, is exceedingly common during intraoperative EP recording, and the time required to obtain a single EP is a major problem in the intraoperative use of this technique.

The amplifiers and electrodes used for EP recordings are similar to those for EEG monitoring, and the same care in electrode placement is mandatory. The bandwidth of the amplifiers used for SEP monitoring is substantially wider than that for EEG monitoring, typically extending from 1 Hz to 1 or 2 kHz. This wider bandwidth increases the potential for electrical noise, and 60 Hz artifact may be particularly troublesome, even though electronic filters (notch filters) are available to reduce the magnitude of this artifact. Such filters not only reduce the artifact, but they also distort the EP by reducing the amplitude of any components with a period of 15–20 milliseconds. As mentioned previously for EEG monitoring, the use of filters to eliminate artifact is far less desirable than is good recording technique.

Compared with the computational requirement of most EEG analysis systems, EP computers are quite simple. They need only to sample the electrical activity at precise times after delivery of the stimulus and to average these samples in order to produce an EP. Automated artifact rejection, usually based on absolute amplitude criteria, is also found in most commercial systems. Although the machines will collect data regardless of the frequency of artifact, good monitoring technique dictates that little reliability is placed on data with high artifact exclusion rates. Although judgment is required in determining excessive artifact rates; certainly, the exclusion of 30–50 percent of stimulus trials due to artifact is sufficient to raise substantial doubts about the validity of the EP that has been recorded.

Ensuring the validity of SEP data in the operating room during a complex and difficult anesthetic (eg, resection of a thoracoabdominal aneurysm) requires the use of many control recordings. First, it must be ensured that the stimulus is actually reaching the afferent nerve and that the electrode has not been dislodged by surgical manipulation. An EP recorded over a proximal portion of a peripheral nerve (eg, popliteal fossa for stimulation over the posterior tibial nerve) will provide evidence of stimulator function and confirm stimulation of the peripheral nerve. Changes in anesthetic concentration and patient temperature will produce similar changes in all SEPs recorded in a patient; thus, an EP derived from the median nerve may serve as a useful control for these variables.[35] Despite the use of such techniques, the interpretation of changes in the EP can be difficult. The identification of peaks is an art, and rigorous criteria have not yet been developed. Thus, it may be difficult to determine if a change represents a reduction in amplitude, an increase in latency, or the total absence of a particular EP. Since treatment may be determined on the basis of such a decision, the problem is a significant one for which there is no simple solution.

Evoked Potentials During Cardiovascular Surgery

Although the SEP is being investigated as a means of assessing neurologic well being during CPB,[36] for theoretical reasons this may not be too helpful. Somatosensory evoked potentials examine the integrity of a small portion of the central nervous system and cannot be expected to identify damage to another part of the brain. In addition, cases have already been reported in which severe cortical damage was not diagnosed by EPs, because much EP activity is subcortical in nature, and subcortical structures are much more resistant to the detrimental effects of hypoxia than is the cerebral cortex. However, Durkin et al[36] and Dolman et al[37] have shown good correlation between the SEP and temperature changes on CPB. However, Dolman et al showed no

correlation between SEP and marked changes in pressure and flow on CPB.[37] It appears that EPs should be used selectively for assessment of pathways at risk, and prime consideration should be given to SEP monitoring during surgery on the descending thoracic aorta (see Chapter 18).

The blood supply to the spinal cord is derived from two sources. The anterior and posterior spinal arteries arise from the vertebral arteries and are supplemented by intercostal and lumbar perforating arteries that anastomose with them. The relative importance of these perforators to the total blood supply of the spinal cord is variable, but the incidence of paraplegia following thoracic aneurysmectomy may be as high as 14 percent,[38] suggesting that in many patients these perforating arteries play a critical role in the maintenance of spinal cord perfusion. Many factors, including location of the aneurysm, extent of the aortic resection, and anatomy of the patient's spinal arteries are all factors in the development of ischemia of the spinal cord. Monitoring of the SEP, which arises as a result of stimulation of the posterior tibial nerve, can provide information regarding ischemic stress being imposed on the spinal cord, and thus allows maneuvers to help prevent postoperative paraplegia.

The technical problems of providing stable conditions during high aortic cross-clamping without the use of halogenated hydrocarbon anesthesia, throughout periods of high blood loss, and without the development of hypothermia are enormous. Even with technical assistance to operate EP equipment, the assessment of the interactive effects of these changes in the patient's condition is difficult. Further complicating this problem is the substantial delay that can occur between aortic cross-clamping and the onset of ischemic changes in the EP. In studies, this delay may be 7–8 minutes in length,[38] and the occurrence of ischemic changes after such a delay may demand substantial modification of the technical procedure in the midst of the surgical repair. Furthermore, it may take many minutes for the EP to return to normal following the augmentation of cord perfusion, and such delayed return does not predict the development of neurologic deficit. Thus, the assessment of individual maneuvers designed to improve perfusion to the spinal cord during the surgical procedure is very difficult.

An additional theoretical problem must be mentioned when considering SEP monitoring during aortic surgery. Somatosensory evoked potentials monitor the function of the posterior column of the spinal cord, but compromise of only the anterior spinal artery (exclusively motor function) is possible during aortic surgery. Thus, even though normal SEPs are present, this does not guarantee the adequacy of motor function following surgical repair, although sustained normal EP activity certainly increases the likelihood of a neurologically satisfactory outcome. It is clear that the application of SEP monitoring to thoracic surgery is more difficult than the application of EEG monitoring to carotid artery surgery. The potential benefits to patients may be more difficult to achieve, and there may be a greater incidence of failure of EP monitoring than of EEG monitoring. Nevertheless, the enormous benefit of preventing paraplegia in a patient undergoing surgery of the thoracic aorta suggests that this monitoring technique be considered whenever possible.

SUMMARY

Neurophysiologic monitoring, whether by processed EEG or SEP, is a high-technology approach to reducing the incidence of neurologic complications during high-risk cardiovascular procedures. Although the placement of electrodes and the recording of electrical activity is of little risk to the patient, the therapeutic maneuvers that are performed as a result of such monitoring are not entirely benign. In most cases, this risk is of acceptable magnitude, but as more aggressive interventions are attempted on the basis of neurophysiologic monitoring, the perspective must remain on the patient as a whole. Myocardial infarction is a more common complication of carotid endarterectomy than is stroke,[33] and the use of deliberate hypertension during carotid cross-clamping may improve cerebral perfusion only by unacceptably exceeding limited cardiac reserves. Exchanging damage of one organ system for the damage of an alternative is not an acceptable use of these complex monitoring techniques. The true value to be obtained from the application of these neurophysiologic monitors lies in the identification and treatment of central nervous system ischemia during cardiovascular surgery in a way that is practical, appropriate, and safe for the patient.

REFERENCES

1. Calvet J, Calvet MC, Scherrer J: Etude stratigraphique corticale de l'activité EEG spontanée. Electroenceph Clin Neurophysiol 17:109–125, 1964
2. Peronnet F, Sindon M, Laviron A, et al: Human cortical electrogenesis: Statigraphy and spectral analysis. In Petsche H, Brazier MAB (eds): Synchronization of EEG Activity in Epilepsies. New York, Springer-Verlag, 1972, pp 235–262
3. DeLucchi MR, Garoutte B, Aird RB: The scalp as an electroencephalographic averager. Electroenceph Clin Neurophysiol 14:191–196, 1962
4. Cooper R, Osselton JW, Shaw JC: EEG Technology. Third Ed. Boston, Butterworths, 1980, p 11
5. Allison T: Calculated and empirical evoked-potential distributions in human recordings. In Otta DA (ed): Multidisciplinary Perspectives in Event-related Brain Potential Research. Washington DC, US Environmental Protection Agency, 1978
6. Pichlmayr I, Lips U, Kunkel H: The Electroencephalogram in Anesthesia. New York, Springer-Verlag, 1984, p 37
7. Obrist WD: The electroencephalogram of normal aged adults. Electroenceph Clin Neurophysiol 6:235–244, 1954
8. Clark DL, Rosner BS: Neurophysiologic effects of general anesthetics. Anesthesiology 38:564–582, 1973

9. Martin JT, Faulconer A, Bickford RG: Electroencephalography in anesthesiology. Anesthesiology 20:359–376, 1959
10. Pichlmayr I, Lips U, Kunkel H: The Electroencephalogram in Anesthesia. New York, Springer-Verlag, 1984, pp 98–121
11. Bimar J, Bellville JW: Arousal reactions during anesthesia in man. Anesthesiology 47:449–454, 1977
12. Jasper HH: The ten-twenty electrode system of the International Federation. Electroenceph Clin Neurophysiol 10:371–375, 1958
13. MacGillivray BB: Handbook of EEG and Clinical Neurophysiology, Vol 3-C. Amsterdam, Elsevier, 1974
14. Bickford RG, Billinger TW, Fleming NI, et al: The compressed spectral array (CSA)—a pictorial EEG. Proc San Diego Biomed Symp 11:365–370, 1972
15. Fleming RA, Smith NT: Density modulation. A technique for the display of three-variable data in patient monitoring. Anesthesiology 50:543–546, 1979
16. Demetrescu TM: The aperiodic character of the electroencephalogram (EEG), new approach to data analysis and condensation. Physiologist 18:189, 1975
17. Davis H, Davis PA: Action potentials of the brain of normal persons and in normal states of cerebral activity. Arch Neurol Psychiat 36:1214–1224, 1936
18. Klein FF: A waveform analyzer applied to the human

EEG. IEEE Trans Biomed Eng BME-23:246–252, 1976

19. Levy WJ, Shapiro HM, Maruchak G, et al: Automated EEG processing for intraoperative monitoring. Anesthesiology 53:223–236, 1980

20. Spackman TN, Faust RJ, Cucchiara RF, et al: A comparison of the Lifescan™ EEG monitor with EEG and cerebral blood flow for detection of cerebral ischemia. Anesthesiology 63:A187, 1985

21. Blackman RB, Tukey JW: The Measurement of Power Spectra. New York, Dover, 1958

22. Chotas HG, Bourne JR, Teschan PE: Heuristic techniques in the quantification of the electroencephalogram in renal failure. Comput Biomed Res 12: 299–312, 1979

23. Smith NT: Monitoring the electroencephalogram in the operating room. In Gravenstein JS, Newbower RS, Ream AK, et al (eds): Monitoring Surgical Patients in the Operating Room. Springfield, Charles C Thomas, 1979, pp 128–130

24. Rampil IJ, Sasse FJ, Smith NT, et al: Spectral edge frequency—a new correlate of anesthetic depth. Anesthesiology 53:S12, 1980

25. Levy WJ: Intraoperative EEG patterns. Implications for EEG monitoring. Anesthesiology 60:430–434, 1984

26. Rampil IJ, Holzer JA, Quest DO, et al: Prognostic value of computerized EEG analysis during carotid endarterectomy. Anesth Analg 62:186–192, 1983

27. Scott JC, Ponganis KV, Stanski DR: EEG quantitation of narcotic effect. The comparative pharmacodynamics of fentanyl and alfentanil. Anesthesiology 62:234–241, 1985

28. Levy WJ: Quantitative analysis of EEG changes during hypothermia. Anesthesiology 60:291–297, 1984

29. Cohen ME, Olszowka JS, Subramanian SE: Electro-encephalographic and neurological correlates of deep hypothermia and circulatory arrest in infants. Ann Thorac Surg 23:238–244, 1977

30. Levy WJ, Shapiro HM, Meathe E: The identification of rhythmic EEG artifacts by power-spectrum analysis. Anesthesiology 53:505–507, 1980

31. Sundt TM Jr: The ischemic tolerance of neural tissue and the need for monitoring and selective shunting during carotid endarterectomy. Stroke 14:93–98, 1983

32. Sebel PS, Bovill JG, Wauquier A: Effects of high-dose fentanyl anesthesia on the electroencephalogram. Anesthesiology 55:203–211, 1981

33. Riles TS, Kopelman I, Imparato AM: Myocardial infarction following carotid endarterectomy. A review of 683 operations. Surgery 85:249–252, 1979

34. Grundy BL: Intraoperative monitoring of sensory-evoked potentials. Anesthesiology 58:72–87, 1983

35. van Rheineck Leyssius AT, Kalkman CJ, Bovill JG: Influence of hypothermia on posterior tibial nerve somatosensory evoked potentials. Anesthesiology 63:A420, 1985

36. Durkin MA, Hume A, Van Ess D, et al: Reliable and reproducible neurologic information using somatosensory evoked potential monitoring during hypothermic cardiopulmonary bypass. Anesthesiology 63:A72, 1985

37. Dolman J, Silvay G, Zappulla R, et al: The effect of temperature, mean arterial pressure, and cardiopulmonary bypass flows on somatosensory evoked potential-latency in man. Thor Cardiovasc Surg 34:217–223, 1986

38. Laschinger JC, Cunningham JN Jr, Cooper MM, et al: Prevention of ischemic spinal cord injury following aortic cross-clamping: Use of corticosteriods. Ann Thoracic Surg 38:500–507, 1984.

PART III

Preoperative Management

Dennis T. Mangano, M.D., Ph.D.

10

Preoperative Assessment

Cardiac disease continues to be a significant problem in the United States. The extent of the problem is indicated by the estimates appearing in Table 10-1.

More than one million patients with heart disease undergo anesthesia and surgery every year.[1] Studies show that patients with a previous myocardial infarction (MI) have an incidence of perioperative MI of about 6 percent, but ranging from 2 to 37 percent.[2-7] Patients undergoing major vascular surgery in the presence of significant coronary artery disease (CAD)[8-10] have an incidence of infarction between 3 and 20 percent.[11-16] Mortality among patients with CAD suffering perioperative MIs is between 38 and 70 percent.[2-7,11-16] Based on these figures, at least 50,000 patients per year are expected to sustain a perioperative MI, leading to more than 20,000 deaths. The financial implications of such statistics are significant when it is realized that the cost of treatment of perioperative cardiac complications is as much as $12,000 per patient,[17] and that the problem is likely to continue into the next several decades. Perioperative cardiac morbidity is likely to rise as the population continues to age and increasingly sophisticated surgery is performed on these higher risk patients.

The present challenge is analogous to that faced by CAD investigators in the 1950s. It was only when predictors of CAD were identified (by studies like that in Framingham[18]) that rational approaches to prevention and treatment could be devised and morbidity thereby reduced. Unfortunately, there are few thorough outcome studies of perioperative cardiac morbidity and only a limited number of predictors are known. One approach to the problem has been to introduce increasingly sophisticated perioperative diagnostic and therapeutic techniques: preoperative exercise[19] and dipyridamole thallium testing;[20] intraoperative peripheral and pulmonary artery monitoring,[7] multiple-lead electrocardiographic monitoring,[21-23] and transesophageal echocardiography;[24] extended postoperative care;[7] and prophylactic therapy.[25] While these techniques help to identify specific patient populations, they may be too costly to apply to large groups of at-risk patients. Identification of populations at risk and preoperative assessment of their disease using routine and non-routine tests is the cornerstone of anesthetic management.

In this chapter, preoperative assessment of the cardiac patient will be reviewed including preoperative predictors of cardiac morbidity, routine and non-routine cardiac tests, and considerations for specific diseases.

CARDIAC ANESTHESIA, SECOND EDITION
ISBN 0-8089-1848-6

Table 10-1

Incidence and Prevalence of Cardiac Diseases
and Therapeutic Procedures

Total number of patients	
with cardiac disease	15,000,000
Number with	
coronary artery disease	10,000,000
valvular heart disease	5,000,000
congenital heart disease	1,000,000
Number with	
previous myocardial infarctions	4,000,000
new myocardial infarctions per	
year	1,300,000
cardiac deaths per year	700,000
Number of	
cardiac catheterizations per year	400,000
cardiac surgeries per year	225,000

PREOPERATIVE PREDICTORS OF CARDIAC MORBIDITY

Certain variables having potential as preoperative predictors have been studied, some of which are, unquestionably, significant predictors of cardiac morbidity, such as recent MI and congestive heart failure. Others, such as angina pectoris, hypertension, and diabetes mellitus are more controversial. Identification of these variables helps to focus preoperative assessment and provide the basis for the selection of preoperative tests. The studies that support or refute current predictor variables are summarized in Table 10-2.

Age

During the next thirty years, a 1.4 percent annual growth rate is projected for the population aged 55 and above; whereas an increase of only 0.5 percent is projected for those aged 16 to 54. By the year 2055, the over-65 age group may constitute 20 percent of the total population.[26] Clearly, an increasing number of patients from this older age group will be presenting for surgical procedures.

Perioperative myocardial infarction is the leading cause of postoperative death.[27] Although resting ejection fraction, end-diastolic volume, and regional wall motion do not appear to be affected by age,[28,29] the response of the elderly heart to different forms of stress, including exercise and catecholamine stimulation, is depressed.[28,30,31] In addition, aged patients incur more surgical complications requiring more intensive and costly hospital care.[32-35] However,

major elective surgery usually can be performed with acceptable risk, indicating that age may be less of a factor than the patient's overall physiologic status.[36,37] Because it is difficult to assess age as a predictor variable independent of associated diseases,[29,38] it is difficult to evaluate its predictive power (Table 10-2).

Previous Myocardial Infarction

Many studies have supported previous myocardial infarction as a risk factor (Table 10-2). The risk of MI after anesthesia and surgery is less than 0.2 percent for the general population.[4,39] However, in patients with previous MI, the perioperative risk is significantly higher; the reinfarction rate is typically between 5 and 8 percent.[2-5] The mortality associated with reinfarction varies between 40 and 70 percent.

The most important predictor appears to be a recent preoperative MI. With recent infarction (within 6 months), the risk of reinfarction varies between 30 and 100 percent.[2-5,40] With infarction occurring from 3 to 6 months before surgery, the reinfarction rate is approximately 15 percent; after 6 months this decreases to approximately 5 percent.

Wells and Kaplan[41] and Rao et al[7] have challenged the above data. In 48 patients who had surgical procedures within 3 months of an infarction, they found that none suffered myocardial reinfarction. Rao et al found that reinfarction occurred in only 1.9 percent of 733 patients who had a previous MI. When the previous infarction was less than 3 months old, perioperative reinfarction occurred in only 5.7 percent of patients. When the previous infarction was 4 to 6 months old, reinfarction occurred in 2.3 percent of patients. These reinfarction rates are significantly lower than those previously reported by most studies and warrant further consideration. Most of the above patients underwent radial and pulmonary artery catheterization. Only patients for whom surgery was expected to last less than 30 minutes, or the interval from infarction to anesthesia was more than 18 months, did not undergo this catheterization. Intraoperative blood pressure and heart rate were not allowed to fluctuate more than 20 percent from preinduction values. Dysrhythmias were treated aggressively, and 596 of the 733 patients were monitored in an intensive care unit for the first 24 to 36 hours following surgery. These results have significant implications, and certainly warrant independent verification. Rao et al suggested that preoperative optimization of the patient's status, aggressive invasive monitoring, and prompt treatment of any hemody-

Table 10-2
Preoperative Risk Factors

Factor	Supported			Refuted		
	Author	*Year*	*Reference*	*Author*	*Year*	*Reference*
Age	Driscoll	1961	241	Mauney	1970	244
	Dack	1963	242	Tarhan	1972	4
	Arkins	1964	243	Steen	1978	5
	Goldman	1977	45	Djokovic	1979	27
	Carliner	1985	69	von Knorring	1981	60
Previous myocardial infarction	Knapp	1962	2	Wells	1981	41
(recent, 6 months)	Topkins	1964	3	Rao	1983	7
	Arkins	1964	243			
	Frazer	1967	246			
	Tarhan	1972	4			
	Hertzer	1981	15			
	Goldman	1977	45			
	Steen	1978	5			
	Eerola	1980	245			
	von Knorring	1981	60			
	Schoeppel	1983	247			
Previous myocardial infarction	Topkins	1964	3	Mauney	1970	244
(old, undetermined)	Sapala	1975	248	Goldman	1977	45
	Cooperman	1978	13	Carliner	1985	69
	von Knorring	1981	60			
	Schoeppel	1983	247			
Location of MI	Arkins	1964	243	Steen	1978	5
Angina	Driscoll	1961	241	Goldman	1977	45
	Tarhan	1972	4	Cooperman	1978	13
	Sapala	1975	248	Steen	1978	5
				von Knorring	1981	60
				Carliner	1985	69
				Wells	1981	41
				Rao	1983	7
Congestive heart failure	Goldman	1977	45			
	Cooperman	1978	13			
	Rao	1983	7			
Dysrhythmia	Goldman	1977	45			
		1978	6			
	Cooperman	1978	13			
Hypertension	Driscoll	1961	241	Goldman	1977	45
	Mauney	1970	244	Riles	1979	14
	Prys-Roberts	1971	250	Cooperman	1978	13

(continued)

Table 10-2

(continued)

Factor	Supported			Refuted		
	Author	*Year*	*Reference*	*Author*	*Year*	*Reference*
Hypertension (*cont.*)	Tarhan	1972	4	Rao	1983	7
	Steen	1978	5			
	Schneider	1979	249			
	von Knorring	1981	60			
Diabetes Mellitus	Driscoll	1961	241	Mauney	1970	244
	Tarhan	1972	4	Goldman	1977	45
	Hertzer	1981	15	Steen	1978	5
				von Knorring	1981	60
Peripheral vascular disease	Driscoll	1961	241	Goldman	1977	45
	Schoeppel	1983	247			
	Jeffrey	1983	88			
	Boucher	1985	20			
Valvular heart disease	Goldman	1977	45			
ECG abnormalities (except dysrhythmias)	Driscoll	1961	241	Goldman	1977	45
	Baers	1965	251			
	Hunter	1968	252			
	Mauney	1970	244			
	Cooperman	1978	13			
	von Knorring	1981	60			
	Carliner	1985	69			
Chest x-ray abnormalities	Goldman	1977	45	Goldman	1977	45
Previous coronary artery bypass grafting surgery/coronary angioplasty	Mahar	1978	253			
	Kimbris	1981	255			
	Schoeppel	1983	247			
	Crawford	1978	254			
	Wells	1981	41			
Risk indices	Vacanti	1970	86 (ASA)	Lewis	1971	87 (ASA)
	Goldman	1977	45 (CRI)	Goldman	1977	45 (ASA)
	Djokovic	1979	27 (ASA)	Jeffrey	1983	88 (CRI)
				Carliner	1985	69 (CRI)
Nonroutine testing	Gage	1977	89	Carliner	1985	69
	Cutler	1979	90			
		1981	19			
	Pasternack	1984	91			
	Boucher	1985	20			

ASA = American Society of Anesthesiologists Classification;
CRI = Cardiac Risk Index.

namic aberration might decrease perioperative morbidity and mortality. However, his study did not address the effect of any of these factors on outcome.

Angina

A history of classical angina is a sensitive and specific predictor for identification of patients with CAD,[42] placing them at higher risk of cardiac complications (sudden death, MI) than the general population. However, stable angina pectoris is not considered a perioperative cardiac risk factor (Table 10-2). Other potential risk factors, such as the severity and stability of angina, have not been studied.

Congestive Heart Failure

In patients with CAD, clinical and radiological evidence of left ventricular failure is associated with a poor prognosis.[43] Patients with ejection fractions of less than 40 percent, determined by radioisotope imaging, have a 1-year cumulative mortality of 30 percent. Patients with compensated left ventricular function (pulmonary capillary wedge pressure less than 15 mm Hg and normal stroke work index) have a 2-year mortality rate of 10 percent. In contrast, patients with elevated filling pressure (greater than 15 mm Hg) and depressed stroke work (less than 20 gm · m/m^2) have a 2-year mortality rate that exceeds 78 percent.[44]

Several studies[7,13,45] have identified preoperative congestive heart failure (CHF) as a risk factor in the surgical population. Two significant signs have prognostic value: a third heart sound (S$_3$) and jugular venous distention. When these signs were excluded, other signs of CHF were not significant.[6] Depressed preoperative ejection fraction (less than 35 percent), determined by radionuclide angiography, has been found to correlate significantly with early perioperative infarction.[46]

Dysrhythmias

In ambulatory patients with significant CAD, dysrhythmias are associated with more serious CAD and ventricular dysfunction. In patients with acute MI, ventricular dysrhythmias or conduction disturbances detected in the late-hospital phase are associated with a poor prognosis.[47,48] Their occurrence in association with left ventricular dysfunction is particularly ominous.[49] For patients with chronic ischemic heart disease, frequent premature ventricular contractions increase risk.

Few data are available regarding preoperative dysrhythmias as a risk factor. Frequent premature ventricular contractions (PVCs) and premature atrial contractions (PACs), as well as rhythms other than normal-sinus or atrial fibrillation, appear to be risk factors.[45] Atrial and ventricular dysrhythmias may be risk factors in patients with peripheral vascular disease undergoing major vascular surgery.[13]

Hypertension

The Framingham Study established the association between hypertension and ischemic heart disease.[50] The importance of this risk factor is relative to the degree of hypertension (both systolic and diastolic) and to the presence of other major risk factors. The risk of fatal and nonfatal MI in patients with diastolic hypertension (greater than 90 mm Hg) is increased, especially in the presence of hypercholesterolemia, cigarette smoking, and electrocardiograph (ECG) abnormalities.[51] However, the importance of preoperative hypertension as a risk factor for postoperative morbidity is controversial (Table 10-2).

Diabetes Mellitus

Coronary artery disease is the leading cause of death in adult diabetics,[52] and it may be difficult to detect in patients with diabetes since painless myocardial infarction frequently occurs. Infarct size is usually larger,[53] and survival rate after infarction is lower than in the general population.[54] In addition, diabetes mellitus may impose as much as a two- to threefold increased risk of clinical atherosclerotic disease.[55] During thallium stress testing, perfusion defects are common in asymptomatic diabetic males.[56] Transient ST depression (ambulatory monitoring) is more frequent in diabetics than in nondiabetics with CAD.[57]

Diabetes is also associated with cerebral atherosclerosis, microangiopathy, surgical and nonsurgical infections, and renal transplant rejections.[58,59] However, perioperative risk in diabetic patients is controversial (Table 10-2), and the data tend to refute diabetes as a major risk factor.[5,45,60]

Peripheral Vascular/Cerebral Vascular Disease

Vascular disease involving the carotid artery, the aorta, and other peripheral circulatory beds is commonly associated with CAD.[8-10] In patients with vascular disease, peripheral vascular surgery is associated with high rates of perioperative MI (up to 20 percent).[12,15,16,61] Although most studies have demonstrated that peripheral vascular disease is a risk factor (Table 10-2), Goldman's study did not support it.[45] In addition, that study found that although aortic operations were associated with the highest risk of postoperative pulmonary edema (11 percent), neither aortic nor peripheral vascular procedures carried an increased risk of postoperative infarction or cardiac death.

Valvular Heart Disease

The presence of associated conditions, such as ventricular dysfunction, dysrhythmias, pulmonary hypertension, and CAD confounds perioperative risk analysis in the patient with valvular heart disease. Few data are available regarding the risk of valvular heart disease in patients undergoing anesthesia and surgery. Skinner and Pearce found that both aortic stenosis and regurgitation were associated with increased perioperative mortality; however, mitral stenosis and regurgitation were not.[62]

In an independent study, Goldman et al found that aortic stenosis was a significant risk factor, with a fourteen-fold greater incidence of perioperative cardiac death, and mitral regurgitation (grade II/VI or greater) was associated with a higher mortality rate.[45] However, in the absence of other risk factors such as an S_3 gallop, jugular venous distention, or recent MI, mitral regurgitation did not add to cardiac risk. Neither aortic regurgitation nor mitral stenosis was associated with increased mortality. However, all four valvular lesions were associated with increased risk of postoperative congestive heart failure.

Cholesterol

There are few data regarding the perioperative risk in patients with hypercholesterolemia. In patients with familial hypercholesterolemia, there is a high incidence of premature CAD.[63,64] These patients are also at risk for both valvular and supravalvular aortic stenosis as well as atherosclerosis of the carotid and femoral arteries. There is a higher-than-expected incidence of proximal lesions in the coronary and in the left main artery in patients with familial hypercholesterolemia.[65]

Cigarette Smoking

The effects of cigarette smoking on perioperative cardiac outcome have not been studied. In the non-surgical population, the Framingham Study demonstrated an increased risk of MI in smokers.[18] A disproportionate number of patients who smoked suffered both infarction and death from CAD.

The effects of acute and chronic cigarette smoking on the cardiovascular system induce significant pathophysiologic responses. Acute effects of smoking include an increased rate-pressure product and increased myocardial oxygen consumption. The direct vasoconstrictor effects of nicotine may cause increased coronary vascular resistance, especially in patients with proximal stenosis of the left anterior descending artery,[66] resulting in an unfavorable myocardial oxygen supply/demand ratio. The increase in carboxyhemoglobin levels, with the resultant decrease in systemic oxygen transport, couples with a decrease in plasma volume and an increase in blood viscosity to further aggravate the supply/demand imbalance. Chronic cigarette use may result in vasoconstriction, enhanced platelet aggregation, and loss of endothelial integrity, leading to accelerated atherosclerosis.[67]

All of these adverse cardiovascular effects, including the well-described detrimental effects on the respiratory system,[68] may put the patient at greater risk for cardiac morbidity, either via direct (coronary vasoconstriction or increased rate-pressure product) or indirect (hypoxemia from respiratory complications as well as carboxyhemoglobin formation) causes.

Electrocardiographic Abnormalities

Several studies (Table 10-2) have suggested ECG abnormalities, excluding dysrhythmias, as preoperative risk factors. Carliner et al found that the preoperative ECG was as predictive of postoperative cardiac complications as abnormal results on exercise stress testing.[69] In contrast, Goldman et al found that ECG abnormalities, including old MI, ST-segment, or T-wave changes, or bundle-branch blocks were not significant risk factors.[45] Few data are available regarding the proper approach to the patient who presents with an abnormal electrocardiogram prior to surgery.

Echocardiographic Abnormalities

Although wall motion abnormalities, detected by ventriculography, are predictive of perioperative ventricular dysfunction,[70] the predictive power of echocardiographic wall motion or other abnormalities has not been studied. The sensitive, dynamic relationship between reduction or cessation of coronary blood flow and the degree of dysfunction of segmental regions of the ventricle is well established.[71,72] The number, type, and degree of segmental wall motion abnormalities (SWMA) dictate the overall degree of ventricular dysfunction,[73] and have prognostic importance for long-term morbidity and mortality.[74] With transmural infarction, some abnormality of left ventricular wall motion can be detected in almost all patients.[73,75-77] With localized ischemia, wall motion and wall thickening changes are segmental and require multiple views to ensure specificity. Changes in wall thickening are believed to be more sensitive predictors of outcome than wall motion abnormalities.[78,79] However, techniques for precise quantitation of the degree of systolic wall thickening and wall thinning using two-dimensional echocardiography are still being developed.

Chest Radiographic Abnormalities

Although the presence of a tortuous or calcified aorta has been found to be a significant risk factor, cardiomegaly has not.[45] However, in patients with CAD, abnormalities in the chest roentgenogram have been shown to be predictive of ventricular function abnormalities detected by ventriculography.[70] The cost-effectiveness of preoperative chest roentgenograms in patients with no cardiac disease and in patients under the age of 60 is questionable.[80-82]

Previous Coronary Artery Bypass Graft Surgery/Coronary Angioplasty

Several studies have suggested that previous coronary artery bypass graft surgery offers protection from perioperative myocardial infarction (Table 10-2). It is speculated that coronary angioplasty also may offer protection.

Risk Indices

A number of risk indices have been suggested for quantitating preoperative risk factors. Among these are the American Society of Anesthesiologists (ASA) Classification,[83] the Cardiac Risk Index (CRI),[45] the New York Heart Association (NYHA) Classification,[84] and the Canadian Cardiovascular Society (CCSC) Classification of Angina.[85] The accuracy of each of these risk indices is controversial (Table 10-2). The ASA Classification has been shown to be useful in predicting perioperative mortality by some researchers[27,86] and not useful by others.[45,87] The CRI compares the patient's preoperative state with the incidence of life-threatening or fatal

postoperative cardiovascular complications. The accuracy of this index has been challenged in the same hospital using the same criteria.[88] A cardiac risk index would be useful if it were generally applicable and consistently accurate.

Predictors From Nonroutine Testing

Several invasive and noninvasive tests have been suggested for preoperative cardiac evaluation and identification of perioperative risk. Some studies have shown that exercise stress testing,[19,89,90] radionuclide angiography,[91] and dipyridamole thallium imaging[20] used to detect evidence of myocardial ischemia or abnormalities of ventricular function are predictive in identifying perioperative morbidity and mortality. In contrast, other studies have demonstrated no significant advantage of exercise testing over the routine preoperative 12-lead ECG.[69] The use of highly sensitive cardiac testing for preoperative identification of perioperative risk is a significant health care cost-containment question.

PREOPERATIVE CARDIAC TESTS

There are routine and nonroutine diagnostic cardiac tests that may be performed prior to anesthesia and surgery. It is often necessary for anesthesiologists to discuss, interpret, or request these tests prior to anesthesia. Therefore, it is necessary to have a knowledge of the individual tests, the specific information they provide, and their role in the preoperative assessment of the patient with cardiac disease.

In this section, the most important components of the preoperative assessment for patients with CAD are discussed. In the final section of this chapter, other diseases are considered.

Clinical History

The clinical history is the focal point, and perhaps the most important part, of the preoperative assessment. Over the past decade there has been an increased emphasis on the use of laboratory and quantitative data derived from specific tests and procedures; however, an in-depth clinical history is essential for interpretation of these tests.

Herberden first described the clinical syndrome of angina pectoris in 1768.[92] Many of the characteristics he described still pertain today, namely, that the pain is of a strangling nature, often occurring with exercise or during meals, and is relieved with rest. During the century that followed Herberden's original description, there were few case reports addressing angina pectoris, leading to the belief that the syndrome was relatively rare. William Osler even described this as a rare condition in 1892. It was not until the 1920s to 1930s that angina pectoris was recognized as an important and relatively common clinical entity.[93,94] It was in the late 1920s that changes in the ECG ST segment were found to occur during episodes of chest pain associated with exercise.[95,96]

Many conditions can mimic the symptoms associated with CAD. Chest pain or discomfort is a major manifestation, not only of effort-related and at-rest angina, but also of such diverse clinical conditions as mitral valve prolapse, esophageal reflux, esophageal spasm, peptic ulcer disease, biliary disease, cervical disease, hyperventilation, musculoskeletal disease, and pulmonary disease. Classically, the duration of anginal pain lasts from 5 to 15 minutes, with longer durations suggestive of unstable angina or MI. Shorter durations of pain, such as transient sharp or stabbing pain, suggest other etiologies, such as musculoskeletal or gastrointestinal disorders. The site of anginal pain was studied by Sampson and Cheitlin in 150 ambulatory patients.[97] Anterior chest pain occurred in 96 percent of the cases, with left arm pain and neck pain occurring in 30 percent and 22 percent of the cases, respectively. Interestingly, right arm pain occurred in 12 percent, back pain in 17 percent, and other pain (chin, forehead, epigastrium) in approximately 18 percent. Typically, anginal pain is related to effort, emotion, sexual intercourse, or eating; although other factors that increase myocardial oxygen consumption, such as fever, hypoglycemia, or exposure to cold air may produce anginal pain as well. Of note is the pain associated with variant angina pectoris, which occurs principally at rest and is usually not associated with physical exertion or emotional stress.

In addition to characterization of chest pain and discomfort for preoperative diagnosis of coronary disease, differentiation of the various types of angina is particularly important. The syndromes of stable angina, unstable angina, and variant angina may carry differing perioperative prognoses, and it is therefore necessary to classify them. Stable angina, as described above, is a substernal discomfort which is precipitated by exertion, relieved by rest and/or nitroglycerin in less than 15 minutes, and has a typical radiation to the shoulder, jaw, or the inner aspect of the arm. At times stable angina may be isolated to the shoulder, jaw, arms, or upper abdomen. Angina is highly specific and sensitive for patients with

CAD,[42] and therefore indicates that these patients are at higher risk of developing cardiac complications (sudden death, MI) than the general population. Surprisingly, therefore, stable angina has been refuted as a risk factor for perioperative cardiac complications (Table 10-2). However, the pattern, severity, and stability of angina have not been studied as potential risk factors.

Unstable angina is defined as: (1) new onset angina, occurring within the past 2 months; (2) progressively worsening angina, occurring with increased frequency, intensity or duration, being less responsive to medicine, or at-rest angina; or (3) angina lasting longer than 30 minutes, exhibiting transient unresponsiveness to standard therapeutic maneuvers, including nitroglycerin and rest, and which is associated with transient ST- or T-wave changes without development of Q waves or diagnostic elevation of enzymes.[85] Although it has been suggested that unstable angina places a patient at higher risk of developing perioperative complications, definitive studies are lacking.

Variant angina pectoris was described in 1959 by Prinzmetal et al.[98] Variant angina usually occurs at rest, is not associated with exercise or emotional stress, and is accompanied by ST-segment elevation. The perioperative risk in patients with variant angina is unknown. However, since this syndrome is associated with a greater incidence of dysrhythmias and conduction abnormalities, it would not be surprising for patients with variant angina to have a higher incidence of perioperative cardiac morbidity than those without cardiac disease.

Although definition of the particular angina characteristics is important for diagnosis, and may be necessary for assignment of perioperative risk, there does not appear to be a significant relationship among these historical characteristics of angina and anatomic coronary artery findings. The duration, location, and precipitating characteristics of angina have not been shown to correlate consistently with the number of vessels involved or the degree of narrowing of these vessels as determined by angiography. It thus remains to be demonstrated whether the clinical syndromes per se or the anatomic description is more predictive of perioperative cardiac morbidity.

In addition to the above syndromes associated with clinically manifest myocardial ischemia, another syndrome has been recently investigated that is not associated with clinical symptoms, ie, silent myocardial ischemia. Silent myocardial ischemia is now recognized as a frequent and potentially serious marker of morbidity. Studies show that 20–30 percent of asymptomatic postinfarction patients have silent ischemia on exercise stress testing.[99] Other studies using frequency-modulated ambulatory ECG ST-segment monitoring have shown that as many as 75 percent of the episodes of significant ST depression are not accompanied by angina and occur at significantly lower heart rates than symptomatic episodes.[100] In contrast, these silent ischemic episodes are very rare in control groups of normal subjects.[101] Silent ischemia appears to be associated with important physiologic changes. Using positron emission tomography with rubidium-82, Deanfield et al have demonstrated that significant decreases in coronary blood flow occur with episodes of asymptomatic ST depression.[102] Electrocardiographic and autopsy studies show that subendocardial and transmural ischemia and MI can occur in the absence of symptoms, especially in patients with diabetes mellitus.[103-108] The mechanism for silent ischemia and infarction is unknown. Sensory neuropathy has been postulated, particularly in diabetics, but this has not been substantiated.[109-112]

During the perioperative period, the incidence of silent ischemia is unknown. It is known that 20–87 percent of postoperative infarctions are painless (Table 10-3). Thus, silent myocardial ischemia during the postoperative period may be a common occurrence and may be a significant risk factor.

After definition of the angina pattern, the next important component of the clinical history is the assessment of ventricular function. Clinical or radiologic evidence of left ventricular failure in patients with CAD is associated with a poor prognosis.[43] Both long- and short-term morbidity and mortality are increased in patients with ventricular dysfunction. Recently, in patients undergoing coronary artery bypass surgery, preoperative ejection fraction and degree of dyssyngery have been shown to be predictive of perioperative right and left ventricular dysfunction.[113] Preoperative evidence of ventricular dysfunction thus places the patient at increased risk for perioperative morbidity and mortality.

The clinical history must include a careful documentation of the symptomatology associated with either right or left ventricular dysfunction both at rest and during exercise. Two standard means of identification of the symptomatology are the New York Heart Association and the Canadian Cardiovascular Society classifications which are shown in Table 10-4. Of particular note is the association of ventricular dysfunction with symptoms of angina (ischemic left ventricular paralysis). With ischemia, incomplete systolic relaxation of the myocardial fibers increases wall tension, intracardiac pressure and, therefore, pulmonary transudation pressure. Congestive symptomatology may ensue. Though transient, this symptomatology is a significant finding since it may place the patient at a substantially higher perioperative risk and may warrant more invasive monitoring of intracardiac pressures.

A history of previous and present cardiac medications and the rationale for their use should be obtained from all patients. Continuation of these medications, as well as alteration of preoperative preparation and treatment during the intra- and postoperative periods, should be based on this history of medications.

The Physical Examination

The general physical examination should look not only for signs specific to CAD, but also for signs

Table 10-3
Silent Postoperative Myocardial Infarction

Study	Year	Reference	Number of patients	Incidence of silent infarction
Wasserman	1955	256	25	17/25 (68%)
Feruglio	1958	257	35	20/35 (57%)
Driscoll	1961	241	12	10/12 (83%)
Dack (review)	1963	242	93	(60–73%)
Baers	1965	251	41	16/41 (39%)
Plumlee	1972	39	24	21/24 (88%)
Tarhan	1972	4	28	6/28 (21%)
Goldman	1978	6	18	9/18 (50%)
Steen	1978	5	28	17/28 (61%)

Table 10-4

Two Methods of Assessing Cardiovascular Disability

Class	New York Heart Association Functional Classification	Canadian Cardiovascular Society Functional Classification
I	Patients with cardiac disease but without resulting limitations of physical activity. Ordinary physical activity does not cause undue fatigue, palpitation, dyspnea, or anginal pain.	Ordinary physical activity, such as walking or climbing stairs, does not cause angina. Angina with strenuous or rapid or prolonged exertion at work or recreation.
II	Patients with cardiac disease resulting in slight limitation of physical activity. They are comfortable at rest. Ordinary physical activity results in fatigue, palpitation, dyspnea, or anginal pain.	Slight limitation of ordinary activity. Walking or climbing stairs rapidly, walking uphill, walking or stair climbing after meals, in cold, in wind, or when under emotional stress, or only during the few hours after awakening. Walking more than two blocks on the level and climbing more than one flight of ordinary stairs at a normal pace and in normal conditions.
III	Patients with cardiac disease resulting in marked limitation of physical activity. They are comfortable at rest. Less than ordinary physical activity causes fatigue, palpitation, dyspnea, or anginal pain.	Marked limitation of ordinary physical activity. Walking one to two blocks on the level and climbing more than one flight in normal conditions.
IV	Patient with cardiac disease resulting in inability to carry on any physical activity without discomfort. Symptoms of cardiac insufficiency or of the anginal syndrome may be present even at rest. If any physical activity is undertaken, discomfort is increased.	Inability to carry on any physical activity without discomfort; anginal syndrome may be present at rest.

of associated and possibly complicating vascular disease. General signs associated with coronary disease such as xanthomas, arcu senilis, and diagonal earlobe creases are noteworthy.

Cardiac examination findings in patients with CAD were thought to be of limited value,[114] but this is incorrect. In addition to manifest signs of left or right ventricular failure, there are several other important signs, summarized in Table 10-5.

A displaced point of maximal impulse (PMI) caused, for example, by cardiomegaly in patients with CAD, usually indicates that the ejection fraction is less than 50 percent, which places the patient at an increased risk.[43,113] With prior MI, an abnormal precordial systolic bulge may occur, indicating a left ventricular wall motion abnormality which is also predictive of perioperative ventricular dysfunction.[113] Altered ventricular compliance can be associated with a fourth heart sound, common in patients with CAD, especially in the presence of a prior MI or acute angina. Third heart sounds, also common, are associated with elevation of the left ventricular end-diastolic pressure, usually with a prior extensive MI. Both third and fourth heart sounds have been shown to be related to hemodynamic and ventriculographic data in patients with CAD. Cohn et al, using a phonocardiogram, found that 42 of 93 patients with CAD had third or fourth heart sounds.[115] The incidence of these heart sounds appears to increase with stress (hand-grip exercise),[116] unstable angina,[117] and

Table 10-5
Cardiac Signs in Patients with Coronary Artery Disease

Finding	Significance	Association
Cardiomegaly	Left ventricular dysfunction (ejection fraction <0.50)	1. Single large infarction 2. Multiple infarctions 3. Complicated infarction 4. Global ischemia
Abnormal precordial systolic bulge	Left ventricular wall motion abnormality	1. Prior myocardial infarction 2. Acute anterior wall ischemia
Third heart sound: S_3	Increased left ventricular end-diastolic pressure	1. Prior extensive myocardial infarction 2. Acute myocardial infarction with ventricular dysfunction 3. Myocardial ischemia
Fourth heart sound: S_4	Decreased left ventricular compliance	1. Prior myocardial infarction 2. Myocardial ischemia
Apical systolic murmur	Papillary muscle dysfunction	1. Prior myocardial infarction 2. Myocardial ischemia

exercise.[118] Although these heart sounds have important diagnostic value, their interpretation is controversial,[119] particularly in the elderly patient population. The finding of an apical systolic murmur, without other signs of valvular heart disease, may indicate papillary muscle dysfunction associated with prior MI or acute angina pectoris.

In addition to these signs, other signs such as rales, cardiomegaly, jugular venous distension, and pulmonary edema have been shown to be risk factors for the development of perioperative cardiac morbidity.[45] Thus, both subtle signs of myocardial ischemia and manifest signs of ventricular dysfunction are important predictors and should be considered in all patients with CAD undergoing anesthesia.

Laboratory Tests

Generally, most preoperative laboratory tests are normal in patients with CAD. With certain diseases, knowledge of the hematocrit or thyroid function may be useful for optimization of the patient's preoperative status and control of myocardial oxygen delivery and consumption. Other laboratory findings, such as hyperlipidemia or carbohydrate intolerance, are predictive of CAD, and are related to coronary angiographic findings. Cohn et al found that 18 percent of patients with cholesterol levels of less than 203 mg/dl had angiographically documented CAD; whereas 80 percent of patients with cholesterol levels greater than 263 mg/dl had CAD.[120] An increase in low density lipoproteins (types 2 or 4) appears to be a strong predictor; whereas the high density lipoprotein:cholesterol ratio appears to correlate with protection from CAD. In contrast, triglyceride levels appear to be relatively unimportant for prediction of CAD.[121] With respect to hematologic function, several studies have demonstrated increased platelet aggregation in patients with CAD, especially during exercise-induced myocardial ischemia.[122]

The most characteristic laboratory changes associated with myocardial ischemia and infarction are cardiac enzyme elevations. With irreversible myocardial cell damage, creatine kinase (CK), glutamic oxaloacetic transferase (GOT), and lactic dehydrogenase (LD) are elevated. GOT levels usually rise above the normal range within 8 to 12 hours following the onset of chest pain, with peak levels occurring 18 to 36 hours after infarction, and return to normal within 3 to 4 days (Fig. 10-1). CK levels rise above normal approximately 6 to 8 hours following infarction, peak at 24 hours, and return to normal within 3 to 4 days. The isoenzymes of CK (MM, BB, and MB), identified by electrophoresis, differentiate tissue extraction from brain and kidney (BB), skeletal muscle (MM), and cardiac muscle (MB). CK-MB is highly specific (greater than 90 percent) and reasonably sensitive (greater than 65 percent) for acute MI. Prediction of infarct size from serial measurements of CK-MB appears to be reasonably accurate.[123-125] Following acute MI, LD rises above the normal range between 24 and 48 hours, peaks between 3 and 6 days, and returns to normal between 8 and 14 days. Both GOT and LD are sensitive but not specific

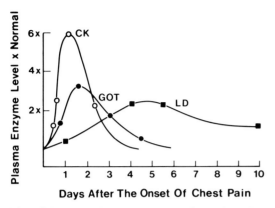

Fig. 10-1. Typical plasma concentrations of cardiac enzymes following the onset of chest pain associated with acute myocardial infarction. Creatine kinase (CK), glutamic oxaloacetic transferase (GOT), and lactic dehydrogenase (LD). (From Hearse DJ: Myocardial enzyme leakage. J Mol Med 2:185, 1977, with permission.)

enzymes, with false positive readings occurring in patients with other noncardiac diseases. The first isoenzyme of LD, LD_1, occurs principally in the heart and rises above normal 8 to 24 hours after infarction. The ratio of LD_1 to LD is abnormal in 95 percent of patients with acute MI.[123,126]

The Chest Radiograph

Although the cost-effectiveness of the routine chest radiograph has recently been ques-

tioned,[80,81,127] this test continues to be used extensively as a preoperative screening test for diagnosis and progression of disease and assessment of the effects of therapy. The routine chest posterior-anterior (PA) and lateral radiographs can provide unique information in selected disease states. For example, in patients with CAD, the chest radiograph has been found to be very specific, with cardiomegaly predicting low ejection fraction.[70] In contrast, in patients with valvular heart disease, a normal chest radiograph is usually associated with normal ventricular function, which is useful in making decisions regarding perioperative monitoring and therapy.

In this section, several important features of the PA and lateral chest radiographs are described, and some examples of radiographic findings in patients with CAD and valvular heart disease are presented.

THE POSTERIOR-ANTERIOR RADIOGRAPH

Radiographic structures can be identified and delineated when the radiodensity of a specific structure is different from that of adjacent structures. Because the chambers, walls, valves, and vascular structures have the same radiodensity as blood, it is difficult to identify intracardiac boundaries and structures unless they are located near the radiolucent lung or are calcified. In Figure 10-2, the posterior-anterior projection of the heart is shown. Two borders of the heart and its vasculature abut against the lung in this view. The right border is in contact with the right

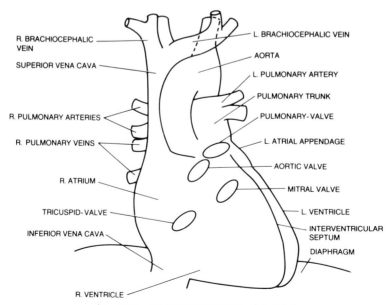

Fig. 10-2. The frontal projection of the heart.

upper and middle lobes of the lung, and the left border, with the left upper lobe and lingular segments. The right border of the heart and its vasculature is formed by the superior vena cava and the right atrium. The left border is formed by the aorta (knob), the main pulmonary artery, the left atrial appendage, and the anterior lateral border of the left ventricle. Right atrial enlargement can be detected by a broadening of the right heart contour. However, right ventricular enlargement is difficult to detect in the PA view. Right ventricular enlargement causes the intraventricular septum to be deviated laterally to the left, causing the left ventricular contour, in turn, to deviate laterally. Differentiation of right versus left ventricular enlargement using the PA view is usually not possible. In certain circumstances, such as in patients with tetralogy of Fallot, the left border of the heart may actually be formed by the right ventricle with the left ventricle rotated posteriorly. Left atrial enlargement causes the left atrial appendage to be displaced laterally and the left bronchus to be displaced upward. Left ventricular enlargement can be readily detected using the PA view, and usually consists of either long-axis enlargement or both long- and short-axis enlargements. For example, with ischemic heart disease both the long and short axis of the left ventricle are elongated, leading to a globular-shaped heart. With aortic or mitral insufficiency, generally only the long axis is elongated, with apical

displacement usually downward and to the left. The intracardiac valves are not normally seen, unless they are significantly calcified. The aortic valve usually lies over the left border of the spine, and although calcification enhances its radiodensity, it is obscured during the entire cardiac cycle by the vertebral bodies of the spine since the aortic valve moves vertically. The mitral valve lies below and to the left of the aortic valve and within the densest part of the cardiac shadow. During the cardiac cycle, the mitral valve moves in a lateral and downward direction, but remains within the dense cardiac shadow. Mild calcification of the mitral valve is usually not perceived in this view, and only with significant calcification can the mitral valve be distinguished from the dense cardiac shadow.

THE LATERAL RADIOGRAPH

The lateral view is most useful for (1) identification of the right ventricle, (2) assessment of left atrial enlargement, (3) differentiation between left atrial and left ventricular enlargement, and (4) identification of calcified mitral and aortic valves.

The lateral projection of the heart is shown in Figure 10-3. Both the anterior and the posterior borders of the heart can be identified in this view. The anterior border structures that are usually identified on the lateral chest radiograph are the superior vena cava, the ascending aorta, the pulmonary trunk

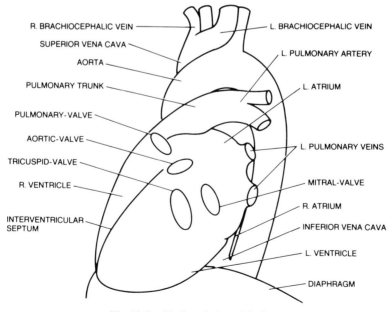

Fig. 10-3. The lateral view of the heart.

(superior to the pulmonary valve), and the right ventricle. The right ventricle usually abuts against the lower third of the sternum, immediately above the diaphragm. With right ventricular enlargement, the retrosternal space along the upper two-thirds of the sternum is encroached upon and obliterated. This sign of right ventricular enlargement is usually accurate. Exceptions are patients with bony thoracic abnormalities (stiff back syndrome) in which the retrosternal space is obliterated, and patients with an abnormally large retrosternal space extending as far as the diaphragm, as found in patients with emphysema. The posterior portion of the heart, consisting of the left atrium and left ventricle, abuts against the esophagus and can be readily identified using dye techniques. The left atrium abuts against the esophagus from the carina to the mid-portion of the esophagus. The left ventricle abuts against the esophagus from the mid-portion of the esophagus to the diaphragm. The left atrium usually can be visualized only via barium swallow, whereas the left ventricle is readily visualized from this lateral view. With left atrial enlargement, the esophagus is displaced posteriorly from the carina to its mid-portion. With left ventricular enlargement, the supradiaphragmatic portion of the esophagus is displaced posteriorly. Calcification of the aortic or mitral valves can be visualized using this view. The aortic valve lies superior to the mitral valve and can be distinguished by a line drawn from the left mainstem bronchus to the anterior costophrenic sulcus. The aortic valve lies above this line and the mitral valve below it.

RADIOGRAPHIC CHANGES WITH SPECIFIC DISEASES

In patients with CAD, the chest radiograph can provide useful information about ventricular function. Four radiographic indices are specific indicators of abnormal ventricular function.[70] The cardiothoracic ratio, total heart volume, left ventricular volume, and signs of congestive heart failure are specific indicators of abnormality of ejection fraction, end-systolic volume, cardiac index, stroke work index, end-diastolic volume, and end-diastolic pressure. The relatively high specificities (68–72 percent) of the radiographic indices indicate that if the chest radiograph is abnormal in a patient with CAD, ventricular function can be assumed to be abnormal. In effect, cardiomegaly predicts a low ejection fraction. In contrast, radiographic findings are not sensitive indicators of ventricular function (sensitivity equals 34–43 percent) in patients with CAD. A normal heart size in a patient may be associated with normal or abnormal function. Thus, not only do signs of congestive heart failure predict poor ventricular function, but so do more subtle signs, such as cardiomegaly, and the routine preoperative chest radiograph, when abnormal, may provide significant information. MI cannot be detected using the chest radiograph unless it is associated with a large aneurysm or significant calcification. Although coronary artery calcification is common in patients with CAD,[128,129] visualization of calcium deposits within the coronary arteries is difficult using chest radiography.

The routine chest radiograph appears to be useful in patients with valvular heart disease as well. However, the specificity and sensitivity findings with valvular heart disease are opposite those found in patients with CAD.[130] Radiographic indices are highly sensitive (0.70), but not specific (0.50) indicators of ventricular dysfunction. A normal chest radiograph in a patient with valvular heart disease is indicative of good ventricular function; however, an abnormal chest radiograph can occur with either good or poor left ventricular function. With valvular heart disease it appears that atrial or ventricular enlargement occurs relatively early in the disease process, and that these enlargements may exist with good ventricular function. If atrial or ventricular enlargement has not occurred, the disease process is in its earliest stages, and ventricular function is likely to be normal.

The individual valvular diseases can be quite distinct in their radiographic presentation. For example, with mitral stenosis, left ventricular size is normal, but left atrial, pulmonary artery, and right ventricular enlargement occur. With mitral insufficiency, both left atrial and left ventricular enlargement occur, eventually resulting in pulmonary hypertension and right ventricular enlargement. Similar to mitral regurgitation is aortic regurgitation, which causes elongation and dilation of the left ventricle. In addition, dilation of the ascending aorta occurs. With aortic stenosis, the concentric hypertrophy is not perceived radiographically. Only with advanced aortic stenosis does dilation or cardiomegaly occur. Calcification of the mitral and aortic valves and their apparati have differing implications depending on the site of calcification. Mitral valve calcification usually signifies mitral stenosis and occurs on the valve leaflets or commissures. When the calcification involves the mitral annulus alone, it is not a sign of mitral stenosis but is usually indicative of an aging valve, found most commonly in older patients. Calcification of the aortic valve usually occurs with aortic stenosis, either congenital or acquired.

In patients with cardiomyopathy, chest radiographic signs depend on whether the cardiomyopathy is dilational, restrictive, or hypertrophic. With dilated cardiomyopathy, moderate-to-marked left ventricular enlargement and pulmonary venous hypertension occur. With restrictive cardiomyopathy, cardiac enlargement is usually mild and accompanied by pulmonary venous hypertension. With hypertrophic cardiomyopathy, cardiac enlargement is mild to moderate and associated with left atrial enlargement. Other specific cardiac diseases and their relationship to radiographic size are summarized in the last section of the chapter.

LIMITATIONS

Radiographic estimation of cardiac function can be affected by several factors. The first limitation is that radiographic indices, such as cardiothoracic ratio and total heart volume, reflect the function of multiple chambers; whereas ventriculographic indices, such as ejection fraction or end-diastolic volume, reflect the function of a single chamber. A second limitation is that radiographic indices are measured at random points of the cardiac cycle, reflecting a combination of systolic and diastolic values. Furthermore, radiographic indices depend on blood volume and flow, which may differ because of changes either in body position (upright versus supine) or the time interval between measurements. Radiographic indices also reflect the external dimensions of the left ventricle, for example. Significant changes in the internal dimensions can occur and cause shifts in the intraventricular septum and not be reflected in the external radiographic measures. Finally, in patients with primary pulmonary disease, changes in pulmonary vascularity, cardiothoracic ratio, or total heart volume may occur even though left ventricular function is unaffected. Thus, although the chest radiograph is useful for identification of compromised ventricular function in patients with CAD or normal ventricular function in patients with valvular heart disease, the limitations of this indirect assessment of ventricular function must be remembered.

CONCLUSIONS

The cost-effectiveness of routine preoperative chest radiography has been justifiably questioned. However, in patients undergoing major abdominal, aortic, thoracic, or cardiac surgery, the routine use of the chest radiograph appears to be well justified. In patients with CAD, even subtle abnormalities of the

chest radiograph, such as cardiomegaly, are indicative of compromised ventricular function and will affect decisions regarding perioperative monitoring, therapeutics, and postoperative care. Furthermore, radiographic identification of compromised ventricular function will limit the number of other costly preoperative tests that might have been used for assessment of ventricular function. In patients with a murmur, the finding of a normal heart size on the preoperative chest radiograph is indicative of good ventricular function, which may indicate that extensive and costly preoperative preparation, intraoperative monitoring, and postoperative care may not be necessary. The routine preoperative chest radiograph thus should be interpreted carefully with respect to both manifest and more subtle signs of ventricular dysfunction, and it should be part of the preoperative assessment in patients with cardiac disease undergoing major surgery.

Electrocardiogram

The resting electrocardiogram (ECG) is normal in 25 to 50 percent of patients with CAD.[131] In an additional 25 percent of patients, the resting ECG may be nondiagnostic because of such conditions as left bundle branch block or Wolff-Parkinson-White syndrome. Despite this, the ECG is one of the most important preoperative tests for patients with CAD. Patterns of ischemia, injury and infarction, conduction changes, and dysrhythmias may have important prognostic significance.

Characteristic patterns describing ischemia, injury and infarction are shown in Figure 10-4. In animals with acute coronary ligation, the T wave becomes positive and peaks and is followed by ST elevation. In humans with subendocardial ischemia, the polarity of the T wave remains upright, since the direction of repolarization is not disturbed, and proceeds from epicardium to endocardium. In contrast, in the case of subepicardial ischemia, repolarization is disturbed and proceeds from endocardium to epicardium, resulting in an inverted T wave. Recovery may be prolonged, resulting in larger, elongated T waves. With myocardial injury, either diastolic or systolic currents of injury may occur. With diastolic currents of injury, the PQ segment is deflected downward, and although the ST segment is isoelectric, it is elevated relative to the depressed baseline. With systolic currents of injury, no baseline (PQ) abnormality occurs; however, the injured area repolarizes more rapidly and ST elevation results. Regardless of the postulated theory, subendocardial injury is detected

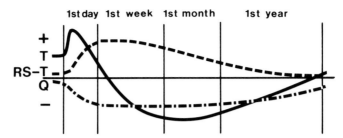

Fig. 10-4. Typical evolutionary changes of the T wave, ST segment, and Q wave following myocardial infarction. (From Lepeschkin E: Modern Electrocardiography. Baltimore, Williams and Wilkins Co., 1951, with permission.)

as ST-segment elevation if the sensing electrode faces the endocardium, or ST-segment depression if the sensing electrode faces the normal epicardium. With subepicardial injury, the opposite occurs.

An MI is classically detected by the occurrence of a Q wave if the infarction is transmural, or by persistent ST elevation over a period of days if the infarction is subendocardial. The sequence of ECG changes with MI appears to be similar in both humans and experimental animals. The earliest change is a T-wave abnormality, with the T wave either being prolonged or magnified, and either being upright or inverted.[132,133] ST-segment elevation occurs in those leads facing the injured area, with ST-segment depression reciprocally occurring in leads facing away from the injured area. The development of significant Q waves (greater than 0.04 seconds and one-third of the height of the R wave) may occur soon thereafter, after a period of days, or never. R wave amplitude may decrease during infarction. Finally, the ST segment becomes isoelectric and the T wave becomes symmetrically inverted.[134] This classical sequence occurs in approximately 50–70 percent of patients sustaining an MI.[135,136] In the remainder, ST- and T-wave changes may be the only manifestation. This classic pattern of T-wave, ST-segment, and Q-wave changes is highly specific for the diagnosis of an acute MI. The more difficult clinical questions occur when nonspecific ST-T wave changes alone are found on the ECG. Early marked ST-segment changes (greater than 2 mm) are highly specific for myocardial injury; however, persistence of such changes over a period of days must occur for diagnosis of infarction. Other conditions are associated with ST elevation or depression, such as Prinzmetal's angina, pericarditis, ventricular aneurysm (ST elevation), and subendocardial injury, or reciprocal changes (ST-segment depression). In addition, even in the case of acute MI, pseudonormalization of

T waves and even ST segments may occur during a true infarction process. These patterns may not represent a normalization of the ischemic process, but may be consistent with a continuation of that process.

Exercise Stress Testing

BACKGROUND

Alteration of the ECG with exercise was first recorded by Einthoven in 1908.[137] Both P- and T-wave amplitude and heart rate increased with stair climbing. The relationship between angina pectoris and the ECG was studied by Feil and Siegel, in 1928, who found ST-T abnormalities in association with at-rest angina as well as with exercise-induced angina.[95] In the following year, Master introduced his two-step exercise technique.[96] The first major application of exercise stress testing to patients with angina pectoris was performed by Goldhammer and Scherf in 1933.[138] Over the next 8 years, Master studied this patient population using refined techniques and adjusted his findings for age, sex, and weight. His standardization of exercise stress testing became the foundation for all future work over the ensuing 50 years. During this period, numerous protocols for exercise stress testing were introduced, including the bicycle ergometer and treadmill testing. The major differences among the protocols are the grade, speed, and duration during each of the stages of the test. The predictive value of these exercise stress tests for CAD has undergone extensive investigation, and considerable controversy has ensued.

PHYSIOLOGY

With exercise, mean arterial blood pressure increases despite significant decreases in systemic vascular resistance due to marked increases in cardiac output, as much as four-fold during maximal exercise.[139] These increases in cardiac output are primarily related to heart rate rather than stroke volume. Stroke volume does increase, but usually not more than 20 percent; whereas heart rate can increase by as much as 300 percent.[140] As heart rate increases, the systolic ejection period decreases. Maintenance of normal end-systolic volume and pressure in the left ventricle is accomplished by an increased rate of tension developed in the myocardial fibers and by an increased contractility of these fibers.[141]

Several of the major determinants of myocardial oxygen consumption are therefore affected by exercise, namely: increases in heart rate, wall tension, and contractility. The myocardial oxygen consumption per contraction has been reported to increase from 1.2×10^{-3} ml/100 gm to 1.9×10^{-3} ml/100 gm per beat. This oxygen demand is met primarily by increases in coronary blood flow, and only secondarily by increases in oxygen extraction. Oxygen extraction usually does not increase significantly with exercise, increasing at most 25–30 percent from the normal value of 11–12 ml/100 ml/min. However, coronary blood flow rises markedly from 60 ml/100 gm at rest to as much as 240 ml/100 gm during vigorous aerobic exercise.[142] This four-fold increase in coronary artery flow is achieved by marked vasodilation of the coronary arterial bed in response to metabolic and other demands during maximal exercise. Coronary vascular reserve, or the potential for vascular dilation, plays a critical role in the ischemic heart's response to exercise. Impairment of vascular reserve during periods of maximal oxygen consumption may lead to myocardial ischemia and its sequelae, dysrhythmias and pump dysfunction.

Exercise-induced ischemia usually occurs in coronary arteries that are moderately or severely obstructed (greater than 75 percent of the cross-sectional area), or in those that develop vasospasm during exercise. However, the degree of coronary artery occlusion necessary to significantly decrease coronary flow and ischemia during exercise is unknown. Reductions in the hyperemic response of the coronary arteries occur with 40–60 percent occlusion; however, more significant reductions in flow (50 percent or greater) require greater degrees of occlusion (70 percent or more of cross-sectional area).[143,144] Both the duration of exercise and the number of ischemic insults may also play a role. With exercise stress testing lasting 10 to 12 minutes or more, smaller reductions in coronary flow may produce an ischemic response.[145,146] Several distinct episodes of smaller reductions in flow, producing repeated episodes of ischemia, may stun the myocardium via a summation effect, producing clinical signs and symptoms of myocardial ischemia.[147] The physiology and pathophysiology of exercise stress testing and its relationship to hemodynamics, myocardial oxygen consumption, and coronary flow and reserve thus are complex, and it is necessary to interpret stress test results and their prognostic implications carefully. The anesthesiologist must apply these stress test results cautiously to patients undergoing anesthesia and surgery where systemic vascular resistance stresses may prevail.

TYPES OF TESTS

All exercise stress test protocols progressively increase myocardial work and allow measurement of signs and symptoms of ischemia, dysrhythmias, and pump dysfunction. Generally, exercise is induced using treadmills, bicycles, or isometric techniques in noninvasive cardiac catheterization or radionuclear laboratories. Outcomes are usually assessed clinically and electrocardiographically. In select circumstances, ventricular function data are obtained using ventriculography or radionuclear imaging. The most familiar treadmill protocols are those introduced by Bruce, Balke, Ellestad, Astrand, Naughton, and Sheffield, several of which are shown in Figure 10-5. In each of these, exercise is performed in stages, defined by treadmill speed and grade, and lasts from 1 to 10 or more minutes. The Balke protocol, for example, consists of stages of one-minute duration, with grade increases of 1 percent per stage, and a constant speed of 3.3 mph. In contrast, the Ellestad protocol consists of two stages, the first of which is limited to 10 minutes. A 10 percent grade is maintained and speed is progressively increased from 1.7 to 5 mph during the first stage and by 1.0 mph every 2 minutes thereafter. The most familiar of these protocols, the Bruce protocol, consists of 3-minute stages which differ in both grade and speed. Stage 1 has a speed of 1.7 mph with a 10 percent grade, and stage 5 (minutes 12–15) has a speed of 5.0 mph with an 18 percent grade. Patients with moderate coronary disease typically exercise to stages 3 and 4 before termination of the test because of symptoms or heart-rate limitations. Well-trained athletes (marathoners) are able to exercise to stages 7 or 8 before exhaustion occurs. Several studies have compared these tests with respect to blood pressure, heart rate, and oxygen uptake. There are no significant differences among these tests; however, difficulties in the performance of these tests exist for patients with impaired cardiac function. For example, the early and abrupt increases in grade using the Balke protocol, occur-

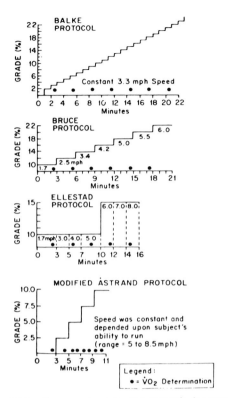

Fig. 10-5. Four exercise stress test protocols demonstrating differences in grade, speed, stage duration, and oxygen consumption determinations. (From Pollock ML, Bohannon RL, Cooper KH, et al: A comparative analysis of four protocols for maximal treadmill stress testing. Am Heart J 92:39, 1976, with permission.)

ring at 1-minute intervals, may represent too significant a stress during the early testing procedure, limiting the usefulness of this test. The same is true for the modified Astrand protocol. The Bruce and the Ellestad protocols, with more gradual increases in workload, appear to be more appropriate. Specifically because of this, the Bruce protocol has become the most widely adopted.

THE ST-SEGMENT RESPONSE

During exercise, and the immediate recovery period, the principal indicator of myocardial ischemia is ECG ST-segment deviation. During the early stage of exercise, heart rate increases and the J point of the ST segment becomes depressed. However, the slope of the ST segment rises and merges with the T wave. This response occurs both in normal individuals and in patients with CAD. With endocardial ischemia, the diastolic injury potential vector becomes opposite that of the QRS, and ST-segment

depression becomes more negative, with a slope that is equal to or less than 0 (flat or downsloping). It is conventionally accepted that downward ST segment deflection is consistent with ischemia when the slope is flat or downsloping. The magnitude of the depression is an important characteristic as well. Although depressions of 1.0 mm (0.1 mv) are usually considered to be the threshhold for diagnosis of ischemia, there are a number of factors that must be considered when interpreting the magnitude of ST depression. Different criteria have been suggested that not only depend upon the lead system used but also on the degree of sensitivity and specificity that is desired. For example, choosing 0.5 mm as the criterion minimizes false negatives (high sensitivity), but produces many false positives (low specificity). In contrast, 2.0 mm is a highly specific index with low sensitivity. Bipolar lead systems are less sensitive than unipolar systems, and a criterion of 2.0 mm deflection has been conventionally accepted. Finally, the Frank leads have increased sensitivity, and a criterion of 0.5 mm is used.

Three types of ST segment exercise and postexercise responses have been described.[148] The first type is characterized by ST depression, with a flat or downsloping segment, occuring during the exercise period, and reverting to normal during the early postexercise period. This response is considered severe when: (1) The magnitude of the depression is greater than 2 mm, (2) depression occurs during the early stages (1–3) of the test, or (3) hypotension occurs during the exercise period. With the second type, the ST depression worsens during the recovery period and is associated with a poor prognosis. The third type of ST response is ST-segment elevation, reportedly occurring in approximately 5 percent of patients undergoing stress testing. The conventionally accepted criterion is a threshhold of elevation of 1.5 mm or more, regardless of slope. This type of response can be associated with fixed coronary lesions, with scarring or dyskinesia due to previous infarction, or with coronary spasm (Prinzmetal's variant angina). Although variant angina usually occurs at rest, exercise stress testing may precipitate this response.

A number of factors affect the interpretation of the ST-segment response. Among these are skin impedance, filter lead systems and signal processing (filter response, amplitude versus frequency modulation). For example, bipolar lead systems (CC_5 or CM_5) record voltages from negative to positive, in contrast to unipolar systems (V_5) which record from ground to positive. The QRS amplitude with bipolar systems is thus larger than that with unipolar systems, and either altered criteria for ST magnitude must be invoked or normalization with respect to R-wave amplitude should be instituted.[149] Interventricular volume increases produce a highly conductive media and augment QRS amplitude. This Brody effect may occur with left ventricular dysfunction, altering the interpretation of the ST response. This noninvasive measure of myocardial ischemia must therefore be carefully interpreted.

Diagnostically, ST-segment depression most likely represents an abnormal relationship between oxygen supply and metabolic demand. It does not necessarily reflect alteration in coronary flow produced by obstruction or spasm of the coronary arteries. Other conditions that independently decrease supply (anemia, hypoxemia, hyperviscosity) or increase metabolic requirement (tachycardia, hyperthermia, increased ventricular mass) may upset the oxygen supply/demand balance and produce ST-segment deviation.

Prognostically, it appears that the ST-segment response is most predictive in those populations who are at risk and who demonstrate significant and early changes during stress testing. In patients with coronary risk factors, the sensitivity of exercise stress testing is approximately 70 percent and the specificity is about 90 percent. With significant exercise or postexercise ST depression, a three-to-sevenfold increased incidence of coronary events occurs from 1 to 5 years after the test.[150-152] In contrast, in asymptomatic patients, use of exercise stress testing as a generalized screening procedure is limited. Erikssen et al studied 2014 healthy men, and found that 75 had ST depression of at least 1.5 mm.[150] Of these, 48 had anatomic CAD evidenced by arteriography. Although this represents a predictive value of 64 percent and identifies patient populations at risk, its usefulness is limited. The Seattle Heart Watch Group found that there was no additional prognostic value afforded by exercise stress testing in asymptomatic individuals without coronary risk factors.[151]

The severity and onset of ST depression appear to correlate with anatomic disease. ST depression of 1 to 3 mm or more, occurring during stages 2 or 3 of a Bruce protocol, is associated with a 67 percent probability of 1 to 3 vessel disease. Changes of 2 mm or more, occurring during stages 1 or 2, are associated with a 90 percent probability of 1 to 3 vessel disease. Furthermore, of patients with ST depression of 3 mm or more, 69 percent had 3 vessel disease and 92 percent had left anterior descending disease.[153] Finally, the occurrence of early ST changes (stage 1 or stage 2) is associated with a poor prognosis. Of patients who developed significant (2 mm or more) ST depression during stage 1 of the Bruce protocol, 40 percent had cardiac events during the first year following their exercise stress testing.[154-156] In contrast, negative tests do not imply lack of disease. Approximately one-third of the patients undergoing coronary artery bypass grafting with demonstrable anatomic lesions have negative exercise stress testing results. Finally, assessment of the location of anatomic lesions from the exercise stress test lead information is controversial.

ADDITIONAL STRESS TESTING RESPONSES

In addition to the ST-segment response, several additional responses are noteworthy, namely: changes in the T wave or R wave, the occurrence of chest pain, alteration in heart rate, hypotension or dysrhythmias. Symmetrical T-wave inversion is usually associated with CAD; however, it is generally considered to be a nonspecific sign during exercise stress testing because of its association with hypertension, electrolyte disturbances, and cardiomyopathy. The QRS magnitude may be a function of the intercavitary left ventricular volume (the Brody effect);[157] with increasing interventricular volume, R wave amplitude increases. In patients with CAD and incomplete systolic emptying (increased end-systolic volume), there is often increased R-wave amplitude which may be associated with myocardial ischemia. Using a bipolar lead system, Bonoris et al found that R wave amplitude remained the same or increased in patients with CAD, but decreased in normal patients.[158,159] In addition, both the specificity and sensitivity increased when using R-wave amplitude versus ST-segment deflection as a measure of myocardial ischemia. Hollenberg et al found that the prognostic value of the ST segment can be increased by incorporating R-wave amplitude into the normalization of the ST-segment response.[149]

The occurrence of angina during exercise stress testing increases the prognostic value of the ST response. Ellestad found that when the ST response was associated with angina, these patients had a twofold increase in outcome events over the 4-year period after the study.[160] The early occurrence of angina also has prognostic significance. Patients with angina occurring at four METS had twice the rate of events as those occurring at twice this energy expenditure later in the test. Hemodynamic changes in heart rate and blood pressure afford additional prognostic significance. Even without an ST-segment response, a subnormal heart rate response may be as predictive as the ST response itself.[160] A subnormal blood pressure response (less than 30 mm Hg during stages 2 or 3) markedly enhances the prognostic value of the ST response. For example, 77 percent of patients with exertional hypotension had significant left main or left main equivalent disease.[161]

With respect to dysrhythmias, exercise stress testing increases the yield of premature ventricular contractions three-fold over the resting ECG, and eight-fold for repetitive forms of ventricular dysrhythmias. Approximately 52 percent of patients with CAD exhibit PVCs on exercise stress testing. These dysrhythmias usually occur not only at peak exercise, but also during the initial three minutes of recovery; in fact, ventricular fibrillation most commonly occurs during the recovery period.

OTHER EFFECTS

Several other effects such as pressure overload, abnormal electrical activation, and pharmacologic effects occur on the stress ECG. Lepeschkin and Surawicz demonstrated that pressure overload of the left ventricle may cause false positive ST segment responses in young patients with hypertension.[162] Mitral valve prolapse patients develop exertional ST segment depression in the absence of CAD. Abnormal activation of the left ventricle, such as with left bundle branch block, Wolff-Parkinson-White syndrome, and, at times, with short P-R intervals without delta waves, alters repolarization and makes interpretation of ST-segment changes difficult. Right bundle branch block appears to decrease the sensitivity of detecting left coronary ischemia.

Pharmacologic agents that most significantly affect the interpretation of the ST-segment response are digitalis, the antidepressants, diuretics, antihypertensives, and beta-adrenergic blockers. Even without resting ECG changes, patients on digitalis may exhibit false positive exertional ST depression.[162] Although unproved, digitalis seems to cause limited ST-segment depression of 2 mm or less; depression in excess of which represents ischemia. Linhart et al have shown that the tricyclic and other antidepressant drugs cause both false positive and false negative ST-segment changes, especially in women.[163] By altering potassium concentrations, diuretics may cause an increased rate of false positive responses.[164] Studies have demonstrated that antihypertensives have an effect on the exercise ECG and make its interpretation difficult. In addition, nitroglycerin and calcium channel blockers (nifedipine) affect exercise stress testing by allowing greater levels of exercise performance before ischemia becomes manifest. Beta-blockers limit the heart rate response during exercise stress testing, and testing must therefore be continued using symptomatic end points.

INDICATIONS AND CONCLUSIONS

Exercise stress testing is a relatively inexpensive, noninvasive test that has its greatest use in patients with chest pain of unknown etiology and for quantitation and prognosis in patients with known CAD. Exercise stress testing has significant prognostic value when the ST changes are characteristic, are of significant magnitude (greater than 1.5 mm), occur during early stages of the test (1–3), are sustained into the recovery period, are associated with subnormal increases in heart rate or blood pressure, and are accompanied by angina or dysrhythmias. It appears to have limited value as a generalized screening procedure in healthy, asymptomatic patients.

Exercise stress testing appears to be relatively safe. Rochmis and Blackburn surveyed 73 exercise stress testing laboratories and found that of 170,000 tests, 16 deaths were reported.[165] Forty additional patients had nonfatal complications requiring hospitalization. The mortality appears to be approximately 1 in 10,000, and morbidity approximately 4 in 10,000.

As a preoperative screening test, exercise stress testing is useful for defining new-onset, atypical chest pain. If new-onset chest pain is demonstrated to be ischemic, perioperative morbidity and mortality may be markedly increased. This unstable angina may develop a crescendo characteristic or may be preinfarction. It is necessary to make assessments prior to anesthesia and surgery to define the chest pain pattern and institute appropriate medical therapy. It is also important to understand exercise stress testing and the interpretation of the results when this information is available prior to surgery. Several of the exercise stress test results are especially important to the anesthesiologist, the first of which is the diagnosis of CAD. It is useful to know the magnitude of the ST response changes, the onset and duration of these changes, and the associated hemodynamic effects. The therapies used during exercise stress testing to reverse ischemia may also be useful for intraoperative treatment of ischemic changes. Dysrhythmias occurring during exercise or the recovery period are useful for treatment of perioperative dysrhythmias. Finally, the heart rate and blood pressure at which ischemic events occur may serve as guidelines for perioperative control of these variables.

Echocardiography

Echocardiography has become an important means of noninvasively assessing regional wall motion and wall thickening, global ventricular function, valvular function, and coronary anatomy. Echocardiography was developed from acoustic research involving submarine detection and materials testing. Over the past decade, significant advances include the refinement of M-mode echocardiography and the introduction of two-dimensional, Doppler and, most recently, contrast echocardiography.

The principle of echocardiography is based on the detection of reflected sound waves from the surfaces of internal organs. In comparison with the audible sound range (20 to 20,000 Hz), frequencies used in echocardiography range from 1 to 7 MHz. At the higher frequencies (5–7 MHz), resolutions of 1 mm are possible, but penetration of surface structures decreases with increasing frequency. At the lower frequencies (1–3 MHz) the resolution is less (2–3 mm), but penetration is improved. Typically, for precordial echocardiography, frequencies of 2 to 3 MHz are used, which allow 2 mm resolution and penetration of the chest wall. With transesophageal echocardiography, penetration is not a difficulty, and higher frequencies (3.5–5 MHz) can be used, thereby achieving excellent resolutions.

In this section, M-mode, two-dimensional, Doppler, and contrast echocardiography are reviewed and the uses of echocardiography for detection of wall motion and wall thickening abnormalities and determination of global ventricular function are discussed (see Chapter 8).

M-MODE ECHOCARDIOGRAPHY

A typical M-mode echocardiogram is shown in Figure 10-6. With the transducer placed on the chest wall, the M-mode (one-dimensional mode) represents an "ice-pick" view of the heart. The tracing represents this one-dimensional view plotted against time. Systolic and diastolic events can be visualized in a single dimension or in multiple dimensions by redirection of the transducer along several lines through the heart. With the patient in the left lateral decubitus position, the transducer is swept along the left parasternal border from the level of the aortic valve to left ventricular cavity. The motion of valves and walls and the linear dimensions of intra- and pericardial structures can be visualized. From these views, linear estimates of end-diastolic and end-systolic left ventricular dimensions can be made and calculations of ejection fraction and fiber shortening derived. Wall motion and wall thickening abnormalities can be estimated as well. In patients with CAD, M-mode echocardiography has limited value because of segmental wall motion abnormalities (dyssynergy). With segmental wall motion abnormalities, estimates for a given segment will accurately reflect the localized changes but cannot be used to estimate global function since other normal contracting and hypercontracting segments will exist and may not be detected. Thus, M-mode linear dimension estimates of intracardiac volumes and ejection fractions are unreliable in this patient population. Despite these limitations, M-mode echocardiography is valuable for diagnosis of a number of other disease states.

TWO-DIMENSIONAL ECHOCARDIOGRAPHY

Real-time cross-sectional, two-dimensional echocardiography was developed from M-mode echocardiography. It enables evaluation of structures perpendicular to the unidimensional beam, characterization of lateral motion, and visual integration of an entire sector of single-dimensional beams. A typical two-dimensional echocardiogram using the parasternal long-axis view is shown in Figure 10-7. Whereas M-mode echocardiography records temporal perturbations of any structure lying parallel to its beam, two-dimensional echocardiography simultaneously scans an entire sector of the field by recording individual B-mode lines on videotape at a sampling rate of 30–60 frames per second (versus 1000 impulses per second with M-mode). With the tip of the transducer stationary, the beam is either mechanically moved through an arc by using an oscillating single transducer or by rotating a series of transducers, or it is steered electronically, using phased-array ultrasonic elements that make up the beam. These scanners are usually referred to as mechanical sector scanners or phased-array scanners.[166,167] The images from both of these scanners are very similar, and both techniques are undergoing rather rapid technological changes.

Two-dimensional echocardiography enables the recording of lateral wall motion, axial motion, and multiple planes. The most common planes visualized are the parasternal long-axis view, the short-axis view at the level of the mitral valve and the papillary muscles, apical, and four-chamber views. In any of these views wall motion and wall thickening during systole and diastole can be quantitated, and estimates of end-diastolic and end-systolic areas can be measured. Echocardiographic measures of global ventricular function correlate well (0.75 or greater) with

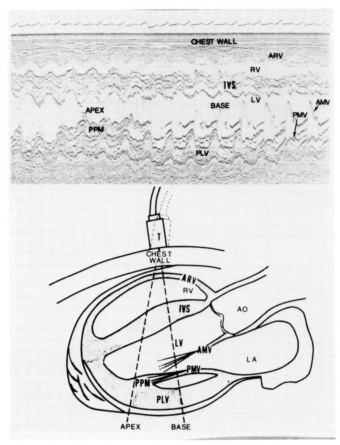

Fig. 10-6. Typical M-mode echocardiogram of the left ventricle with a pictorial display. The transducer is swept from base to apex at the level of the posterior papillary muscle. With systolic contraction the posterior papillary muscle and posterior left ventricular wall move toward the interventricular septum. AMV = anterior mitral valve leaflet; AO = aorta; ARV = anterior right ventricular wall; IVS = interventricular septum; LA = left atrium; LV = left ventricle; PLV = posterior left ventricular wall; PMV = posterior mitral valve leaflet; RV = right ventricle; PPM = posterior papillary muscle; T = transducer. (From Corya BC: Applications of echocardiography in acute myocardial infarction. Cardiovasc Clin 2:113, 1975, with permission.)

radiographic and angiographic techniques. However, for accurate estimation of these volume measurements, multiple parallel planes are necessary.[168,169]

TRANSESOPHAGEAL TWO-DIMENSIONAL ECHOCARDIOGRAPHY

Transesophageal echocardiography is a technique that was developed in Europe during the last decade and is used in Europe in both anesthetized and awake (lightly sedated) patients. In the United States, it is used in anesthetized patients. Using a 9-mm gastroscope with a transducer placed at its distal end, this echoprobe is readily passed into the esophagus and advanced to obtain aortic valve, four-chamber, mitral valve (papillary muscle), and apical views. Because the transducer is nearly in direct contact with the heart and the sound waves do not have to penetrate chest wall or lung structures, higher frequency transducers (3.5–5 MHz) enable 1-mm resolution and very high quality images.

DOPPLER ECHOCARDIOGRAPHY

Doppler echocardiography is based on the physical characteristics of sound waves: when a sound wave of a particular frequency is transmitted and reflected off of a moving object, the frequency differ-

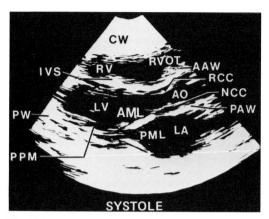

Fig. 10-7. Typical two-dimensional echocardiogram illustration demonstrating the parasternal long-axis view of the heart in systole. AAW = anterior aortic wall; AML = anterior mitral leaflet; AO = aorta; CW = chest wall; IVS = interventricular septum; LA = left atrium; LV = left ventricle; NCC = noncoronary cusp; PAW = posterior aortic wall; PML = posterior mitral leaflet; PPM = posteromedial papillary muscle; PW = posterior wall (left ventricle); RCC = right coronary cusp; RV = right ventricle; RVOT = right ventricular outflow tract. (From Talano JV: Cardiac Ultrasound Workbook. Orlando, FL, Grune & Stratton, 1982, with permission.)

ence between the transmitted and reflected waves is proportional to the velocity of the moving object and the angle at which the transmitted wave strikes the object. Given this angle and the Doppler shift frequency difference, the velocity of the moving object can be calculated. It is possible to calculate velocities of cardiac valves, ventricular walls and, most commonly, red blood cells. When the transmitted signal is a continuous wave, the technique is referred to as "continuous wave" Doppler. Using continuous wave Doppler, blood flow can be accurately quantitated in superficial arteries and veins[170-173] and estimated in central arteries such as the aorta or common carotid artery. Absolute values for central blood flow are more difficult to obtain; however, accuracy appears to be improving with newer techniques.

The most recent advances in Doppler technology incorporate continuous wave Doppler with pulsed ultrasound used for cardiac imaging. Using this combination of techniques, cardiac structures can be imaged, flows across these structures can be quantitated, and valve orifice size estimated. Because the Doppler shift is in the audible range, Doppler echocardiography can enhance clinical diagnosis. In addition, from time-interval histogram displays, differentiation of laminar flow from turbulent flow

through or across intracardiac structures, such as valves, can be made. With laminar flow, the velocities detected are approximately equal; however, with turbulent flow, Doppler signals are scattered and represent a combination of multiple velocities and directions of flow.

Doppler technology is increasing rapidly. A number of technical problems exist, such as aliasing with pulsed Doppler, spatial localization with continuous wave Doppler, and quantitation of velocities with both techniques. Intraoperative Doppler echocardiography, using a precordial or transesophageal approach, will offer significant potential for characterizing the dynamic state of the circulation.

CONTRAST ECHOCARDIOGRAPHY

Injection of a liquid into the circulation creates microbubbles that can be visualized using echocardiography. Intraatrial and ventricular septal defects producing right-to-left shunts have been diagnosed using this form of contrast echocardiography. A variety of contrast agents have been used, including saline, dye, carbon dioxide, and hydrogen peroxide. This technique is gaining popularity and may offer significant potential for visualizing intracardiac and even coronary artery structures; over the next five years significant advances will be made.

During the intraoperative period, this technique has been used to identify patients with right-to-left shunts, which is especially useful during sitting craniotomies. Several preliminary reports have demonstrated that contrast echocardiography enables visualization of septal defects using the transesophageal approach, making it potentially useful as a monitor in such situations.

VISUALIZATION OF CORONARY ARTERIES

During the past decade, a small group of investigators has used echocardiography to identify coronary arteries. Block and Popp recently demonstrated adequate visualization of the coronary arteries in 37 of 50 patients; in 4 of 5 patients, left main CAD was correctly identified.[174] In the future, refinements such as strobe freeze-frame analysis, digital grayscale analysis, and advanced signal processing techniques[174-176] will enable more extensive use of this technique.

EVALUATION OF WALL MOTION AND WALL THICKENING

Studies in animals have demonstrated that soon after coronary occlusion, the ischemic myocardium develops wall motion and wall thickening abnormalities. Both systolic shortening and thickening of the myocardial fibers become impaired. The regional effects on contractility produce dyssynergy, abnormal contractions of the wall. These local segmental effects often occur before reductions in local ATP are evident, possibly suggesting the early role played by calcium. With depletion of ATP, impairment of contraction becomes complete. Wall thickening may be a more specific index of ischemia than wall motion. In the area of acute MI, segmental lengths of the involved tissue are increased, paradoxical bulging is noted, and systolic thinning of the wall occurs. Transition regions between the area of infarction and normal tissue show similar abnormalities, but to a lesser degree. Normal regions of the myocardium compensate for these changes with shortened fiber length and increased wall thickening during systolic contraction.

Two-dimensional echocardiography appears to have a significant advantage over M-mode echocardiography for detection of wall motion and wall thickening abnormalities. With M-mode, only an "ice-pick" view of the ventricle is provided, and regions of segmental wall motion abnormality may be missed. Using two-dimensional echocardiography, segmental wall motion abnormalities can be described both qualitatively and quantitatively. Qualitative assessment of wall motion is described as hyperkinetic (greater than normal), normal, hypokinetic (normal direction but reduced motion), akinetic (absent motion), or dyskinetic (paradoxic motion). Wall motion abnormalities may be quantitated using several methods. One specific method, adapted from Heger et al, is shown in Figure 10-8.[75] In this commonly used method, the ventricle is divided into nine segments of approximately equal size, and the segments are defined with respect to fixed anatomic landmarks. For each segment, wall motion can be quantitated by measuring the degree of radial shortening and the amount of wall thinning occurring during systole. One commonly used system classifies a segment as normal if the radius shortens by more than 30 percent and wall thickening occurs with systole. Hypokinesis is radial shortening of less than 30 percent, with wall thickening. Akinesis is radial shortening of less than 10 percent, without wall thickening during systole. Dyskinesis is defined by radial lengthening and wall thinning. Segmental wall motion abnormalities have been considered a gold standard for definition of myocardial ischemia; however, other factors can affect wall motion and endocardial excursion and, thereby, make interpretation difficult. A normal variation in the degree of endocardial excursion with systole

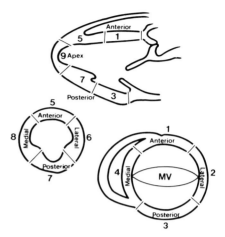

Fig. 10-8. A typical method for defining specific left ventricular segments for wall motion analysis. (From Heger JJ, Weyman AE, Wann SL, et al: Cross-sectional echocardiography in acute myocardial infarction. Detection and localization of regional left ventricular asynergy. Circulation 60:531, 1979, with permission.)

makes absolute quantification difficult. Temperature, intracardiac volume, ventricular interference, and abnormalities of electrical conduction may affect wall motion. Wall thickening may be a better indicator of myocardial ischemia because it is less affected by spatial motion of the ventricle or alterations in ventricular shape. The ventricular wall thickens during systole by approximately 14–57 percent (an average of 36 percent).[177] Decreases in wall thickening occur with acute ischemia and where there is a scar from a previous MI. Wall thinning with systole appears to occur only with acute myocardial ischemia and infarction.[178–180] Mean wall thickening decreases by approximately 50 percent with MI when 20 percent of the myocardium is infarcted, and infarctions of greater than 20 percent are associated with wall thinning.[181] Two-dimensional echocardiography appears to be particularly advantageous for detection of wall thickening changes. In the future, improved methods of endocardial mapping, using advanced data processing techniques, will enable characterization of wall thickening changes, thus enabling quantitative assessment of acute ischemic and infarction changes.

GLOBAL VENTRICULAR FUNCTION

The effects of ischemia on global contractility are complex and depend on a number of factors: the degree of ischemia, the type of wall motion abnormality (akinetic versus dyskinetic), and the amount and performance of the remaining normally functioning myocardial fibers. Quantitative assessment of left ventricular function in normal ventricles can be performed using both M-mode and two-dimensional echocardiography. However, in patients with ventricular dysfunction with wall motion abnormalities, M-mode echocardiography is inaccurate. With two-dimensional echocardiography, ejection fraction, velocity of circumferential fiber shortening, and ventricular volumes can be estimated. This quantitation relies on adequate visualization of the endocardial surface, reproducible transducer positioning, and imaging of the maximum cavity size from each position. Given these constraints, ejection fraction and volumes can be calculated, and correlate well with those derived from ventriculography or radionuclear techniques. However, precise estimation of ejection fractions and ventricular volumes from the single-plane, two-dimensional echocardiogram is limited. Multiple planes (3–4) are necessary for precise estimation of ventricular volumes and ejection fractions using two-dimensional echocardiography.[182-184] The echocardiographic volumes consistently underestimate true ventricular cavity volume because of endocardial interference, which broadens the echoes, failure to include the cavity volume contained within the trabeculae, artifactual diastolic or systolic reduction of wall motion through the scan plane, and other technical considerations.[185-188] In contrast, the angiographically obtained volumes consistently overestimate true volume because of inclusion of papillary muscle and mitral valve apparatus in the calculated volumes, silhouette formatting, which maximizes the projected area, and inclusion of the trabeculae. In comparison with the angiographic technique, end-systolic volumes determined echocardiographically are more accurate than end-diastolic volumes because of the improved definition of the endocardial surface at end-systole. Finally, the accuracy of any of these quantitative ventricular function techniques is related to the choice of applied formulae, the frequency of sampling, and the configuration of the ventricle. The most accurate technique appears to be Simpson's rule, which uses sections spaced 3 mm apart (see Chapter 8).

CONCLUSIONS

As a preoperative test, precordial echocardiography is a noninvasive, relatively inexpensive test, which has specific advantages in several clinical situations. First, it is useful for the diagnosis of an acute MI when other techniques, such as the ECG, are uninterpretable (because of left bundle branch block, Wolff-Parkinson-White syndrome). Second, for assessment of global ventricular function, two-dimensional echocardiography provides useful information on ejection fraction (correlation of 0.78 to 0.94), end-systolic and end-diastolic volumes, and circumferential wall motion and ventricular mass. This may be particularly useful in patients undergoing major third-space surgery or surgery involving aortic cross-clamping, in whom the degree of ventricular dysfunction is not apparent from routine clinical tests. Third, in patients with a questionable anginal pattern, wall motion and wall thickening changes, assessed echocardiographically either at rest or during exercise, can provide both qualitative and quantitative information. In patients undergoing extensive surgery, this technique may be useful for deciding optimal preoperative management and perioperative monitoring and care. Finally, echocardiography is useful for definition of left ventricular (LV) aneurysms, septal rupture, papillary muscle abnormalities, and mural thrombus formation.

Nuclear Imaging

Over the past half century, and particularly over the past two decades, nuclear imaging of the cardiovascular system has made significant advances. It is now a safe and accurate method for assessment of myocardial perfusion and infarction, and ventricular function. One of the earliest descriptions of the use of nuclear imaging was in 1927 when radioactive radon was injected intravenously and circulation time measured using a modified Wilson cloud chamber.[189] Imaging of the heart using radiocardiograms was first described in 1949 by Prinzmetal and Corday. Despite these early accomplishments, it has been only within the last 20 years that significant advances in cardiac perfusion and function measurements have been made. The instrumentation, radiopharmaceuticals, techniques for MI and perfusion imaging, and the evaluation of cardiac performance will be described.

INSTRUMENTATION

The scintillation camera, also known as the Anger or gamma camera, detects gamma rays from an injected radiopharmaceutical, converts the energy to electrical energy, and displays this representation of radioactivity. It consists of a collimator that absorbs gamma rays and passes them through multiple channels or holes. The gamma rays are, in effect, focused by the collimator to a receiving crystal that converts the gamma ray energy to light. The crystal is a position-sensitive detector made of sodium iodine. The light energy is enhanced and converted into electrical energy by photomultiplier tubes that are packed tightly against the crystal. The electrical signals are then electronically processed by the detector, and the energy from the original gamma rays is calculated and spatially described. Several types of collimators are used for different cardiology studies. Most of these are parallel-hole collimators, which enable detection of only those gamma rays that are emitted perpendicular to the crystal. There is a trade-off between resolution and sensitivity; high-resolution collimators have a lower sensitivity and vice versa. For time-dependent studies, such as exercise thallium-201 and gated blood pool imaging, general-purpose collimators, which have moderate sensitivity and resolution, are used. High-resolution collimators are used when sensitivity is not of primary importance, such as in studies at rest. High-sensitivity collimators are used in first-pass radionuclide angiography when photon count may be limited.

A second type of camera, the multicrystal scintillation camera, has 294 sodium iodide crystals and 35 photomultiplier tubes associated with the crystal array. Signal processing of photomultiplier row and column tubes allows spatial identification of scintillation events. Because of its design, count rates of 500,000 events per second can be recorded. Thus, the multicrystal camera can be used for dynamic studies, such as first-pass radionuclide angiography.

In addition to the gamma and multicrystal cameras, a third type of detector, the single-probe scintillation detector, allows measurement of ejection fraction, cardiac output, pulmonary transit time, and other measures of global left ventricular function. Its significant advantages are that it is small and portable and can be used in a large number of environments. The actual probe is approximately 3 inches in diameter by 2 inches in depth, and uses a variety of collimators. The most common crystal used is sodium iodide; however, cadmium telluride crystals have recently been used and allow sequential measurement over prolonged periods. After injection of the radiopharmaceutical, such as technetium-99m, passage through the right heart, pulmonary circulation, and the left heart can be recorded by measuring count rates during the systolic and diastolic cycles (first-pass angiography). The radiopharmaceuticals may also be used to label albumin or red blood cells and the study gated to the ECG following equilibration (equilibration radionuclide angiography). From the time-activity curves, end-systolic and end-diastolic counts, ejection fraction, cardiac output, and pulmonary transit time may be measured.

In addition to these detectors, a fourth type of system uses tomography. Tomography, using single-photon or positron-emission, offers significant advantages by enabling resolution of adjacent structures and background noise. Although both limited-angle and transaxial tomography are used, it appears that only transaxial tomography provides the necessary depth resolution required. Positron-transaxial tomography is currently being used in studies of regional myocardial metabolism and perfusion.

MYOCARDIAL INFARCTION IMAGING

Diagnosis of an acute MI using historical, electrocardiographic, and enzymatic data is not always possible. For example, diabetics or the elderly may be asymptomatic, the ECG may be uninterpretable (in about 25 percent of the population with left bundle branch block, Wolff-Parkinson-White syndrome), or cardiac enzymatic changes may be masked by other tissue effects, such as skeletal muscle destruction during surgery. Use of nuclear imaging techniques to determine the presence and extent of MI can significantly enhance the diagnosis.

For diagnosis of MI, two types of imaging exist. The principal method, infarct-avid myocardial scintigraphy (hot-spot imaging), uses technetium-99m pyrophosphate as the radionuclide. The infarcted segment of the myocardium has a selective affinity for technetium. Once taken up, the increased activity of the area, referred to as a hot-spot, can be detected using a gamma camera. Normal tissue or areas of old scarring and infarction do not have an affinity for technetium, and these areas are not visualized. The uptake in acute MI depends on the regional blood flow, the concentration of calcium in the myocardium, the reversibility of the myocardial injury, and the time of infarction. The earliest detectable images are seen from 12 to 16 hours following the event, but maximum abnormality occurs from 48 to 72 hours afterwards. After 5–7 days, the intensity of the image returns toward normal (Fig. 10-9).

Technetium pyrophosphate is a readily available radionuclide with favorable photon energies (140 kev) and a short half-life (6 hours). After injection into a peripheral vein, 50 percent of the dose is extracted by bone and the remainder is rapidly excreted through the kidneys, with 5 percent of the injected dose remaining in the blood 90 minutes following injection. With acute coronary occlusion in animals, the infarcted area concentration is approximately 20 times that of normal tissue. Because a minimal coronary blood flow of 20–40 percent to the infarcted area is necessary for adequate uptake, false negatives exist. In addition, endocardial concentrations appear to be significantly less than epicardial

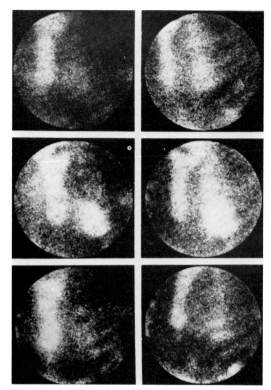

Fig. 10-9. A typical technetium pyrophosphate image in a patient with an acute transmural myocardial infarction. (Top) A faintly positive image is seen lateral to the sternum over the left ventricle, approximately 10 hours after myocardial infarction. (Middle) A more intense image 3 days after infarction. (Bottom) Marked reduction of the myocardial uptake of technetium 7 days following infarction. (From Willerson JT, Parkey RW, Bonte FJ, et al: Technetium stannouspyrophosphate myocardial scintigrams in patients with chest pain of varying etiology. Circulation 51:1046, 1975, with permission.)

concentrations, and subendocardial MIs may not be detected. It is estimated that at least 5 gm of infarcted tissue is necessary for adequate detection. Following binding of the isotope to the infarcted tissue, the radionuclide emits photons which allow detection and localization by the gamma camera. The mechanism by which the infarcted tissue binds this radioisotope is unknown, but it appears to be related to myocardial calcium. With myocardial necrosis, intracellular calcium deposition has been shown to occur and may complex with the radionuclide.[190]

Technetium pyrophosphate imaging has been shown to have a sensitivity of greater than 90 percent in the detection of acute MI.[191] In dogs, infarcts can be detected when as little as 2 percent of the ventricular mass has been affected. A strong correlation has been demonstrated among technetium, infarcted areas, ECG Q waves, and myocardial perfusion scintigraphy defects. Infarct size assessment using this technique remains investigational.

A second nuclear imaging technique is available for MI imaging, namely perfusion scintigraphy or cold-spot imaging. Using radioactive potassium and rubidium, it was found that areas of the heart with normal perfusion and function would take up these isotopes and allow imaging of normal myocardium.[192,193] Defects in the normal pattern, known as cold-spots, would represent areas of decreased flow or function, possibly associated with ischemia, as well as acute or old myocardial infarction. The cold-spot technique is highly sensitive for detection of MI (greater than 90 percent), but not as specific as technetium pyrophosphate hot-spot imaging.

Because of the high photon energies associated with radioactive potassium and rubidium, thallium-201 was developed and is currently the radiopharmaceutical of choice for myocardial perfusion scintigraphy. After this potassium analogue is injected into a peripheral vein, it is extracted by normal myocardium (85 percent extraction), and images can be obtained within minutes of the intravenous injection. Thallium is distributed within the myocardium in proportion to the regional myocardial blood flow when flow is low-to-normal. At higher flow rates, its uptake is no longer linear, and substantial stress is required to achieve adequate imaging. Thallium uptake is also related to myocardial function and adenosine triphosphatase. With normal flow and function, the thallium image appears doughnut shaped. The central zone of decreased uptake reflects the ventricular cavity. Normally, all walls demonstrate activity; however, in approximately 20 percent of normal patients, the apical views will demonstrate a perfusion defect although function and flow are normal in this area. With alteration of coronary flow or function during ischemia or infarction, areas of decreased perfusion or cold-spots are visualized (Fig. 10-10). It has been shown that thallium imaging is highly specific if performed within 6 hours of an acute MI.[194] However, this specificity decreases dramatically after approximately 24 hours following infarction, particularly in cases where less than 5 gm of infarcted tissue is involved. A comparison between hot-spot and cold-spot imaging is shown in Table 10-6.

MYOCARDIAL PERFUSION IMAGING

Myocardial perfusion imaging using thallium-201 provides information regarding the extent, local-

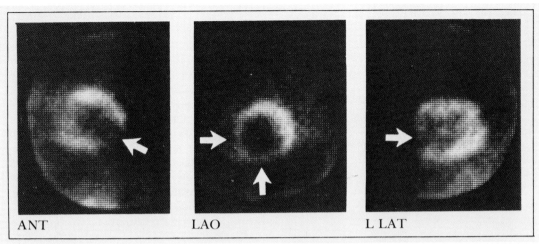

Fig. 10-10. Resting thallium-201 myocardial perfusion scintigraphy shown in the anterior (ANT), left anterior oblique (LAO), and left lateral (L LAT) positions in a patient with a recent transmural myocardial infarction. Perfusion defects as seen in the apical (ANT), inferior, and septal (LAO) regions. (From Cohn PF: Diagnosis and Therapy of Coronary Artery Disease. Boston, Little, Brown, 1979, with permission.)

ization, reversibility and stress response of the coronary circulation. It enables a quantitative assessment of the functional significance of CAD. Quantitation of the functional impairment associated with myocardial ischemia requires significant increases in coronary blood flow to effect visible changes in thallium uptake. In the absence of MI, coronary blood flow, even with stenoses of up to 75 percent, is relatively homogeneous throughout the ventricle. In the resting state, only with severe coronary stenosis (greater than 90 percent) will perfusion defects be detected using thallium imaging. As such, resting perfusion scans are of limited value. However, because stenotic vessels have limited coronary vascu-

lar reserve in response to metabolic stress, the normal resting homogeneous pattern of coronary perfusion can be altered and made heterogeneous during metabolic stress. Injection of the isotope during maximal stress will allow visualization of perfusion heterogeneities reflecting areas of ischemia. Because of the rapid myocardial clearance rate of thallium-201, redistribution of thallium occurs quickly, allowing visualization of the reperfusion process.

After injection of thallium-201 during maximal exercise or infusion of a coronary vasodilator such as dipyridamole, imaging is performed within 5 to 10 minutes. Perfusion defects, or cold-spots, will last

Table 10-6
Hot-Spot Versus Cold-Spot Radionuclear Imaging

	"Hot-spot" Imaging	"Cold-spot" Imaging
Radionuclide	Technetium-99m pyrophosphate	Thallium-201
Uptake by	Infarcted tissue	Normal tissue (normal perfusion and metabolism)
Positive with	Acute MI (5 gm infarct)	Acute MI (5 gm infarct) Old MI Ischemia
Timing:		
Earliest positive test	12–16 hours (post MI)	Immediately
Most sensitive	48–72 hours	24 hours
Other uses	RV MI	Chamber size
	Subendocardial MI	LVH, RVH, ASH
	Infarct size (+)	Stress testing

LVH = left ventricular hypertrophy; RVH = right ventricular hypertrophy; ASH = assymetric septal hypertrophy.

approximately 30 to 60 minutes, and redistribution usually occurs during the next 2 to 3 hours. Repeat imaging is performed approximately 3 to 4 hours after the initial injection. The initial perfusion defects will either persist or disappear. Those that persist are indicative of infarction or prolonged ischemia (unlikely). Those that disappear are indicative of a reversible perfusion defect or transient myocardial ischemia without infarction (Fig. 10-11). It is also possible that the perfusion defect will worsen, which is consistent with previous infarction with superimposed new myocardial ischemia. The highest sensitivities reported with this technique are 90 percent,[195-197] but sensitivities as low as 60 percent in patients with single vessel disease involving the circumflex or right coronary arteries have been reported. Specificities are greater than 90 percent, with few false positives noted.

Dipyridamole thallium scintigraphy is useful in predicting outcome events in patients undergoing vascular surgery procedures.[20] Dipyridamole (Persantine, Boehringer Ingelheim Ltd., Ridgefield, CT) is a coronary vasodilator that simulates the effects of exercise. In patients with marked peripheral vascular disease who are incapable of maximal or submaximal exercise, dipyridamole offers significant potential. Although this study demonstrated that dipyridamole has prognostic value, the costs and morbidity associated with this technique warrant further study to justify its use in this large patient population.

TOMOGRAPHY

The advantages of tomography over the previously described scintigraphic techniques are that it enables differentiation of different regions of the myocardium and isolation of background noise. Of the two forms of tomography available, limited-angle and transaxial computed, only the latter appears to offer a significant advantage at present. With transaxial-computed tomography, the gamma camera is rotated through 180 or 360 degrees about the patient, making 32 or 64 stops at 20- to 40-second intervals. These data are processed, averaged, and summed, and images in multiple planes are produced. In a normal patient the left ventricle appears to be horseshoe-shaped, with the open end of the horseshoe corresponding to the region of the aortic valve. Distribution of thallium-201 is homogeneous throughout the septum, anterior, and lateral walls. As with thallium scintigraphy, the central perfusion defect represents the ventricular cavity.

Perfusion defects are more easily detected using tomography since there is no overlap in the images of the normally perfused and hypoperfused myocardium, as there is with thallium perfusion scintigraphy. Differentiation of myocardial tissue from other tissues, such as lung, is enhanced using tomography. It appears that this technique offers significant potential for precise definition of infarct size or degree of perfusion defect. This technique has been used for verification of ambulatory ECG changes in studies of silent myocardial ischemia, and it holds particular promise as a gold standard for verification of other clinical measures of ischemia.

RADIONUCLEAR EVALUATION OF CARDIAC MECHANICS

Two radionuclear techniques are presently available for evaluation of cardiac mechanics: first-pass

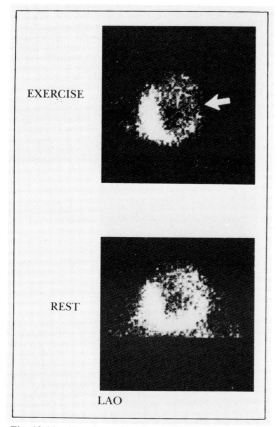

EXERCISE

REST

LAO

Fig. 10-11. Exercise and resting thallium-201 myocardial perfusion scintigrams in the left anterior oblique (LAO) position in a patient with a reversible diffusion defect. During exercise a lateral wall perfusion defect is noted (arrow) that resolves with rest, consistent with transient myocardial ischemia. (From Cohn PF: Diagnosis and Therapy of Coronary Artery Disease. Boston, Little, Brown, 1979, with permission.)

radionuclide angiography and gated blood pool imaging. Both provide ventricular function information, including ejection fraction, end-systolic and end-diastolic volumes, cardiac output, pulmonary transit time, and intracardiac shunt. First-pass radionuclide angiography and gated blood pool imaging are both useful and have distinct advantages.

FIRST-PASS RADIONUCLEAR ANGIOGRAPHY

First-pass radionuclear angiography allows a temporal separation of the right and left sides of the heart, as well as the lung. With this technique, a bolus of the radiopharmaceutical, usually technetium-99m, is injected into a peripheral or central vein, and the radioactivity is counted as this bolus passes through the central circulation. The entire sequence is measured over 10 to 15 seconds and allows acute assessment of cardiac performance, particularly in unstable patients. Repeat assessments can be made at multiple time intervals thereafter and require repeated injections of the radiopharmaceutical.

The scintillation counters employed in this technique are usually multicrystal digital cameras, allowing for the rapid acquisition and measurement of high radioisotope count rates necessary for this technique. Ejection fraction, cardiac output, end-diastolic volume, pulmonary transit time, and shunt calculations can be performed using this technique.

A representative time-activity curve showing the transit of the radioisotope through the right and left ventricles is presented in Figure 10-12. Only the initial transit of the radioisotope is measured, which allows anatomic separation of the right and left ventricles. With each cardiac cycle, the measured activities at end-diastole and end-systole are proportional to the respective ventricular volumes. The maximum

count rates during a cycle correspond to end-diastole, and the minimum to end-systole. Ejection fraction can be computed by the difference between the end-diastolic and end-systolic count rates, divided by the end-diastolic count, subtracted from the background count. Typically, the ejection fraction is computed over 3 to 5 cycles and averaged. This first-pass ejection fraction technique correlates well with contrast angiography ($r = 0.94$ to 0.97).[198-200]

Right ventricular ejection fraction has been measured using a similar technique. This technique is particularly useful since the geometry of the right ventricle is variable and complex, making other techniques using geometric calculations less precise. Using the first-pass technique, right ventricular ejection fraction has been shown to have a mean normal value of 0.55, with a lower normal limit of 0.45.[201] Right ventricular ejection fraction has been measured using this technique for several clinical disorders, including chronic obstructive pulmonary disease,[201-203] cystic fibrosis,[202] and during MI.[204,205]

The first-pass technique can also be used for calculation of end-diastolic volume,[183] left ventricular ejection phase indices such as ejection rate,[198] and peak diastolic filling rate.[206] These indices are difficult to validate, however, and only measurement of relative changes appears to be useful.

The detection of intracardiac shunts, using first-pass radionuclide angiography, has been shown to be a sensitive technique, with some studies reporting the detection of shunt as small as 1.1:1.[207] When the radioisotope is introduced into the venous system in normal patients, passage through the right ventricle, the lungs, and the left ventricle produces a distinct pattern. Approximately 15 seconds following the first-pass, recirculation occurs. In patients with a left-to-right shunt, recirculation occurs much earlier,

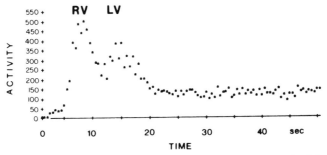

Fig. 10-12. A normal time-activity curve demonstrating the first transit of the radiotracer through the right ventricle (RV) and the left ventricle (LV). (From Ashburn WL, Schelbert HR, Verba JW, et al: Left ventricular ejection fraction. A review of several radionuclide angiographic approaches using the scintillation camera. Prog Cardiovasc Dis 20:267, 1978, with permission.)

and causes the right heart, lung, and left heart distinct activity curves to merge. A left-to-right shunt can be quantified from the activity curves. This technique allows detection of the shunt; however, quantification of the shunt is not precise. Furthermore, if the injection technique is not rapid, if pulmonary or tricuspid regurgitation occur, or if pulmonary transit time is prolonged (pulmonary arterial disease), false positive results can be produced. Right-to-left shunt cannot be detected using this technique.

GATED BLOOD-POOL IMAGING.

The second radionuclide imaging technique for assessment of ventricular performance is gated blood-pool imaging. Unlike the first-pass technique, the radionuclude is used to label blood products that remain within the intravascular space and create an equilibrium state. Radiopharmaceuticals such as technetium-99–labeled human serum albumin or technetium-99–labeled red blood cells are presently used. Following equilibrium of the radionuclide in the intravascular space, the gamma camera accumulates activity over the region of interest, and identifies end-systole and diastole by gating to a physiologic marker, usually the R wave of the ECG. Data from 300 to 500 cardiac cycles are averaged to produce count rates of approximately 300,000 over the 2- to 10–minute imaging time. Because of this high number of counts, the resolution of the radionuclide angiocardiogram is high. Background activity

is measured by selecting a noncardiac area (lung), and this activity is subtracted from the measured cardiac volumes to produce a relative ventricular volume. As with the first-pass technique, ejection fraction is computed as the ratio of the difference between end-diastolic and end-systolic volumes to the end-diastolic volume.

Regional ejection fraction and wall motion may be measured using a series of geometrical models and processing algorithms.[208-210] Absolute determinations are difficult to validate, but relative changes in these indices provide useful information.

In addition to ejection fraction and ventricular volume, a measure of valvular regurgitation can be calculated as well. The ratio of the right-to-left ventricular stroke counts has been used as an index of valvular regurgitation, but although the presence of regurgitation may be detected, quantitation remains a problem.[211]

First-pass and gated-pool radionuclide imaging provide accurate assessment of global left ventricular ejection fraction, and the correlation between these methods is high (r = 0.87–0.89).[212,213] However, several important differences between these techniques exist and are summarized in Table 10-7. Gated-pool imaging is particularly advantageous when higher count rates are necessary, such as for estimation of regional wall motion. In studies where background plays a significant role, such as with edge detection, first-pass studies using lesser activity

Table 10-7
First-Pass Versus Gated-Pool Radionuclear Angiography

	First-Pass	Gated-Pool
Radionuclide	Any technetium (99m)-labeled pharmaceutical	Technetium (99m)-labeled albumin or RBC
Type of technique	Transient (30 seconds) Multiple injections/hour	Steady state (6 hours) Single injection/hour
EF Correlation with angiography	>0.90	>0.90
Uses	LVEF Exercise testing Dyskinesis RVEF Intracardiac shunt	LVEF Exercise testing Dyskinesis
Geometric assumptions	None	Several

EF = ejection fraction; LVEF = left ventricular ejection fraction; RVEF = right ventricular ejection fraction.

are more accurate. For monitoring clinical function over a period of up to 4 hours, gated-pool imaging is superior. For interventional studies requiring multiple measurements, first-pass techniques are more suitable, although accumulation of background activity with each bolus injection limits the number of repeated studies using the first-pass technique.

CONCLUSIONS

Radionuclear imaging provides unique information regarding detection of MI, quantification of myocardial perfusion abnormalities, and calculation of ventricular performance and wall motion indices. Knowledge of the techniques and the ability to interpret the results are important to anesthesiologists in order to enhance the preoperative assessment of MI and quantification of ventricular function. The results of these studies can affect decisions regarding preoperative preparation, intra- and perioperative monitoring, and choice of therapeutics.

Cardiac Catheterization

Cardiac catheterization has a rich history, starting in about 1844 with Claude Bernard, who is credited with catheterizing the left and right ventricles of a horse using a retrograde approach from the jugular vein and the carotid artery. The most significant events are summarized below.

1844 Bernard: First catheterization of the right and left ventricles (horse).
1929 Forssmann: First catheterization of the right ventricle in humans.
1930 Kline: Catheterization of the right ventricle in 11 patients with measurement of cardiac output using the Fick technique.
1941 Cournand and Richards: Studies on right-heart physiology in humans.
1947 Dexter: Studies of congenital heart disease, and first use of the pulmonary artery wedge position to obtain pulmonary capillary bed measurements.
1949 Dexter, Lagerlof, and Werko: First measurement of pulmonary artery wedge pressures.
1950 Zimmerman and Lason: Retrograde left-heart catheterization.
1953 Seldinger: Percutaneous technique for catheterization of the left and right heart chambers.
1959 Ross: Transseptal left-heart catheterization.
1959 Sones: Selected coronary arteriography.

1970 Swan and Ganz: Introduction of the balloon-tipped flow-guided catheter.
1977 Gruentzig: Transluminal coronary angioplasty.

Regional ejection fraction and wall motion may be measured using a series of geometrical models and processing algorithms. Absolute determinations are difficult to validate, but relative changes in these indices provide useful information.

INDICATIONS

The indications for cardiac catheterization and coronary arteriography vary widely. In patients with chest pain as the predominant symptom, cardiac catheterization is performed when angina is unstable, medically refractory, atypical (Prinzmetal's angina) or recurrent, and following cardiac surgery. In the absence of chest pain, cardiac catheterization is performed in patients with pump failure (usually following infarction), for evaluation of valvular or congenital heart disease, or for evaluation of the coronary circulation following coronary bypass.

COMPLICATIONS

In 89,079 patients, Adams and Abrams summarized the overall complication rate associated with cardiac catheterization and arteriography.[214] The overall mortality from these procedures was 0.14 percent. In order of decreasing incidence, the morbid outcomes were contrast reactions (1.08 percent), ventricular fibrillation (0.76 percent), thrombosis (0.67 percent), MI (0.18 percent), hemorrhage (0.09 percent), cerebral embolus (0.09 percent), and pseudoaneurysm (0.04 percent). The only significant difference between the brachial and femoral approaches was the incidence of thrombosis, being 1.13 percent with the brachial approach, versus 0.20 percent with the femoral approach.

TECHNIQUES

The patient undergoing cardiac catheterization is usually fasting and premedicated. Prior to catheterization, the patient is anticoagulated with heparin (5000 units IV). In sequence, hemodynamic measurements, ventriculography, and coronary arteriography are performed.

Hemodynamic Measurements

After catheterization of the brachial or femoral artery, the catheter is advanced into the aorta and left ventricle. Coronary arteriography is performed using multiple views. For the left coronary artery, the left anterior oblique, anteroposterior, and right anterior oblique views are routinely used. At times, the left lateral projection is used for further visualization of the left anterior descending coronary artery. To separate the proximal portions of the left circumflex and left anterior descending arteries, hemiaxial views, with a left anterior oblique rotation and cranial-caudal angulation, is performed. Visualization of the right coronary artery is accomplished using right anterior oblique and left anterior oblique views. The most commonly used contrast agent for arteriography and ventriculography is meglumine diatrizoate. The use of this contrast agent has significantly decreased the incidence of ventricular fibrillation and asystole. However, contrast reactions occur in approximately 1 percent of patients and result in hypotension, bradycardia, and T-wave changes on the ECG. Injections into the right coronary artery characteristically produce T-wave inversions in lead II, while left coronary artery injection produces T-wave peaking. The usual amount of contrast agent used is 10–20 ml for visualization of the coronary arteries, two-thirds of which is used for visualization of the left coronary arteries.

A series of hemodynamic measurements and calculations are made, including: systemic, pulmonary, and intracardiac pressure measurements, calculation of cardiac output, vascular resistance, oxygen consumption and arteriovenous oxygen difference, and valve areas. Right-heart measurements are also usually performed, via a catheter placed in the brachial or femoral vein. Normal values for these hemodynamic measurements are shown in Table 10-8 (see Chapter 6).

CARDIAC OUTPUT

Cardiac output can be calculated using the Fick oxygen method, the indicator-dilution technique, or from ventriculography measurements. The Fick oxygen method is based on the principle that total uptake

Table 10-8
Normal Resting Hemodynamic Values

	Pressure		
	Systolic	*Diastolic*	*Mean*
	mm Hg		
Right atrium	—	—	−2–6
Right ventricle	15–30	0–8	5–15
Pulmonary artery	15–30	0–12	5–18
Pulmonary wedge			0–12
Left atrium			0–12
Left ventricle	100–140	60–90	70–105
Volume			
Left ventricle			
end-diastolic	70–95 ml/m^2		
end-systolic	24–36 ml/m^2		
Performance			
Cardiac index	2.5–4.2 l/min/m^2		
Stroke volume index	50–70 ml/m^2		
Ejection fraction	0.67 ± 0.08 (SD)		
Resistance			
Pulmonary vascular	20–120 dynes-sec-cm^{-5}		
Systemic vascular	770–1500 dynes-sec-cm^{-5}		
Oxygen measurements			
Oxygen consumption	110–150 ml/min/m^2		
Arteriovenous oxygen			
difference	3–5 ml/100 ml blood		
Valve measurements			
Aortic valve area	2.6–3.5 cm^2		
Mitral valve area	4.0–6.0 cm^2		

or release of any substance by an organ is the product of the blood flow to the organ and the arteriovenous concentration difference of the substance. By measurement of the arteriovenous oxygen difference across the lungs and the oxygen consumption, pulmonary blood flow can be calculated. Given that there is no intracardiac shunt, and pulmonary blood flow is equal to systemic blood flow, systemic blood flow can be derived. The following formula is used:

$$\text{Cardiac index (liters/min/m}^2) = \frac{\text{O}_2 \text{ consumption (ml/min/m}^2)}{\text{arteriovenous O}_2 \text{ difference (ml/l)}}.$$

OXYGEN CONSUMPTION AND SATURATION

Oxygen consumption is measured by collecting expired air over a 3-minute period. The oxygen content is calculated from the ratio of the partial pressure of oxygen to the corrected barometric pressure. Oxygen content is then calculated from the product of the expired air oxygen consumption and minute ventilation. Arteriovenous oxygen difference is calculated from the oxygen content, which can be measured using a variety of techniques. The time-consuming technique of van Slyke and Neill[215] has generally been replaced by reflectance oximetry for the measurement of oxygen saturation. Oxygen content is calculated from the product of hemoglobin concentration and saturation. The indicator-dilution method, first introduced in 1897,[216] is similar to the Fick method introduced 27 years earlier. With the indicator-dilution method, indocyanine green dye is commonly used as the indicator. It is rapidly injected as a bolus into the right heart, and its concentration is recorded from a systemic artery (brachial, femoral, or radial). From the arterial concentration curve (concentration versus time), the cardiac output is calculated:

$$\text{Cardiac output} = V_i/(C \times T),$$

where V_i is the volume of dye injected, C is the average concentration of the indicator during its first pass, and T is the total duration of the curve. C and T may be calculated from the curve by using planimetry or, more conveniently, by using electronic signal processing techniques. The Fick method is analogous to this, but uses oxygen as the dye. When cardiac output measurements are normal or elevated, there is excellent agreement between the indicator-dilution method and the Fick method. However, when cardiac outputs are low, or when valvular regurgitation

or intracardiac shunt exists, the indicator-dilution method becomes inaccurate. The third, and most commonly used, method of computing cardiac output is ventriculography. By quantitation of the end-diastolic and end-systolic images, volumes can be approximated. The difference between the end-diastolic and end-systolic volumes, or the stroke volume, multiplied by the heart rate, equals the cardiac output. This method, although less accurate than the Fick method, yields acceptable cardiac output measurements, except when aortic or mitral regurgitation or atrial fibrillation is present.

VASCULAR RESISTANCE

Systemic and pulmonary vascular resistance (SVR, PVR) are calculated from the measurements of the pressures and cardiac output as follows:

$$\text{SVR (dynes} \cdot \text{sec} \cdot \text{cm}^{-5}) = \frac{80 \times (\overline{\text{BP}} - \overline{\text{RA}})}{\dot{Q}_s} \quad (10\text{-}1)$$

$$\text{PVR (dynes} \cdot \text{sec} \cdot \text{cm}^{-5}) = \frac{80 \times (\overline{\text{PA}} - \overline{\text{LA}})}{\dot{Q}_p}$$

where $\overline{\text{BP}}, \overline{\text{RA}}, \overline{\text{PA}}, \overline{\text{LA}}$ are the mean aortic, right atrial, pulmonary artery, and left atrial blood pressures in mm Hg, and $\dot{Q}_s$ and $\dot{Q}_p$ are the systemic and pulmonary blood flows in liters/min. The normal range for these values is shown in Table 10-8.

SHUNT

Intracardiac shunts are calculated from pulmonary and systemic blood flows using the Fick principle. Pulmonary blood flow is defined as:

$$\dot{Q}_p \text{(liter/min)} = \frac{\text{O}_2 \text{ consumption (ml/min)}}{\text{PV O}_2 \text{ content} - \text{PA O}_2 \text{ content (ml/liter)}} \quad (10\text{-}2)$$

where PV and PA are the pulmonary venous and pulmonary arterial values.

Systemic blood flow is defined as:

$$\dot{Q}_s \text{(liter/min)} = \frac{\text{O}_2 \text{ consumption (ml/min)}}{\text{A O}_2 \text{ content} - \text{PA O}_2 \text{ content (ml/liter)}} \quad (10\text{-}3)$$

where A refers to the arterial blood. With a left-to-right shunt (atrial septal defect, ventricular septal defect, patent ductus arteriosus), pulmonary blood flow is greater than systemic blood flow, and pulmonary oxygen saturation is greater than mixed-venous saturation. From the oxygen saturation measurements sampled in the cardiac chambers, shunts can be localized anatomically. This technique is generally sensitive except when shunts are small, ($\dot{Q}_p/\dot{Q}_s$ ≥ 1.3). Smaller shunts may be detected from hydrogen gas measurements, using a right heart hydrogen-sensitive electrode to measure direct current voltage changes. Right-to-left shunts can be detected clinically and may be detected from relative desaturations. Small right-to-left shunts can be detected using indocyanine dye injections.

VALVE AREA

The orifice area of the aortic and mitral valves is calculated from the flow through the valve and the pressure gradient across it.[217-219] The following formulae are used:

$$\text{Aortic valve area (cm}^2) = \frac{F}{44.5 \times \sqrt{\Delta P}} \qquad (10\text{-}4)$$

$$\text{Mitral valve area (cm}^2) = \frac{F}{38.0 \times \sqrt{\Delta P}} \qquad (10\text{-}5)$$

where F is the flow through the orifice in ml/sec, and P is the mean pressure gradient across the orifice in mm Hg. The constants 44.5 and 38.0 incorporate the effects of the viscous resistance to flow and turbulent flow. The flow through the valve is calculated from:

$$\text{Flow (ml/sec)} = \frac{\text{cardiac output (ml/min)}}{\text{DFP (sec/min) or SEP (sec/min)}} \qquad (10\text{-}6)$$

where DFP is the diastolic filling period and SEP is the systolic ejection period.

REGURGITANT FRACTION

The aortic or mitral valve regurgitant fraction can be calculated from the ventriculographic stroke volume and the Fick stroke volume. The ventriculographic stroke volume, derived from the difference between the end-diastolic and end-systolic volumes, represents the total stroke volume, or the combination of the forward and regurgitant volumes. The Fick stroke volume represents the forward stroke volume. The difference between the ventriculographic volume and the Fick volume is the regurgitant stroke volume. The regurgitant fraction (RF) is defined as:

$$RF = \frac{\text{Ventriculographic SV} - \text{Fick SV}}{\text{Ventriculographic SV}} \qquad (10\text{-}7)$$

Regurgitant fractions greater than 30 percent have been considered to be hemodynamically important.

CORONARY SINUS FLOW

Coronary sinus blood flow may be calculated using thermodilution.[220] The thermodilution catheter is advanced into the coronary sinus from the right antecubital vein. From temperature measurements of the injectate, the downstream blood, and the body, flow can be determined using standard formulae.[220] Coronary sinus flow can also be determined using inert gases (xenon-133) injected into the coronary artery and recording the radioactivity washout with a scintillation camera. Regional myocardial blood flow can be derived from the radioactivity curve, the partition coefficient of the isotope in myocardial tissue, and the specific gravity of the myocardial tissue.

Ventriculography Measurements

Left ventriculography is usually performed following hemodynamic measurements and prior to coronary arteriography. With the catheter positioned beneath the mitral valve leaflets, a test injection of approximately 10–15 ml of contrast is given over a 1-second period. The ventriculogram is then performed in either the 30° right anterior oblique projection alone, or in combination with a 60° left anterior oblique projection. Approximately 35 ml of contrast material, containing diatrizoate meglumine, and diatrizoate sodium (Renografin-76, E.R. Squibb & Sons, Princeton, NJ) is injected into the left ventricle over 3 to 4 seconds. The diastolic and systolic phases of the ventricular cycle are recorded on 35 mm cine film.

End-diastolic and end-systolic volume measurements can be made using the area-length method, based on formulae developed by Dodge.[221] Both single-plane and biplane volume determinations can be measured using:

$$V = \frac{4}{3} \times \frac{L}{2} \times \frac{D_a}{2} \times \frac{D_b}{2} \qquad (10\text{-}8)$$

where V is volume (ml), L is the major axis length (cm), and D_a and D_b are the minor axis lengths (cm) in the right or left anterior oblique projections. A number of modifications of this formula are used and are summarized by Rackley.[221] Ventriculographic stroke volume can be calculated as the difference between the end-diastolic and the end-systolic volumes. Cardiac output is the product of stroke volume times heart rate, and ejection fraction is the ratio of stroke volume to end-diastolic volume. The normal values for these variables are shown in Table 10-8.

Ventriculography is also used to estimate the velocity of circumferential fiber shortening, the mean ejection rate, wall thickness, left ventricular mass, and stress.[221,222]

Segmental wall motion abnormalities are visualized and may be quantitated from ventriculography. Ventricular dyssynergy includes a number of abnormal contraction patterns, namely, hypokinesis, akinesis, dyskinesis, and hyperkinesis. These abnormalities are shown in Figure 10-13. Quantitation of these abnormalities can be performed using several techniques, including calculation of hemiaxial shortening, "area" ejection fraction, and the percentage of dyssynergic segments.[221,223] These methods involve the superposition of the ventricular silhouettes at end-systole and end-diastole, and can be performed manually or with computerized image processing systems.[224] An example of axis-shortening calculations is shown in Figure 10-14.

Biplane ventriculography is performed in patients who have had a previous MI, cardiomegaly, or congestive heart failure, since these patients have a greater number of wall motion abnormalities and require more comprehensive wall motion studies. Intervention ventriculography (two-state or dynamic ventriculography) is performed to determine latent ventricular dysfunction or contractile reserve. Latent ventricular dysfunction is assessed by inducing myocardial ischemia using atrial pacing or dynamic

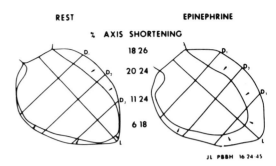

Fig. 10-14. The change in axis shortening with administration of epinephrine is demonstrated. The percent axial shortening is shown for three minor axes (D_1, D_2, and D_3) and the long axis (L). (From Horn HR, Teichholz LE, Cohn PF, et al: Augmentation of left contraction pattern in coronary artery disease by an inotropic catecholamine. The epinephrine ventriculogram. Circulation 49:1063, 1974, with permission.)

or static exercise. With myocardial ischemia, new segmental wall motion abnormalities occur and may cause decreased left ventricular performance (depressed ejection fraction). The hemodynamic significance of an obstructive coronary artery lesion can be assessed using this technique. The contractile reserve of the left ventricle can be assessed using inotropic stimulation (catecholamine infusion, postextrasystolic potentiation) or by decreasing preload (nitroglycerin). Following the infusion of epinephrine, a second ventriculogram is performed, and wall motion contractile patterns are compared. Postextrasystolic potentiation is performed by inducing a premature contraction via manipulation of the right heart catheter, or by pacemaker R wave triggering. Ventricular unloading is assessed using 0.4 mg of nitroglycerin sublingually to determine the reversibility of dyssynergy.

COMPARISON OF MEASURES OF MYOCARDIAL FUNCTION

The relative specificity and sensitivity of these measurements has been studied in 317 patients with CAD, but not valvular heart disease.[225] The most specific indices were, in order of decreasing specificity, the ejection fraction, degree of dyssynergy, stroke work, end-diastolic volume, end-systolic volume, cardiac index, and end-diastolic pressure. The specificity was greater than 0.80 for all of these indices, with the exceptions of the cardiac output (0.59–0.77) and the end-diastolic pressure (0.53–0.59). In contrast, the sensitivity of these indices, with the exception of ventricular dyssynergy, was low (less than 0.50). From these data, it appears that ventricu-

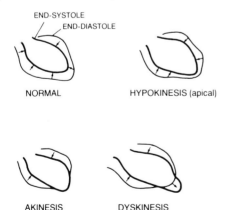

Fig. 10-13. Segmental wall motion abnormalities contrasting normal wall motion with apical hypokinesis, akinesis, and dyskinesis.

lar dysfunction is best predicted by the ejection fraction and the degree of dyssynergy, with abnormalities of these variables commonly associated with abnormalities in ventricular output (cardiac output, stroke work), filling (end-diastolic volume, end-diastolic pressure), and ejection (end-systolic volume). Abnormality of the stroke work index, end-diastolic volume, and end-systolic volume appear to be good indicators of ventricular dysfunction. Cardiac output is a marginal index, being associated with normality of the other indices 23–41 percent of the time.

Coronary Arteriography

After ventriculography, the catheter is removed and is replaced by either a Sones or Judkins catheter. With the Sones technique, the catheter is advanced into the aorta via a right brachial arteriotomy; with the Judkins technique, the femoral artery is directly punctured using a Seldinger needle, and the catheter is advanced into the aorta. Typical arteriograms are

illustrated in Figure 10-15 for four standard views. The normal dimensions of the right coronary artery are 3.7 ($\pm$1.1) mm by 2.4 ($\pm$0.9) mm. The dimensions of the left coronary artery are 4.7 ($\pm$1.2) mm by 3.2 ($\pm$1.1) mm. Lesions involving less than 50 percent of the luminal diameter (approximately 75 percent of the cross-sectional area) are usually not hemodynamically significant. Those involving 75 percent or more of the luminal diameter are considered significant. However, White has recently questioned the accuracy of coronary artery visualization.[226]

The degree of stenosis can be estimated by comparison of the vessel widths of the stenotic and prestenotic (normal) segments, using angled projections to enhance visualization of the coronary system. A number of quantification and coding systems have been developed, and computer-assisted programs have been introduced.[227]

Coronary collaterals are usually not detected in normal hearts. Coronary arteries typically lie freely on the epicardial surface of the heart. Coronary anas-

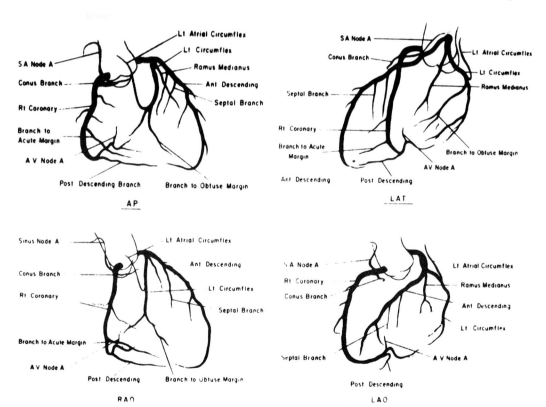

Fig. 10-15. An illustration of normal coronary arteriograms in four standard views: Anteroposterior (AP), lateral (LAT), right anterior oblique (RAO), and left anterior oblique (LAO). (From Abrams H, Adams DF: The coronary arteriogram: Structural and functional aspects. N Engl J Med 281:1277, 1969, with permission.)

tomoses, when visualized, are either intercoronary or intersegmental. An intercoronary anastomosis usually involves two of the three principal coronary arteries, while the intersegmental anastomosis joins two points along the same artery.

INTERVENTIONAL TECHNIQUES

Coronary artery spasm may be induced using ergonovine maleate, as well as morphine, alpha- and beta-stimulants and blockers, and cholinergic and anticholinergic agents.

Coronary artery spasm was first noted in 1960 by Prinzmetal,[98] who described spontaneous spasm and resolution of that spasm with the administration of sublingual nitrate. In addition to Prinzmetal's angina, spasm may also occur with fixed coronary obstructions, or it may be iatrogenically produced by catheter manipulation.

Intracoronary thrombolysis was first induced in 1976, with the administration of fibrinolysin during an acute MI.[228,229] Later, streptokinase was introduced for use in thrombotic occlusion during the evolving stage of an acute MI. Rentrop reported recanalization of occluded arteries in over 75 percent of patients during the acute stages of an MI.[230] Schwarz et al demonstrated that the success of this procedure is related to the duration of ischemia, and suggested that early recognition and prompt treatment enhance the success.[231]

Transluminal coronary angioplasty was first developed by Gruentzig et al in 1977.[232] The technique appears to be most useful in patients with recent onset angina and a single, proximal concentric stenosis of a major epicardial coronary artery. More recently, higher risk subgroups have undergone angioplasty, including those with multivessel disease, distal stenoses, eccentric and calcified lesions, and those with prior coronary bypass surgery or an evolving MI.[232-236] A typical technique involves pretreatment with nifedipine (20 mg sublingual) for coronary spasm, and advancement of the #8 French catheter into the coronary ostium. Following diagnostic angiograms, intracoronary nitroglycerin (200 μg) is injected. Anticoagulation is monitored throughout the procedure to prevent thrombotic complications. Following insertion of the guiding catheter, a dilating catheter system is introduced. The inflated balloon diameter varies from 2.0 to 4.0 mm in diameter, and is usually 25 mm in length. The initial inflations are performed for 10 to 20 seconds. Patients are monitored, and signs of chest pain or ST elevation are noted. Repeat inflations are performed with increasing pressures until hemodynamic and angiographic results occur. A gradient across the stenosis of 15 mm Hg or less is attempted.

Dorros et al studied 3079 patients undergoing coronary angioplasty.[237] The mean age of the population was 54 years, with 26 percent of the patients in Canadian heart-class IV and 37 percent in Canadian heart-class III. Of the patients, 73 percent had single-vessel disease, with 64 percent of these involving the left anterior descending artery. The success rate was 65 percent, the complication rate was 20 percent, and the mortality rate was 0.8 percent. The morbid outcomes included coronary dissection, occlusion or spasm (10.4 percent), MI (5.5 percent), ventricular tachycardia (2.3 percent), and prolonged angina (6.7 percent). One year after angioplasty, 72 percent, or 1397 patients, exhibited a successful result and did not require repeat angioplasty or coronary artery bypass; 12 percent of these patients required repeat dilation.

Magnetic Resonance Imaging

Magnetic resonance imaging, used to characterize molecular structures, has recently been shown to provide high-resolution tomographic and three-dimensional images of the heart. In addition, spectroscopic information can quantify metabolic derangements. Although this method is costly, it is a safe form of imaging since it does not require the use of ionizing radiation.

Certain nuclei with an odd number of protons and neutrons have an intrinsic net nuclear spin. The spinning charged nucleus generates a magnetic field, which can be imaged. Photons, carbon-13, sodium-23, and phosphorus-31 nuclei exhibit such magnetic moments and are used for magnetic imaging. The concentration of these magnetic nuclei in a sample can be determined by placing the sample in an external magnetic field. Prior to placement in the magnetic field, the magnetic moments are randomly oriented. After placement, magnetic moments are aligned either in the same or opposite direction as the field. This results in a macroscopic magnetic moment, whose magnitude is related to the concentration of the magnetic nuclei (such as phosphorus-31) in the sample.

Magnetic resonance imaging, unlike computed tomography, can be gated to the cardiac cycle, allowing assessment of left ventricular function.[238] Ischemic insults to the heart may also be detected since prolonged ischemia affects proton relaxation parameters. Increased signal intensities in ischemic regions appear to be associated with lipid accumulation, edema, and fibrosis. Magnetic resonance may allow characterization of ischemia and quantification of its extent. Recent advances include a proton imaging technique, which allows acquisition of the entire image in less than 100 msec;[239] and sodium-23 images, characterizing the blood pool in the isolated beating rat heart.[240] Phosphorus-31 spectroscopy will enable quantitation of the turnover of high-energy phosphates and the accumulation of inorganic phosphorus in acutely ischemic tissue.

Magnetic resonance imaging is of particular interest at present, and it is feasible that several noninvasive tests will be performed using this approach, including quantification of ventricular volumes and mass, coronary angiography, myocardial perfusion imaging, and metabolic assessment of ischemic segment function, using high-energy phosphate turnover and intracellular pH calculations.

APPENDIX A

Preoperative Tests: Indications And Findings For Specific Diseases

In the previous section, the most important findings of the preoperative tests for ischemic heart disease were discussed in detail. In this section, the specific findings of the preoperative tests for selected other cardiac diseases are detailed (valvular heart disease, mitral valve prolapse, cardiomyopathy, adult congenital heart disease, pulmonary thromboembolism, and pericardial effusion). In addition, the general features of these tests for ischemic heart disease are outlined for completeness. For those tests that are nonroutine (exercise stress testing, echocardiography, radionuclide imaging, and cardiac catheterization), specific indications are outlined.

ISCHEMIC HEART DISEASE

Clinical history
1. Stability of angina
   a. stable versus unstable (new, crescendo, rest)
   b. exercise tolerance
   c. maintenance medications
2. Ventricular dysfunction
   a. NYHA classification
   b. exercise tolerance
3. Associated cardiovascular diseases
   a. cerebral, carotid, aortic
   b. low output syndromes
   c. dysrhythmia symptoms (palpitations)

4. Medications
   a. history
   b. current medications
   c. effectiveness
Physical examination
1. Vital signs
   a. blood pressure (orthostatic changes, extremity variation)
   b. pulse (radial, carotid, femoral; regularity)
2. Cardiac examination
   a. Displaced PMI: Cardiomegaly (decreased ejection fraction)
   b. S_3, S_4: S_3 (increased LVEDP), S_4 (decreased compliance)
   c. Apical systolic murmur: papillary muscle dysfunction (infarction, ischemia)
   d. Precordial systolic bulge: Left-ventricular wall motion abnormality (ischemia, infarction)
   e. Other ventricular dysfunction signs: Mitral regurgitation, JVD, HJ reflux, pulmonary signs
Laboratory
1. CK, LD: Rule-out myocardial infarction
2. Associated diseases: Diabetes, thyroid
Chest radiograph
1. Cardiomegaly (decreased ejection fraction)
2. Signs of ventricular dysfunction
   a. increased pulmonary vascular markings
   b. edema (interstitial, alveolar)
   c. effusions
3. Complicating diseases
   a. hypertension
   b. calcified aorta, valves, coronaries
   c. cardiomyopathy
   d. pulmonary disease
Electrocardiogram
1. Previous myocardial infarction
   a. Q waves (significance, location)
   b. persistent ST depression (location, extent)
   c. new LBBB
2. Myocardial ischemia
   a. comparison with previous ECG
   b. ST-T wave (character, location, reciprocal changes)
   c. ST elevation (Prinzmetal's angina, aneurysm, pericardial disease)
3. Conduction abnormalities
   a. LBBB
   b. Mobitz 2
   c. third-degree heart block, complete heart block
   d. multifascicular blocks

4. Dysrhythmias
   a. comparison with previous ECG, rhythm strip, ambulatory monitor, stress test
5. Ventricular hypertrophy
   a. voltage
   b. strain criteria
6. Effects of medications
   a. digitalis
   b. propranolol
   c. nitrates
   d. calcium channel blockers

Ambulatory monitoring: indications
1. Dysrhythmias
   a. supraventricular and ventricular tachycardias, multifocal PVCs on ECG or rhythm strip
   b. hypoperfusion symptoms
2. Myocardial ischemia
   a. unstable angina
   b. silent ischemia (preoperative ECG)

Information
1. Dysrhythmias
   a. type
   b. incidence
   c. symptoms
   d. response to therapy
2. Ischemia
   a. incidence
   b. symptoms
   c. relation to exercise

Exercise stress testing: indications
1. Atypical chest pain: Confirmation of ischemic heart disease
2. Progression of ischemic heart disease: Comparison with prior tests when symptoms worsen
3. Medical therapy: Effectiveness of pharmacologic treatment

Information
1. Positiveness of test
   a. duration
   b. ST response
   c. symptoms
   d. hypotension
   e. recovery characteristics
   f. termination (heart rate versus symptoms)
2. Heart rate and blood pressure during symptoms: Maximum tolerated heart rate and blood pressure for perioperative guidelines
3. LV dysfunction: Hypotension or congestion with exercise or ischemia (systolic versus diastolic dysfunction)
4. Dysrhythmias
   a. exercise versus recovery
   b. response to medications

5. Medications: Effective therapies for treatment of ischemia, dysfunction, and dysrhythmia complications

Echocardiography: Indications
1. Myocardial infarction: For diagnosis when ECG/enzymes are noninterpretable
2. Ventricular function: When function is unknown especially prior to aortic (major third space) surgery

Information
1. Segmental wall motion abnormalities—diagnosis of MI
   a. type (hypokinesis, akinesis, dyskinesis)
   b. location (anterior, septal, lateral, apical, inferior, posterior)
2. Wall thickening abnormalities—diagnosis of MI
   a. degree (decreased thickening versus thinning)
   b. location
3. Ejection fraction, V_{cf}: Quantitation of ventricular function
4. Associated diseases
   a. ventricular hypertrophy
   b. valvular
   c. pericardial

Nuclear imaging: indications
1. Myocardial infarction—diagnosis: Principal tests when ECG, history and enzymes are equivocal
2. Myocardial ischemia—Stress testing: Thallium-201
3. Ventricular function: When function is unknown (major third space, aortic surgery)
4. Prediction of surgical outcome: Dipyridamole thallium (selected major aortic surgery)

Information
1. Perfusion abnormality: Thallium-201 diagnosis of myocardial infarction
   Uptake abnormality: Technetium pyrophosphate diagnosis of myocardial infarction
2. Reperfusion abnormality: Dipyridamole thallium: Reversibility of ischemia (degree, location)
3. Ejection fraction, end-diastolic/systolic volumes: Determination of ventricular function

Cardiac catheterization: indications
1. Progressive angina
   a. unstable
   b. medically refractory
2. Chest pain
   a. atypical
   b. Prinzmetal's

3. Ventricular dysfunction: With ischemic heart disease (with/without symptoms)
4. Left main coronary disease
5. Post-cardiac surgery
6. Interventional techniques
   a. angioplasty
   b. thrombolysis

Information
1. Atherosclerotic lesions
   a. lesion extent
   b. occlusion degree
   c. location
   d. collateral flow
   e. vessel dominance

Ventricular function
1. EF, ESV, EDV
2. ΔEDP, SW, CO, EDP (all obtained at a specific EDV, SVR, HR)
3. Segmental wall motion abnormalities—diagnosis of myocardial infarction/new ischemia
   a. extent
   b. location
   c. response to therapy
4. Associated diseases
   a. valvular
   b. cardiomyopathy

VALVULAR HEART DISEASE

Five types of valvular heart disease are outlined: mitral stenosis (MS), mitral regurgitation (MR), mitral valve prolapse (MVP), aortic stenosis (AS), and aortic regurgitation (AR). For each of these, the typical findings of the preoperative cardiac tests will be presented.

Clinical history
MS: Dyspnea, orthopnea, hemoptysis, thromboembolism, infective endocarditis
MR: Fatigue, dyspnea, orthopnea
MVP: Usually asymptomatic; anxiety, palpitations, chest discomfort, fatigue (with MR)
AS: Angina, syncope, dyspnea, orthopnea
AR: Fatigue, dyspnea, orthopnea, palpitations

Physical examination
MS: Increased JVP a wave (sinus rhythm), RV lift; increased P_2; diastolic murmur—low pitched, and rumbling murmur at apex; opening snap
MR: Cardiomegaly; hyperdynamic PMI; holosystolic murmur—blowing high-pitched, loudest at apex; radiation to axilla
MVP: Marfanoid, systolic click (nonejection), holosystolic murmur (with severe regurgitation)

AS: Pulsus parvus, tardus, alternans; increased JVP a wave; sustained PMI; midsystolic ejection murmur—at base transmitted along carotid vessels and to apex
AR: De Musset's sign (head bob), Corrigan's pulse (water hammer), bisferians pulse, cardiomegaly, diffuse—hyperdynamic PMI, holodiastolic murmur—left sternal border, Austin Flint murmur (mid-to-late diastolic decrescendo rumble)

Laboratory
1. No specific laboratory findings unless associated diseases are present (thromboembolism, coagulation abnormalities).

Chest radiograph
MS: Enlarged atrial appendage—left atrium (lateral film), pulmonary hypertension, interstitial edema (Kerley B lines), right ventricular enlargement
MR: Cardiomegaly, left atrial enlargement, interstitial edema, calcification of mitral annulus
MVP: Signs with MR (see above)
AS: Mild cardiomegaly, post-stenotic dilation of ascending aorta, calcification of aortic valve
AR: Cardiomegaly, dilation of the ascending aorta

Electrocardiogram
MS: Left atrial enlargement ($P > 0.12$ seconds—lead II), atrial fibrillation, right ventricular hypertrophy (axis > 80 degrees, $R/S > 1.0$ in V_1)
MR: Left atrial enlargement, atrial fibrillation
MVP: Usually normal; ST-T wave abnormalities in II, III, and aVF; paroxysmal supraventricular tachycardia, other dysrhythmias
AS: Left ventricular hypertrophy, pseudoinfarction pattern.
AR: Left axis deviation, pseudoinfarction pattern in I, aVL, $V_3 - V_6$ (Q waves), intraventricular conduction defects, 1st degree AV block (inflammatory AR)

Ambulatory monitoring
Useful for delineation of dysrhythmias, particularly with mitral valve disease

Exercise stress testing
Not routinely useful

Echocardiography
MS: M-mode: Annular calcification
    2-D: Orifice size, left atrial enlargement, normal or decreased left ventricular cavity, left atrial thrombus

2-D: Left atrial enlargment, left ventricular enlargement, etiology (rheumatic versus chordae tendinae damage, MVP, flail leaflets, vegetations), calcification

Pulsed Doppler: Regurgitant flow, orifice size

MVP: M-mode: Abrupt posterior leaflet motion, question mark sign, hammock sign

2D: Diagnosis—leaflet position and motion, left atrium (four chamber view)

AS: M-mode: Thickened leaflets, diminished orifice, calcific size (multiple echos)

2D: Severity (wall thickness/chamber radius)

Doppler: Flow, severity of the stenosis

AR: M-mode: Increased end-diastolic and systolic shortening

2D: Increased septal and posterior wall motion, etiology

Doppler: Flow, regurgitant orifice size

Nuclear imaging

MS: RV function, pulmonary transit time

MR: End-systolic volume, regurgitant fraction

MVP: Exercise thallium imaging (stress scintigraphy) for atypical chest pain

AS: Associated coronary artery disease

AR: End-systolic volume, regurgitant fraction

Cardiac catheterization

MS: Valve area, pulmonary hypertension, right ventricular function

MR: End-systolic volume, regurgitant fraction, left atrial compliance, pulmonary hypertension, right ventricular involvement

MVP: Only with severe MR (See above)

AS: Valve area, ventricular function, associated coronary artery disease

AR: End systolic volume, regurgitant fraction

CONGENITAL HEART DISEASE IN THE ADULT

Three congenital heart diseases in the adult will be considered—atrial septal defect (ASD), ventricular septal defect (VSD) and pulmonic stenosis (PS). Considerations for aortic stenosis are outlined above, and considerations for other congenital diseases in adults and children are discussed in Chapter 17.

Clinical history

ASD: Fatigue, dyspnea

VSD: Fatigue, dyspnea

PS: Fatigue, dyspnea, chest pain

Physical examination

ASD: Prominent RV impulse, mid-systolic pulmonary ejection murmur, split-second heart sound

VSD: Harsh holosystolic murmur (left sternal border) 5th interspace, transmitted over entire precordium

PS: Cardiomegaly, RV parasternal lift, increased JVP a wave, S_4, systolic ejection murmur (upper left sternal border—expiration)

Laboratory tests

Not specific

Chest radiograph

ASD: Prominent peripheral pulmonary vascular bed; late—pulmonary hypertension and decreased peripheral bed, calcification of pulmonary artery

VSD: Usually normal with large VSD; increased pulmonary vascular markings; late—pulmonary hypertension

PS: Post-stenotic dilation of pulmonary arteries, RA and RV enlargement

Electrocardiogram

ASD: Atrial fibrillation, atrial flutter, PAT, first-degree AV Block, right ventricular hypertrophy (with pulmonary hypertension)

VSD: Usually normal; with large VSD—left ventricular hypertrophy

PS: Right axis deviation, right ventricular hypertrophy (QR, T inversion, ST depression in V_1, V_2; rSR$'$ in V_1; increased P in II, V1)

Ambulatory monitoring

Not routinely performed

Exercise Stress Testing:

Not routinely performed

Echocardiography

ASD: M-mode: RV dilation, decreased LV size, MVP (occasionally detected)

2D: Anatomic type via intraatrial septal imaging

Contrast Echo: Shunt detection

VSD: M-mode: Nondiagnostic

2D: Diagnosis, position of defect

Pulse Doppler: Position, flow

PS: Technically difficult

Nuclear imaging

ASD: Quantification of pulmonary-systemic blood flow

VSD: Quantification of pulmonary-systemic blood flow

PS: Not routinely performed

Cardiac catheterization
ASD: Performed with atypical physical findings; direction of shunt, RV size, degree of pulmonary hypertension
VSD: Direction of shunt, RV size, degree of pulmonary hypertension
PS: Site of obstruction, degree of stenosis, RV function, associated anatomic malformations

CARDIOMYOPATHIES

The preoperative tests for dilated (DCM), restrictive (RCM), and hypertrophic (HCM) cardiomyopathies are outlined in this section.
Clinical history
DCM: Fatigue, LV failure symptoms, embolic symptoms
RCM: Fatigue, RV failure symptoms, systemic disease symptoms (eg, amyloidosis)
HCM: Fatigue, dyspnea, angina, syncopy, palpitations
Physical examination
DCM: Cardiomegaly, S_3, S_4, MR
RCM: Moderate cardiomegaly, S_3, S_4, Kussmaul's sign
HCM: Mild cardiomegaly, apical systolic thrill, S_4, systolic murmur with Valsalva
Laboratory
No specific findings
Chest radiograph
DCM: Cardiomegaly (moderate to severe, increased LV size), pulmonary venous hypertension, congestion
RCM: Cardiomegaly (mild to moderate), pulmonary venous hypertension
HCM: Cardiomegaly (mild), left atrial enlargement
Electrocardiogram
DCM: Sinus tachycardia, dysrhythmias, IV conduction defects, ST-T wave abnormalities
RCM: Low voltage, conduction defects (IV, AV)
HCM: LVH, pseudoinfarction (Q waves), ST-T wave abnormalities, dysrhythmias
Ambulatory monitoring
Not routinely performed
Exercise stress testing
Not routinely performed
Echocardiography
DCM: LV dilation, dysfunction; MR
RCM: Increased LV wall thickness, mass; normal-to-small LV cavity, normal systolic function, pericardial effusions
HCM: Decreased LV outflow, ASH, normal-to-

small LV cavity, abnormal mitral valve motion
Nuclear imaging
DCM: RV dilation, dysfunction
RCM: Normal LV size, function; myocardial infiltration with thallium imaging
HCM: Normal-small LV cavity, enhanced systolic function, ASH
Cardiac catheterization
DCM: LV enlargement, dysfunction; MR, TR; LV failure (increased LVEDP, increased CVP, decreased CO)
RCM: Normal systolic function; decreased compliance (increased LVEDP)
HCM: Enhanced systolic function, MR, decreased LV compliance, dynamic LV outflow gradient

ASSYMETRIC SEPTAL HYPERTROPHY (ASH, IHSS)

See above findings for hypertrophic cardiomyopathy

PULMONARY THROMBOEMBOLISM

Clinical history
Chest pain, dyspnea, apprehension, cough; less frequent—hemoptysis, diaphoresis, syncopy
Physical examination
Tachypnea, rales, increased P_2, tachycardia, fever; less frequent—diaphoresis, phlebitis, cyanosis
Laboratory
Nondiagnostic
Chest radiograph
Usually normal, loss of lung volume (elevated diaphragm), peripheral oligemia, increase in vessel size, tapering of occluded vessel, RV dilation, parenchymal consolidation (infarction)
Electrocardiogram
Conduction disturbances, ST-T wave changes, T wave inversion
Ambulatory monitoring
Not routinely performed
Exercise stress testing
Not routinely performed
Echocardiography
Useful for identification of right atrial or right ventricular thrombus
Nuclear imaging
Not routinely performed; markedly prolonged pulmonary transit time, right ventricular dysfunction
Cardiac catheterization (pulmonary angiography)
The most specific test for diagnosis of pulmonary thromboembolism: Pulmonary arterial cut-off, filling defects in larger arteries, hypovascularity, decreased pulmonary flow

PULMONARY HYPERTENSION

The findings associated with secondary pulmonary hypertension (such as associated with mitral stenosis or congenital heart disease) are discussed above. The following findings refer specifically to primary pulmonary hypertension.

Clinical history

Fatigue, dyspnea, syncopy, chest pain, palpitation; less frequent—cough, hemoptysis

Physical examination

Increased JVP a wave, decreased carotid upstroke, right ventricular lift, systolic ejection murmur, ejection click, S_4; late—hepatomegaly, peripheral edema, ascites, cyanosis

Laboratory

Late—hypercoagulability, abnormal platelet function, abnormal liver function tests

Chest radiograph

Enlargement of the main pulmonary artery and branches, decreased peripheral vessels, RA and RV enlargement

Electrocardiogram

RA and RV enlargement

Ambulatory monitoring

Not routinely performed

Exercise stress testing

At times performed to quantitate the functional significance by the measurement of lactate production during exercise

Pulmonary function tests

Usually normal; arterial blood gas—hyperventilation, PO_2 normal or slightly decreased

Echocardiography

Increased RA, RV, decreased LV, thickened intraventricular septum, abnormal septal motion, MVP (occasional)

Nuclear imaging

Lung scan—usually normal, subsegmental defects occasionally noted.

REFERENCES

1. Hospital Statistics: Data from the American Hospital Association 1981 Annual Survey, Chicago: American Hospital Association, 1982
2. Knapp RB, Topkins MJ, Artusio JF: The cerebrovascular accident and coronary occlusion in anesthesia. JAMA 182:322, 1962
3. Topkins MJ, Artusio JF: Myocardial infarction and surgery: A five-year study. Anesth Analg 43:716, 1964
4. Tarhan S, Moffitt E, Taylor WF, et al: Myocardial infarction after general anesthesia. JAMA 220:1451, 1972
5. Steen PA, Tinker JH, Tarhan S: Myocardial reinfarction after anesthesia and surgery. JAMA 239:2566, 1978
6. Goldman L: Supraventricular tachyarrhythmias in hospitalized adults after surgery. Chest 73:450, 1978
7. Rao TK, Jacobs KH, El-Etr AA: Reinfarction following anesthesia in patients with myocardial infarction. Anesthesiology 59:499, 1983
8. Crawford SE, Bomberger RA, Glaeser DH, et al: Aortoiliac occlusive disease. Factors influencing survival and function following reconstructive operation over a twenty-five year period. Surgery 90:1055, 1981
9. Brown OW, Hollier LH, Pairolero PC, et al: Abdominal aortic aneurysm and coronary artery disease. Arch Surg 116:1484, 1981
10. Rokey R, Rolak LA, Harati Y, et al: Coronary artery disease in patients with cerebrovascular disease. A prospective study. Ann Neurol 16:1, 1984
11. Hicks GL, Eastland MW, DeWeese JA, et al: Survival improvement following aortic aneurysm resection. Ann Surg 181:863, 1975
12. Young AE, Sandberg GW, Couch NP: The reduction of mortality of abdominal aortic aneurysm resection. Am J Surg 134:585, 1977
13. Cooperman M, Pflug B, Martin EW Jr, et al: Cardiovascular risk factors in patients with peripheral vascular disease. Surgery 84:505, 1978
14. Riles TS, Kopelman I, Imparato AM: Myocardial infarction following carotid endarterectomy. A review of 683 operations. Surgery 85:249, 1979
15. Hertzer NR: Fatal myocardial infarction following lower extremity revascularization. Two hundred seventy-three patients followed six to eleven postoperative years. Ann Surg 193:4, 1981
16. Hertzer NR: Myocardial ischemia. Surgery 93:97, 1983
17. Harrison DC: Cost containment in medicine: Why cardiology? Am J Cardiol 56:10C, 1985
18. Kannel WB, McGee D, Gordon T: A general cardiovascular risk profile: The Framingham Study. Am J Cardiol 38:46, 1976
19. Cutler BS, Wheeler HB, Paraskos JA, et al: Applicability and interpretation of electrocardiographic stress testing in patients with peripheral vascular disease. Am J Surg 141:501, 1981

20. Boucher CA, Brewster DC, Darling CR, et al: Determination of cardiac risk by dipryridamole-thallium imaging before peripheral vascular surgery. N Engl J Med 312:389, 1985

21. Kaplan JA, King SB: The precordial electrocardiographic lead (V5) in patients who have coronary artery disease. Anesthesiology 45:570, 1976

22. Kotrly KJ, Kotter GS, Mortara D, et al: Intraoperative detection of myocardial ischemia with an ST segment trend monitoring system. Anesth Analg 63:343, 1984

23. Slogoff S, Keats AS: Does perioperative myocardial ischemia lead to postoperative myocardial infarction? Anesthesiology 62:107, 1985

24. Schluter M, Hinrichs A, Thier W, et al: Transesophageal two-dimensional echocardiography. Comparison of ultrasonic and anatomic sections. Am J Cardiol 53:1173, 1984

25. Coriat P, Daloz M, Bousseau D, et al: Prevention of intraoperative myocardial ischemia during noncardiac surgery with intravenous nitroglycerin. Anesthesiology 61:193, 1984

26. U.S. Department of Health and Human Services. The National Institute on Aging Macroeconomic-Demographic Model. Population Estimates, 1984, pp 59–62

27. Djokovic JL, Hedley-Whyte J: Prediction of outcome of surgery and anesthesia in patients over 80. JAMA 242:2301, 1979

28. Port S, Cobb FR, Coleman RE, et al: Effect of age on the response of the left ventricular ejection fraction of exercise. N Engl J Med 303:1133, 1980

29. Fleg HR, Gerstenblidth G, Lakatta EG: Pathophysiology of the aging in heart and circulation. In Messerli F (ed): Cardiovascular Disease in the Elderly. Boston, Martinus Nijhoff, 1984, pp 11–34

30. Weisfeldt ML: Aging of the cardiovascular system. N Engl J Med 303:1172, 1980

31. Bertrand YM, Boelens D, Collin L, et al: Preoperative assessment in geriatric patients for elective surgery. Acta Anaesthesiol Belg 35 (Suppl): 155, 1984

32. Drucker WR, Gavett JW, Kirshner R, et al: Toward strategies for cost containment in surgical patients. Ann Surg 198:284, 1983

33. Harbrecht PJ, Garrison RN, Fry DE: The impact of demographic trends on hospital surgical care. Am Surg 50:270, 1984

34. Cullen DJ, Ferrara LC, Briggs BA, et al: Survival hospitalization charges and follow-up results in critically ill patients. N Engl J Med 294:982, 1976

35. Roberts AJ, Woodhall DD, Conti CR, et al: Mortality, morbidity, and cost-accounting related to coronary artery bypass graft surgery in the elderly. Ann Thorac Surg 39:426, 1985

36. Greenberg AG, Saik RP, Pridham D: Influence of age on mortality of colon surgery. Am J Surg 150:65, 1985

37. Mohr DN: Estimation of surgical risk in the elderly: A correlative review. J Am Geriatr Soc 31:99, 1983

38. Gerstienblidth G, Lakatta EG, Weisfeldt ML: Age changes in myocardial function and exercise response. Prog Cardiovasc Dis 19:1, 1976

39. Plumlee JE, Boetner RB: Myocardial infarction during and following anesthesia and operation. South Med J 65:886, 1972

40. Goldman L: Cardiac risks and complications of noncardiac surgery. Ann Intern Med 98:504, 1983

41. Wells P, Kaplan JA: Optimal management of patients with ischemic heart disease for noncardiac surgery by complementary anesthesiologist and cardiologist interaction. Am Heart J 102:1029, 1981

42. Diamond GA, Forrester JS: Analysis of probability as an aid in the clinical diagnosis of coronary artery disease. N Engl J Med 300:1350, 1979

43. Cohn PF, Gorlin R, Cohn LH, et al: Left ventricular ejection fraction as a prognostic guide in surgical treatment of coronary and valvular heart disease. Am J Cardiol 34:136, 1979

44. Moraski RE, Russell RO, Smith M, et al: Left ventricular function in patients with and without myocardial infarction and one, two or three vessel coronary artery disease. Am J Cardiol 35:1, 1975

45. Goldman L, Caldera DL, Nussbaum SR, et al: Multifactorial index of cardiac risk in noncardiac surgical procedures. N Engl J Med 297:845, 1977

46. Pasternack PF, Imparato AM, Riles TS, et al: The value of radionuclide angiogram in prediction of perioperative myocardial infarction in patients undergoing lower extremity revascularization procedures. Circulation 70:II–163, 1984

47. Schultz RA, Strauss HW, Pitt B: Sudden death in the year following myocardial infarction. Relation to ventricular premature contractions in the last hospital phase and left ventricular ejection fraction. Am J Med 62:192, 1976

48. Vismara LA, Amsterdam EA, Mason DT: Relation of ventricular arrhythmias in the late hospital phase of acute myocardial infarction to sudden death after hospital discharge. Am J Med 59:6, 1975

49. Olson HG, Lyons KP, Troope P, et al: The high-risk acute myocardial infarction patients at 1-year follow-up: Identification at hospital discharge by ambulatory electrocardiography and radionuclide ventriculography. Am Heart J 107:358, 1984

50. Kannel WB, Sorlie P: Hypertension in Framingham. In Paul O (ed): Epidemiology and Control of Hypertension. Miami, FL: Symposia Specialist, 1975, pp 553–593

51. Pooling Project Research Group: Relationship of blood pressure, serum cholesterol, smoking habit, relative weight and ECG abnormalities to incidence of major coronary events. Final report of the Pooling Project. J Chronic Dis 31:201, 1978

52. Waller BF, Palumbo PJ, Lie JT, et al: Status of the coronary arteries at necropsy in diabetes mellitus

with onset after age 30 years: Analysis of 229 diabetic patients with and without clinical evidence of coronary heart disease and comparison to 183 control subjects. Am J Med 69:498, 1980

53. Rennart G, Saltz-Rennart H, Wanderman K, et al: Size of acute myocardial infarcts in patients with diabetes mellitus. Am J Cardiol 55:1629, 1985

54. Beard OW, Hipp HR, Robins M, et al: Survival in myocardial infarction. Am Heart J 73:317, 1967

55. Kannel WB, McGee DL: Diabetes and cardiovascular risk factors: The Framingham Study. Circulation 59:8, 1979

56. Abenavoli T, Rubler S, Fisher VJ, et al: Exercise testing with myocardial scintigraphy in asymptomatic diabetic males. Circulation 63:1, 1981

57. Chiarello M, Indolfi C, Cotecchia MR, et al: Asymptomatic transient ST changes during ambulatory ECG monitoring in diabetic patients. Am Heart J 110:539, 1985

58. Cruse PJ, Foord R: A 5-year prospective study of 23,649 surgical wounds. Arch Surg 107:206, 1973

59. Anderson RJ, Schafer LA, Olin DB: Infectious risk factors in the immunosuppressed host. Am J Med 54:453, 1973

60. Von Knorring JV: Postoperative myocardial infarction: A prospective study in a risk group of surgical patients. Surgery 90:55, 1981

61. Hertzer NR: Fatal myocardial infarction following peripheral vascular operations: A study of 951 patients followed 6 to 11 years postoperatively. Cleve Clin Q 49:1, 1982

62. Skinner JF, Pearce ML: Surgical risk in the cardiac patient. J Chronic Dis 17:57, 1964

63. Jensen D, Blankenhorn DH, Kornerup V: Coronary disease in familial hypercholesterolemia. Circulation 36:77, 1967

64. Goldstein JL, Brown MS: The LDL receptor defect in familiar hypercholesterolemia: Implications for pathogenesis and therapy. Med Clin North Am 66:335, 1982

65. Forman MB, Kinsley RH, Duplessis JP: Surgical correction of combined supravalvular and valvular aortic stenosis in homozygous familial hypercholesterolemia. S Afr Med J 61:579, 1982

66. Nicod P, Rehr P, Winniford MD, et al: Acute systemic and coronary hemodynamic and serologic responses to cigarette smoking in long-term smokers with atherosclerotic coronary artery disease. J Am Coll Cardiol 4:964, 1984

67. Klein LW: Cigarette smoking, atherosclerosis and the coronary hemodynamic response: A unifying hypothesis. J Am Coll Cardiol 4:972, 1984

68. Pearce AC, Jones RM: Smoking and anesthesia. Preoperative abstinence and perioperative morbidity. Anesthesiology 61:576, 1984

69. Carliner NH, Fisher ML, Plotnick GD, et al: Routine preoperative exercise testing in patients undergoing major norcardiac surgery. Am J Cardiol 56:51, 1985

70. Mangano DT, Hedgcock M, Wisneski JA. Predictive value of the chest radiograph in patients with coronary artery disease. Anesthesiology (In press).

71. Weyman AE, Franklin TD, Egenes KM, et al: Correlation between extent of abnormal regional wall motion and myocardial infarct size in chronically infarcted dogs. Circulation 56:72, 1977

72. Ross J: Myocardial ischemia. In Rosen MR, Hoffman BF (eds): Cardiac Therapy. Boston, Martinus Nijhoff, 1983, pp 45-71

73. Heger JJ, Weyman AE, Wann SL, et al: Cross-sectional echocardiographic analysis of the extent of left ventricular asynergy in acute myocardial infarction. Circulation 61:1113, 1980

74. Burggraf GW, Parker JO: Prognosis in coronary disease: Angiographic, hemodynamic and clinical factors. Circulation 51:146, 1975

75. Heger JJ, Weyman AE, Wann LS, et al: Cross-sectional echocardiography in acute myocardial infarction. Detection and localization of regional left ventricular asynergy. Circulation 60:531, 1979

76. Bloch A, Morard J, Mayor C, et al: Cross-sectional echocardiography in acute myocardial infarction. Am J Cardiol 43:387, 1979

77. Drobar M: Complicated acute myocardial infarction. The importance of two-dimensional echocardiography. Am J Cardiol 43:387, 1979

78. Topol EJ, Weiss JL, Guzman PA, et al: Immediate improvement of dysfunctional myocardial segments after coronary revascularization: Detection by intraoperative transesophageal echocardiography. J Am Coll Cardiol 4:1123, 1984

79. Lieberman AN, Weiss JL, Jugdutt B, et al: Two-dimensional echocardiography and infarct size: Relationship of regional wall motion and thickening to the extent of myocardial infarction in the dog. Circulation 63:739, 1981

80. Neuhauser D: Cost-effective clinical decision making. Pediatrics 60:756, 1977

81. Sagal SS, Evens RG, Forrest JV, et al: Efficacy of routine screening and lateral chest radiographs in a hospital-based population. N Engl J Med 291:1001, 1974

82. Rees AM, Roberts CJ, Bligh AS: Routine preoperative chest radiography in noncardiopulmonary surgery. Br Med J 1:1333, 1976

83. Dripps RD, Lamont A, Eckenhoff JE: New classification of physical status. Anesthesiology 24:111, 1963

84. Braunwald E: The history. In Braunwald E (ed): Heart Disease: A Textbook of Cardiovascular Medicine. Philadelphia, W.B. Saunders, 1984, pp 1-13

85. Coronary Artery Surgery Study (CASS): Manual of Operations II: Data Collection and Storage. Collaborative Studies in Coronary Artery Surgery. Washington, D.C.: National Heart, Lung and Blood Institute, prepared by the CASS Coordinating Center, University of Washington, Seattle, 1978

86. Vacanti CJ, Van Houten RJ, Hill RC: A statistical

analysis of the relationship of physical status to post-operative mortality in 68,388 cases. Anesth Analg 49:564, 1970

87. Lewin I, Lerner AG, Green SH: Physical class and physiological status in the prediction of operative mortality in the aged sick. Ann Surg 174:217, 1971

88. Jeffrey CC, Kunsman J, Cullen DJ, et al: A prospective evaluation of cardiac risk index. Anesthesiology 58:462, 1983

89. Gage AA, Bhayana JN, Balu V, et al: Assessment of cardiac risk in surgical patients. Arch Surg 112:1488, 1977

90. Cutler BS, Wheeler HB, Paraskos JA, et al: Assessment of operative risk with electrocardiographic exercise testing in patients with peripheral vascular disease. Am J Surg 137:484, 1979

91. Pasternack PF, Imparato AM, Bear G: The value of radionuclide angiography as a predictor of perioperative myocardial infarction in patients undergoing abdominal aortic aneurysm resection. J Vasc Surg 1:320, 1984

92. Herberden W: Some account of a disorder of the breast. Med Trans Roy Coll Physicians (Lond.) 2:59, 1772

93. Wearn JT: Thrombosis of the coronary arteries, with infarction of the heart. Am J Med Sci 165:250, 1923

94. Mackenzie J: Angina Pectoris. London, Oxford University Press, 1923, pp 115–118

95. Feil H, Siegel ML: Electrocardiographic changes during attacks of angina pectoris. Am J Med Sci 175:255, 1928

96. Master AM, Oppenheimer ET: A simple exercise tolerance test for circulatory efficiency with standard tables for normal individuals. Am J Med Sci 177:223, 1929

97. Sampson JJ, Cheitlin, MD: Pathophysiology and differential diagnosis of cardiac pain. Prog Cardiovasc Dis 13:507, 1971

98. Prinzmetal M, Kennamer R, Merliss R, et al: A variant form of angina pectoris. Am J Med 27:375, 1959

99. Cohn PF: Silent myocardial ischemia as a manifestation of asymptomatic coronary artery disease: What is appropriate therapy? Am J Cardiol 56:28D, 1985

100. Deanfield JE, Selwyn AP, Chierchia S, et al: Myocardial ischemia during daily life in patients with stable angina: Its relation to symptoms and heart rate changes. Lancet II:753, 1983

101. Deanfield JE, Ribiero P, Oakley K, et al: Analysis of ST segment changes in normal subjects: Implication for ambulatory monitoring in angina pectoris. Am J Cardiol 54:1321, 1984

102. Deanfield JE, Shea M, Ribiero P, et al: Transient ST-segment depression as a marker of myocardial ischemia during daily life. Am J Cardiol 54:1195, 1984

103. Boyd LD, Werblos SC: Coronary thrombosis without pain. Am J Med Sci 194:814, 1937

104. Lindberg HA, Berkson DM, Stamler J: Totally asymptomatic myocardial infarction: An estimate of its incidence in the living population. Arch Intern Med 106:628, 1960

105. Friedman GD, Kannel WB, Dawber TR: An evaluation of follow-up methods in the Framingham Heart Study. Am J Public Health 57:1015, 1967

106. Gordon T, Moore FE, Shurtleff D: Some methodologic problems in the long-term study of cardiovascular disease: Observation on the Framingham Study. J Chronic Dis 10:186, 1959

107. Johnson WJ, Achor RWP, Burchell HB: Unrecognized myocardial infarction. Arch Intern Med 163:253, 1954

108. Kennedy JA: The incidence of myocardial infarction without pain in autopsied cases. Am Heart J 14:703, 1937

109. Cohn PF: Severe asymptomatic coronary artery disease. A diagnostic, prognostic and therapeutic puzzle. Am J Med 62:565, 1977

110. Gorham LW, Martin SJ: Coronary artery occlusion with and without pain. Arch Intern Med 112:821, 1938

111. Herrick JB: Clinical features of sudden obstruction of the coronary arteries. JAMA 59:2015, 1912

112. Stroud WD, Wagner JA: Silent or atypical coronary occlusion. Ann Intern Med 15:25, 1941

113. Mangano DT: Biventricular function after myocardial revascularization in humans: Deterioration and recovery patterns during the first 24 hours. Anesthesiology 62:571, 1985

114. Cheng TO: Physical diagnosis of coronary artery disease. Am Heart J 80:716, 1970

115. Cohn PF, Vokonas PS, Williams RA, et al: Diastolic heart sounds and filling waves in coronary artery disease. Circulation 44:196, 1971

116. Cohn PF, Thompson P, Strauss W: Diastolic heart sounds during static (handgrip) exercise in patients with chest pain. Circulation 47:1217, 1973

117. Fischl S, Gorlin R, Herman MV: The intermediate coronary syndrome: Clinical, angiographic and therapeutic aspects. N Engl J Med 288:1193, 1973

118. Martin CE, Shaver JA, Leonard JJ, et al: Physical signs, apexcardiography, phonocardiography and systolic time intervals in angina pectoris. Circulation 46:1098, 1972

119. Spodick DH, Quarry VM: Prevalence of the fourth heart sound by phonocardiography in the absence of cardiac disease. Am Heart J 87:11, 1974

120. Cohn PF, Gabbay SI, Weglicki WB: Serum lipid levels in angiographically defined coronary artery disease. Ann Intern Med 84:241, 1976

121. Gotto AM, Gorry GA, Thompson JR, et al: Relationship between plasma lipid concentration and coronary artery disease in 496 patients. Circulation 56:875, 1977

122. Marcella JJ, Nichols AB, Johnson LL, et al: Exercise-induced myocardial ischemia in patients with coronary artery disease. Lack of evidence for platelet activation or fibrin formation in peripheral venous blood. J Am Coll Cardiol 1:1185, 1983

123. Sobel BE, Shell WE: Serum enzyme determination in the diagnosis and assessment of myocardial infarction. Circulation 45:471, 1972

124. Shell WE, Kjekshus JK, Sobel BE: Quantitative assessment of the extent of myocardial infarction in the conscious dog by means of analysis of serial changes in serum creatine phosphokinase activity. J Clin Invest 50:2614, 1971

125. Grande P, Hansen BF, Christiansen C: Estimation of acute myocardial infarct size in man by serum CK-MB measurements. Circulation 65:756, 1982

126. Weidner N: Laboratory diagnosis of acute myocardial infarct. Usefulness of determination of lactate dehydrogenase (LDH)-1 level and the ratio of LDH-1 to total LDH. Arch Pathol Lab Med 106:375, 1982

127. Collen MF, Feldman R, Sieglaub AB, et al: Dollar cost per positive test for automated multiphasic screening. N Engl J Med 283:459, 1970

128. Bartel AG, Chen JT, Peter RH, et al: The significance of coronary calcification detected by fluoroscopy. A report of 360 patients. Circulation 49:1247, 1974

129. Hamby RI, Tabrah F, Wisoff BF, et al: Coronary artery calcification. Clinical implications and angiographic correlates. Am Heart J 87:565, 1974

130. Mangano DT, Hedgcock MD, Wisneski J: Noninvasive prediction of ventricular dysfunction. Valvular heart disease. Anesthesiology 63(3A):A65, 1985

131. Gorlin R: Coronary Artery Disease. Philadelphia, WB Saunders, 1976, p 177

132. Madias JE: The earliest electrocardiographic sign of acute transmural myocardial infarction. J Electrocardiol 10:193, 1977

133. Dressler W, Roesler H: High T waves in the earliest stage of myocardial infarction. Am Heart J 34:627, 1947

134. Pardee HEB: An electrocardiographic sign of coronary artery obstruction. Arch Intern Med 26:244, 1920

135. Abbott JA, Scheinman MM: Nondiagnostic electrocardiogram in patients with acute myocardial infarction. Clinical and anatomic correlations. Am J Med 55:608, 1973

136. Autenrieth G, Surawicz B, Kuo CS, et al: Primary T wave abnormalities caused by uniform and regional shortening of ventricular monophasic action potential in dog. Circulation 51:668, 1975

137. Einthoven W: Weiteres uber das Elektrokardiogramm. Arch Disch Ges Physiol 172:517, 1908

138. Goldhammer S, Scherf D: Elektrokardiographische Untersuchungen Bei Kranker mit Angina Pectoris ("Ambulatorischer Typus"), Zschr Klin Med 045 122:134, 1933

139. Epstein SE, Beiser GD, Stampfer M, et al: Characterization of the circulatory response to maximal upright exercise in normal subjects and patients with heart disease. Circulation 35:1049, 1967

140. Astrand P, Rodahl K: Evaluation of physical work capacity on the basis of tests. In Textbook of Work Physiology (ed 2). New York, McGraw-Hill, 1977, pp. 331–366

141. Braunwald E, Ross J Jr, Sonnenblick ES: Mechanism of Contraction of the Normal and Failing Heart (ed 3). Boston, Little Brown, 1976, pp 166–200

142. Cannon PJ, Weiss MB, Sciacca RR: Myocardial blood flow in coronary artery disease. Studies at rest and during stress with inert gas washout techniques. Prog Cardiovasc Dis 22:95, 1977

143. Gould KL, Hamilton GW, Lipscomb K, et al: Method for assessing stress-induced regional malperfusion during coronary arteriography. Experimental validation and clinical application. Am J Cardiol 34:557, 1974

144. Logan SE: On the fluid mechanics of human coronary artery stenosis. IEEE Trans Biomed Eng 22:327, 1975

145. Wyatt HL, Forrester JS, Tyberg JV, et al: Effect of graded reductions in regional coronary perfusion on regional and total cardiac function. Am J Cardiol 36:185, 1975

146. Waters DD, Da Luz P, Wyatt HL: Early changes in regional and global left ventricular function induced by graded reduction in regional coronary perfusion. Am J Cardiol 39:537, 1977

147. Braunwald E, Kloner RA: The stunned myocardium. Prolonged postischemic ventricular dysfunction. Circulation 66:1146, 1982

148. Sheffield LT: Exercise stress testing. In Braunwald E (ed): Heart Disease: A Textbook of Cardiovascular Medicine. Philadelphia, WB Saunders, 1984, pp 267–268

149. Hollenberg M, Go M, Massie BM, et al: Influence of R wave amplitude on exercise-induced ST depression: Need for a "gain factor" correction when interpreting stress electrocardiograms. Am J Cardiol 56:13, 1985

150. Erikssen J, Rasmussen K, Forfany K, et al: Exercise ECG and case history in the diagnosis of latent coronary heart disease among presumably healthy middle-aged men. Eur J Cardiol 5:463, 1977

151. Bruce RA, DeRouen TA, Blake B: Maximal exercise predictors of coronary heart disease events among asymptomatic men in Seattle Heart Watch. Circulation 56 (suppl 3):15, 1977

152. Froelicher VF Jr, Yanowitz FG, Thompson AJ, et al: The correlation of coronary angiography and the electrocardiographic response to maximal treadmill testing in 76 asymptomatic men. Circulation 48:597, 1973

153. Goldman S, Tselos S, Cohn K: Marked depth of ST-segment depression during treadmill exercise testing. Indicator of severe coronary artery disease. Chest 69:729, 1976

154. Dagenais GR, Rouleau JR, Christen A, et al: Sur-

vival of patients with a strongly positive exercise electrocardiogram. Circulation 65:452, 1982

155. Weiner DA, McCabe CH, Ryan TJ: Prognostic assessment of patients with coronary artery disease by exercise testing. Am Heart J 105:749, 1983

156. Schneider RM, Seaworth JF, Dohrmann ML, et al: Anatomic and prognostic implications of an early positive treadmill exercise test. Am J Cardiol 50:682, 1982

157. Brody DA: A theoretical analysis of intracavitary blood mass influence on the heart-lead relationship. Circ Res 4:731, 1956

158. Bonoris P, Greenberg PS, Castellanet M, et al: Significance of changes in R wave amplitude during treadmill testing. Angiographic correlation. Am J Cardiol 41:846, 1978

159. Bonoris PE, Greenberg PS, Christison GW, et al: Evaluation of R wave amplitude changes versus ST-segment depression in stress testing. Circulation 57:904, 1978

160. Ellestad MH: Stress Testing: Principles and Practice. Philadelphia: Davis, 1975

161. Morris SN, McHenry PL: Incidence and significance of decreases in systolic blood pressure during graded treadmill exercise testing. Am J Cardiol 41:221, 1978

162. Lepeschkin E, Surawicz B: Characteristics of true-positive and false positive results of electrocardiographic Master two-step exercise tests. N Engl J Med 258:511, 1958

163. Linhart JW, Laws JG, Satinsky JD: Maximum treadmill exercise electrocardiography in female patients. Circulation 50:1173, 1974

164. Riley CP, Oberman A, Shelfield LT: Electrocardiographic effects of glucose ingestion. Arch Intern Med 130:703, 1972

165. Rochmis P, Blackburn H: Exercise tests. A survey of procedures, safety and litigation experience in approximately 170,000 tests. JAMA 217:1061, 1971

166. Feigenbaum H: Echocardiography (ed 3). Philadelphia, Lea and Febiger, 1981

167. Helak JW, Plappert T, Muhammad A: Two dimensional echocardiographic imaging of the left ventricle: Comparison of mechanical and phased array systems in vitro. Am J Cardiol 48:728, 1981

168. Eaton LW, Maughan WL, Shoukas AA, et al: Accurate volume determination in the isolated ejecting canine left ventricle by two-dimensional echocardiography. Circulation 60:4, 1979

169. Folland ED, Parisi AF, Moynihan PF: Assessment of left ventricular ejection fraction and volumes by real-time, two-dimensional echocardiography. Circulation 60:4, 1979

170. Rushmer RF, Baker DW, Stegal HF: Transcutaneous Doppler flow detection as a non-destructive technique. J Appl Physiol 21:554, 1966

171. Lavenson GS, Rich NM, Baugh JH: Value of ultra-sonic flow detection in the management of peripheral vascular disease. Am J Surg 120:522, 1970

172. Sigel B, Popley GL, Boland J, et al: Augmentation of flow sounds in the ultrasonic detection of venous abnormalities. Invest Radiol 2:256, 1967

173. Strandness DE, McCutcheon EP, Rushmer RF: Application of a transcutaneous Doppler flow meter in evaluation of occlusive arterial disease. Surg Gynecol Obstet 122:1039, 1966

174. Block PJ, Popp RL: Two-dimensional echocardiographic assessment of left main coronary artery disease in man (abstract). Circulation 68 (Suppl II): 1463, 1983

175. Rink LD, Feigenbaum H, Godley RW, et al: Echocardiographic detection of left main coronary artery obstruction. Circulation 65:719, 1982

176. Friedman MJ, Sahn DJ, Goldman S, et al: High predictive accuracy for detection of left main coronary artery disease by antilog signal processing of two-dimensional echocardiographic images. Am Heart J 103:194, 1982

177. Corya BC, Rasmussen S, Feigenbaum H, et al: Systolic thickening and thinning of the septum and posterior wall in patients with coronary artery disease, congestive cardiomyopathy and atrial septal defect. Circulation 56:109, 1977

178. Corya B, Rassmussen S, Knoebel SB, et al: Echocardiocardiography in acute myocardial infarction. Am J Cardiol 36:1, 1975

179. Pandian N, Kerber R: Ultrasonic sonomicrometers vs 2-D echocardiography in the detection of transient myocardial dyskinesis. Circulation 62:III, 329, 1980

180. Laurenceau J, Turcot J, Dumesnit J: Echocardiographic evaluation of ventricular wall thickness during acute coronary occlusions in dogs. Circulation (suppl), 59, 60:II, 1979

181. Weiss JL, Becker LC, Bulkley BH, et al: Relationship of systolic thickening to transmural extent of myocardial infarction in the dog. Circulation 62:III, 328, 1980

182. Dodge HT, Sandler H, Ballen DW, et al: The use of biplane angiocardiography for the measurement of left ventricular volume in man. Am Heart J 60:762, 1960

183. Sandler H, Dodge HT: The use of single plane angiocardiograms for the calculation of left ventricular volume in man. Am Heart J 75:325, 1968

184. Dodge HT, Sandler H, Bailey WA, et al: Usefulness and limitations of radiographic methods for determining left ventricular volume. Am J Cardiol 18:10, 1966

185. Carr KW, Engler RL, Forsythe JR, et al: Measurement of left ventricular ejection fraction by mechanical cross-sectional echocardiography. Circulation 59:1196, 1979

186. Wyatt HL, Heng MK, Meerbaum S, et al: Cross-sectional echocardiography: II. Analysis of mathe-

matic models for quantifying volume of formalin fixed left ventricle. Circulation 61:1119, 1980

187. Schiller NB, Acquatella H, Ports TA, et al: Left ventricular volume from paired biplane two-dimensional echocardiography. Circulation 60:547, 1979

188. Rakowski H, Martin RD, Popp RL: Left ventricular function: Assessment by wide angle two-dimensional ultrasonic sector scanning. Acta Med Scand 626 (suppl):104, 1978

189. Blumgart HC, Weiss S: Studies on the velocity of blood flow. VII. The pulmonary circulation time in normal resting individuals. J Clin Invest 4:399, 1927

190. Buja LM, Parkey RW, Dees JH, et al: Morphologic correlates of technetium-99m stannous pyrophosphate imaging of acute myocardial infarcts in dogs. Circulation 52:596, 1975

191. Stokely EM, Buja LM, Lewis SE, et al: Measurement of acute myocardial infarcts in dogs with 99m Tc-stannous pyrophosphate scintigrams. J Nucl Med 17:1, 1975

192. Martin ND, Zaret BL, McGowan RL, et al: Rubidium-81, a new myocardial scanning agent: Noninvasive regional myocardial perfusion scans at rest and exercise and comparison with potassium-43. Radiology 111:651, 1974

193. Zaret BL, Strauss HW, Martin ND, et al: Noninvasive regional myocardial perfusion with radioactive potassium: Study of patients at rest, with exercise and during angina pectoris. N Engl J Med 288:809, 1973

194. Wackers F, Sokole FB, Samson G, et al: Value and limitations of thallium-201 scintigraphy in the acute phase of myocardial infarction. N Engl J Med 295:1, 1976

195. Bailey IK, Griffith LS, Rouleau J, et al: Thallium-201 myocardial perfusion imaging at rest and during exercise: Comparative sensitivity to electrocardiography in coronary artery disease. Circulation 55:79, 1977

196. Ritchie JL, Trobaugh, GB, Hamilton GW, et al: Myocardial imaging with thallium-201 at rest and during exercise. Circulation 56:66, 1977

197. Botvinick EH, Taradash MR, Shames DM: Thallium-201 myocardial perfusion scintigraphy for the clinical clarification of normal, abnormal and equivocal electrocardiographic stress tests. Am J Cardiol 41:43, 1978

198. Marshall RC, Berger HJ, Costin JC, et al: Assessment of cardiac performance with quantitative radionuclide angiocardiography: Sequential left ventricular ejection fraction, normalized left ventricular ejection rate and regional wall motion. Circulation 56:820, 1977

199. Schelbert HR, Verba JW, Johnson AD, et al: Nontraumatic determination of left ventricular ejection fraction by radionuclide angiocardiography. Circulation 51:902, 1975

200. Jengo JA, Mena J, Blaufuss A, et al: Evaluation of left ventricular function (ejection fraction and segmental wall motion) by a single pass radioisotope angiography. Circulation 57:326, 1978

201. Berger HJ, Matthay RA, Loke J, et al: Assessment of cardiac performance with quantitative radionuclide angiocardiography. Right ventricular ejection fraction with reference to findings in chronic obstructive pulmonary disease. Am J Cardiol 41:897, 1978

202. Matthay R, Berger HJ, Loke J, et al: Right and left ventricular performance in cystic fibrosis: Assessment by noninvasive radionuclide angiocardiography. Chest 72:407, 1977

203. Matthay R, Berger H, Gottschalk A, et al: Effects of aminophylline on right and left ventricular performance in chronic obstructive pulmonary disease: Assessment by quantitative radionuclide angiocardiography. Am J Med 65:903, 1978

204. Reduto L, Berger H, Cohen LS, et al: Sequential radionuclide assessment of left and right ventricular performance after acute transmural myocardial infarction. Ann Intern Med 89:441, 1978

205. Cohn JN, Guiha NH, Border MI, et al: Right ventricular infarction. Clinical and hemodynamic features. Am J Cardiol 33:209, 1974

206. Polak JF, Kemper AJ, Bianco JA, et al: A sensitive index of myocardial dysfunction in patients with coronary artery disease. J Nucl Med 23:471, 1982

207. Alazraki NP, Ashburn WL, Hagan A, et al: Detection of left-to-right cardiac shunts with the scintillation camera pulmonary dilution curve. J Nucl Med 13:142, 1972

208. Papapietro SE, Yester MV, Logic JR, et al: Method for quantitative analysis of regional left ventricular function with first pass and gated blood pool scintigraphy. Am J Cardiol 47:618, 1981

209. Ratib O, Henze E, Schon H, et al: Phase analysis of radionuclide ventriculograms for the detection of coronary artery disease. Am Heart J 104:1, 1982

210. Vos PH, Vossepoel AM, Pauwels EKJ: Quantitative assessment of wall motion in multiple-gated studies using temporal fourier analysis. J Nucl Med 24:388, 1983

211. Lam W, Pavel D, Byron E, et al: Radionuclide regurgitant index: Value and limitations. Am J Cardiol 47:292, 1981

212. Ashburn WL, Schelbert HR, Verba JW: Left ventricular ejection fraction: A review of several radionuclide angiographic approaches using the scintillation camera. Prog Cardiovasc Dis 20:267, 1978

213. Slutsky R, Karliner J, Ricci D, et al: Response of left ventricular volume to exercise in man assessed by radionuclide equilibrium angiography. Circulation 60:565, 1979

214. Adams DF, Abrams HL: Circulation 52 (suppl): 27, 1975

215. Van Slyke DD, Neill JM: The determination of gases in blood and other solutions by vacuum extraction

and manometric measurements. J Biol Chem 8:654, 1962

216. Stewart GN: Researches on the circulation time and on the influences which affect it. IV. The output of the heart. J Physiol 22:159, 1897

217. Grossman W: Cardiac Catheterization and Angiography. 2nd Ed. Philadelphia, Lea and Febiger, 1980

218. Cohen MV, Gorlin R: Modified orifice equation for the calculation of mitral valve area. Am Heart J 84:839, 1972

219. Gorlin R, Gorlin G: Hydraulic formula for calculation of area of stenotic mitral valve, other valves and central circulatory shunts. Am Heart J 41:1, 1951

220. Ganz W, Tamura K, Marcus HS, et al: Measurement of coronary sinus blood flow by continuous thermodilution in man. Circulation 44:181, 1971

221. Rackley CE: Quantitative evaluation of left ventricular function by radiographic techniques. Circulation 54:862, 1976

222. Karliner JS, Peterson KL, Ross J Jr: Myocardial mechanics: Assessment of isovolumic and ejection phase indices of left ventricular performance. In Grossman W (ed): Cardiac Catheterization and Angiography. Philadelphia, Lea & Febiger, 1974, pp 188–206

223. Cohn PF, Gorlin R, Adams DF, et al: Comparison of biplane and singleplane left ventriculography in patients with coronary artery disease. Am J Cardiol 33:1, 1974

224. Bove AA, Kreulen TH, Spann JF: Computer analysis of left ventricular dynamic geometry in man. Am J Cardiol 41:1239, 1978

225. Mangano DT: Preoperative assessment of cardiac catheterization data: Which are the most important parameters? Anesthesiology 53(3S):S105, 1980

226. White CW, Wright CB, Doty DB, et al: Does visual interpretation of the coronary arteriogram predict the physiologic importance of a coronary stenosis? N Engl J Med 310:819, 1984

227. Alderman EL, Hamilton KK, Silverman J, et al: Anatomically flexible, computer-assisted reporting system for coronary angiography. Am J Cardiol 49:1208, 1982

228. Chazov EI, Matveeva LS, Mazaev AV, et al: Intracoronary administration of fibrinolysin in acute MI. Ter Arkh 4:8, 1976

229. Chazov EI, Lakin KM: Anticoagulants and fibrinolytics. Chicago, Yearbook Medical Publishers, 1980

230. Rentrop R: Mortality and functional changes after intracoronary streptokinase infusion: Circulation 66:II-335, 1982

231. Schwarz F, Schuler G, Katus H: Intracoronary thrombolysis in myocardial infarction. Duration of ischemia as a major determinant of late results after recanalization. Am J Cardiol 50:933, 1982

232. Gruentzig AR, Senning A, Siegenthaler WE, et al: Nonoperative dilatation of coronary artery stenosis by percutaneous transluminal coronary angioplasty. N Engl J Med 301:61, 1979

233. Goldberg S, Urban P, Greenspan A: Combination therapy for evolving myocardial infarction: Intracoronary thrombolysis and percutaneous transluminal angioplasty. Am J Med 72:994, 1982

234. Meyer J, Merz W, Schmitz H: Percutaneous transluminal coronary angioplasty immediately after intracoronary streptolysis of transmural myocardial infarction. Circulation 66:905, 1982

235. Hartzler GO, Rutherford BD, McConhay DR: Percutaneous transluminal coronary angioplasty with and without thrombolytic therapy for treatment of acute myocardial infarction. Am Heart J 1067, 965, 1983

236. Cowley MJ, Vetrovec GW, Lewis SA, et al: Coronary angioplasty of multiple vessels: Acute and long-term results. Circulation 70 (Suppl II):322, 1984 (abstr)

237. Dorros G, Cowley MJ, Simpson J, et al: Percutaneous transluminal coronary angioplasty. Report of complications from the National Heart, Lung, and Blood Institute PTCA Registry. Circulation 67:723, 1983

238. Higgins CB, Lanzer P, Stark D, et al: Imaging by nuclear magnetic resonance in patients with chronic ischemic heart disease. Circulation 69:523, 1984

239. Ordidge RJ, Mansfield P, Doyle M, et al: "Real-time" moving images by NMR. In Wicofski RL, Karstaedt N, Partain CL (eds): Proceedings of the International Symposium in NMR Imaging. Winston-Salem, NC, Bowman Gray School of Medicine Press, 1982, pp 80–92

240. DeLayre JL, Ingwall JS, Malloy C, et al: Gated sodium-23 nuclear magnetic resonance images of an isolated perfused working rat heart. Science 212:935, 1981

241. Driscoll AC, Hobika JH, Etsten BE, et al: Clinically unrecognized myocardial infarction following surgery. N Engl J Med 264:633, 1961

242. Dack S: Symposium on cardiovascular-pulmonary problems before and after surgery: Postoperative problems. Am J Cardiol 12:423, 1963

243. Arkins R, Smessaert AA, Hicks RG: Mortality and morbidity in surgical patients with coronary artery disease. JAMA 190:485, 1964

244. Mauney MF Jr, Ebert PA, Sabiston DC Jr: Postoperative myocardial infarction: A study of predisposing factors, diagnosis and mortality in a high-risk group of surgical patients. Ann Surg 172:497, 1970

245. Eerola M, Erola R, Kaukinen S, et al: Risk factors in surgical patients with verified preoperative myocardial infarction. Acta Anaesthesiol Scand 24:219, 1980

246. Frazer JG, Ramachandran MB, Davis HS: Anesthesia and recent myocardial infarction. JAMA 199:96, 1967

247. Schoeppel LS, Wilkinson C, Waters J, et al: Effects

of myocardial infarction on perioperative cardiac complications. Anesth Analg 62:493, 1983

248. Sapala JA, Ponka JL, Duvernoy WF: Operative and nonoperative risks in the cardiac patient. J Am Geriatr Soc 23:529, 1975

249. Schneider AJL: Assessment of risk factors and surgical outcome. Surg Clin N Am 63:1113, 1983

250. Prys-Roberts C, Meloche R, Foex P: Studies of anesthesia in relation to hypertension: Cardiovascular responses of treated and untreated patients. Br J Anaesthesiol 43:122, 1971

251. Baers S, Nakhjavan F, Kajani M: Postoperative myocardial infarction. Surg Gynecol Obstet 120:315, 1965

252. Hunter PR, Endrey-Walder P, Bauer GE, et al: Myocardial infarction following surgical operations. Br Med J 4:725, 1968

253. Mahar LJ, Steen PA, Tinker JH, et al: Perioperative myocardial infarction in patients with coronary artery disease with and without aorta-coronary artery bypass grafts. J Thorac Cardiovasc Surg 76:533, 1978

254. Crawford ES, Morris GC, Howell JF, et al: Operative risk in patients with previous coronary artery bypass. Ann Thorac Surg 26:215, 1978

255. Kimbris D, Segal BL: Coronary disease progression in patients with and without saphenous vein bypass surgery. Am Heart J 102:811, 1981

256. Wasserman F, Bellet S, Saichek RP: Postoperative myocardial infarction; report of 25 cases. N Engl J Med 252:967, 1955

257. Feruglio G, Bellet S, Stone H: Postoperative myocardial infarction. Arch Intern Med 102:345, 1958

Edward D. Miller, Jr., M.D.

11

Antihypertensive Therapy

Over the past 20 years there has been a large amount of information generated that suggests that early detection and treatment of hypertension can have a marked effect on morbidity and mortality in the adult population. A major emphasis in the United States has been to apprise the general public of the importance of hypertension and its subsequent treatment. A variety of factors are known to be important in maintaining blood pressure at elevated levels with subsequent detrimental effects on several organs. This chapter examines general considerations regarding a patient with hypertension, as well as the basic underlying pathophysiology. With this as a basis, the various modes of drug therapy are examined in detail, and their relationship to anesthesia and surgery is defined.

DEFINITION OF HYPERTENSION

The World Health Organization defined *hypertension* as a single sitting or recumbent blood pressure exceeding 160/95 mm Hg.[1] Values that were below 140/90 mm Hg were considered to be normotensive. Blood pressures between 140/90 and 160/95 mm Hg have subsequently been regarded as borderline hypertension. These are rather arbitrary defini-

tions and rely on the accuracy of the blood pressure determinations. There is a spectrum of hypertension, and these arbitrary classifications are only guidelines in attempting to quantify a heterogenous population.

The entire issue of systolic hypertension (systolic blood pressure greater than 160 mm Hg with a normal diastolic pressure) is an area of considerable controversy.[2] The clinical contention that the diastolic pressure is more important for prognostic purposes than the systolic pressure has not proved to be correct. The Framingham Study showed that systolic pressure is as good a predictor of cardiovascular disease in men as is the diastolic pressure and, in some instances, is better (Fig. 11-1).[3] However, systolic blood pressure is relatively more dependent on the compliance of the aorta, and a raised systolic pressure with a normal or low diastolic pressure indicates disease of the large arteries. Systolic hypertension is not of equal importance in women or in the elderly. Systolic blood pressure is known to rise with age, averaging about a 1 mm Hg rise each year between the ages of 40 and 55, and rising more rapidly thereafter. In women, this increase is greater, averaging 1–2 mm Hg each year. It is this gradual rise with age that creates a problem in trying to decide whether or not treatment of systolic hypertension is warranted, since treatment of hypertension is not without com-

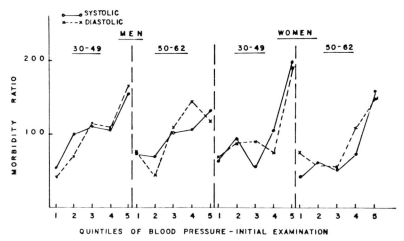

Fig. 11-1.   Risk of coronary heart disease (14-year follow-up) according to systolic and diastolic blood pressures. (From Kannel WB, Gordon T, Schwartz MH: Systolic vs diastolic blood pressure and risk of coronary heart disease: The Framingham Study. Am J Cardiol 27:335–346, 1971, with permission.)

plications. More data are still needed before a large program to treat systolic hypertension can be undertaken in this country.

TYPES OF HYPERTENSION

Hypertension may be divided into two broad categories: primary or essential hypertension and secondary hypertension. Secondary hypertension includes hypertension due to identifiable factors such as primary aldosteronism, stenosis of a renal artery resulting in renal vascular disease, parenchymal renal disease such as nephrosclerosis, and other disorders (Table 11-1).

Secondary hypertension comprises only about 10 percent of all cases of hypertension. Specific treatment of the underlying condition often results in complete cure of the hypertension. While patients with secondary hypertension represent only a small percentage of all hypertensive patients, an understanding of their basic pathophysiology may be helpful in the diagnosis and treatment of patients with essential hypertension. A few of the more common examples of secondary hypertension are reviewed below.

Primary aldosteronism is one of the few conditions in human beings in which an accompanying hypertension can be completely cured. The syndrome results from a single abnormality: inappropriate overproduction of aldosterone, the potent mineralcorticoid that is secreted normally by the zona glomerulosa of the adrenal cortex. The excess secretion of aldosterone results in almost complete reabsorption of all sodium that reaches the distal tubule of the kidney. There is also a decrease in loss of sodium in sweat, saliva, and intestinal fluid. The result of this increase in aldosterone is that extracellular sodium is increased and the extracellular fluid is kept isotonic by an accompaning retention of water. Not only is sodium reabsorbed, but the excess aldosterone also increases the secretion of potassium at all of the sites in which sodium reabsorption is enhanced. Aldosterone also increases renal tubular

Table 11-1

Classification of Hypertension

  I. Essential or primary hypertension

 II. Renal

    A. Parenchymal: eg, acute glomerulonephritis, chronic glomerulonephritis, and pyelonephritis

    B. Renovascular: eg, fibromuscular arterial stenosis and atherosclerotic arterial stenosis

III. Endocrine

    A. Adrenal

      1. Pheochromocytoma

      2. Primary aldosteronism

      3. Cushing's disease

IV. Neurogenic

 V. Toxemia of pregnancy

VI. Exogenous: eg, poisoning and medications

The Renin-Angiotensin System

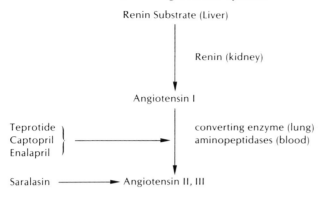

Renin Substrate (Liver)

Renin (kidney)

Angiotensin I

Teprotide
Captopril   } ⟶   converting enzyme (lung)
Enalapril   aminopeptidases (blood)

Saralasin   ⟶   Angiotensin II, III

vascular smooth muscle contraction
aldosterone secretion
thirst
CNS pressor system
potentiation and release of catecholamines

Fig. 11-2. The renin-angiotensin system, demonstrating the major components of this cascade of peptides and some of their potential effects. The left side illustrates some of the inhibitors of the system and their sites of action.

secretion of hydrogen, which escapes mainly as an ammonium ion. The alkalosis that ensues correlates with the degree of potassium depletion.[4] The resulting manifestations of the disease are hypertension, hypokalemia, and low plasma renin activity secondary to volume expansion.[5] In sum, the steps of primary aldosteronism are as follows:

1. Excess production of aldosterone
2. Reabsorption of sodium by distal tubule
3. Water retention and excess extracellular volume
4. Decreased renin with increased potassium loss

The mechanism for the hypertension in primary aldosteronism is related to the volume expansion that occurs early in the disease. It appears that the sodium is deposited within the vascular tree, making the vascular smooth muscle more responsive to exogenous stimuli. Once a diagnosis of primary aldosteronism has been made, localization of the adenoma to one adrenal gland or the other is accomplished with a computerized tomography (CT) scan or the administration of radiolabeled cholesterol, which is visualized by photoscanning. Preoperative preparation of the patient can be facilitated by the use of spironolactone, a nonspecific aldosterone-blocking diuretic.[6] Attention to serum potassium, magnesium, and

sodium is essential prior to operative removal of the adenoma.

Stenosis of one or both renal arteries may result in hypertension. In younger individuals, the stenosis is often due to fibromuscular thickening of the renal artery, while in older patients it is due to atherosclerosis. The stenosis causes a decrease in pressure within the kidney. Initially, flow to the kidney may remain normal, but the decreased pressure is sensed by the kidney, resulting in the release of renin from the juxtaglomerular apparatus in the afferent arterioles of the kidney.[7] Renin, a protolytic enzyme, acts on a plasma protein to form angiotensin I. Angiotensin I is then converted to angiotensin II by a single passage through the pulmonary circulation. Angiotensin II is a potent vasoconstrictor, as well as a stimulus to aldosterone secretion (Fig. 11-2).[8] These two factors work in concert to raise arterial blood pressure. With a correction of the stenosis either by removal of the offending kidney or by a bypass graft, renin production decreases and blood pressure returns toward control levels.[9] However, if the hypertension has persisted for a long period of time, there is an apparent resetting of the baroreceptor mechanism. Blood pressure may return toward control levels but never achieve normotensive levels without the use of antihypertensive medications. In sum, the steps of renovascular hypertension are as follows:

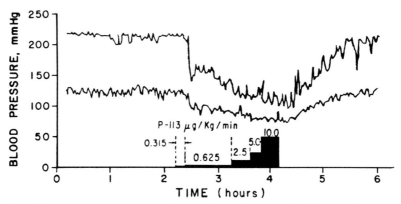

Fig. 11-3. Blood pressure recording during infusion of saralasin (P-113) in a patient with renal artery stenosis and high plasma renin activity. Blood pressure fell as the dose of P-113 was increased from 0.315 to 10.0 μg/kg/min. (From Streeton DHP, Anderson GH, Freiberg JM, et al: Use of an angiotensin II antagonist (saralasin) in the recognition of "angiotensinogenic" hypertension. N Engl J Med 292:657–661, 1975, with permission.)

1. Decreased renal artery pressure
2. Increased renin release and angiotensin II
3. Increased aldosterone stimulated by angiotensin II
4. Increased arterial pressure

Disease processes that involve the kidneys often result in increased arterial blood pressure.[10] Many patients who have a loss of nephrons and a resulting decrease in renal function will become hypertensive. The hypertension that is seen in patients with markedly decreased renal function is due to volume expansion.[11] Since the patient is unable to excrete solutes because of the renal dysfunction, there is an increase in the extracellular volume. With dialysis, the patient's blood pressure can be adequately controlled, often without the use of antihypertensive drugs. However, some patients with renal parenchymal disease have hypertension that is dependent on the renin-angiotensin system and have been effectively treated with drugs that inhibit it (Fig. 11-3).[12]

Management of a patient with a pheochromocytoma is still an anesthetic challenge. In the past, operative mortality for removal of this tumor was high, but with better understanding of the underlying pathophysiology and improvement in drug therapy, this is no longer true. A pheochromocytoma is a catecholamine-producing tumor of neuroectodermal origin that is made up of chromaffin cells. Tumors are usually located within the sympathetic nervous system, and roughly 95 percent of them are found in the adrenal medulla. Another 2 percent of the tumors are located at various sites within the abdomen, and 3 percent are extra-abdominal.[13]

Hypertension is the clinical hallmark of a pheochromocytoma. Fifty percent of the patients have sustained hypertension, and many of the other patients have paroxysmal hypertension. Most tumors secrete both norepinephrine and epinephrine, but norepinephrine-secreting tumors predominate. Smaller tumors usually cause more signs and symptoms than do large tumors, and diagnosis is suspected because of these signs and symptoms, which include headache, nervousness, palpitations, weight loss, and diaphoresis. Rarely, the diagnosis may be made during surgery with a sudden onset of severe hypertension at the time of abdominal exploration. Preoperative antihypertensive therapy is aimed at decreasing the alpha- and beta-agonist properties of the excess norepinephrine- or epinephrine-secreting tumors. This can be accomplished with the use of phenoxybenzamine, an alpha-blocking agent, with or without propranolol. More recently, metyrosine (alphamethyltyrosine, an inhibitor of tyrosine hydroxylase) has been used as a preoperative drug instead of phenoxybenzamine (Fig. 11-4).[14] Whichever drug therapies are used preoperatively, it appears important to restore plasma volume and to continue the treatment of the hypertension up to and during the operative procedure.[15]

PATHOPHYSIOLOGY OF ESSENTIAL HYPERTENSION

The regulation of blood pressure in normotensive patients is influenced by a variety of factors. The central sympathetic nervous system plays an impor-

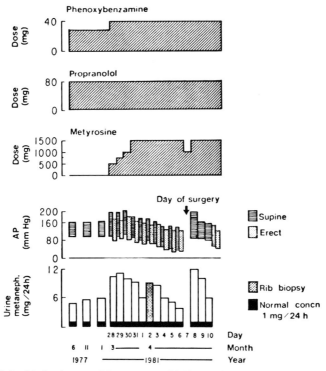

Fig. 11-4. Medication, arterial pressure, and 24-hour urine metanephrine concentration before and during operation. (From Triner L, Baer L, Gallagher R, et al: Use of metyrosine in the anaesthetic management of patients with catecholamine-secreting tumors. Br J Anaesth 54:1333–1336, 1982, with permission.)

tant role in maintaining moment-to-moment blood pressure control. Equally important, however, are the peripheral mechanisms, which often send afferent impulses into the central nervous system so that appropriate sympathetic responses can be initiated. The baroreceptors, renin-angiotensin system, peripheral sympathetic nervous system, antidiuretic hormone, serum sodium concentration, and atrial natriuretic factor all contribute to the regulation of blood pressure in the normotensive range. Structural alterations of the vascular tree, which occur with either increased blood pressure or with aging, also have an important role to play in blood pressure regulation. Many of the factors that have been studied in the control of normal blood pressure have also been investigated in regard to producing hypertension. While no one theory is conclusive, there are pieces of information from several sources to suggest that hypertension is a composite disease. Small disorders in one system may have important effects on another system, with the resultant effect of an increase in arterial blood pressure. Following is a brief review of

some of the factors that have been studied in order to better explain how antihypertensive therapy is directed:

1. Pathogenic role of sodium
2. Membrane defects
3. Sympathetic nervous system
4. Renin-angiotensin system
5. Microcirculation

Mechanisms of Hypertension

PATHOGENIC ROLE OF SODIUM

The relationship between salt and hypertension centers on the fact that blood pressure can be lowered with diets that are very low in sodium chloride. Kempner first noted that patients with kidney disease and hypertensive vascular disease could be treated with a rice diet.[16] This type of diet contains little sodium chloride. Subsequently, there has been a variety of epidemiologic and laboratory investigations examining the role of sodium. In rats, hypertension can be induced with high-sodium feedings.[17] It has been found that there are strains of rats that are either salt sensitive or salt resistant. These two strains of rats have normal blood pressures when they are young, as long as their sodium intake is low. With adulthood, however, the salt-sensitive strain has a pressure approximately 15 mm Hg higher than the resistant strain.[18]

It appears that sodium has an important role in modulating blood pressure control. When all of the population studies are reviewed, it is noted that areas with very high salt intakes have a very high incidence of hypertension. If the sodium intake is less than 4 g/day, there is a very low incidence of hypertension, and blood pressure does not rise with increasing age. It may be that in humans there are salt-sensitive and salt-resistant individuals. The identification of such individuals has important therapeutic implications in the development and treatment of hypertension.

MEMBRANE DEFECTS

Considerable controversy exists concerning the role of cell membranes in hypertension. A genetic link with hypertension has often been sought, since it is known that hypertension has a tendency to occur more frequently in the offspring of hypertensive patients than in the offspring of normotensive persons. Recent evidence from several laboratories has shown that patients with essential hypertension, but not secondary hypertension, have a defect in their red cell membranes. In patients with essential hypertension, Garay et al showed that cotransport, a transport system of red cells, was unable to excrete sodium from the interior of the red cell.[19] Subsequent work by other investigators has examined different transport systems of the red cell and of other cellular components of the body and has found defects.[20] The data are still too incomplete to say definitively that patients have essential hypertension because of membrane defects. It is intriguing to speculate on the interrelationship between membrane defects and sodium sensitivity, however, since defects that are found in red cells may also be found in other important structures such as vascular smooth muscle or the sympathetic nervous system.

SYMPATHETIC NERVOUS SYSTEM

Indirect evidence suggests that the sympathetic nervous system is altered in essential hypertension. DeChamplain et al found elevated levels of serum catecholamines in patients with essential hypertension.[21] Hypertensive patients subjected to mental stress or postural changes had urinary norepinephrine excretion greater than in control subjects. Several therapeutic interventions of hypertension are directed at inhibiting the sympathetic nervous system in order to control blood pressure. Whether the differences in sympathetic nervous system function observed in the hypertensive patient are the cause or the effect of the disease process has not been clearly defined.

The spontaneously hypertensive rat, a specific strain developed over the past 20 years, is cited by some authors as the best model for essential hypertension.[22] Biochemical evidence suggests that, in the early development of hypertension in these rats, there is a decrease in norepinephrine content in selected brain areas and activation of the peripheral sympathetic nervous system. In the adult hypertensive rat, changes in the brain norepinephrine persist, and signs of increased peripheral sympathetic nervous system activities subside.[23] Physiologic studies also implicate the sympathetic nervous system in the established phase of hypertension in these spontaneously hypertensive rats. Cardiac output is normal, but there is a marked increase in total peripheral resistance.[24] Both the biochemical and the physiological evidence demonstrate the derangement in the sympathetic nervous system in the spontaneously hypertensive rat; it must be concluded that the sympathetic nervous system plays an important role either in the initiation or the maintenance of hypertension.

RENIN-ANGIOTENSIN SYSTEM

In 1934, Goldblatt et al demonstrated that hypertension could be produced in the dog by constriction of the renal artery.[25] Renin release from the kidney was first demonstrated by Kohlstaedt and Page in 1940.[26] Subsequent to this, various workers have demonstrated that the initiation and maintenance of renal vascular hypertension are due to the release of renin from the kidney. Through the use of inhibitors, the role of the renin-angiotensin system and blood pressure control in both normotensive and pathologic states has been more clearly defined (Figs. 11-2 and 11-5).[27]

While many had thought that the role of the renin-angiotensin system was as a peripheral mechanism alone, it is now known that the renin-angiotensin system exists intact in the central nervous system and may play an important role in blood pressure control.[28] The demonstration that captopril is effective in the treatment of patients with essential hypertension who have low or normal plasma renin activity further substantiates the role of the renin-

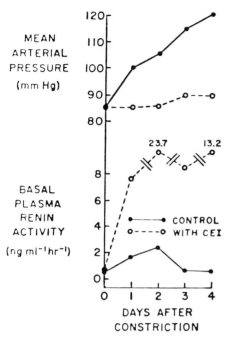

Fig. 11-5. Comparison of changes in mean arterial pressure and basal renin activity induced by renal artery constriction in the same dog without converting enzyme inhibitor (CEI) and during chronic infusion of CEI. (From Miller ED, Samuels A, Haber E, et al: Inhibition of angiotensin conversion: Effect of initiation and maintenance of renal hypertension. Am J Physiol 228:448–453, 1975, with permission.)

angiotensin system in the development and maintenance of hypertension.[29]

MICROCIRCULATION

Microcirculatory alterations accompany hypertension (whether these are cause or effect remains to be established) and may be broadly classified into two categories: (1) anatomical changes and (2) functional changes.

Anatomical changes consist of either a reduced density (the number of arterioles in each volume of tissue) or a reduced internal diameter of the vessels. In either case, there is an increase in vascular resistance. Recent studies of the microcirculation of the conjunctiva of hypertensive patients reveal a 20 percent reduction in arteriolar density and a 5 percent reduction in arteriolar caliber as compared with those in age- and sex-matched normotensive control subjects.[30]

Folkow et al have emphasized the relationship between the microvascular wall thickening and

microvascular function.[31] They proposed that a fundamental defect in hypertension was an increased ratio of wall thickness to lumen diameter, resulting in an increase in vascular reactivity in the hypertensive animal. They emphasized that the sensitivity (threshold) to humoral agents was not altered by hypertension, but the reactivity (intensity of constriction) was increased as a result of the altered microvascular anatomy. Whatever the mechanism, there is evidence that the microvasculature responds differently in hypertensive people as compared with normotensive people. While there is considerable debate concerning the Folkow hypothesis, the general scenario of hypertension appears to be one of both an altered microvascular response to vasoactive agents, and, perhaps, an increased circulating amount of vasoactive agents, leading to an alteration of the microvascular control in the hypertensive patient.

The preceding is only a small example of some of the areas that have been investigated as possible primary mechanisms responsible for an elevation in arterial blood pressure. Certainly, none of these is mutually exclusive; it is more likely that the interaction of a defect in one system may play an important role in generating a defect in another. From all of the studies, there are certain salient features that can be stressed. First, in essential hypertension there is an increase in peripheral vascular resistance, and cardiac output remains normal. Second, sympathetic nervous system activity is increased, most likely at times of increased stress. Third, the vasculature of the hypertensive patient responds in a more vigorous manner than in the normotensive patient (Fig. 11-6). The therapy of chronic hypertension is based on these findings and is aimed at decreasing peripheral resistance, sympathetic nervous system activity, and the reactivity of the vasculature.

MEDICAL TREATMENT OF HYPERTENSION

The medical treatment of hypertension has been shown to be extremely effective in decreasing morbidity and mortality. In the Veterans Administration Cooperative Study, 380 patients with diastolic pressures between 90 and 114 mm Hg were randomized into the trial.[32] Of this number, 186 received active treatment and 194 were given placebos. Fifteen percent of the 380 randomized patients dropped out of the study, an equal number in both groups. The estimated risk of developing a morbid event over a 5-year period was reduced from 55 percent to 18 percent by treatment. Thirty-five patients died in the

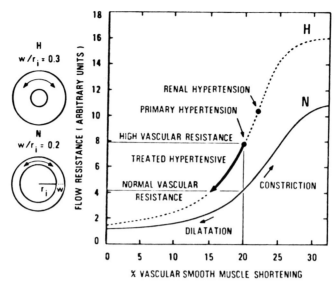

Fig. 11-6. Relationship between flow resistance in arterioles as a function of the muscle tone in the arteriolar smooth muscle in normotensive (N) and hypertensive (H) patients. The curve for treated hypertensive patients is superimposed on that for untreated hypertensives, either primary or renal. Treated hypertensive patients have lower arterial pressures as a result of decreased vascular smooth muscle shortening (ie, vasodilatation). (From Prys-Robert C: Chronic antihypertensive therapy. *In* Kaplan JA (ed): Cardiac Anesthesia: Volume 2, Cardiovascular Pharmacology. Orlando, FL, Grune & Stratton, 1983, p 346.)

control group, as compared with 9 patients in the treated group. With such strong evidence from studies like this, it is not surprising that there is a large variety of antihypertensive drugs available that can effectively decrease arterial pressure.

Diuretics

The introduction of chlorothiazide in 1957 was an extremely important advance in antihypertensive treatment. This oral diuretic adequately controls blood pressure in many hypertensive patients and remains the initial line of treatment for patients with hypertension. Not only does the diuretic help decrease blood pressure by itself, but it also potentiates other antihypertensive drugs (Table 11-2).

Chlorothiazide is a benzothiadizine derivative, and so are most of the other oral diuretics synthesized after 1957. The diuresis caused by chlorothiazide comes about by inhibiting sodium reabsorption in the cortical segment of the ascending loop of Henle, and it can result in a maximum excretion of between 10

and 15 percent of the filtered sodium load. Such a diuresis also produces hypovolemia and alkalosis, because more sodium is reabsorbed in the distal con-

Table 11-2
Diuretics

	Recommended Dosage (mg/day)
Thiazides and related agents	
Chlorothiazide (Diuril)	250–1000
Hydrochlorothiazide (Hydrodiuril)	25–150
Methylclothiazide (Enduron)	2.5–10.0
Trichlormethiazide (Naqua)	2–4
Chlorthalidone (Hygroton)	50–150
Metolazone (Zaroxolyn)	1–5
Loop diuretics	
Furosemide (Lasix)	40–200
Ethacrynic acid (Edecrin)	50–100
Potassium-sparing diuretics	
Spironolactone (Aldactone)	50–100
Triamterene (Dyrenium)	100–300

Table 11-3

Incidence of Intraoperative Dysrhythmias

	Hypokalemic Group		Normokalemic Group		
	2.6–2.9 *(mEq/l)*	3.0–3.4 *(mEq/l)*	3.5–3.9 *(mEq/l)*	4.0–4.4 *(mEq/l)*	4.5–5.2 *(mEq/l)*
Number	21	41	39	32	17
Premature atrial contractions	14% (3)	10% (4)	13% (5)	16% (5)	6% (1)
Premature ventricular contractions	10% (2)	17% (7)	21% (8)	34% (11)	18% (3)
Bigeminy	0 (0)	7% (3)	3% (1)	0 (0)	0 (0)
Junctional	10% (2)	17% (7)	13% (5)	31% (10)	12% (2)
Sinus tachycardia	0 (0)	2% (1)	10% (4)	19% (6)	18% (3)
Total dysrhythmias	29% (6)	39% (16)	41% (16)	59% (19)	47% (8)

voluted tubule in exchange for potassium and hydrogen ion excretion. Although the term "diuretic" is used, the major hypotensive effect of chronic administration of thiazides appears to be due to vasodilatation rather than to sodium or free-water loss.[33] However, these changes in the peripheral vasculature may be due to a loss of sodium from the vascular smooth muscle.

Furosemide was introduced in 1963 and is referred to as a *loop diuretic* because of its extensive action on the ascending loop of Henle. Furosemide is more effective than the thiazide diuretics in promoting diuresis because it inhibits sodium reabsorption in the medullary and cortical segments of the ascending loop of Henle.[34]

The major toxicity of loop diuretics is related to electrolyte depletion. A hypokalemic metabolic alkalosis (contraction alkalosis) frequently results. Hyperuricemia and, rarely, hyperglycemia have been reported with these diuretics.[35]

Potassium-sparing diuretics, such as spironolactone and triamterene, have also been used in the treatment of hypertension. Spironolactone is a competitive antagonist of aldosterone and is very effective in the treatment of patients with primary aldosteronism.[36] It is also used in patients who are unable to maintain an adequate serum potassium level with other types of diuretics.

Drug interactions with the diuretics are important considerations. The two main concerns are interactions with nonsteroidal anti-inflammatory drugs and potassium homeostasis.

Nonsteroidal anti-inflammatory drugs inhibit the biosynthesis of the prostaglandins and related compounds. Since prostaglandins play an important role in the regulation of renal blood flow, glomerular filtration, renin secretion, tubular ion transport, and water metabolism, it is not surprising that the response to thiazides may be altered. Patients who are taking thiazides and then concurrently start with a nonsteroidal anti-inflammatory drug may have a loss in the control of blood pressure.[37]

Potassium homeostasis is also impaired by diuretics. There is a chronic loss of potassium because of the actions of diuretics, and total body potassium may be severely depleted. The need for routine potassium supplementation for hypertensive patients receiving diuretic therapy remains extremely controversial.[38] In various studies examining a possible interaction between low potassium and morbidity and mortality, the data still remain obscure. Cardiac dysrhythmias do not appear more common in chronic potassium depletion. Studies are currently in progress to try to define whether additional potassium supplementation should be required in patients who take diuretics. Anesthesiologists are frequently confronted with patients who have taken diuretics and whose serum potassium level is between 3 and 3.5 mEq/l. Acute therapy of this deficit does not seem justified since total body potassium will not be replaced. A recent study suggests that chronic hypokalemia does not result in an increased incidence of intraoperative dysrhythmias and that routine surgical postponement and acute potassium replacement may be unnecessary practices in patients with chronic hypokalemia (Table 11-3).[39]

Central Nervous System Adrenergic Neuron Inhibitors

This group of drugs comprises a relatively new approach to the therapy of hypertension. Alpha-methyldopa, clonidine, and guanabenz are drugs that act on central alpha$_2$-receptors. It is thought that their antihypertensive effects are due to stimulation of these receptors, with a resulting decrease in sympa-

Table 11-4

Central-Acting Antihypertensive Agents

	Recommended Dosage (mg/day)
Methyldopa (Aldomet)	250–1000
Clonidine (Catapres)	0.2–0.8
Guanabenz (Wytensin)	4–32

thetic tone from the central nervous system to the peripheral sympathetic system (Table 11-4).

METHYLDOPA

Methyldopa is one of the oldest and most widely used of all antihypertensive drugs. Early theories on the mechanism of action of methyldopa centered on the possibility that a false neurotransmitter was produced, stored, and released in place of norepinephrine. Currently it is believed that alpha-methyldopa exerts its antihypertensive effect by virtue of its conversion to alpha-methylnorepinephrine, a potent alpha$_2$–adrenergic agonist. This concept is supported by the observation that inhibition of decarboxylation of methyldopa centrally, but not in the periphery, blocks the hypotensive effect of the drug. Furthermore, the effects of methyldopa on blood pressure do not correlate with reductions in the concentrations of norepinephrine within the central nervous system.[40]

Methyldopa reduces total peripheral resistance without much of a change in cardiac output or rate. If used alone, methyldopa results in fluid retention and weight gain and, therefore, is commonly used with a diuretic. It has been shown that treatment with methyldopa may significantly reduce left ventricular hypertrophy within 12 weeks after institution of therapy; interestingly, this occurs without any apparent relationship to the degree of change in blood pressure.[41]

The side effects recorded with methyldopa are usually sedation, postural hypotension, dizziness, dry mouth, and headache. These undesirable side effects are one reason for poor compliance with the drug. There are more serious side effects, though, including hemolytic anemia, thrombocytopenia, leukopenia, hepatitis, and a lupus-like syndrome. With prolonged therapy 10–20 percent of patients may develop a positive direct Coombs' test, and in 5 percent of these patients hemolytic anemia may occur. The Coombs' test may remain positive for several months after discontinuation of therapy with methyldopa.[42]

CLONIDINE

Clonidine is a recently synthesized central antihypertensive drug that stimulates alpha$_2$–adrenergic receptors within the central nervous system; its actions, thereby, resemble the actions of methyldopa.[43] Acute oral administration of clonidine results in a reduction in heart rate, stroke volume, and total peripheral resistance. Long-term results with clonidine are not as clear-cut. Cardiac index and heart rate usually decrease more than does total peripheral resistance. The hypotensive effects of the drug appear to parallel reductions in circulating norepinephrine.

Clonidine is not available in a parenteral form at the present time; therefore, it has caused problems in the perioperative period. Sudden withdrawal of oral clonidine may produce a hypertensive crisis that can be life-threatening.[44] The syndrome has been reported in patients who are receiving as little as 0.2 mg of clonidine each day,[45] and usually begins 8–20 hours after the last dose. The anesthesiologist must be aware of this potentially critical problem and make plans for appropriate treatment in the postoperative period. It should be emphasized that severe rebound hypertension is the exception and not the rule with withdrawal therapy, but it is difficult to define which patient will have these exaggerated responses.

GUANABENZ

Guanabenz is another centrally acting alpha$_2$–adrenergic agonist that has properties similar to clonidine. Guanabenz appears to have fewer side effects, such as sodium and water retention, mental depression, sexual dysfunction, or a positive Coombs' test, but it does seem to produce a greater overall incidence of drowsiness and weakness. As with clonidine, there is concern for acute rebound hypertension after sudden withdrawal of the drug.[46]

Beta-Blockers

The antihypertensive effects of beta-adrenergic receptor blocking drugs were accidentally discovered by Pritchard in 1964 in patients being treated for angina pectoris.[47] Since then, many beta-blocking agents have become available for clinical use in the management of patients with angina pectoris and hypertension, and they are often prescribed in conjunction with diuretics or other antihypertensive drugs.

Beta-blockers competitively block the effect of endogenous catecholamine release at the nerve endings or circulating in the blood. How they reduce blood pressure is not totally known, but several mechanisms have been proposed. A reduction in cardiac output has been proposed as one mechanism for the decrease in blood pressure.[48] Other studies have not been able to substantiate this, and the decrease in cardiac output does not seem to be a major mechanism responsible for the decrease in blood pressure.[49] Modulation of the renin-angiotensin system is another mechanism thought to play an important role in blood pressure regulation in hypertensive patients. Propranolol is known to decrease basal renin release from the kidney, as well as to decrease stimulated renin release. Since plasma renin activity would be decreased by beta-blockers, the production of aldosterone would also be decreased, therefore providing another salutary effect on decreasing blood pressure.[50] The central effects of beta-blockers have also been considered to be responsible for their antihypertensive effects. However, drugs like atenolol, which penetrate the blood–brain barrier poorly, argue against this belief.[51] Other possible mechanisms involve adaptation of the peripheral circulation,[52] modulation of prostaglandin release, and resetting or readjustment of baroreceptor sensitivity.[53]

Despite the differences in the pharmacologic properties of the various beta-blockers that are now available, it is known that all beta-blockers reduce blood pressure to a similar extent when given in equipotent doses. These drugs are most commonly used with diuretics and/or vasodilating agents for maximum effectiveness in the treatment of hypertension:

1. Beta-blockers: propranolol, metoprolol, and atenolol
2. Alpha-adrenergic antagonists: prazosin
3. Mixed antagonists: labetalol
4. Adrenergic neuron-blocking agents: guanethidine and reserpine

Sympatholytic Agents

PRAZOSIN

Prazosin is an alpha-blocking drug that has specific alpha$_1$-adrenergic antagonist properties. Prazosin competitively blocks the vascular postsynaptic alpha$_1$-adrenergic receptor.[54] While both alpha$_1$- and alpha$_2$-receptors are found postsynaptically in vascular smooth muscle, the ratio of these two receptor subgroups determines the effect of the drug. Since alpha$_2$-receptors are not blocked, the normal inhibi-

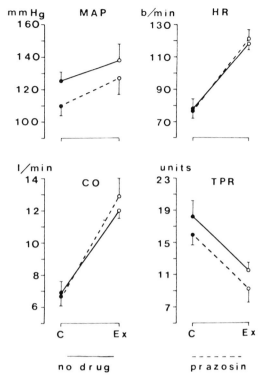

Fig. 11-7. Hemodynamic effects of dynamic exercise before and during treatment with prazosin. Responses to exercise before and during prazosin are not different. (From Mancia G, Ferrari A, Gregorini L, et al: Effect of prazosin on autonomic control of circulation in essential hypertension. Hypertension 2:700–707, 1980, with permission.)

tory function of these alpha$_2$-receptors on norepinephrine release is not affected.

Prazosin reduces mean arterial blood pressure and peripheral resistance but produces little or no tachycardia, in contrast to peripheral vasodilators. Although blood pressure does decrease with prazosin, cerebral and renal blood flow are well maintained, and glomerular filtration rate is not altered. Prazosin appears to be very effective in treating patients who have hypertension and associated renal failure (Fig. 11-7).[55]

Prazosin does not produce adverse metabolic effects and is now used as a first alternative in patients who cannot tolerate diuretics due to gout or hyperglycemia; it also replaces beta-blockers in patients with an underlying history of asthma or congestive heart failure. Prazosin is used to treat mild-to-moderate hypertension and is more effective when combined with a diuretic and/or beta-blocker.

RESERPINE

The class of drugs coming from plants called *Rauwolfia* has long been used for the treatment of hypertension. In 1931, treatment of psychosis and hypertension with *Rauwolfia* compounds was first described; later, the ability of these compounds to deplete biogenic amines from storage sites within the body initiated a great number of investigations. Reserpine depletes stores of catecholamines and serotonin in many organs, including the brain and the adrenal medulla.[56] Reserpine causes a slowly developing decrease in blood pressure, frequently associated with bradycardia. The chronic administration of reserpine usually results in a reduced cardiac output and partial inhibition of some cardiovascular reflexes.[57]

Reserpine acts centrally to produce a state of sedation, and it is thought that its effects are due to depletion of both catecholamines and serotonin within the brain. One of the major drawbacks of reserpine has been its ability, even in small doses, to produce a considerable incidence of nightmares and psychic depressions, sometimes severe enough to require hospitalization or even to end in suicide. It is for these reasons, as well as development of newer modes of therapy, that the drug is not used as frequently as in the past.

GUANETHIDINE

Guanethidine has an interesting property of interfering with postganglionic adrenergic nerve endings and decreasing blood pressure through this mechanism. The major effect of guanethidine is to inhibit responses that are normally seen with sympathetic nervous system stimulation. Guanethidine is taken up and stored in the adrenergic nerves, and this accumulation is essential for its action. Guanethidine displaces norepinephrine from these intraneuronal storage granules and is released by nerve stimulation.[58]

Guanethidine is used only in patients with severe hypertension and is not as frequently used today as it was in the past. The drug does not enter the CNS in significant amounts and, therefore, may be used in some patients in whom the central effects of other sympatholytics are not tolerated.

LABETALOL

Labetalol is an antihypertensive drug that has both beta- and alpha-adrenergic blocking properties, which are useful for the therapy of hypertension.[59] It is approximately one-tenth as potent as phentolamine in its ability to block alpha-receptors. Labetalol's beta-blocking properties appear to be one-third as pronounced as those of propranolol. When given as an oral or intravenous dose, the preponderant effect is beta-blockade rather than alpha-blockade.[60] Its role in the treatment of hypertension on a chronic basis needs to be fully evaluated.

Peripheral Vasodilators

HYDRALAZINE

Hydralazine has been used in clinical practice for over 30 years and has gained in popularity recently because of its combined use with beta-adrenergic antagonists. Hydralazine causes direct relaxation of the vascular smooth muscle, producing a decrease in peripheral vascular resistance and concomitant increases in heart rate and contractility.[61] These latter effects can be offset by the use of a beta-adrenergic antagonist. The drug itself decreases diastolic pressure more than systolic blood pressure, and it causes preferential dilatation of the arterioles rather than the veins. Since hydralazine is available both orally and parenterally, it is extremely useful in controlling blood pressure in the perioperative period.

The major problems with hydralazine include headache, nausea, vomiting, and tachycardia. A more disturbing side effect of the drug is a lupus-like syndrome that develops in less than 10 percent of the patients taking the drug.[62]

MINOXIDIL

Minoxidil is a potent vasodilator with a mode of action similar to hydralazine. As with hydralazine, there is a reflex increase in heart rate and cardiac index.[63] The most common side effects of minoxidil therapy are fluid retention and hypertrichosis. The drug increases sodium reabsorption in the proximal tubule, and furosemide is usually given to patients taking minoxidil to avoid weight gain.[64] Hypertrichosis occurs in nearly all patients treated with minoxidil for more than 4 weeks. Due to this side effect, many patients refuse the drug. Studies are still incomplete as to the efficacy of this agent as a topical preparation to treat severe alopecia.[65]

CALCIUM CHANNEL BLOCKERS

The use of calcium channel blockers for the treatment of hypertension is presently in the investigative stage. It has been found that patients receiving these drugs for angina pectoris also have a significant reduction in their blood pressure.[66] Calcium channel blockers are potent arterial vasodilators. What role these agents will eventually play in the long-term control of hypertensive patients remains to be decided. There appears to be minimal postural hypotension and, therefore, good acceptance by patients. The overall clinical studies to date suggest that the direct peripheral vasodilator effect lowers the peripheral resistance but does not affect the physiologic reflexes that help maintain blood pressure during exertion.

The Renin-Angiotensin System

Since Goldblatt's discovery of the importance of renal artery stenosis in causing hypertension, the renin-angiotensin system has often been a focus of research involved with control of blood pressure. With improved knowledge of the renin-angiotensin system, specific inhibitors have been developed. The first of these inhibitors was saralasin, a competitive inhibitor of angiotensin II (Fig. 11-2).[67] This agent allowed specific information to be gained concerning how angiotensin II controlled blood pressure in both normotensive and hypertensive subjects. Since saralasin is a peptide, it cannot be used in an oral preparation. At the time that saralasin was developed, a converting enzyme inhibitor called teprotide was also developed. It also was a peptide and blocked the conversion of angiotensin I to angiotensin II. With a better understanding of how teprotide inhibited the converting enzyme in the lung, a new drug was synthesized that was not a peptide. This oral drug, captopril, has been used in many clinical situations.[68]

CAPTOPRIL

There are now a multitude of reports evaluating the effectiveness of captopril in various forms of hypertension. Captopril effectively decreases blood pressure in patients with renal vascular hypertension; however, probably more importantly, it is also effective in decreasing blood pressure in patients with essential hypertension.[69] Surprisingly, there has been no correlation between the pretreatment plasma renin activity and the decline in arterial pressure in patients with essential hypertension.

Captopril decreases blood pressure by decreasing total peripheral resistance with little effect on cardiac output. Plasma renin activity increases sharply because the negative feedback inhibition of angiotensin II is no longer present. Since angiotensin II is a potent stimulus of aldosterone secretion, there is also a marked drop in plasma aldosterone. Circulating plasma norepinephrine is unchanged and

responds appropriately when the patient assumes an upright posture.

The mechanism of action of captopril is complex. Certainly, the decrease in angiotensin II resulting from converting enzyme inhibition is one important component. However, converting enzyme is also responsible for the inactivation of bradykinin. With inhibition of this enzyme, plasma levels and, perhaps more importantly, tissue levels of bradykinin may increase. The possibility also exists that captopril reaches sites within vascular smooth muscle or the central nervous system that have significant influences on blood pressure.[70]

Clinical trials with captopril suggest that side effects are very low when compared with those of other antihypertensive drugs. Fear was raised concerning proteinuria and membranous glomerulonephritis in the initial studies; however, with increased use of the drug, these concerns have decreased markedly and a variety of patients have been treated with captopril who had borderline renal function. This drug is only available in an oral preparation, which has led several manufacturers to examine other ways to inhibit converting enzyme activity.

ENALAPRIL

Enalapril (MK422) is a long-acting nonsteroidal angiotensin-converting enzyme inhibitor that is well-absorbed after oral administration and then hydrolized to its bioactive form, enalaprilic acid.[71] It is similar to captopril in many regards except that it appears to be a more specific inhibitor of converting enzyme. The bioactive form of the drug has also been produced and is available for intravenous administration. The ability to administer either an oral or intravenous preparation has distinct advantages for patients at the time of surgery. This drug has only been released for clinical use in the United States.

ANTIHYPERTENSIVE THERAPY AND ANESTHESIA

Antihypertensive medications should be continued up to the night before surgery and given in the morning prior to the surgical procedure. While the views of the 1960s encouraged the withdrawal of antihypertensive medications, there is no evidence that anesthetic agent–antihypertensive medication interactions are detrimental. On the contrary, the sudden withdrawal of antihypertensive medication has led to severe postoperative hypertension.[72] Most of the common antihypertensive drugs have a sufficient length of action so that they may be restarted the morning after surgery. Another reason to continue antihypertensive agents, especially beta-adrenoreceptor antagonist drugs, is to protect the patient's heart from responding to noxious stimuli during the operative procedure.

Clonidine and captopril arc two drugs that need special attention, since there are no intravenous preparations. Therefore, the anesthesiologist must decide preoperatively how to manage these patients postoperatively. Many of these patients will be able to take oral medications the next morning. If not, the placement of the tablets (crushed) down a nasogastric tube is also effective. If neither of these options is available, a decision to change medication preoperatively should be made so that postoperative hypertension does not become a problem.

The decision to postpone elective surgery because of inadequately controlled hypertension should be based on sound reasons. The anesthesiologist must be convinced that intraoperative and postoperative mortality can be significantly decreased by such a decision. A diastolic blood pressure of greater than 120 mm Hg carries a significant risk of intraoperative myocardial ischemia and dysrhythmias and, therefore, should be considered sufficient reason to postpone elective surgery.[73] The data concerning patients whose blood pressure is lower than this remain controversial. Goldman and Caldera examined patients with mild hypertension and found no evidence to suggest that elective operations should be postponed in such patients.[74] They cautioned, however, that their findings were predicated on the fact that close intra- and postoperative monitoring was done and that sudden increases in blood pressure were rapidly treated. Further studies are necessary to define more precisely which patients would benefit most from postponement of elective surgery.

Intraoperative management of the hypertensive patient is difficult at best. Because of the increased reactivity of the vasculature, a "roller coaster" anesthetic may result. No particular anesthetic technique or specific drug combinations have been shown to be superior to others in the hypertensive patient. Some would suggest that a large-dose, narcotic-based anesthetic technique could provide a more "stress-free" state while ventricular function remains intact.[75] However, not all studies have found that intraopera-

tive arterial pressure control is adequate using a large-dose fentanyl technique.[76]

Volatile anesthetics have been advocated as a better method of blood pressure control.[77] In normotensive humans, isoflurane has been shown to have a greater peripheral vasodilating effect with minimal effect on cardiac output.[78] In experimental animals with hypertension, however, cardiac output is depressed by isoflurane, which is in marked contrast to the results found in the age-matched normotensive control animals.[79] Studies in hypertensive humans on the effects of isoflurane are necessary since extrapolation of data from normotensive to hypertensive humans cannot be made. When the effect of other volatile anesthetic agents on other organs is examined, it would appear that no one agent is superior. Blood flow to various organs, while altered by these agents, does not appear to be so severely affected as to compromise organ function.[80]

Perhaps the main goal of intraoperative management of the hypertensive patient should not be choosing the perfect anesthetic agent but rather attenuating the noxious stimuli in the intraoperative period. Laryngoscopy and intubation remain a time of intense stimulation, and a variety of techniques have been advocated to diminish the cardiovascular response.[81] Endotracheal extubation should be performed early so that the patient does not strain and cough at the end of the procedure. Relief of pain in the early postoperative period is also essential to decrease paroxysms of hypertension and tachycardia.

Monitoring in the postoperative period is an important component of the satisfactory management of the hypertensive patient. Increases in blood pressure should be treated with vasodilators and beta-blocking drugs. Attention to ventilation, oxygenation, and pain relief, however, are necessary prior to antihypertensive therapy.

The main aim of antihypertensive therapy is to lower systemic arterial pressure toward the normal range. The aim in the perioperative period should be the same. Because hypertension leads to organ dysfunction, the anesthesiologist must have an increased awareness of the potential problems that may occur in the anesthetic management of the hypertensive patient. Only by maintenance of adequate antihypertensive medication throughout the perioperative period can some of the potential problems be minimized.

REFERENCES

1. World Health Organization: Tech Rep 168, 1958
2. Amery A, Fagard R. Lijnen P, et al: Influence of hypotensive drug treatment on morbidity and mortality in elderly hypertensives—Review of the published trials. Acta Med Scand 678(suppl):64–85, 1983
3. Kannel WB, Gordon T, Schwartz MH: Systolic vs diastolic blood pressure and risk of coronary heart disease: The Framingham Study. Am J Cardiol 27:335–346, 1971
4. Kassier JP, Appleton F, Chagon J: Aldosterone in metabolic alkalosis. J Clin Invest 46:1558–1571, 1967
5. Conn JW, Rovner DR, Cohen EL: Normal and altered function of the renin-angiotensin-aldosterone system in man. Applications in clinical and research medicine. Ann Intern Med 63:266–284, 1965
6. Brown JJ, Davies DL, Ferriss JB, et al: Comparison of surgery and prolonged spironolactone therapy in patients with hypertension, aldosterone excess and low plasma renin. Br Med J 2:729–734, 1972
7. Gutmann FD, Tagawa H, Haber E, et al: Renal arterial pressure, renin secretion, and blood pressure control in trained dogs. Am J Physiol 224:66–72, 1973
8. Kaufman WB, Steiner B, Durr F, et al: Aldosteronstoffwechsel bei Nierenarterienstenose. Klin Wochenschr 45:966–976, 1967
9. Stanley JC, Fry WJ: Surgical treatment of renovascular hypertension. Arch Surg 112:1291–1299, 1977
10. Weiss S, Parker F: Pyelonephritis: Its relation to vascular lesions and to arterial hypertension. Medicine 18:221–234, 1939
11. Kim KE, Onesti G, Schwartz J, et al: Hemodynamics of hypertension in chronic end-stage renal disease. Circulation 46:456–464, 1972
12. Streeton DHP, Anderson GH, Freiberg JM, et al: Use of angiotensin II antagonist (saralasin) in the recognition of "angiotensinogenic" hypertension. N Engl J Med 292:657–661, 1975
13. van Heerden JH, Sheps S, Hamberger B, et al: Pheochromocytoma: Current status and changing trends. Surgery 91:367–373, 1982
14. Triner L, Baer L, Gallagher R, et al: Use of metyrosine in the anaesthetic management of patients with catecholamine-secreting tumors. Br J Anaesth 54:1333–1336, 1982
15. Bravo EL, Tarazi RC, Fouad FM, et al: Blood pressure regulation in pheochromocytoma. Hypertension 4(suppl II):193–199, 1982
16. Kempner W: Treatment of kidney disease and hypertensive vascular disease with rice diet. NC Med J 5:125–130, 1944
17. Tobian L, Ishii M, Duke M: Relationship of cytoplasmic granules in renal papillary interstitial cells to "post salt" hypertension. J Lab Clin Med 73:309–316, 1969
18. Dahl LK, Heine M, Tassinari L: Effects of chronic salt ingestion. Evidence that genetic factors play an important role in susceptibility to experimental hypertension. J Exp Med 115:1173–1178, 1962
19. Garay RP, Dagher G, Pernollet MG, et al: Inherited defect in a Na+, K+ cotransport system in erthyrocytes from essential hypertensive patients. Nature 284:281–283, 1980
20. Canessa M, Bize I, Solomon H, et al: Na countertransport and cotransport in human red cells: Function, dysfunction, and genes in essential hypertension. Clin Exp Hypertens 3:783–795, 1981
21. DeChamplain J, Farley L, Cousineau D, et al: Circulating catecholamine levels in human and experimental hypertension. Circ Res 38:109–117, 1976
22. Yamori Y, Okamoto K: Spontaneous hypertension in the rat: A model of "essential" hypertension. Verh Dtsch Ges Inn Med 80:168–175, 1974
23. Saavedra JM, Grobecher H, Axelrod J: Changes in central catecholaminergic neurons in the spontaneously (genetic) hypertensive rat. Circ Res 42:529–534, 1978
24. Miller ED, Beckman JJ, Althaus JS: Hormonal and hemodynamic responses to halothane and enflurane in spontaneously hypertensive rats. Anesth Analg 64:136–142, 1985
25. Goldblatt H, Lynch J, Hanzal RF, et al: Studies on experimental hypertension: Production of persistent elevation of systolic blood pressure by means of renal ischemia. J Exp Med 59:347–355, 1934
26. Kohlstaedt KG, Page IH: Liberation of renin by perfusion of kidneys following reduction of pulse pressure. J Exp Med 72:201–207, 1940
27. Miller ED, Samuels A, Haber E, et al: Inhibition of angiotensin conversion: Effect of initiation and maintenance of renal hypertension. Am J Physiol 228:448–453, 1975
28. Husain A, Bumpus FM, Soneby RR, et al: Evidence for the existence of a family of biologically active angiotensin I-like peptides in the dog central nervous system. Circ Res 52:460–464, 1983
29. Hutchinson JS, Mendelsohn FAO, Doyle AE: Blood pressure responses of conscious normotensive and spontaneously hypertensive rats to intracerebroventricular and peripheral administration of captopril. Hypertension 2:546–550, 1980
30. Hutchins PM, Darnell AE: Observation of a decreased number of small arterioles in spontaneously hypertensive rats. Circ Res 34(suppl 1):I-161–168, 1974
31. Folkow B, Hallback M, Lundgren Y, et al: Importance of adaptive changes in vascular design for establishment of primary hypertension studied in man and spontaneously hypertensive rats. Circ Res 32–33(suppl 1):2–10, 1973
32. Freis ED: Effects of treatment of morbidity in hyper-

tension II. Results in patients with diastolic blood pressure averaging 90 through 114 mm Hg. JAMA 213:1143–1148, 1970

33. DeCarvalho JGR, Dunn FG, Lohmoller G, et al: Hemodynamic correlates of prolonged thiazide therapy: Comparison of responders and nonresponders. Clin Pharmacol Ther 22:875–880, 1977

34. Stason WB, Cannon PJ, Heinemann HO: Furosemide: A clinical evaluation of its diuretic action. Circulation 34:910–917, 1966

35. Breckenridge A, Welbron TA, Dolley CT: Glucose tolerance in hypertensive patients on long-term diuretic therapy. Lancet 1:61–66, 1967

36. Johnston LC, Greible HG: Treatment of hypertensive disease with diuretics. V. Spironolactone, an aldosterone antagonist. Arch Intern Med 119:225–232, 1967

37. Clive DM, Staff JS: Renal syndromes associated with nonsteroidal anti-inflammatory drugs. N Engl J Med 310:563–572, 1984

38. Harrington JT, Isner JM, Kassirer JP: Our national obsession with potassium. Am J Med 73:155–159, 1982

39. Vitez TS, Soper LE, Wong KC, et al: Chronic hypokalemia and intraoperative dysrhythmias. Anesthesiology 63:130–133, 1985

40. Langer SZ, Cavero I, Massingham R: Recent developments in noradrenergic neurotransmission and its relevance to the mechanism of action of certain antihypertensive agents. Hypertension 2:372–382, 1980

41. Fouad FM, Nakashima Y, Tarazi RC, et al: Reversal of left ventricular hypertrophy in hypertensive patients treated with methyldopa: Lack of association with blood pressure control. Am J Cardiol 49:795–801, 1982

42. Gilman AF, Goodman LS, Rall TW, et al: The Pharmacological Basis of Therapeutics (ed 7). New York, MacMillan, 1985, p 789

43. Isaac L: Clonidine in the central nervous system: Site of mechanism of hypotensive action. J Cardiovasc Pharmacol 1:515–519, 1980

44. Bruce DL, Croley TF, Lee JS: Preoperative clonidine withdrawal syndrome. Anesthesiology 51:90–92, 1979

45. O'Connor DE: Accelerated acute clonidine withdrawal syndrome during coronary artery bypass surgery. Br J Anaesth 53:431–433, 1981

46. Holmes B, Brogden RN, Heel RC, et al: Guanabenz. Drugs 26:212–229, 1983

47. Pritchard BNC: Hypotensive action of pronethalol. Br Med J 1:1227–1228, 1964

48. Lund-Johansen P: Hemodynamic changes at rest and during exercise in long-term beta-blockade therapy of essential hypertension. Acta Med Scand 195:117–121, 1974

49. Tarazi RC, Dustan HP: Beta-adrenergic blockade in hypertension. Practical and theoretical implications of long-term hemodynamic variations. Am J Cardiol 29:633–640, 1972

50. Morgan TO, Roberts R, Carney SL, et al: Beta-adrenergic receptor blocking drugs, hypertension and plasma renin. Br J Clin Pharmacol 2:159–164, 1975

51. Scales B, Cosgrove MD: The metabolism and distribution of the selective adrenergic beta-blocking agent, practolol. J Pharmacol Exp Ther 175:338–344, 1970

52. Langer SZ: Presynaptic receptors and their role in the regulation of transmitter release. Br J Pharmacol 60:481–487, 1977

53. Simon G, Kiowski W, Julius S: Effects of beta-adrenoreceptor antagonists on baroreceptor reflex sensitivity in hypertension. Clin Pharmacol Ther 22:293–298, 1977

54. Scivoletto R, Toledo AJO, Gomes da Silva AC: Mechanism of the hypotensive effect of prazosin. Arch Int Pharmacodyn Ther 223:333–338, 1976

55. Mancia G, Ferrari A, Gregorini L, et al: Effect of prazosin on autonomic control of circulation in essential hypertension. Hypertension 2:700–707, 1980

56. Iggo A, Vogt M: Preganglionic sympathetic activity in normal and reserpine-treated cats. J Physiol (Lond) 154:114–119, 1960

57. Sannerstedt R, Conway J: Hemodynamic and vascular responses to antihypertensive treatment with adrenergic blocking agents: A review. Am Heart J 79:122–127, 1970

58. Kirpekar SM, Furchgott RF: Interaction of tyramine and guanethidine in the spleen of the cat. J Pharmacol Exp Ther 180:38–46, 1972

59. Weber MA, Drager JI, Kaufman CA: The combined alpha- and beta-adrenergic blocker labetalol and propranolol in the treatment of high blood pressure: Similarities and differences. J Clin Pharmacol 24:103–112, 1984

60. Richards DA: Pharmacological effects of labetalol in man. Br J Clin Pharmacol 3:721–723, 1976

61. Ablad B: A study of the mechanism of the hemodynamic effects of hydralazine in man. Acta Pharmacol Toxicol 20(suppl 1):1–15, 1963

62. Perry HM: Late toxicity to hydralazine resembling systemic lupus erythematosus or rheumatoid arthritis. Am J Med 54:58–64, 1973

63. Pettinger WA: Minoxidil and the treatment of severe hypertension. N Engl J Med 303:922–926, 1980

64. Zins GR: Alterations in renal function during vasodilator therapy. In Wesson LG, Fanelli GM (eds): Recent Advances in Renal Physiology and Pharmacology. Baltimore, University Park Press, 1974, pp 165–186

65. Weiss VC, West DP, Mueller CE: Topical minoxidil in alopecia areata. J Am Acad Dermatol 5:224–226, 1981

66. Gould BA, Mann S, Kieso H, et al: The role of a slow channel inhibitor, verapamil, in the management of hypertension. Acta Med Scand 681(suppl):117–123, 1984

67. Laragh JH, Case DB, Wallace JM, et al: Blockade of renin or angiotensin for understanding human hyper-

tension: A comparison of propranolol, saralasin and converting enzyme blockade. Fed Proc 36:1781–1787, 1977

68. Vidt DG, Bravo EL, Fouad FM: Captopril. N Engl J Med 306:214–218, 1982

69. Frohlich ED, Cooper RA, Lewis EJ: Review of the overall experience of captopril in hypertension. Arch Intern Med 144:1441–1444, 1984

70. Antonaccio MJ: Angiotensin converting enzyme inhibitors. Annu Rev Pharmacol Toxicol 22:57–87, 1982

71. Gomez HJ, Cirillo VJ, Jones KH: The clinical pharmacology of enalapril. J Hypertens 1(suppl 1):65–70, 1983

72. Katz JD, Croneau LH, Barash PG: Postoperative hypertension: A hazard of abrupt cessation of antihypertensive medication in the postoperative period. Am Heart J 92:79–80, 1976

73. Prys-Roberts C, Foex P, Greene LT, et al: Studies of anaesthesia in relation to hypertension. IV. The effect of artificial ventilation on the circulation and pulmonary gas exchange. Br J Anaesth 44:335–349, 1972

74. Goldman L, Caldera DL: Risks of general anesthesia and elective operation in the hypertensive patient. Anesthesiology 50:285–292, 1979

75. Stanley TH, Philbin DM, Coggins CH: Fentanyl-oxygen anesthesia for coronary artery surgery: Cardiovascular and antidiuretic hormone responses. Can Anaesth Soc J 26:168–172, 1979

76. Waller JL, Hug CC, Nagle DM, et al: Hemodynamic changes during fentanyl-oxygen anesthesia for aortocoronary bypass operations. Anesthesiology 55:212–217, 1981

77. Hamilton WK: Do let the blood pressure drop and do use myocardial depressants. Anesthesiology 45:273, 1976

78. Graves CL, McDermott RW, Bidwai A: Cardiovascular effects of isoflurane in surgical patients. Anesthesiology 41:486–489, 1974

79. Seyde WC, Longnecker DE: Normotension versus hypertension: Does isoflurane influence hemodynamics differently? Anesthesiology 63:A13, 1985

80. Miller ED, Beckman JJ, Althaus JS: Hormonal and hemodynamic responses to halothane and enflurane in spontaneously hypertensive rats. Anesth Analg 64:136–142, 1985

81. Barash PG, Giles R, Marx P, et al: Intubation: Is low-dose fentanyl really effective? Anesth Analg 61:S168–S169, 1982

Richard F. Davis, M.D.

12

Etiology and Treatment of Perioperative Cardiac Dysrhythmias

Cardiac dysrhythmias are among the most frequent perioperative cardiovascular abnormalities. In 1936, Kurtz et al reported that, in over 100 patients studied, sinus arrhythmias, premature ventricular contractions (PVCs), and "downward displacement" of the pacemaker were the most common rhythm disturbances; the total frequency of dysrhythmias was 79 percent.[1] A summary of the literature in 1970 revealed that the incidence of cardiac dysrhythmias during anesthesia and operation ranged from 16.3 to 61.7 percent;[2] however, subsequently, an even higher incidence of dysrhythmias (84 percent) was recorded via Holter monitoring.[3] On the other hand, in a series of 5012 patients undergoing halothane anesthesia, the incidence of "serious" dysrhythmias was only 0.9 percent.[4] Understanding the etiology and treatment of perioperative dysrhythmias is, therefore, essential to the safe use of anesthesia; this applies equally to patients with and without cardiac disease and to those having noncardiac as well as cardiac operations. This chapter reviews the basic electrophysiology of the heart, origins of cardiac dysrhythmias in both the electrophysiologic and the clinical framework, and pharmacologic agents used to treat dysrhythmias.

CARDIAC ELECTROPHYSIOLOGY

Knowledge of the normal electrical activity of myocardial cells is required in order to understand the abnormal electrical activity that produces the various dysrhythmias seen clinically. For practical purposes the myocardium can be considered as being comprised of two cell types: the working myocardial cells and the conduction system cells. Working myocardial cells have the specialized ability to shorten against a load when electrically stimulated; this is the property that forms the basis of cardiac contraction. The process of electrical stimulation, depolarization, changes the physical properties of the myocardial cell membrane; the altered permeability of the membranes, in turn, changes transmembrane ionic gradients so that calcium can enter the cell and subsequently activate the contractile apparatus. The contractile efforts of individual working myocardial cells must be coordinated in order to effect contraction; it is this coordination that is performed by the cells of the cardiac conduction system, which spontaneously produce depolarization and transmit the resulting electrical activity to the working myocardial

CARDIAC ANESTHESIA, SECOND EDITION
ISBN 0-8089-1848-6

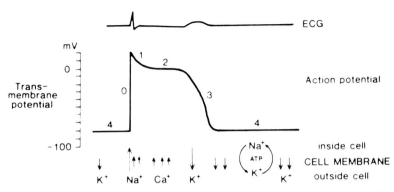

Fig. 12-1. Schematic representation of the action potential in a ventricular myocardial cell as it correlates with the electrocardiogram (ECG). Arrows indicate times of major ionic movement across the cell membrane. (From Lewis AJ: Monitoring and dysrhythmia recognition in advanced cardiac life support. *In* McIntyre KM, Lewis AJ (eds): Textbook of Advanced Cardiac Life Support. Dallas, American Heart Association, 1983, with permission.)

cells in a specific, coordinated time sequence. Any disturbance of these functions (formation and conduction of the impulse and the depolarization and repolarization of working myocardial cells) potentiates cardiac dysrhythmias.

Action Potential

The electrical events during depolarization and repolarization can be demonstrated for single myocardial cells by means of microelectrodes that penetrate the cell membrane and record the electrical potential that exists across the membrane. In working myocardial cells at rest, this electrical potential is stable, the cell interior being negative relative to the exterior by approximately 90 mv; the *resting potential* in working myocardial cells is approximately −90 mv. This resting potential is determined by the transmembrane distribution of electrolytes, notably sodium and potassium. When an electric current passes through the cell, the membrane becomes highly permeable to sodium, which rapidly enters the cell and makes the cell interior positive relative to the exterior by approximately 20 mv. Depolarization and repolarization, when recorded from microelectrodes and displayed on an oscilloscope, produce the characteristic *action potential* (AP) waveform.

In working myocardial cells, the AP is subdivided into five distinct periods (Fig. 12-1).[5] An external stimulus, which reduces the resting membrane potential to a certain level termed the *threshold potential,* normally about −65 mv, produces the AP. The AP is propagated by the flow of electrical current into adjacent nondepolarized areas of the membrane, which lowers that local membrane potential to threshold and, thereby, produces further depolarization.[6]

Depolarization itself is initiated by a 1-msec change in the permeability of the cell membrane to sodium and calcium.[7] Two specific transmembrane channels for ion movement have been described. The fast channel permits rapid entry of sodium into the cell and has a threshold of approximately −60 mv.[8] The slow channel has a threshold of −30 mv and allows the slow entry of calcium into the cell.[9] A large amount of evidence indicates that these two channels are not just conceptual but, in fact, represent physical structures in the membrane. Sodium conductance (but not that of calcium) is blocked by tetrodotoxin,[10] while calcium conductance is inhibited by other divalent ions, such as manganese, lanthanum, and cobalt, and by calcium channel blocking drugs such as verapamil, diltiazem, and nifedipine. Also, the myocardial contractile response to membrane depolarization, which requires extracellular calcium, is slight until the threshold of calcium conductance is reached at about −30 mv,[11] despite a large increase in sodium conductance at more negative (−65 mv) membrane potentials.

During the resting phase (phase 4) of the action potential, sodium and potassium are distributed across the membrane such that sodium concentration is higher outside than inside, while potassium is higher inside than outside. This distribution is governed by the properties of the cell membrane, and is described by the Nernst equation:

$$E = (R/NF) \cdot \log_N (C_o/C_i)$$

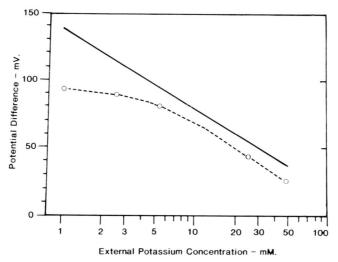

Fig. 12-2. Transmembrane potential of cardiac muscle fiber varies inversely with the potassium concentration of the external medium (dashed curve). The continuous line represents the change in transmembrane potential predicted by the Nernst equation for E_K. (From Page E: Circulation 26:582, 1962, with permission.)

where E = membrane potential, R = gas constant, N = valency of ion, F = Faraday, and Co and Ci = ion concentrations outside and inside the membrane, respectively. For the normal outside-to-inside concentration gradient of potassium, the equation predicts a transmembrane potential of −90 mv. The directly measured potential varies inversely with the external concentration of potassium (Fig. 12-2).[12] In contrast, extracellular sodium concentration has little influence on resting potential but does critically influence AP amplitude.[12]

At the onset of depolarization, the fast sodium channel opens briefly and sodium flows down its concentration gradient into the cell. This influx of sodium rapidly depolarizes the membrane, which makes the inside of the cell positive relative to the exterior by 20 mv. This is phase 0 of the AP, which, in the working myocardium, coincides with the QRS complex of the surface electrocardiogram (ECG). Repolarization begins with the closing of the fast sodium channel, which produces a brief period when the membrane potential rapidly returns toward 0 (phase 1 of the AP). Calcium entry into the cell via the slow channel keeps the cell isoelectric but depolarized during phase 2 of the AP, which corresponds in time to the ST segment of the surface ECG. Potassium efflux from the cell is primarily responsible for the majority of repolarization, which occurs during phase 3, when the membrane potential returns to the resting level of −90 mv. Although

repolarization is complete at this point, the normal ionic gradient across the membrane has not yet been reestablished. During phase 4 of the AP, specialized membrane-bound enzyme systems (the sodium–potassium pump) effectively remove sodium from the cell interior and return potassium into the cell. This pumping action involves ionic transport against concentration gradients and is, therefore, a high-energy process that depends on an abundant supply of adenosine triphosphate (ATP).

The AP recorded from cells in the conduction system, especially in the sinoatrial (SA) and atrioventricular (AV) nodes, differs from that in the working cells (Fig. 12-3). In these cells, the resting potential (phase 4) is not isoelectric; rather, there is a slow spontaneous depolarization of the membrane, a property termed *automaticity*. This depolarization (spontaneous diastolic depolarization) is due to a low membrane permeability to potassium and a high resting permeability to calcium.[7] When this diastolic depolarization reaches threshold potential, an AP is propagated. Phase 0 of the AP recorded from cells in the SA and AV nodes is due primarily to entry of calcium (and possibly sodium) through the slow channel. The slope of phase 0 in these cells is less than that in working cells both because of a dependence on slow channel activity and because of onset at a less negative transmembrane potential.

The rate at which spontaneous diastolic depolarization or automaticity produces the AP is influenced

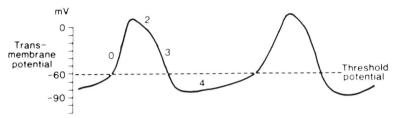

Fig. 12-3. Schematic representation of pacemaker cell action potential and phases 0–4. (From Lewis AJ: Monitoring and dysrhythmia recognition in advanced cardiac life support. *In* McIntyre KM, Lewis AJ (eds): Textbook of Advanced Cardiac Life Support. Dallas, American Heart Association, 1983, with permission.)

by a variety of factors. The slope of spontaneous depolarization in SA nodal cells is closely controlled by autonomic nervous system activity. Sympathetic activity, initiated predominantly by the right sympathetic chain (or circulating catecholamines through beta$_1$-agonist effects), increases the slope and thereby both decreases the time to reach threshold potential and increases the frequency of depolarization (Fig. 12-4). Vagal activity, in contrast, decreases the frequency of depolarization, which occurs because acetylcholine (1) increases K$^+$ conductance, which produces a hyperpolarization of the membrane; (2) decreases the slope of phase 4; and (3) increases threshold potential (Fig. 12-4).[13] Typically, cells of the SA node exhibit the highest spontaneous frequency of depolarization, and, therefore, the SA

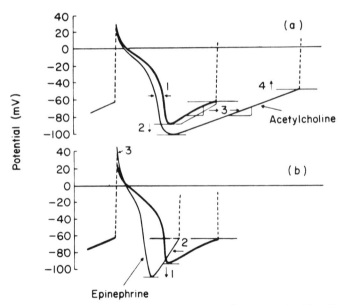

Fig. 12-4. Changes of pacemaker potential in a Purkinje fiber as a result of the effects of acetylcholine (a) and epinephrine (b). Acetylcholine shortens action potential duration (1), hyperpolarizes the membrane (2), decreases the slope of phase 4 diastolic depolarization (3), and increases threshold potential (4). Epinephrine produces hyperpolarization of the cell (1), increases the slope of phase 4 diastolic depolarization (2), and increases the overshoot in the action potential phase 0 (3). In each panel, the normal action potential is indicated by the dense solid line. (Based on material from Noble D: The Initiation of the Heart Beat. Oxford, Oxford University Press, 1975. From Prys-Roberts C: Electrophysiology—The origin of the heart beat. *In* Prys-Roberts C (ed): The Circulation in Anaesthesia. Applied Physiology and Pharmacology. London, Blackwell Scientific, 1980, with permission.)

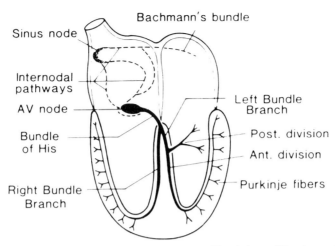

Fig. 12-5. Diagram of cardiac conduction system (abbreviations: AV, atrioventricular; post., posterior; ant., anterior). (From Lewis AJ: Monitoring and dysrhythmia recognition in advanced cardiac life support. In McIntyre KM, Lewis AJ (eds): Textbook of Advanced Cardiac Life Support. Dallas, American Heart Association, 1983, with permission.)

node is the dominant pacemaker for the heart with resting frequencies from 60 to 100 per minute. Spontaneous depolarization in the AV node and the Purkinje system is masked by the conducted impulse from the SA node. However, these areas may be conceptualized as "escape" or back-up pacemakers with intrinsic rates of 40–60 and 20–40 per minute in the AV node and Purkinje system, respectively.

Two important concepts for understanding the development of dysrhythmias are refractoriness and excitability. Excitability is the property of cardiac tissue to depolarize to a given stimulation. Increased excitability, which indicates responsiveness to a lesser stimulus or a greater response to any given stimulus, is an important cause of dysrhythmias.[6] During depolarization and the early part of repolarization (ie, phases 0, 1, and 2 through the initial part of phase 3 of the AP), the cell cannot depolarize and produce another AP. This time interval is termed the *absolute refractory period.* During the latter portion of phase 3, a stronger-than-usual impulse can produce a propagated AP, and this interval is the *relative refractory period;* the sum of these two periods is termed the *effective refractory period* (ERP). The relative refractory period is also termed the *vulnerable period* because an impulse occurring at this time will reach areas of the heart that are at various stages of repolarization, and this increases the likelihood of producing repetitive but dyssynchronous depolarization, such as in ventricular fibrillation.

Conduction System Anatomy

An AP is conducted from its origin in the SA node to its end point in the ventricular myocardium by discrete specialized tissue pathways (Fig. 12-5). The impulse is conducted from the SA node to the AV node by at least three discrete pathways.[14] Conduction to the left atrium is mediated by the anterior interatrial myocardial band (Bachmann's bundle).[15] Conduction through the atria to the AV node is rapid, on the order of 800–1000 mm/sec. The AV node is located anatomically at the inferior margin of the right atrium in the septal wall anterior to the orifice of the coronary sinus and just above the tricuspid valve.[16] Conduction velocity through the AV node is about 20–25 percent of that through the atria (200 mm/sec). Conceptually, this conduction delay is analogous to a capacitor in an electrical circuit and allows completion of both atrial activation and contraction before ventricular activation.

At its inferior margin, the AV node merges into the AV bundle of His, which penetrates the annulus fibrosis. At the upper margin of the muscular interventricular septum, the AV bundle divides into the left and right bundle branches. The left bundle divides early in its course in many directions, but divisions are commonly grouped into the anterior and posterior fascicles; the anterior division supplies the anterior interventricular septum (IVS), anterior papillary muscle, and anterior left ventricle; the posterior division supplies the posterior IVS, posteromedial papillary muscle, and posterior left ventricle. The right bundle supplies the IVS near the apex and the right ventricle. Conduction velocity through the bundles and the Purkinje system is the most rapid of the conduction system at 4000 mm/sec, a feature that assures rapid synchronous activation of the ventricle but preserves the activation sequence necessary for optimal efficiency. The IVS and papillary muscles are the first portion of the ventricle to depolarize and contract; this, in effect, provides a skeleton for ventricular contraction and prevents prolapse and regurgitation of the AV valves. Subsequent ventricular activation is earliest at the apical endocardium and latest at the basal epicardium, a sequence producing an apical-to-basal, spiraling contraction pattern by which the heart "wrings" out its stroke volume.

MECHANISMS OF DYSRHYTHMIA FORMATION

Electrophysiologic Context

For conceptual purposes, the origins of the electrical impulses producing normal and abnormal cardiac activation can be grouped as automaticity, conductivity, or combinations of the two.[7] Automaticity regulates normal heart rate and the frequency of lower pacemakers in the event of SA node or conduction failure and may also produce dysrhythmias. The speed of impulse conduction (conductivity or *dromotropism*) is an important parameter of the spread of activation. Disturbed conductivity (either slower or faster than normal) may either be primarily responsible for dysrhythmias or may set the stage for another mechanism, reentry.

Abnormal automaticity is a common source of perioperative dysrhythmias. Simple examples are sinus tachycardia or sinus bradycardia. More localized disturbances of automaticity may be responsible for isolated premature depolarizations or cyclic rhythms originating at any point in the conduction system. Examples are junctional or ventricular ectopy, either as isolated contractions or as sustained rhythms such as nodal or ventricular tachycardia. Causes of abnormal automaticity may be grouped as *after-potentials, oscillation, incomplete repolarization,* or *triggered automaticity.* An after-potential is a transient decrease in membrane potential during phase 4, which, if threshold is reached, can produce a propagated wave of depolarization. Oscillation refers to the occurrence of multiple after-potentials, which produce an oscillating rather than a stable

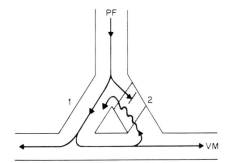

Fig. 12-6. A single branched Purkinje fiber (PF) terminates on a strip of ventricular muscle (VM) by one of two branches. The shaded area in branch 2 represents an area of unidirectional block produced by abnormal repolarization. A single impulse propagated through the Purkinje fiber will reach the ventricular muscle via path 1 and then be conducted retrograde along path 2. If the normal pathway has recovered excitability, the retrograde impulse from path 2 will reexcite the normal pathway and produce an ectopic impulse. (From Bigger JT, Hoffman BF: Antiarrhythmic drugs. *In* Gilman AG, Goodman LS, Rall TW, et al. (eds): The Pharmacologic Basis of Therapeutics (ed 7). New York, Macmillan, 1985, with permission.)

phase 4 potential. Incomplete repolarization, by creating a potential difference between adjacent groups of cells, can produce enough current to cause depolarization. A common clinical correlate of incomplete repolarization is myocardial ischemia. Triggered automaticity refers to the production of an automatic focus within the myocardium, which depends on an antecedent premature beat for initiation.

Abnormal conductivity produces dysrhythmias through a mechanism termed *reentry,* which may occur at any level in the conduction system and may produce isolated ectopic contractions or repetitive dysrhythmias. Conceptually, reentry requires local areas of myocardium with both depressed conductivity and either delayed repolarization or prolonged refractoriness (Fig. 12-6). Normal impulse conduction provides equally rapid spread of depolarization in adjacent areas of the conduction system. An area of delayed repolarization will effectively block normal antegrade conduction through that area; however, the impulse may proceed at a normal rate down adjacent pathways, which have normal repolarization and conduction, through cardiac muscle, and then retrograde through the pathway with delayed repolarization. Such a retrograde impulse would normally be extinguished in the refractory area of the abnormal pathway. However, if conduction of the impulse down the "normal" pathway is slowed but not blocked (abnormal conductivity), then the impulse will arrive retrograde at the previously blocked site after the refractory period in that area and will be conducted through the abnormal area to produce antegrade but premature depolarization of the original pathway. Thus, a "unidirectional" block is produced by the interaction of the disparity of refractory period duration between normal and abnormal pathways and abnormal conductivity. A similar mechanism has been evoked to account for "circus movement,"[17] which may account for atrial fibrillation and flutter.[18-20]

Parasystole, another mechanism of dysrhythmia formation, is due to simultaneously activated but independently fired impulses that compete to activate the myocardium.[21] Like reentry, parasystole depends on altered conductivity, but abnormal automaticity creates the abnormal parasystolic impulse. This impulse can partially activate the myocardium independently of the normal impulse. The area producing the parasystolic impulse is protected by a unidirectional "protection block," which is simply the refractory period produced by the parasystolic impulse. Diagnosis of parasystole is based on demonstrating independence of the ectopic from the normal rhythms by showing (1) variable intervals between the normal complex and the abnormal complex (coupling interval), (2) a constant shortest interectopic complex interval, or (3) frequent fusion complexes.[22,23]

Clinical Context

A sound understanding of the electrophysiologic mechanisms of dysrhythmia formation is important; however, equally important is an understanding of the clinical conditions that predispose to dysrhythmias. Inhalational anesthetic agents, acid-base and electrolyte alterations, temperature abnormalities, and myocardial ischemia or infarction are common clinical correlates of perioperative dysrhythmias.

INHALATIONAL ANESTHETIC AGENTS

The ability of halogenated hydrocarbon anesthetic agents to potentiate the dysrhythmogenic effect of circulating catecholamines and to produce dysrhythmias, either independently or through interactions with other drugs, is well recognized.[13,24,25]

One of the most widely appreciated electrophysiologic effects of inhalational anesthetics is the potentiation of the dysrhythmogenic effects of catecholamines. In a review of interactions of inhalational anesthetics and adrenergic drugs, halothane produced

no effect on resting membrane potential but did decrease the difference between threshold potential and maximal (most negative) diastolic potential and the rate of spontaneous diastolic depolarization.[26,27] The decreased potential required to reach threshold (produced by halothane) and the increase in rate of phase 4 depolarization (produced by epinephrine) was hypothesized to account for the potentiation of the dysrhythmogenic effects of epinephrine by halothane. This potentiation has also been ascribed to slower conduction velocity, briefer refractory period, and decreased action potential duration (APD), and the disparity between refractory period durations of Purkinje and ventricular muscle fibers.[28] Despite more recent studies documenting the influence of inhalational anesthetics on slow channel inward currents,[29-31] the precise electrophysiologic mechanism of the dysrhythmogenicity of the catecholamine-inhalational anesthetic interaction remains obscure.

There are significant differences among the inhalational anesthetics with regard to this catecholamine interaction. Earlier observations of currently unused or little-used anesthetics, such as diethyl ether, cyclopropane, methoxyflurane, and fluroxene were reviewed by Katz and Epstein.[24] The degree of sensitization to catecholamine dysrhythmogenicity among currently used anesthetics is greatest with halothane and least with enflurane (Fig. 12-7).[32,33] However, the catecholamine dose–response curve is nonlinear with enflurane.[34] This relationship (although the calculated ED_{50} for enflurane is greater than for isoflurane or halothane) makes prediction of the response with enflurane for a given catecholamine dose unreliable. Children, in contrast to adults, have a higher dysrhythmic threshold to epinephrine during halothane anesthesia. In a series of 83 pediatric patients, no ventricular dysrhythmias were reported during anesthetia maintained with halothane despite the administration of epinephrine by submucosal or subcutaneous injection up to 15.7 μg/kg.[35]

The injected dose of catecholamine is only one parameter of the interaction; plasma concentrations of epinephrine that produced dysrhythmias in anesthetized dogs were reported to be 38.7 ng/ml (a dose of 2.18 μg/kg/min for 10 minutes) with halothane (0.87 percent), 206 ng/ml (a dose of 11.4 μg/kg/min for 10 minutes) with enflurane (2.2 percent), and 296.5 ng/ml (15.3 μg/kg/min) with pentobarbital (30 mg/kg, IV).[36] These results for pentobarbital contrast with another study in which a 20 mg/kg dose of sodium thiopental potentiated the halothane–epinephrine interaction in dogs.[37]

The conclusion is that the prudent practitioner

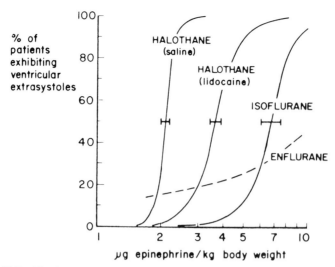

Fig. 12-7. The dose-response curves for the dysrhythmogenicity of increasing doses of epinephrine in the presence of halothane, halothane with lidocaine, isoflurane, and enflurane. The curves for halothane and isoflurane are parallel although the ED_{50} differs significantly. The curve for enflurane is markedly flattened, and, although the ED_{50} is greater with enflurane, the response is less predictable. (From Johnston RR, Eger EI II, Wilson C: A comparative interaction of epinephrine with enflurane, isoflurane, and halothane in man. Anesth Analg 55:709–712, 1976, with permission.)

should not use inhalational anesthetics, especially halothane, when a catecholamine infusion is required for hemodynamic stability. Concurrent use of submucosal or subcutaneous epinephrine and inhalational anesthetics should be guided by the known dose–response curves for each agent (halothane, ED_{50} 2.11 ± 15 μg/kg; isoflurane, ED_{50} 6.72 ± 0.66 μg/kg; and enflurane, ED_{50} 10.9 ± 8.9 μg/kg)[33] and by the flat slope of the curve for enflurane.

Another clinical factor that potentiates the dysrhythmogenic catecholamine–inhalation anesthetic interaction is fasting. Miletich et al reported that fasting significantly lowered the dysrhythmic threshold for epinephrine in rats during 2 percent halothane anesthesia.[38] In those rats that were not fasted, the threshold was 10.9 μg/kg, but after a 24-hour fast, the threshold decreased to 2.2 μg/kg and stabilized at that point with longer fasting. The fasted thresholds correspond closely to those observed clinically. The effect of fasting was mimicked by infusing lipids in nonfasted animals, which may indicate that the increase in fatty acid concentration that accompanies fasting can alter cardiac cell membrane sensitivity to beta-adrenergic stimulation.[39] However, halothane does not affect the affinity of canine cardiac beta-adrenergic receptors for either dihydroalprenolol or L-isoproterenol.[40]

Other concomitantly administered drugs influence the inhalational anesthetic–catecholamine interaction. Drugs that produce catecholamine release or block catecholamine removal through degradation or reuptake, and drugs that inhibit phosphodiesterase activity enhance sensitivity to epinephrine dysrhythmogenicity during inhalation anesthesia. Cocaine, which inhibits neuronal uptake of catecholamines; tropolone, which inhibits catechol-O-methyl transferase; aminophylline, which inhibits phosphodiesterase; and ketamine all decrease the dysrhythmic threshold with epinephrine during halothane anesthesia.[41]

The dysrhythmogenic interaction of inhalational anesthetics and catecholamines notwithstanding, the inhalational anesthetics themselves depress cardiac membrane activity and, therefore, tend to be intrinsically antiarrhythmic. Halothane decreases the rate of spontaneous phase 4 depolarization and increases the maximal diastolic potential of the SA node at 2 MAC.[29] These effects appear to be due primarily to an interference with slow channel (Ca^{++}) conduction. Isoflurane may differ from halothane in this regard. Isoflurane depresses the maximal rate of depolarization ($\dot{V}max$) of the slow-channel AP less than does halothane at anesthetically equivalent concentrations; however, both agents similarly depress the development of late after-potentials.[31] Although these effects have been studied primarily with regard to excitation-contraction coupling, they may also have implications for the mechanism of the observed differences in conduction effects of the two agents. Halothane increases conduction time from the SA node to the His bundle (A-H interval) in dogs, primarily by slowing AV nodal conduction.[42] Isoflurane in equivalent concentrations does not interfere with AV conduction or prolong the A-H interval. Halothane and isoflurane, therefore, have different effects on AP generation, impulse conduction, and sensitization of the myocardium to catecholamines. Whether the electrical effects of the two agents, which differ at the cellular level, produce the differences in the conduction effects and catecholamine interactions is not definitely known but seems likely. Nevertheless, both halothane and isoflurane possess some effects similar to class IV antiarrhythmic agents, and both anesthetics have antifibrillatory properties during reperfusion after myocardial ischemia.[43]

ELECTROLYTE ABNORMALITIES

Potassium. Because of the close relationship between extracellular pH and potassium,[44] the primary mechanism of a pH-induced dysrhythmia may be alteration of potassium concentration. Potassium is undoubtedly the electrolyte most commonly associated with dysrhythmias. Both hypo- and hyperkalemia are associated with cardiac dysrhythmias; however hypokalemia is more common perioperatively in cardiac surgical patients. Decreasing extracellular potassium concentration increases the peak negative diastolic potential, which would appear to decrease the likelihood of spontaneous depolarization. However, because the permeability of the myocardial cell membrane to potassium is directly related to extracellular potassium concentration, hypokalemia decreases cellular permeability to potassium, prolonging the AP by slowing repolarization. This effect both slows conduction and increases the dispersion of recovery of excitability, which, in turn, causes a predisposition to dysrhythmias. Electrocardiographic correlates of hypokalemia include appearance of a U wave and increased P wave amplitude.[45] The dysrhythmias most commonly associated with hypokalemia are premature atrial contractions (PACs), atrial tachycardia, and supraventricular tachycardia (SVT). Hypokalemia also accentuates the toxicity of cardiac glycosides.

Moderate hyperkalemia, on the other hand,

increases membrane permeability to potassium, which increases the speed of repolarization and decreases AP duration, thereby decreasing the tendency to dysrhythmias. An increased potassium concentration also affects pacemaker activity. The increased potassium permeability caused by hyperkalemia decreases the rate of spontaneous diastolic depolarization, which slows heart rate and, in the extreme case, can produce asystole. The repolarization abnormalities of hyperkalemia lead to the characteristic ECG findings of T wave peaking, prolonged P-R interval, decreased QRS amplitude, and a widened QRS complex.[6] Both atrioventricular and intraventricular conduction abnormalities result from the slowed conduction and uneven repolarization.

Treatment of hyperkalemia is based on its magnitude and clinical presentation. For life-threatening, hyperkalemia-induced dysrhythmias, the principle is rapid reduction of extracellular potassium concentration without necessarily decreasing total body potassium content, at least initially. Calcium chloride, 10–20 mg/kg, given by intravenous infusion, will antagonize the effects of potassium on the cardiac cell membranes. Sodium bicarbonate, 1–2 mEq/kg, or a dose calculated from acid–base measurements to produce moderate alkalinity (pH approximately 7.45–7.50), will shift potassium intracellularly. A change in pH of 0.1 unit produces a 0.5–1.5 mEq/l change of potassium concentration in the opposite direction. An intravenous infusion of glucose and insulin has a similar effect; glucose at a dose of 0.5–2 g/kg with insulin in the ratio of 1 unit:4 g of glucose is appropriate. Sequential measurement of serum potassium is important with this treatment because marked hypokalemia can result. Loop diuretics and potassium-binding resins, such as Kayexalate, promote excretion of potassium, although the effects are less rapid than with the previously mentioned modalities.

The treatment of hypokalemia is more straightforward than that of hyperkalemia; potassium deficiency is countered by potassium administration. However, with chronic potassium deficiency, the plasma deficit poorly reflects the total body deficit. Since only 2 percent of total body potassium is in plasma, and total body potassium stores may be 2000–3000 mEq, a 25 percent decline in serum potassium from 4 to 3 mEq/l indicates an equilibrium total body deficiency of 500–800 mEq, for which replacement should be undertaken slowly.

Acute hypokalemia occurs frequently after cardiopulmonary bypass, due to hemodilution, urinary losses, and intracellular shifts,[46] the latter perhaps relating to abnormalities of the glucose–insulin system seen with nonpulsatile cardiopulmonary bypass.[47] With frequent assessment of serum potassium concentrations and continuous ECG monitoring, as is routine in postoperative cardiac surgical units, potassium infusion at rates of up to 0.25–0.33 mEq/kg/hr may be administered to combat or prevent serious hypokalemia.

Sodium. Although transmembrane flux of sodium is fundamentally important to the electrical activity of the myocardium, there is little information regarding clinically significant dysrhythmias produced by abnormal serum sodium concentrations. Theoretically, the extremes of both hypo- and hypernatremia should be associated with electrophysiologic abnormalities. In one report, however, a patient with a serum sodium of 210 mEq/1 had no rhythm disturbance.[48] The author of that report also stated that severe hyponatremia should have an effect similar to that of marked hypernatremia.

Calcium and magnesium. Because of its ubiquitous role in excitation and contraction of cardiac muscle, calcium balance would be expected to be associated significantly with cardiac rhythm. In fact, although ECG abnormalities due to both hypo- and hypercalcemia are well recognized, clinically significant dysrhythmias due to an abnormal calcium concentration are much less common than those due to potassium abnormalities.

Electrocardiographic correlates of hypercalcemia include shortening of the Q-T interval and, less commonly, of the P-R interval and QRS duration.[49] Premature ventricular contractions (PVCs), tachycardia, and fibrillation may occur in relation to hypercalcemia. The synergistic interaction of cardiac glycosides and calcium deserves emphasis in this regard because hypercalcemia has been implicated in sudden death due to ventricular fibrillation (VF) in association with digitalis intoxication.

In contrast to hypercalcemia, hypocalcemia is relatively common among cardiac surgical and other critically ill patients.[50-53] The hemodynamic effects of hypocalcemia in relation to cardiopulmonary bypass and rapid blood transfusion are well recognized and are primarily those of myocardial depression. The ECG abnormality most commonly associated with hypocalcemia is a prolonged Q-T interval due to lengthening of the ST segment.[6] Other findings include tachycardia and decreased T-wave amplitude or T-wave inversion.[54]

Magnesium deficiency is also a relatively common electrolyte abnormality in critically ill patients, especially in chronic situations. Hypomagnesemia is associated with a variety of cardiovascular disturbances, including dysrhythmias.[55,56] Sudden death from ischemic heart disease, alcoholic cardiomyopathy, and congestive heart failure (CHF) may involve magnesium deficiency.[55-57] Functionally, magnesium is required for the membrane-bound, sodium-potassium ATPase, which is the principal enzyme that maintains normal intracellular potassium concentration. Not surprisingly, the ECG findings seen with magnesium deficiency mimic those seen with hypokalemia: prolonged P-R and Q-T intervals, increased QRS duration, and ST-segment abnormalities. In addition, as with hypokalemia, magnesium deficiency predisposes to the development of the dysrhythmias produced by cardiac glycosides.[58,59] Dysrhythmias induced by magnesium deficiency may be refractory to treatment with antiarrhythmic drugs and either electrical cardioversion or defibrillation. For this reason, adjunctive treatment of refractory dysrhythmias with magnesium has been advocated even when magnesium deficiency has not been documented.[60] Other important considerations with magnesium deficiency in critically ill patients have recently been reviewed by Chernow et al.[61]

Lithium. Although this electrolyte does not occur naturally in the body, its therapeutic use for psychiatric disorders is common and its potential to produce dysrhythmias warrants discussion. The cardiac action of lithium is related to its substitution for other cations, notably sodium and potassium.[62] Lithium displaces some intracellular potassium, and its ECG effects may resemble those of hypokalemia. Additionally, lithium interferes with adenyl cyclase and, thus, with catecholamine activity in the heart. Electrophysiologic effects of lithium include decreased spontaneous depolarization and decreased conduction velocity at the AV nodal and ventricular levels.[63] Reports of dysrhythmias during lithium therapy include increases in both SA node recovery time and ventricular dysrhythmias,[64] as well as development of a paroxysmal left bundle branch block.[65] Lithium therapy should thus be considered a risk factor for perioperative development of dysrhythmias.

TEMPERATURE

Metabolic and hemodynamic effects of profound hypothermia in cardiac surgical patients are widely appreciated. From the standpoint of routine clinical

Table 12-1

Incidence of Dysrhythmias and Atrioventricular Conduction Abnormalities
in Inferior (Diaphragmatic) and Anterior Myocardial Infarctions

	Inferior Myocardial Infarction	Anterior Myocardial Infarction
Dysrhythmia		
Atrial	Uncommon	Uncommon
Ventricular	Common	Common
Intraventricular block	Uncommon	Common
Atrioventricular block		
First degree	Common	Rare
Second degree		
Mobitz I	Common	None
Mobitz II	None	Common
Third degree		
Incidence	7–27 percent	1–5 percent
Site	Atrioventricular nodal	Infranodal
Escape rate	45–60 percent	25–40 percent
Duration	Transient	Permanent
Mortality	20–40 percent	>75 percent

Source. Modified from Chung EK: Principles of Cardiac Arrhythmias (ed 2). Baltimore, Williams & Wilkins, 1977.

practice, even moderate hypothermia can significantly affect the incidence and severity of cardiac dysrhythmias. In one early study, heart rate decreased progressively as temperature decreased.[66] Subsequent clinical observations have verified this finding.[67] Hypothermia decreased conduction velocity in all areas of the conduction system, which increases P-R and Q-T intervals and QRS duration. The ST segment is altered in a way that suggested ischemia to earlier workers;[68] this ST-segment change consists of a steeply inclined portion, which has been termed a *J loop, J deflection,* or *Osborn wave.*[69–71]

Ventricular fibrillation threshold is decreased with hypothermia, and this is the effect of greatest clinical concern. The electrophysiologic explanation of the increased risk of VF at low temperatures is unclear but may relate to decreased conduction velocity. Ventricular fibrillation becomes increasingly likely after temperature has decreased to approximately 30°C. Treatment of VF during hypothermia is difficult, and pharmacologic therapy is largely ineffective. Common Class I antiarrhythmic agents, such as lidocaine and procainamide, actually increase the mean lethal temperature.[72] Certainly the best treatment is prevention or early correction of hypothermia. In the context of the cardiac surgical patient, adequate rewarming before termination of

bypass and the prevention of rebound hypothermia is essential.

Hyperthermia is less frequently encountered. Sinus tachycardia is the earliest indicator of the increased metabolic state associated with hyperthermia. Associated increases in plasma catecholamines may exacerbate the development of dysrhythmias, especially in conjunction with inhalational anesthetics. Anesthetic problems due to dysrhythmias are likely in the case of severe temperature elevation, as may be seen with malignant hyperthermia, or with more moderate hyperthermia in association with cardiac pathology.

MYOCARDIAL ISCHEMIA AND INFARCTION

The final clinical context to be discussed in which cardiac dysrhythmias are likely to be a clinical anesthetic problem is myocardial ischemia. Virtually every type of dysrhythmia has been described in conjunction with cardiac ischemia. The location of the ischemic or infarcted portion of myocardium has a direct bearing on the type and the severity of dysrhythmia likely to occur. There are distinct differences in the type and severity of dysrhythmia between inferior wall or diaphragmatic myocardial infarction and anterior wall myocardial infarction (Table 12-1).[6] The types of dysrhythmias produced

Table 12-2
Classification of Antiarrhythmic Drugs

	Class			
Effect	I (Membrane Stabilizers)	II (Beta-Adrenergic Receptor Antagonists)	III (Drugs Prolonging Repolarization)	IV (Calcium Antagonists)
Pharmacologic	Fast channel (Na) blockade	Beta-adrenergic receptor blockade	Uncertain: possible interference with Na and Ca exchange	Decreased "slow-channel" calcium conductance
Electrophysiologic	Decreased rate of $\dot{V}$max	Decreased $\dot{V}$max, increased APD, increased ERP, and increased ERP:APD ratio	Increased APD, increased ERP, increased ERP:APD ratio	Decreased slow-channel depolarization; decreased APD

Abbreviations: $\dot{V}$max, rapid depolarization; APD, action potential duration; and ERP, effective refractory period.

during regional ischemia may also follow a similar distribution.

The mechanism of formation and the locus of dysrhythmias during acute ischemia or in the early phase of myocardial infarction are different from those of dysrhythmias that occur later in the course of infarction. During the acute phase of infarction, dysrhythmias are commonly due to reentry mechanisms originating in the ischemic epicardial regions.[73] In contrast, later in the infarction process, dysrhythmias originate as ectopic foci from surviving endocardial Purkinje fibers within the infarcted tissue. This difference, together with altered pharmacokinetics of antiarrhythmic drugs in ischemic myocardial tissue, may have therapeutic importance.

Aggressive treatment and prophylaxis of ischemia-related dysrhythmias are fundamental to the care of patients with myocardial infarction. Treatment of even relatively minor supraventricular and ventricular dysrhythmias may prevent subsequent occurrence of life-threatening dysrhythmias such as ventricular tachycardia (VT) or VF. For example, antiarrhythmic treatment is recommended when PVCs occur more frequently than six each minute, are in close proximity to the T wave, appear in groups of two or more, or have multiple ECG forms, since, for each condition, the frequency of VT or VF is increased.[74-80]

ANTIARRHYTHMIC DRUGS

Perhaps the most widely used electrophysiologic and pharmacologic classification of antiarrhythmic drugs is that proposed by Vaughan Williams (Table 12-2).[81] There is, however, substantial overlap in pharmacologic and electrophysiologic effects of specific agents among the classes. Likewise, especially in Class I, there may be considerable diversity within a single class. Moreover, other classes may be added to the list as evidenced by the report that alinidine, an experimental negative chronotropic drug, may exert its effect through restriction of anionic currents.[82]

Cardiac Glycosides

One difficulty with the Vaughan Williams classification scheme is that it fails to incorporate the considerable antiarrhythmic effects of cardiac glycosides (digitalis). Although, undoubtedly, the primary therapeutic use of this group of drugs is to increase the force of cardiac contraction, a very useful secondary effect is the slowing of the ventricular response rate during atrial fibrillation or flutter. As with the positive inotropic effect, the antiarrhythmic effect of digitalis is a complex combination of direct and indirect actions.

The primary direct pharmacologic effect of digitalis is inhibition of the membrane-bound Na^+-K^+-dependent ATPase. This enzyme provides the chemical energy necessary for the transport of sodium (out) and potassium (in) during repolarization phases. Digitalis binds to the enzyme in a specific, saturable way that inhibits enzyme activity and impairs the active transport of sodium and potassium. The net result is a slight increase in intracellular sodium and a corresponding decrease in intracellular potassium concentration.

In Purkinje fibers, digitalis increases the slope of

phase 4 depolarization and decreases resting potential or maximal diastolic potential so that the initiation of depolarization (phase 0) begins at a less negative potential; therefore, both the $\dot{V}$max and conduction velocity are lower. The phase 4 effect is inversely related to extracellular potassium concentration. At low concentrations of potassium, the increased rate of phase 4 depolarization is augmented and automaticity increases, which may partially explain the increased risk of digitalis-related toxicity during hypokalemia or pronounced potassium fluxes, such as during cardioversion or in the period surrounding cardiopulmonary bypass. At concentrations approaching toxicity, digitalis produces delayed after-potentials, which may be sufficient to reach threshold and trigger depolarization.[83-85] The direct action of therapeutic concentrations of digitalis in Purkinje fibers therefore decreases conduction velocity and increases ERP.

In specialized conduction fibers in the SA and AV nodes, similar electrophysiologic effects occur; in both of these regions, however, the dominant effects are indirect and mediated by the autonomic nervous system. In atrial and ventricular muscle, direct effects resemble those in Purkinje fibers. The indirect effects of digitalis, by decreasing APD, account for the decreased Q-T interval in the ECG; effects of this drug during phases 2 and 3 of the AP account for the characteristic downward convexity of the ST segment.[86]

Indirect effects of digitalis are in part due to the inhibition of reflex responses elicited by cardiac failure, because the positive inotropic effect of the drug decreases the degree of cardiac failure. Digitalis also increases vagal efferent activity, the origin of which may relate to increased sensitivity of arterial baroreceptors, to increased carotid sinus nerve activity, or to an effect on the central vagal nuclei and the nodose ganglion.[87-89] In addition, SA node sensitivity to acetylcholine may be enhanced by digitalis. In high concentrations, digitalis may decrease SA and AV nodal sensitivities to catecholamines and sympathetic stimulation, although this may be due to increased sympathetic efferent activity[90] produced by both the central nervous system (CNS) (medulla) effects of digitalis and the inhibition of norepinephrine uptake at peripheral sympathetic nerve terminals.[88,89] The decreased sinus rate seen with digitalis is, therefore, due in part to both increased vagal efferent activity and decreased sympathetic tone.

The AV node is the portion of the conduction system most strongly influenced by both the direct and indirect effects of digitalis. Conduction through the AV node is slowed, and the ERP of the AV node is lengthened by digitalis. In toxic concentrations, digitalis can effectively block AV nodal transmission.

In atrial tissue, the direct and indirect (vagal) effects of digitalis are opposed. The direct effect is an increase in APD, but the indirect effect (mediated by acetylcholine release) is a marked decrease in APD and ERP. At therapeutic concentrations, the indirect effect predominates, which makes the atria responsive to higher stimulation frequencies.[86] The effectiveness of digitalis in reducing the ventricular response rate in cases of atrial fibrillation and atrial flutter is, therefore, in part, a paradox. The frequency of atrial impulses arriving at the AV node is generally increased, which leads to frequent partial depolarization (termed *concealed conduction*). This effect, plus the increased AV nodal ERP (due to direct effects, vagal effects, and sympatholytic effects), results in a net decrease in the frequency of impulses that successfully traverse the AV node to depolarize the His–Purkinje system.

Numerous preparations of cardiac glycosides are available, but those most commonly used for acute, parenteral (intravenous), rapid digitalization, especially in the perioperative period, are digoxin, ouabain, and deslanoside, the first being the most widely used of the three but the slowest acting. The usual initial intravenous dose of ouabain is 0.25–0.5 mg, the onset of activity occurring between 3 and 10 minutes, and the peak effect at 30 minutes. Subsequent to the initial dose, 0.1-mg increments can be given at 30-minute intervals; the total dose within the first 24 hours should not exceed 1.2 mg.[91] Deslanoside has a slower onset than ouabain; its peak effect occurs within 2–3 hours after an intravenous dose. For previously undigitalized patients, appropriate initial doses of this drug are 0.8–1.6 mg. Digoxin reaches peak effects in 1.5–2 hours but has a significant effect within 5–30 minutes. For undigitalized patients, the initial dose is 0.5–1.0 mg of digoxin with subsequent doses of 0.25–0.5 mg. The usual total digitalizing dose ranges from 0.5 to 2.0 mg by the intravenous route. Digoxin is approximately 25 percent protein bound, and the therapeutic range of plasma concentrations is 0.5–2.0 ng/ml.

Class I: Membrane Stabilizers

Although a pharmacologically diverse group, Class I drugs have the common property of inhibiting the fast inward depolarizing current carried by sodium. Interestingly, at sufficient concentrations, all drugs of this class have membrane-stabilizing

Table 12-3
Subgrouping of Class I Antiarrhythmic Drugs

	Subgroup		
	IA	IB	IC
Electrophysiologic activity			
Phase 0	Depressed	Slight effect	Marked depression
Depolarization	Prolonged	Slight effect	Slight effect
Conduction	Decreased	Slight effect	Marked decrease of velocity
Effective refractory period (ERP)	Increased	Slight effect	Slight prolongation
Action potential duration (APD)	Increased	Decreased	Slight effect
ERP:APD ratio	Increased	Decreased	Slight effect
QRS duration	Increased	No effect during sinus rhythm	Marked increase
Prototype drugs	Quinidine, procainamide, disopyramide, diphenylhydantoin	Lidocaine, mexiletine, tocainide	Lorcainide, encainide, flecainide, aprinidine

effects, and this class of antiarrhythmic drugs is sometimes labeled "local anesthetics."[92] Because of the diversity of other effects of these Class I drugs, a subgrouping of the class has been proposed (Table 12-3).[93]

Whether the depression of fast inward current of the sodium channel produces the primary antiarrhythmic effect of all Class I drugs is controversial. Other proposed mechanisms involve abolishing reentry by improving conduction in the reentry pathway;[94] however, shortening the APD in ventricular pathways and improving conduction of premature impulses by shortening the refractory period of the AP also could decrease the potential for reentry.[95,96]

Class I drugs also have additional clinically important properties. The anticholinergic action seen with quinidine and disopyramide is responsible for many of the noncardiac antimuscarinic effects such as bladder outlet obstruction with disopyramide and gastrointestinal symptoms with quinidine. Moreover, the anticholinergic action, by removing tonic vagal activity at the AV node, may prevent a therapeutic effect in supraventricular tachyarrhythmias by facilitating AV nodal conduction. Conversely, in the absence of a significant underlying vagal effect, both drugs can produce AV nodal block.[97]

With some Class I drugs, CNS toxicity is prominent. For example, CNS abnormalities, including convulsions, are the primary toxic effect of lidocaine and its close chemical relatives, tocainide and mexiletine. Metabolism, excretion, and pharmacologic

activity of metabolites are other sources of variability among Class I drugs. For instance, the rapid hepatic metabolism of lidocaine and the accumulation and toxicity of its primary metabolites have prevented its oral use.[98] The individual electrophysiologic effects of Class I drugs are summarized in Table 12-3.

CLASS IA

Quinidine. In addition to the electrophysiologic effects summarized in Table 12-3, quinidine decreases the slope of phase 4 diastolic depolarization at a low concentration and increases threshold potential at a high concentration.[99] Quinidine depresses cardiac contractility, which, in combination with an indirect alpha-adrenergic blockade, can reduce arterial pressure. This hypotensive effect is the principal limitation to intravenous administration of quinidine.

Electrocardiographic effects of quinidine include an increase in sinus rate, which is perhaps a reflex response both to vasodilatation and to cardiac depression. Conduction through the AV node may be enhanced or depressed or may not change depending on the interplay of the direct effect (depression) and the anticholinergic effect (enhancement) of quinidine. Infranodal conduction is slowed, and, at high concentrations, bundle branch block, complete AV block, or asystole may result. The Q-T interval is prolonged.

Clinically, quinidine is used primarily in oral form to treat both atrial and ventricular dysrhythmias; when used alone, however, quinidine may substantially accelerate the ventricular response rate in atrial fibrillation or lower the blockade ratio with atrial flutter. Its use in these conditions, therefore, should be preceded by beta-blockade or digitalization. This acceleration of ventricular response rate is a function of the direct slowing of the atrial rate produced by quinidine and its indirect anticholinergic effects. The decreased frequency of atrial depolarization allows a greater percentage of impulses to be conducted through the AV node to depolarize the His bundle. The beneficial interaction of digitalis and quinidine in atrial fibrillation is, therefore, a function of the vagolytic effect of quinidine, which decreases the acetylcholine effect at the AV node and thereby increases AV nodal ERP, the direct effect of quinidine to increase nodal ERP, and the direct effect of digitalis to decrease AV nodal conduction.

Quinidine may be administered orally or parenterally, but the former is preferred because of the acute hemodynamic effects of the parenteral route. The gastrointestinal absorption of quinidine is good, and plasma levels peak 1–2 hours after oral administration. Quinidine has an elimination half-life of 6–7 hours; therefore, a dose every 6 or 8 hours is appropriate, although shortening the dosage interval may more effectively maintain a stable plasma concentration than increasing the dosage. Typical maintenance doses are 300–600 mg, and therapeutic plasma concentrations range from 2 to 6 μg/ml.[100] Recommended intravenous dosages of either quinidine gluconate or quinidine sulfate range from 0.2 to 0.4 mg/kg/min up to a total dose of 4–10 mg/kg titrated to the antiarrhythmic effect.[6,92,101]

Quinidine is 70–80 percent protein bound in plasma, with much of that due to hemoglobin.[102] A well-described drug interaction occurs between quinidine and digoxin; administration of quinidine substantially increases the plasma concentrations of digitalis, probably by releasing the glycoside from protein-binding sites.[103] Elimination of quinidine is primarily by hepatic metabolism (hydroxylation), although about 20 percent is excreted unchanged by the kidney. Renal excretion is by both glomerular filtration and tubular secretion and depends on urinary pH; excretion is decreased up to 50 percent when urine is alkaline.[104]

The most serious toxic effect of quinidine is cardiac and is largely a function of its conduction effects. Monitoring both the QRS duration and Q-T interval is a useful guide to therapy; a 50 percent increment in either should prompt a reduction in dose. Various degrees of conduction block at both the atrial and ventricular levels may occur, including asystole. "Quinidine syncope" probably relates to a ventricular tachyarrhythmia produced by Q-T interval prolongation and may not be dose related.[105] Symptoms of tinnitus, visual disturbance, and gastrointestinal irritation progressing to severe CNS symptoms (headache, diplopia, photophobia, confusion, or psychosis) are part of the spectrum of "cinchonism" produced by quinidine, by other cinchona alkaloids such as quinine, and by salicylates. Thrombocytopenia may occur with quinidine, and hypersensitivity to quinidine may appear as fever, anaphylaxis, or bronchospasm, which can be severe.

Procainamide. Electrophysiologic effects of procainamide (decreased $\dot{V}$max and amplitude during phase 0, decreased rate of phase 4 depolarization, and prolonged ERP or APD) are similar to those of quinidine. Clinically, procainamide prolongs conduction and increases ERP in atrial and His–Purkinje portions of the conduction system, which may prolong P-R and QRS durations; however, the Q-T interval is lengthened less than with quinidine. As with quinidine, AV nodal ERP may be decreased by indirect anticholinergic side effects.

While sharing with quinidine both a supraventricular and ventricular antiarrhythmic spectrum, procainamide is more commonly used for the latter. If used for supraventricular dysrhythmias, especially atrial fibrillation or flutter, an increased ventricular response rate will be seen (as with quinidine) unless AV nodal conduction is suppressed. Most commonly, procainamide is used to treat ventricular dysrhythmias, especially those unresponsive or incompletely responsive to lidocaine. It is very useful for chronic suppression of PVCs but may be supplanted in this use by newer Class IB drugs, such as tocainide and mexiletine. Both quinidine and procainamide are reported to reduce the frequency of short coupling-interval (less than 400 msec) PVCs and thereby to reduce the frequency of VT or VF created by the R-on-T phenomenon.[106]

Administered intravenously, procainamide is an effective emergency treatment for ventricular dysrhythmias, especially after lidocaine failure. By this route, dosage is 100 mg, or approximately 1.5 mg/kg, given at 5-minute intervals until the therapeutic effect is obtained, up to a total dose of 1 g. Arterial pressure and ECG should be monitored continuously during this loading-dose technique and administration stopped if significant hypotension occurs or if the QRS complex is prolonged by 50 percent or more. Maintenance infusion rates are 20–80 μg/kg/min to maintain therapeutic plasma concentrations of 4–8 μg/ml.[107] A double infusion technique has been described in which 17 mg/kg is infused initially over 1 hour (remarkably similar to loading a 70-kg patient with 1 g given at 20 mg/min for 50 minutes) followed by a maintenance infusion of 2.8 mg/kg/hr.[108]

Oral administration of procainamide has a 75–95 percent absorption rate, and plasma levels peak after 1–2 hours.[109] The elimination half-life of procainamide is 3–4 hours, and the oral dosage interval is similar; however, sustained release preparations are available. Oral dose requirements are on the order of 50 mg/kg/24 hr or 500–600 mg every 3–4 hours.[110] As with quinidine, decreasing the dosage interval rather than increasing the dose may be a better method of producing a stable increase in plasma concentrations without creating peak levels that are toxic.

Procainamide has both hepatic and renal routes of elimination, with each route approximately equal in magnitude. Hepatic metabolism is by acetylation and, therefore, will be either fast or slow in individual patients due to genetic variation.[111] The primary metabolite, N-acetyl procainamide, has antiarrhythmic effects as well as toxic side effects and is excreted almost entirely by the kidney.[112] The clinical importance is that patients with impaired hepatic or renal function, or with diminished perfusion of either organ, as in CHF, will have markedly impaired elimination of procainamide. Recommended dosages with renal impairment or CHF are a loading dose of 12 mg/kg given over 1 hour, with a maintenance dose of 1.4 mg/kg/hr.[113]

Toxic side effects of procainamide appear to be dose related and are primarily related to plasma concentration, a function of both total dose and rate of administration during the loading technique. Serious cardiac toxicity generally requires plasma concentrations over 12 μg/ml. The likelihood of producing VT or VF due to Q-T prolongation (Torsade de pointes) is less with procainamide than with quinidine.[114] Procainamide may also produce gastrointestinal disturbances, CNS symptoms (headache and sleep disturbance), rash, and agranulocytosis. Among patients receiving procainamide chronically, antinuclear antibodies develop in 50–70 percent, and approximately half will suffer fever, myalgia, rash, pleuritis, or pericarditis similar to lupus erythematosus, although renal and CNS effects are rare.[115] These reactions are due to the parent compound, not metabolites, since N-acetyl procainamide given

chronically does not produce the syndrome.[116] They are also more common among patients who are slow acetylators. After discontinuation of the drug, lupus symptoms resolve slowly.

Intramyocardial distribution of procainamide, especially during ischemia or infarction, is an important component of its therapeutic effect. In a canine infarction model, procainamide increased ERP more in ischemic than in nonischemic myocardium.[117] The pharmacokinetics of procainamide have been shown to differ between ischemic and nonischemic regions of myocardium; tissue concentrations of procainamide decline more rapidly in the latter.[118] Moreover, during constant infusion of procainamide, there is a concentration of the drug relative to regional perfusion in ischemic regions of the myocardium; myocardium having blood flow rates of only 10 percent of normal retained procainamide concentrations of 42 percent of normal.

Disopyramide. Although disopyramide is chemically different from quinidine and procainamide, electrophysiologic effects of the three drugs are similar. Conduction through the AV node may be facilitated slightly by disopyramide due to its indirect vagolytic effect.[119] Accessory pathway conduction may be slowed in patients with Wolff-Parkinson-White (WPW) syndrome.[120] Disopyramide is a potent negative inotropic drug, and, after intravenous use, systemic vascular resistance reflexly increases.[121]

Disopyramide is therapeutically effective against supraventricular and ventricular tachyarrhythmias. However, as with quinidine and procainamide, disopyramide should not be used for ventricular tachyarrhythmias due to prolonged repolarization (long Q-T syndrome). The marked negative inotropic and anticholinergic effects limit the usefulness of the drug.

When given orally, 80 percent of disopyramide is absorbed, and steady-state therapeutic plasma concentrations of 2–4 μg/ml can be achieved with 100–200 mg orally every 6 hours.[122] The elimination half-life is approximately 7 hours and occurs equally by hepatic and renal mechanisms; hepatic or renal insufficiency may necessitate smaller doses.[123] Disopyramide is approximately 30–50 percent protein bound at plasma concentrations of 3 μg/ml.[124]

Toxicity of disopyramide is most frequently anticholinergic in origin with symptoms of gastrointestinal upset, visual disturbance, and urinary tract obstruction, which may be marked in elderly men with prostatic hypertrophy. Unless there is left ventricular failure, cardiovascular complications are infrequent; however, in up to 50 percent of patients with a history of CHF, it may recur.[121] Conduction system toxicity resembles that with quinidine.

Diphenylhydantoin. Diphenylhydantoin (DPH), or phenytoin, is unique among Class IA drugs in that it has a potent central sympatholytic effect that decreases cardiac sympathetic efferent nerve activity.[125,126] Its electrophysiologic effect in many ways bridges the IA and IB classification. In normal conduction system cells, DPH decreases $\dot{V}$max and amplitude of phase 0, but this effect is weaker than with other Class IA drugs,[127] and clinically DPH does not decrease intraventricular conduction. Diphenylhydantoin shortens APD as does lidocaine, the prototype Class IB drug.[128] Also, DPH can effectively abolish the delayed after-potentials associated with digitalis intoxication, and this effect may be its primary therapeutic use.[129,130] In cells partially depolarized from cold, hypoxia, or cardiac glycoside administration, DPH increases maximal diastolic potential, $\dot{V}$max of phase 0, and the conduction velocity.[131] Thus, DPH exerts its antiarrhythmic effect by increasing the ERP:APD ratio and by decreasing automaticity, both of these effects being enhanced in partially depolarized cells.

Clinically, the primary use of DPH is to treat the atrial and ventricular dysrhythmias produced by cardiac glycoside toxicity. It is less effective for other supraventricular dysrhythmias and for suppressing chronic ventricular ectopy. The drug is also useful in children to prevent late postoperative dysrhythmias after surgical correction of congenital heart disease.[132]

Intravenous loading of DPH is accomplished in much the same way as with procainamide. Doses of 50–100 mg (0.5–1.5 mg/kg) are given at 5-minute intervals until therapeutic effects are obtained up to a total dose of 1 g (15 mg/kg); the usual therapeutic plasma concentration is 8–10 μg/ml.[133] Excretion of DPH is preceded by hepatic metabolism, and urinary excretion of unchanged DPH accounts for only 5 percent of the total dose.[134] Hepatic metabolic capability is approximately 10 mg/kg/24 hr.[135] Patients with impaired hepatic or renal function should be expected to have higher plasma concentrations of DPH for a given dose; therefore, the dose should be reduced to prevent toxicity.

With DPH administration, especially via the intravenous route, a depressor effect is seen together with decreased contractile function and a moderate increase of left ventricular end-diastolic pressure (LVEDP).[136,137] These effects may, in part, be due to the solvents used for the injectable preparation, propylene glycol and ethyl alcohol.[138] Infusion rates over 50 mg/min in adults have produced cardiovascular collapse, VF, and death.[139] Other side effects include visual disturbances (nystagmus and blurring), nausea, dysarthria, and cerebellar ataxia. Chronic DPH use produces gingival hyperplasia, macrocytic anemia, and dermatologic disorders.

CLASS IB

Lidocaine. Among class IB drugs (lidocaine, tocainide, and mexiletine), and probably among all antiarrhythmic drugs, lidocaine is the most widely used. First introduced as an antiarrhythmic drug in the 1950s,[140-143] lidocaine has become the clinical standard for the acute treatment of ventricular dysrhythmias of virtually all types except those precipitated by an abnormally prolonged Q-T interval. Lidocaine may, in fact, be one of the most useful drugs in clinical anesthesia because it has both local and general anesthetic properties,[144] in addition to an antiarrhythmic effect.

The direct electrophysiologic effects of lidocaine produce virtually all of its antiarrhythmic action, because lidocaine lacks the autonomic side effects of the Class IA drugs. Therapeutic blood concentrations of lidocaine depress the slope of phase 4 diastolic depolarization in Purkinje fibers,[145] but only interfere with SA nodal activity when there is pre-existing SA node disease.[146] Lidocaine increases ventricular fibrillation threshold.[147] In Purkinje fibers, lidocaine increases transmembrane potassium conductance but does not affect resting membrane potential or threshold potential.[148] At less negative (partially depolarized) initial membrane potentials, lidocaine decreases fast channel (Na^+) responses due to an increase in background outward potassium flux, an effect directly related to extracellular potassium concentration.[149,150] Lidocaine may be ineffective in hypokalemic patients.[151]

Conduction velocity is not affected by lidocaine in normal tissue, but it is significantly decreased in ischemic tissue.[152] The effects of lidocaine on APD vary by conduction system location. In atrial tissues, there is little or no effect. In contrast, in Purkinje fibers, APD is markedly decreased, and the magnitude of the decrease is directly proportional to normal APD; preterminal or gate regions of the Purkinje system normally have significantly longer APD and are the site of the predominant lidocaine effect.[153] This effect has led to the assertion that the decreased disparity in the recovery of excitability produced by

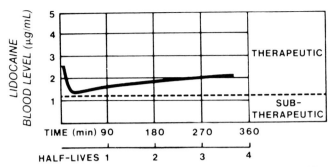

Fig. 12-8. Estimated blood levels of lidocaine hydrochloride following a 100-mg bolus injection and a 2-mg/min infusion in a normal, average-weight human. (From White RD: Cardiovascular pharmacology: Part 1. *In* McIntyre KM, Lewis AJ (eds): Textbook of Advanced Cardiac Life Support. Dallas, American Heart Association, 1983, with permission.)

lidocaine is an important aspect of its antiarrhythmic effect, although the therapeutic significance of this effect is discounted by Vaughan Williams.[96] Since lidocaine decreases APD, its antiarrhythmic effect also has been attributed to improved conduction in ectopic foci, which would decrease the likelihood of reentry;[154] however, it has been shown that lidocaine slows conduction in these areas and decreases reentrant ventricular ectopy after experimental infarction.[155]

The regional pharmacokinetics of lidocaine may have an important bearing on its antiarrhythmic effect during myocardial ischemia. The concentration of lidocaine achieved in ischemic myocardium determines its antiarrhythmic effect, while that in arterial or venous plasma or normal myocardium does not.[156] There is a threshold for lidocaine concentration in ischemic myocardium of 1.0 $\mu g/g$, below which an antiarrhythmic effect is unlikely.[156] In addition, regional perfusion and lidocaine concentration in ischemic areas are significantly related.[156] While decreased washout of lidocaine from ischemic tissue due to low blood flow may be a factor in these observations,[157] other factors also are likely to be operative, since during the acute phase of myocardial infarction, constant lidocaine infusion produces higher concentrations in ischemic than in normal myocardium.[158] An ion-trapping mechanism produced by the lower pH in ischemic than in normal myocardium has been proposed to account for these observations.[156] A similar mechanism has been proposed to explain the increased fetal-maternal lidocaine ratio associated with fetal acidosis[159] and the increased urinary excretion in response to urinary acidification produced by lidocaine;[160] however, no pH-related effect has been shown for the cardiovascular effects of lidocaine.[161] Regardless, regional myocardial distribution of lidocaine (and perhaps other antiarrhythmic drugs) is an important aspect of the antiarrhythmic effect, especially during acute ischemia.

Clinically, lidocaine is indicated for the treatment of PVCs that (1) occur more frequently than five each minute; (2) are closely coupled to the T wave; (3) originate in multiple foci (or have multiple ECG forms); or (4) appear in groups of two or more (ventricular tachycardia).[113] Lidocaine is useful when used prophylactically for acute myocardial infarction to prevent life-threatening ventricular dysrhythmias such as VT and VF.[162]

The clinical pharmacokinetics of lidocaine are well-described. Both distribution and elimination half-lives of lidocaine are short, approximately 60 seconds and 100 minutes, respectively.[163] Hepatic extraction of lidocaine is about 60–70 percent, and essentially all lidocaine is metabolized, as the urine contains negligible amounts of unchanged lidocaine.[101] Hepatic metabolism produces monoethylglycine-xylidide and glycine-xylidide, both of which possess antiarrhythmic effects. Metabolic products are eliminated by the kidney, and accumulation of the monoethyl metabolite is related to the toxicity of intravenous lidocaine.[164–166] In patients with impaired hepatic function or blood flow (eg, those with CHF), the dose requirement is approximately 50 percent of that in the healthy person (Figs. 12-8 and 12-9).

Therapeutic plasma levels of lidocaine range from 1.5 to 5 $\mu g/ml$; signs of toxicity are frequent with concentrations above 9 $\mu g/ml$.[165] Various intravenous dosages can be used, but the important factor is to achieve steady-state therapeutic plasma concen-

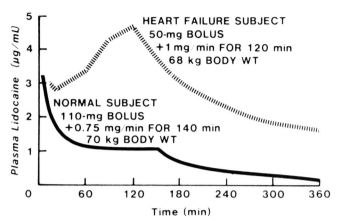

Fig. 12-9. The difference between plasma level responses to infused lidocaine in a normal subject (solid line) and a subject with heart failure (broken line). The accumulation of lidocaine in patients with depressed hepatic metabolism is illustrated dramatically. (From White RD: Cardiovascular pharmacology: Part 1. *In* McIntyre KM, Lewis AJ (eds): Textbook of Advanced Cardiac Life Support. Dallas, American Heart Association, 1983, with permission.)

trations rapidly. Thus, an initial bolus dose of 1–1.5 mg/kg should be followed immediately by a continuous infusion of 20–50 μg/kg/min in order to prevent the "therapeutic hiatus" produced by the rapid redistribution half-life of lidocaine (Fig. 12-8).[113] Likewise, infusion increments should be accompanied by additional bolus doses to immediately increase plasma level. When used for prophylaxis against VF, the same dosage considerations apply, and ectopy need not be totally abolished in order to produce a significant prophylactic effect.

The major toxic effect of lidocaine is associated with the CNS and is manifested by drowsiness and disorientation, which progress to agitation, muscle twitching, and hearing abnormalities, and culminate in seizures. With regard to CNS toxicity, it is important to note that lidocaine and other local anesthetics can be effective general anesthetic agents; cases of coma and apparent brain death, corroborated by electroencephalographic findings, have been produced by an overdose of lidocaine and have resolved completely on discontinuation of the drug. Interestingly, the direct CNS effect of lidocaine and other local anesthetics is anticonvulsant.[167-169] Local anesthetic-induced seizures do not produce permanent damage to the CNS system as long as cardiovascular and respiratory complications of the seizure are prevented. Pharmacologically, benzodiazepines are superior to barbiturates (eg, thiopental) for stopping seizure activity. Drug therapy alone is insufficient, however; airway control, ventilation, and especially

oxygenation are paramount to prevent CNS morbidity.

Tocainide and mexiletine. Both of these drugs were developed specifically for oral administration. Although they each have intravenous preparations and have been used by that route clinically, neither has provided any additional effect or advantage over lidocaine.[170-174]

Tocainide and mexiletine have electrophysiologic effects similar to those of lidocaine (decreases in APD and ERP but little effect on conduction); tocainide may also increase the Q-T interval.[175] Hemodynamic effects of both drugs are minor and consist primarily of small decreases of LV dP/dt and increases of LVEDP.[176] Small decreases of cardiac output, vascular resistance, and arterial pressure have been reported; however, even in patients with coronary artery disease, acute myocardial infarction, or valvular heart disease, hemodynamic effects are clinically insignificant.[177-180]

The antiarrhythmic effects of both drugs are likewise similar; both decrease the frequency of ventricular ectopy. Mexiletine may decrease symptomatic dysrhythmias in patients not responding to other therapy[181-183] and may be more effective than lidocaine when used intravenously to suppress PVCs and VT in acute myocardial infarction.[184] Mexiletine, administered orally, also may be effective prophylaxis for PVCs and VT, but it may suppress closely coupled PVCs less effectively.[185-187]

Tocainide produces a dose-related (and plasma concentration-related) suppression of PVCs. Plasma concentrations less than 3.4 μg/ml suppress PVCs by less than 50 percent, while concentrations over 8.5 μg/ml are over 90 percent effective; however, higher levels produce little additional effect.[188] Oral tocainide is also effective against recurrent VT or VF and may be effective when other oral therapy has failed.[189-191] A response to intravenous lidocaine may predict a therapeutic response to tocainide.[189] Tocainide suppresses PVCs in acute myocardial infarction, and prophylactic use decreases the incidence of frequent PVCs and VT during the first 24 hours after myocardial infarction.[192-194] Chronic use of tocainide prevents the increased frequency of PVCs that occurs when normal activity is resumed after myocardial infarction.

Pharmacokinetics of orally administered mexiletine and tocainide are similar with regard to bioavailability (85 percent for mexiletine and 95 percent for tocainide); however, the volume of distribution of mexiletine is 2.5 times that for tocainide.[195] Tocainide is eliminated by both renal excretion (unchanged drug in urine accounts for approximately 40 percent of an administered dose) and hepatic metabolism. Elimination half-life is 15 hours for tocainide and 11 hours for mexiletine; thus, both are suitable for b.i.d. or t.i.d. dosage regimens.[196] Elimination of tocainide is decreased in renal dysfunction, with its half-life increasing to 30 hours, although hepatic dysfunction has little effect, except in the case of acute hepatic necrosis.[197,198] Mexiletine is eliminated primarily by hepatic metabolism, which is accelerated with microsomal enzyme induction and predictably decreased with hepatic disease but unaffected by renal failure.[199,200]

The usual dosage of tocainide is 1200–1800 mg/24 hr, while the upper limit for mexiletine is 2400 mg. Effective plasma level of mexiletine ranges from 1 to 2 μg/ml, but there is wide individual variation of the dose required to achieve that concentration.[201] Adverse effects of tocainide are nausea (14.3 percent), dizziness (12.5 percent), paresthesia (6.5 percent), tremor (5.9 percent), vomiting (5 percent), and sweating (5 percent); these adverse effects occur in 25 percent of patients with plasma levels over 11 μg/ml.[189] Convulsions, dysrhythmias, and significant hypersensitivity are rare, but rashes occur in 1–3 percent of patients receiving tocainide. Adverse reactions to mexiletine, which tend to be gastrointestinal and neurologic, are dose related. The incidence of minor reactions is 30 percent, and the incidence of severe reactions (dysrhythmias, vomiting, confusion,

and hypotension) is 19 percent when the plasma concentration is over 2 μg/ml.[201]

CLASS IC

This subgrouping of Class I drugs, consisting of aprinidine, encainide, flecainide, and lorcainide, is based on their very potent suppression of phase 0 activity and the resultant markedly decreased conduction velocity, which is a common property of these drugs.

Aprinidine. Aprinidine has an antiarrhythmic effect in supraventricular and ventricular dysrhythmias. It is reported to be remarkably effective in controlling VT occurring in association with mitral valve prolapse.[202] In patients with WPW syndrome who develop excessively rapid ventricular rates due to accessory pathway conduction during atrial fibrillation or flutter, aprinidine is useful.[203] Electrophysiologic effects of aprinidine are depression of phase 0 and, to a lesser extent, spontaneous phase 4 depolarization and increases of both APD and ERP. Interference with slow channel activity has also been reported,[204] and clinical studies have shown prolonged A-H and H-V intervals and QRS duration.

Aprinidine is well absorbed after oral administration; typical oral doses of 100–150 mg daily produce therapeutic plasma concentrations of 1–2 μg/ml. Aprinidine is metabolized to a great extent, and its plasma half-life is approximately 60 hours.[205] The usefulness of aprinidine is limited by its narrow therapeutic ratio. Neurologic (dose-related) side effects occur in over 50 percent of patients and include vertigo, tremor, ataxia, and hallucinations.[123] Idiosyncratic reactions, such as agranulocytosis and cholestatic jaundice, have been reported.[206]

Encainide. This drug is effective for both supraventricular and ventricular dysrhythmias. Electrophysiologic effects include marked phase 0 depression but minimal APD and ERP effects.[207] Clinically, encainide increases P-R and H-V intervals and QRS duration, but atrial effects (SA node recovery time and A-H interval) are less.[208,209] Prolongation of the Q-T interval occurs with long-term therapy, an effect that may represent activity of an accumulated metabolite.[209] Hemodynamic effects of encainide are slight even with LV dysfunction, although mild negative inotropic effects have been shown.[210,211]

Encainide absorption is variable and its half-life is approximately 3 hours. The elimination rate may be dose dependent, and metabolism produces two active metabolites, which accumulate during chronic treatment.[212] The usual dosage is 75–300 mg/24 hr in four to six divided doses; however, because of active metabolite accumulation, the frequency of dose is less important with chronic therapy.

Encainide has a high therapeutic ratio, and adverse effects (primarily neurologic and gastrointestinal) are relatively uncommon. Polymorphic VT without Q-T prolongation has been reported with a frequency of 11 percent in patients with histories of VT or VF.

Flecainide. Relatively less data are available for flecainide than other Class IC drugs. Electrophysiologically, flecainide depresses phase 0, delays repolarization in canine ventricular muscle, and increases intracardiac monophasic APD in humans. Therefore, the drug has both Class IC and Class III properties.[213] Flecainide decreases LV dP/dt and cardiac output experimentally.[214] Clinical studies have shown no effects of oral flecainide on arterial pressure, echocardiographic parameters, or exercise tolerance.[215-217] Flecainide is well absorbed after oral administration; it has a plasma half-life of 20 hours, and effective plasma concentrations range from 245 to 980 ng/ml. Dosages range from 100 to 300 mg b.i.d. Chronic clinical studies have shown that PVCs and VT are suppressed effectively.[217] Adverse effects are usually minor at doses that have a significant therapeutic effect, but the Q-T interval has been prolonged with induction of polymorphic VT.[218]

Lorcainide. This new Class IC antiarrhythmic, currently undergoing clinical trials, appears to have wide efficacy for ventricular dysrhythmias. Electrophysiologic effects of lorcainide include a decrease of $\dot{V}$max of the AP, with decreased conduction velocity and increased APD and ERP. Ventricular conduction is affected more than is atrial or AV nodal.[219]

Clinical data show that the oral and intravenous forms have different effects due to the high degree of hepatic metabolism with oral administration of the drug; oral lorcainide increases A-H conduction time and ERP (atrial and ventricular) more than the intravenous form.[220] Both dosage forms of lorcainide increase P-R, QRS, and Q-T intervals; likewise the ERP of the accessory pathway in WPW is increased.[221,222] The VF threshold is increased; lorcainide is more potent in this regard than lidocaine.[223] Lorcainide doses greater than 2 mg/kg intravenously may produce a third-degree AV block and may worsen SA node dysfunction.[222]

Hemodynamic effects of lorcainide include mild depressor effects and significant depression of LV dP/dt (-27 percent) in dogs 2 hours after a single 10 mg/kg oral dose.[224] Clinically, single intravenous doses of 2 mg/kg infused over 5 minutes decreased ejection fraction by 5 percent; circumferential shortening velocity was decreased similarly, but cardiac output and systemic pressure were not significantly affected.[225] In acute myocardial infarction, however, lorcainide decreased the cardiac index by about 10 percent and increased wedge pressure from 6.6 to 8.4 mm Hg.[226]

After oral administration, lorcainide is metabolized into nor-lorcainide, which accumulates in plasma to a concentration nearly twice that of the parent compound.[227] This metabolism (dealkylation) is hepatic, has a very high first-pass effectiveness, and is saturable.[228] Hydroxylated metabolites are inactive.[229] The dealkylated metabolite is not measurable in plasma after acute intravenous administration in humans.[230] Lorcainide and nor-lorcainide have similar electrophysiologic profiles and, with combined administration of the two, their effects are additive.

Bioavailability of unchanged lorcainide during chronic therapy approaches 100 percent; however, acute bioavailability is highly dose dependent. An initial 100 mg dose has a bioavailability of only 2 percent, but bioavailability is approximately 50 percent for a 300-mg dose.[231,232] These findings indicate a substantial first-pass hepatic metabolism that is saturated by increasing dose or by long-term treatment. Free lorcainide in plasma has been reported to be 15–27 percent.[228,232] After intravenous administration, lorcainide has an elimination half-life of 7.8 hours, but this is markedly prolonged with hepatic disease.[233,234] Therapeutic plasma concentrations of lorcainide are 40–200 ng/ml (80–330 ng/ml for nor-lorcainide), although, in one study, whether the suppression of ectopy correlated best with the parent compound or the metabolite could not be assessed.[235] Suppression of complex dysrhythmias correlates well with suppression of PVCs. The variability of both bioavailability and effective plasma concentration makes it advisable to begin treatment with lorcainide at lower doses (100 mg b.i.d. orally) with long intervals between dose increases. Additionally, because of the active metabolite, some patients failing to respond to intravenous administration may respond to a low oral dose. Adverse effects of lorcainide are relatively minor and include sleep disturbance (which is easily treated with benzodiazepines), gastrointestinal abnormalities, and headache.

Class II: Beta-Adrenergic Receptor Antagonists

This group of antiarrhythmic agents has a much more concise effect than the Class I drugs. Class II drugs produce their antiarrhythmic effect by competitive blockade of beta-adrenergic receptors. Beta-blockers have diverse therapeutic uses, the most prominent of which are antihypertensive and anti-anginal therapy. This section focuses on the antiarrhythmic usefulness of three drugs that are strictly beta-adrenergic receptor blockers (propranolol, metoprolol, and esmolol) and one drug with mixed alpha- and beta-receptor–blocking properties (labetalol). The use of beta-blockers to treat hypertension and ischemic heart disease is discussed in Chapters 11 and 13, respectively.

Based on the differences observed among catecholamines with regard to smooth muscle tone, in 1948 Ahlquist proposed the categorization of adrenergic receptors as alpha and beta.[236] The beta-receptors are found throughout the body and have been subgrouped as beta$_1$ and beta$_2$.[237] Cardiac beta-receptors and those in fat cells comprise the beta$_1$ subgroup, while smooth muscle and glandular receptors are designated beta$_2$. There is significant anatomic overlap of receptor distribution, however, and many tissues contain both types but in different proportions. For example, in the rat, the ratio of beta$_1$ to beta$_2$ receptors is 4:1 in the heart and 1:5 in the lung.

PROPRANOLOL

This was the first beta-receptor–blocking drug to be used clinically and it remains the most widely used. Propranolol is very potent but nonselective for beta-receptor subtypes. It possesses essentially no intrinsic sympathomimetic activity. Because it interferes with the bronchodilating actions of epinephrine and the sympathetic stimulating effects of hypoglycemia, propranolol is less useful in patients with diabetes or bronchospasm. These difficulties with propranolol stimulated the search for beta-receptor–blocking drugs with receptor subtype specificity. Although several beta$_1$-selective agents exist (metoprolol, atenolol, acebutolol, and tolamolol), only metoprolol is available in this country as an injectable preparation.

The electrophysiologic effects of beta-receptor antagonism are decreased automaticity, increased APD, primarily in ventricular muscle, and a substantially increased ERP in the AV node. Beta-blockade decreases the rate of spontaneous (phase 4) depolarization in the SA node; the magnitude of this effect

depends on the background sympathetic tone. Although resting heart rate is decreased by beta-blockade, the inhibition of the increase of heart rate in response to exercise or emotional stress is much more marked. Automaticity in the AV node and more distal portions of the conduction system is also depressed. Beta-blockade affects the VF threshold variably, but it consistently reverses the fibrillation-threshold–lowering effect of catecholamines. Perhaps the predominant antiarrhythmic effect of beta-blockade is an increase of ERP in the AV node.

In addition to beta-blockade, propranolol also possesses two properties that are important to its antiarrhythmic effect. Propranolol decreases the background outward current of potassium and, at higher concentrations, also inhibits inward sodium current. Because of similarity to Class I activity, these effects have been termed a *membrane-stabilizing activity* (MSA) or quinidine-like effects. In very high concentrations (1000–3000 ng/ml), this effect increases depolarization threshold in Purkinje fibers.[238] Although effective beta-blockade is achieved at propranolol concentrations of 100–300 ng/ml, concentrations of 1000 ng/ml may be required to control ventricular dysrhythmias.[239] In acutely ischemic myocardium, propranolol decreases intramyocardial impulse conduction but does not do so in normal myocardium.[240]

The overall antiarrhythmic effect of propranolol is multifactoral. AV nodal reentry often causes paroxysmal supraventricular tachycardia (PSVT), and, in such cases, the increased AV nodal ERP caused by beta-blockade may abolish the reentry. At the ventricular level, propranolol abolishes catecholamine-induced after-potentials and decreases Purkinje fiber response by means of MSA. Myocardial metabolic effects of beta-blockade may be indirectly antiarrhythmic by decreasing the severity of ischemia.

Pharmacokinetics of propranolol are well understood. Absorption after oral administration is virtually 100 percent, but bioavailability is impaired by an extensive first-pass hepatic metabolism of about two-thirds of the administered dose. The degree of hepatic extraction is highly variable, which probably accounts for the great variability of the plasma concentration produced by a given oral dose of propranolol. As with lorcainide, the hepatic extraction of propranolol is a saturable process, and bioavailability improves with increased oral dose or with chronic therapy.[241] Propranolol is 90–95 percent protein bound in plasma, which further confounds the use of plasma concentration as a guide to therapy.[242] Propranolol is metabolized before excretion; one product, 4-hydroxypropranolol, has a beta-blocking potency similar to that of propranolol, but a short half-life prevents this metabolic product from contributing significantly to the therapeutic effect of propranolol.[243] The elimination half-life of orally administered propranolol is 3–4 hours, but it is increased during chronic therapy due to saturation of hepatic metabolic processes.[244] Cardiopulmonary bypass alters the kinetics of propranolol. Heparinization doubles the free fraction of propranolol, which reverses after protamine is administered. This effect is thought to be due to an increase of free fatty acid concentration produced by heparin, which decreases the protein binding of propranolol.[245]

Major toxic side effects of propranolol relate to beta-blockade per se. Cardiac toxicity includes CHF (uncommon without other causes of ventricular dysfunction) and depressed AV conduction. Both complete heart block and asystole have occurred in patients with pre-existing AV nodal or intraventricular conduction abnormalities. In contrast, sudden discontinuation of beta-blockade therapy may precipitate a withdrawal syndrome of excessive beta-adrenergic activity, due to the denervation hypersensitivity associated with chronic blockade; responses to normal levels of sympathetic activity are exaggerated as the beta-blockade declines.[246,247] The existence of such a withdrawal syndrome, however, has been challenged by studies unable to demonstrate increased sensitivity to adrenergic stimulation after abrupt withdrawal of propranolol.[248] Increased airway resistance results from beta$_2$-receptor blockade by propranolol, and this can precipitate severe pulmonary compromise in the asthmatic patient. The hypoglycemic action of insulin is accentuated by propranolol, since the sympathomimetic effect of hypoglycemia is blocked. Side effects perhaps not related to beta-receptor blockade include CNS disturbances such as insomnia, hallucinations, depression, dizziness, and minor allergic manifestations such as rash, fever, and purpura.

A common clinical problem associated with chronic propranolol therapy is inability to continue oral administration after intra-abdominal surgical operations. Intermittent intravenous bolus dosage makes it difficult to obtain stable plasma concentrations. However, an appropriate intravenous dose for acute control of dysrhythmias is 0.5–1.0 mg titrated to therapeutic effect up to a total of 0.1–0.15 mg/kg. Stable therapeutic plasma concentrations of propranolol can be obtained with continuous intravenous infusion, and effective beta-blockade may be obtained with a continuous infusion approximating 3 mg/hr in adult postoperative patients previously receiving chronic treatment.

METOPROLOL

This agent is a relatively selective beta$_1$-receptor antagonist that is without any significant agonist properties. The beta$_1$-blockade produced by metoprolol has the same spectrum as that described for propranolol. The potency of metoprolol for beta$_1$-receptor blockade is equal to that of propranolol, but metoprolol exhibits only 1–2 percent of the effect of propranolol at beta$_2$-receptors.[249]

Like propranolol, metoprolol is rapidly and efficiently absorbed after oral administration; however, its first-pass extraction by the liver is lower, and 40 percent of the administered dose reaches the systemic circulation. Plasma half-life after oral administration is approximately 3 hours. Metoprolol is 90 percent metabolized, with hydroxylation and o-demethylation being the primary pathways. The metabolites lack beta-receptor effects. As with acetylation of procainamide, however, the rate of hydroxylation of metoprolol is genetically determined. "Slow hydroxylators" show a markedly prolonged elimination of the parent drug and higher plasma concentrations.[250]

Toxicity of metoprolol is related primarily to its limited beta$_2$ activity. Metoprolol increases airway resistance and decreases forced expiratory volume in 1 second in asthmatic patients, although less than does propranolol at equipotent beta$_1$-antagonist doses. In contrast to propranolol, metoprolol does not inhibit the bronchodilation of isoproterenol. Metoprolol may impair beta-receptor-mediated insulin release, and the signs of hypoglycemia will be masked as with propranolol. Other side effects of metoprolol are similar to those of propranolol.

Metoprolol is useful for treating the same spectrum of dysrhythmias for which propranolol is useful. The primary utility of metoprolol is its relative lack of most, but not all, of the bronchoconstrictive effects of propranolol in patients with chronic obstructive pulmonary disease. Acute intravenous dosage is the same as for propranolol (0.5–1.0 mg titrated to therapeutic effect up to 0.1–0.15 mg/kg).

ESMOLOL

Esmolol is a cardioselective (beta$_1$) receptor antagonist with an extremely brief duration of action. Its pharmacokinetics and therapeutic uses were the subject of a recent symposium.[251] In anesthetized dogs, esmolol infused at 50 μg/kg/min produced a steady-state beta-blockade that was completely reversed 20 minutes after stopping the infusion.[252] Esmolol has only minimal intrinsic sympathomimetic effects and MSA, and, in conscious dogs, it has no effect on LVEDP, arterial pressure, heart rate, cardiac output, or peripheral resistance, but, at 5–60 μg/kg/min, it does decrease LV dP/dt. The decreased contractility, however, fully resolves by 20 minutes after the infusion. Esmolol has no demonstrable alpha-adrenergic receptor effects.

Electrophysiologic effects of esmolol are those of beta-adrenergic receptor antagonism. In open-chest dogs, esmolol infused at 300 μg/kg/min increased SA node recovery time and A-H conduction interval but not H-V interval. Effective refractory period was increased in the AV node, but this effect does not occur in vitro at beta-blocking concentrations.

Esmolol is rapidly metabolized in blood by hydrolysis of its methyl ester linkage; its half-life in whole blood is 12.5 and 27.1 minutes in dogs and humans, respectively. The acid metabolite possesses a slight degree (1500 times less than esmolol) of beta antagonism. Esmolol is not affected by plasma cholinesterase; the esterase responsible is located in erythrocytes and is not inhibited by cholinesterase inhibitors such as neostigmine, physostigmine, edrophonium, or echothiopate, but it is deactivated by sodium fluoride. Of importance to clinical anesthesia, no metabolic interactions between esmolol and other ester molecules are known. Specifically, esmolol doses up to 500 μg/kg/min have not modified neuromuscular effects of succinylcholine.[253]

Clinically, in asthmatic patients, esmolol (300 μg/kg/min) increases airway resistance only slightly. Also, in patients with chronic obstructive pulmonary disease who received esmolol, no adverse pulmonary effects occurred.[254] In a multicenter trial, in a comparison with propranolol for the treatment of PSVT, esmolol was equally efficacious and had the advantage of a much faster termination of the beta-blockade.[255] Thus, esmolol may prove to be useful in the perioperative period, a time when a titratable and brief beta-blockade is desirable.

LABETALOL

Labetalol is a drug with the unique pharmacologic properties of combined alpha$_1$-receptor and nonselective beta-receptor blockade. In vitro, the alpha-adrenergic receptor antagonism by labetalol is about 10–15 percent of that of phentolamine, while its beta-antagonism is 5–10 percent of that of propranolol.[256] Beta agonist activity in human myometrium has also been reported.[257] The ratio of alpha to beta-blockade is 1:7 with intravenous administration, but 1:3 with oral administration, and the drug is effective by both routes.

Labetalol is used both acutely and chronically, primarily as an antihypertensive drug (see Chapter 11). Studies of its use in anesthetized patients are limited, but a 25-mg intravenous dose during steady-state 1 percent halothane anesthesia was shown to decrease arterial pressure from a mean of 71 mm Hg before administration to 53 mm Hg.[258] Pressure declined rapidly, but the new lower level was stable for 15 minutes. Heart rate, peripheral resistance, and stroke volume either decreased slightly or were unaffected. Since the hemodynamic effects of labetalol in anesthetized patients are not yet fully documented, labetalol should be given in small doses (eg, 5–10 mg in an adult) and titrated to therapeutic effect. The use of labetalol as an antiarrhythmic agent is largely untested. With regard to perioperative use, however, its pharmacologic properties of combined alpha- and beta-blockade would theoretically make it a good drug with which to treat dysrhythmias associated with the catecholamine–inhalational anesthetic interaction discussed earlier. Other antiarrhythmic effects would appear to depend on beta-receptor antagonism and have a spectrum similar to propranolol.

Class III: Antifibrillatory Agents

An important distinction in antiarrhythmic therapy is that between antiectopic and antifibrillatory effects. The latter have been defined as primarily increasing electrical stability in contrast to decreasing frequency of ectopic depolarization (antiectopic effect).[259] While these effects overlap as exemplified by lidocaine, which has both antifibrillatory and antiectopic activities, the two prototype drugs in Class III, bretylium and amiodarone, exhibit prominent antifibrillatory effects, although only bretylium is marketed specifically for that purpose.

BRETYLIUM

Bretylium is a quarternary ammonium compound that produces a biphasic cardiac response after acute intravenous administration. Initially, norepinephrine is displaced from adrenergic nerve endings, and there are attendant increases in arterial pressure, vascular resistance, and cardiac automaticity. After 20–30 minutes, this response wanes and the adrenergic blocking effects of bretylium predominate.[260-262] These latter effects depend on uptake of bretylium by adrenergic neurons; however, inhibition of its adrenergic blocking effects does not impair the antiarrhythmic effect.

The direct electrophysiologic effect of bretylium is prolongation of the ventricular ERP. In this regard, the electrophysiologic effect correlates with the myocardial rather than the plasma concentrations of bretylium,[263] as has been reported for the antiarrhythmic effect of lidocaine. Bretylium delays conduction of premature impulses from normal myocardium to the border of ischemic zones and decreases the disparity between the excitation thresholds of adjoining zones of ischemic and normal myocardium. Bretylium increases the electrical current required to induce VF and may spontaneously convert VF to sinus rhythm.[264] The antiarrhythmic effect of bretylium is undiminished by cardiac denervation or by chronic reserpine treatment, which indicates that the antiarrhythmic effects are dissociated from the antiadrenergic effects.[265,266] Bretylium also decreases the amount of electrical current required to produce defibrillation.[267]

Results of clinical trials of bretylium in acute cardiac arrest are inconsistent. In one study in which it was compared with lidocaine, bretylium neither had a better antiarrhythmic effect, improved resuscitation, nor lowered mortality.[268] In contrast, in another study, bretylium (10 mg/kg) was used as a first-line treatment for out-of-hospital VF and significantly improved the outcome from resuscitation; lidocaine administered after bretylium also decreased the incidence of recurrent VF.[269] In the acute setting, bretylium is effective prophylaxis against VF.[270–274]

Clinical indications for bretylium include refractory VT or VF. For VF, bretylium is administered as a 5–10 mg/kg intravenous bolus, which can be repeated to a total dose of 30 mg/kg if fibrillation persists. The antifibrillatory effect may require some time to develop, so full resuscitative efforts should continue for at least 20–30 minutes after bretylium has been administered. Administration for recurrent VT is similar to that for VF. Continuous infusion of 2 mg/min may be used to maintain plasma levels. As with VF, the effect of bretylium in VT may take 20–30 minutes to manifest.

Adverse reactions to bretylium include nausea and vomiting in conscious patients. During chronic therapy, postural hypotension may develop, but it is reduced by tricyclic drugs, which block uptake of bretylium by adrenergic neurons.

AMIODARONE

Amiodarone is a benzofuran derivative initially introduced as an antianginal drug. It was subsequently noted to be a very effective antiarrhythmic agent and to have a wide spectrum of effectiveness, including supraventricular[275] and ventricular dysrhythmias[276,277] and preexcitation of the WPW syndrome.[278] This drug also may be effective against VT and VF refractory to other treatment.[279]

Electrophysiologic effects of amiodarone are complex and differ for acute and chronic therapy. Amiodarone used in vitro in an isolated rabbit SA node preparation increased APD and decreased the slope of diastolic (phase 4) depolarization, which depressed SA node automaticity.[280] Amiodarone prolongs repolarization and refractoriness in the SA node, in atrial and ventricular myocardium, in the AV node, and in the His–Purkinje system.[281] Resting potential and myocardial automaticity are minimally affected,[275] but both ERP and absolute refractory period are prolonged. In vitro, amiodarone blocks inactive sodium channels in Purkinje fibers, which significantly depresses phase 0.[282] In anesthetized dogs, amiodarone decreases AV junctional as well as SA node automaticity, and prolongs intranodal conduction.[283]

There are substantial differences in the electrophysiologic effects of acute and chronic amiodarone administration. Acutely, the drug slightly increases ERP of the His–Purkinje system and ventricular myocardium. The corrected Q-T interval (Q-Tc) is not prolonged by acute intravenous administration of amiodarone despite myocardial concentrations similar to those with chronic oral therapy.[284] However, chronic oral administration significantly increases Q-Tc.[285] Although AV nodal ERP increases with acute intravenous amiodarone therapy, the increase is greater following chronic use. In other cardiac tissue, there is little or no change in ERP following intravenous administration; however, after chronic oral use, ERP is increased globally and both A-H and H-V conduction times are increased clinically.[286]

The electrophysiologic effects of chronic amiodarone treatment mimic those of thyroid ablation.[287] Moreover, the repolarization effects of the drug are reversed by tri-iodothyronine (T$_3$) administration. This suggests that among the basic effects of amiodarone is the blockade of the cardiac effect of T$_3$; this mechanism has been proposed as an alternative to the active-metabolite–accumulation theory to account for the slow onset of the antiarrhythmic effect of amiodarone.[286]

Another electrophysiologic effect of amiodarone is an increase in the amount of electric current required to elicit VF (an increase in VF threshold). In most patients, refractory VT is suppressed by acute intravenous use of amiodarone. This effect has been attributed to a selectively increased activity in diseased tissue as has been seen with lidocaine.[288] Amiodarone also has an adrenergic receptor (alpha and beta) antagonistic effect produced by a noncompetitive mechanism; the contribution of this effect to the antiarrhythmic action of the drug is not known.[101]

Hemodynamic effects of intravenous amiodarone (10 mg/kg) include decreased LV dP/dt, maximal negative dP/dt, mean aortic pressure, heart rate, and peak LV pressure after coronary artery occlusion in dogs. Cardiac output was increased despite the negative inotropic effect due to the more marked decrease of LV afterload.[289] Clinical effects are similar; a 5-mg/kg intravenous dose during cardiac catheterization decreased arterial pressure, LVEDP, and systemic vascular resistance and increased cardiac output, but it did not affect heart rate. Chronic amiodarone therapy is not associated with clinically significant depression of ventricular function in patients without LV failure. Hemodynamic deterioration may occur in patients with compensated CHF, however, perhaps because of the antiadrenergic effects of the drug, although, in one study, chronic oral amiodarone therapy had no effect on ejection fraction.[290]

Pharmacokinetics of amiodarone are notable for the low bioavailability, very long elimination half-life, relatively low clearance, and large volume of distribution. Oral absorption of amiodarone is slow, peak plasma levels occurring 3–7 hours after ingestion.[291] Bioavailability is variable and low, ranging from 22 to 50 percent. The hepatic extraction ratio, however, is only 0.13, so that the major limit to bioavailability may be incomplete absorption. Amiodarone has a large volume of distribution, variably estimated as 1.3–65.8 1/kg; plasma clearance rates range from 0.14 to 0.60 1/min.[292] Plasma half-life following chronic oral therapy is variably reported from 14 to 107 days; therapeutic and steady-state plasma concentrations are slowly achieved with maintenance oral administration at 9.5 and 30 days, respectively.[293]

Because steady-state plasma levels are achieved slowly, loading techniques have been developed. Patient-specific pharmacokinetic data have been used to prescribe loading infusion rates from 0.5 to 3.9 mg/min and maintenance rates of 0.43–0.84 mg/min to produce plasma levels of 2.6 ± 0.6 μg/min during maintenance infusion; this dosage reduced VT by 85 percent, paired PVCs by 74 percent, and isolated PVCs by 60 percent.[294] A comparison of onsets of antiarrhythmic effect of oral loading (800 mg/day for 7 days, then 600 mg/day for 3 days) and intravenous (5 mg/kg for 30 min) plus oral (as for oral alone)

administration demonstrated that the combined intravenous and oral loading technique had a more rapid therapeutic effect (20 ± 18 days versus 105 ± 83 days, $\pm$SD) with a lower total amiodarone dose (10 ± 8 versus 48 ± 39 mg, respectively).[295]

Adverse reactions to amiodarone are numerous. Photosensitivity of the skin occurs in 57 percent of patients without apparent relation to dose or plasma level.[296] Other skin manifestations include abnormal pigmentation (slate gray) and an erythematous, pruritic rash. Corneal microdeposits occur in most patients taking amiodarone chronically, although visual symptoms are uncommon.

Pulmonary side effects are more severe.[297-300] Clinical features include exertional dyspnea, cough, and weight loss. Hypoxia may occur; pulmonary function studies show decreased total lung capacity and diffusion rate. Chest roentgenogram findings are diffuse bilateral interstitial infiltrates, which histologically may be fibrosing alveolitis. Pulmonary effects may resolve with discontinuation of treatment or with dose reduction. The pathophysiologic mechanism of these pulmonary effects is not known but may relate to abnormal production of phospholipid. The overall incidence of pulmonary toxicity is up to 6 percent, with a mortality rate in those affected of 20–25 percent.

Thyroid abnormalities are associated with amiodarone; the frequencies of hyper- and hypothyroidism range from 1 to 5 and 1 to 2 percent, respectively.[301] Amiodarone contains two iodine atoms per molecule, or 75 mg of organic iodide per 200 mg of drug, and 10 percent of that amount may become free iodine. The iodine alone does not account for the thyroid abnormalities because intake of an amount of inorganic iodine equivalent to that ingested with chronic amiodarone intake does not have the same effect. Heart rate is not increased during hyperthyroidism associated with amiodarone, probably because of its antiadrenergic effects. Amiodarone therapy increases both thyroxine (T_4) and reverse T_3 but only slightly decreases T_3.[302,303] As discussed previously, one explanation of the slowly developing antiarrhythmic effect is an interference with cardiac effects of T_3 by blocking peripheral conversion of T_4 to T_3.[287]

Despite relatively widespread use of amiodarone, anesthetic complications have been infrequently reported. In two case reports, bradycardia and hypotension were prominent.[304,305] One of the reports described profound resistance to the vasoconstrictive effects of alpha-adrenergic agonists.[305] The slow decay of amiodarone in plasma and tissue makes such adverse reactions possible long after discontinuing its administration. Since T_3 is reported to reverse electrophysiologic effects of amiodarone, T_3 could possibly be used to reverse hemodynamic abnormalities, such as those described in these two case reports,[304,305] although this theory has not been tested.

Class IV: Calcium Channel Antagonists

The final class of antiarrhythmic agents to be reviewed is comprised of drugs that inhibit the inward flux of calcium across cellular and intracellular membranes during depolarization and excitation–contraction coupling. This class of drugs is discussed in the context of anti-ischemic therapy in Chapter 13; therefore, this discussion focuses on the properties pertinent to the antiarrhythmic effects. In this regard, while the principal direct electrophysiologic effects of the three main chemical groups of calcium antagonists (verapamil, a benzoacetonitrite; nifedipine, a dihydropyridine; and diltiazem, a benzothiazepine) are similar, verapamil is the prototype antiarrhythmic agent of the group. Several excellent recent reviews of the general properties of the calcium channel itself and calcium antagonists are available.[306-309]

As with other transmembrane ionic channels, the calcium channel is conceptualized as macromolecular protein that spans the ion-impermeable lipid bilayer of the membrane (Fig. 13-26). Such ion-impermeable channels exhibit selectivity both for a particular ionic species and for specific transmembrane electrical potential ranges to control the permeability of the pore.[308] The decreased membrane potential produced by depolarization increases the permeability of the Ca^{++} channel for Ca^{++}, which permits Ca^{++} to pass down its concentration gradient into the cell. Conversely, the "gate" closes on repolarization This mechanism has been termed the *voltage-dependent channel*. In cardiac tissue, the Ca^{++} channel is also controlled by membrane beta-adrenergic receptors; activation of beta$_1$-receptors recruits additional Ca^{++} channels to the open or active state,[310] and such channels are termed *receptor-operated channels*.

Based on studies with the sodium channels in the giant axons of squid, three different activity states of the Ca^{++} channel have been distinguished: resting, open, and inactive. The resting state of the Ca^{++} channel is characterized by a closed d gate on the external surface of the membrane and an opened f gate on the internal surface (Fig. 12-10).[311] Depolarization triggers the open state when the d gate relaxes to permit Ca^{++} influx, and also triggers the slower closure of the f gate, which, when complete, blocks further Ca^{++} influx; the resulting "inactive" state persists until complete repolarization resets both gates. For the Ca^{++} channel, the time constant for the transition from the resting to the open state is 5–20 msec, from the open to the inactive state 30–300 msec, and from the inactive to the resting state also 30–300 msec.[312]

The "use dependence" noted with Ca^{++} antagonists is the direct relation between the antagonist effect and the frequency of tissue activation. Thus, in cardiac tissue, the negative inotropic and Ca^{++}-blocking properties of verapamil depend on both transmembrane potential and stimulation frequency; the inhibitory activity increases with increased frequency and with partial depolarization.[313] Such findings may indicate that verapamil interacts primarily with the inactive (depolarized) state of the Ca^{++} channel. In contrast, the activation state of the membrane is less important for the inhibitory action of nifedipine.

The lipophilic nature of Ca^{++} antagonists is important to their effect. In skinned cardiac cells, D600, a cogener of verapamil, is ineffective, which would seem to indicate a primary effect of the drug at the plasma membrane.[314] Likewise, quarternary ammonium derivatives of D600 and nifedipine, which are highly ionized and therefore less lipophilic, are also less effective Ca^{++} antagonists.[313] Such data indicate that perhaps the locus of activity of these Ca^{++} antagonists is the internal surface of the channel or within the membrane itself.

In general, the drugs commonly classified as Ca^{++} antagonists, typified by verapamil, diltiazem, and nifedipine, exhibit specificity for vascular smooth muscle and cardiac tissues; however, within the group, specificity for these tissues varies. Nifedipine (and its other dihydropyridine relatives) is more potent in smooth muscle than cardiac tissue, while verapamil and diltiazem, in contrast, are more potent in cardiac tissue.[315,316] Although Ca^{++} channel antagonism is the dominant effect of these agents, at sufficiently high (greater than 10^{-6} M) concentrations, other effects become notable. For example, verapamil and D600 at concentrations greater than 10^{-6} M inhibit sodium channel activity and receptor binding at muscarinic, adrenergic, and opiate receptors.[317] These latter effects do not exhibit stereoselectivity as do Ca^{++} channel–specific action.[318]

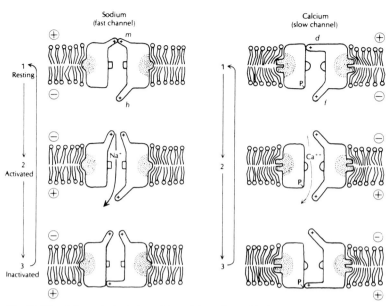

Fig. 12-10. Schematic depiction of the calcium channel in the sarcolemmal membrane. The upstroke (Phase 0) of the action potential, which allows rapid entry of sodium into the cell, produces the opening of the activation gates (m) in the sodium channel. The resulting change in transmembrane potential closes the inactivation gate (h), which stops sodium influx but maintains a refractory state in the cell membrane until repolarization. Similar processes occur in the calcium channel [activation gate (d) and inactivation gate (f)] except that at least some of the steps in slow channel activation require phosphorylation (P) by a cAMP protein kinase. Changes in the conformation of the channel proteins provide the three functional states of the channel: (1) resting, ie, closed and able to open; (2) activated, ie, open; and (3) inactivated, ie, closed and unable to open in response to depolarization. (From Katz AM, Messineo FC: Lipids and membrane function: Implications in arrhythmias. Hosp Prac 16:49–59, 1981, with permission.)

VERAPAMIL

As the prototype antiarrhythmic agent among the Ca^{++} blockers, verapamil has extensive utility in the treatment of supraventricular tachycardias, atrial fibrillation, and atrial flutter. Verapamil is especially effective at preventing or terminating PSVT. This effect is mediated by blocking impulse transmission through the AV node by prolonging AV nodal conduction and refractoriness.[319] Verapamil is also useful in the treatment of atrial fibrillation and flutter in order to decrease the ventricular response rate by decreasing AV conduction. In the case of atrial fibrillation, verapamil may (1) decrease the frequency of random impulse conduction through the AV node; (2) "regularize" AV conduction at a slower rate; or (3) convert to sinus rhythm (least common). The effect on ventricular response rate is similar to that of the cardiac glycosides, although the onset is more rapid, which makes verapamil more acutely effective for control of the abnormal physiology produced by

tachycardia in patients with highly rate-dependent lesions.[320,321] In the perioperative period, verapamil may be a useful antiarrhythmic agent. In one study of anesthetized patients, it successfully controlled a variety of supraventricular and ventricular dysrhythmias.[321] However, verapamil should be used cautiously intraoperatively because, in conjunction with inhalational anesthetics, significant cardiac depression may occur.[322,323]

A significant precaution in the use of verapamil to treat PSVT involves preexcitation of the AV node in WPW. If PSVT is orthodromic (anterograde conduction through the AV node and retrograde over the accessory pathway), then verapamil has a high success rate by blocking anterograde AV nodal conduction. If the PSVT is antidromic (anterograde conduction through accessory pathway and retrograde over the AV node), successful blockade with verapamil is unlikely, because it has little effect on refractoriness or conduction in accessory pathways.

Atrial flutter and fibrillation also may occur in WPW. In this setting, agents that shorten the ERP of the accessory pathway or increase the ERP in the AV node (ie, digitalis, verapamil, and beta-blockers) will often increase ventricular response and may precipitate VF.[324] Type I and III drugs, such as procainamide and disopyramide or amiodarone, are more effective.

Electrophysiologic effects of verapamil are seen predominantly in tissues in which phase 0 or phase 4 depolarization is calcium dependent, namely SA and AV nodes. Discharge rate and recovery time in the SA, AV conduction time, and AV node ERP are prolonged. Clinically, the QRS and Q-Tc intervals are not significantly affected, while A-H (but not H-V) conduction time is prolonged. Electrophysiologic effects of verapamil have been shown experimentally (in anesthetized dogs) to relate to plasma concentration; the A-H interval was prolonged at lower concentrations than were necessary to slow the SA node or to produce AV block.[325]

As with several other antiarrhythmic drugs, the pharmacokinetics of intravenously and orally administered verapamil differ. The hepatic extraction of orally administered verapamil is extensive; as a result, its bioavailability, which is normally low, is increased significantly by liver disease.[326] After intravenous administration of verapamil, plasma clearance approximates splanchnic blood flow rate, and, because of its lipophilic nature, the apparent volume of distribution is large. Elimination half-life of verapamil is approximately 5 hours, but it may be longer with chronic administration, perhaps due to saturation of hepatic metabolic pathways. Also, a principal metabolite, nor-verapamil, is biologically active, accumulates to concentrations equal to those of verapamil during chronic therapy, and has a longer half-life (8–13 hours).[327] Excretion of verapamil after metabolism is renal (65–70 percent), but 3–4 percent is excreted unchanged.[324] Metabolism involves n-dealkylation and o-demethylation with nor-verapamil (one eighth of the Ca^{++} channel–blocking potency of verapamil) as the major metabolite.[328] Verapamil and metabolites are highly protein bound (90 percent).

Verapamil dosage for acute intravenous treatment of PSVT is 0.07–0.15 mg/kg over 1 minute with the same dose repeated after 30 minutes if the initial response is inadequate (10 mg maximum). Since the cardiovascular depressant effects of the inhalational anesthetics involve inhibition of calcium-related intracellular processes, the interaction of verapamil and these anesthetics is synergistic. In a large clinical series, verapamil given during steady-state halothane anesthesia transiently decreased blood pressure and produced a 4 percent incidence of P-R interval prolongation.[329] In laboratory studies, verapamil interacts similarly with halothane, enflurane, and isoflurane to mildly depress ventricular function and to slow AV conduction (P-R interval).[322] AV block can occur, however, and may be refractory.

Another adverse effect of verapamil is the potentiation of neuromuscular blockade. In two laboratory studies, verapamil depressed twitch height response to indirect stimulation.[330,331] Although the exact presynaptic versus postsynaptic site of the block was not determined, the qualitative similarity of the effect to that of pancuronium suggested an effect at the neuromuscular junction. At clinically relevant doses of verapamil, the effect is slight, but the clinical potential for synergistic interaction with residual muscle relaxants seems substantial. Cautious clinical attention to neuromuscular function is necessary to safely use verapamil in patients who are receiving or have recently received muscle relaxants.

SUMMARY

Cardiac dysrhythmias occur frequently in the perioperative period, but severe rhythm disturbances are uncommon (0.9 percent). Causes of perioperative dysrhythmias include intrinsic cardiac disease (such as coronary artery disease), interaction between anesthetic agents and catecholamines (exogenous or endogenous), anesthetic effects on electrophysiologic properties of the heart (predominantly Ca^{++} related), and abnormalities of electrolyte concentration and body temperature. Initial treatment of dysrhythmias should be based on an accurate assessment of the underlying cause unless the severity of the situation mandates immediate treatment.[332,333]

Antiarrhythmic drugs are grouped according to major pharmacologic and electrophysiologic effects. Class I agents interfere with the fast channel of sodium conductance; typical Class I drugs are quinidine, procainamide, and lidocaine. Class II drugs block the beta-adrenergic receptor, and the two principal agents for acute use are propranolol and metoprolol. Class III drugs prolong repolarization and possess significant antifibrillatory power. Amiodarone and bretylium are examples of such drugs. Finally, Class IV drugs are calcium channel antagonists, among which verapamil has the most pronounced antiarrhythmic effect.

REFERENCES

1. Kurtz CM, Bennett JH, Shapiro HH: ECG studies during surgical anesthesia. JAMA 106:434–440, 1936

2. Katz RL, Bigger JT Jr: Cardiac arrhythmias during anesthesia and operation. Anesthesiology 33:193–213, 1970

3. Bertrand CA, Steiner NV, Jameson AG, et al: Disturbances of cardiac rhythm during anesthesia and surgery. JAMA 216:1615–1617, 1971

4. Vanik PE, Davis HS: Cardiac arrhythmias during halothane anesthesia. Anesth Analg 47:299–307, 1968

5. Hoffman BF, Cranefield PF, Wallace AG: Physiological basis of cardiac arrhythmias. Parts I and II. Mod Concepts Cardiovasc Dis 35:103, 1966

6. Chung EK: Principles of Cardiac Arrhythmias (ed 2). Baltimore, Williams & Wilkins, 1977, pp 25, 32, 570, 651–660, 668, 672

7. Lewis AJ: Monitoring and dysrhythmia recognition in advanced cardiac life support. In McIntyre MC, McIntyre KM, Lewis HA (eds): Textbook of Advanced Cardiac Life Support. Dallas, American Heart Association, 1983, pp 60, 61

8. Noble D: A modification of the Hodgkin-Huxley equations applicable to Purkinje fiber action and pacemaker potentials. J Physiol 160:317, 1962

9. Reuter H: The dependence of slow inward current in Purkinje fibers on the extracellular calcium concentration. J Physiol 192:497, 1967

10. Noble D: Cardiac action potentials and pacemaker activity. In Linden RJ (ed): Recent Advances in Physiology. London, Churchill, 1974

11. Davis LD, Temte JV, Murphy QR: Epinephrine-cyclopropane effects on Purkinje fibers. Anesthesiology 30:369–377, 1969

12. Berne RM, Levy MN: Cardiovascular Physiology. St. Louis, CV Mosby, 1967, pp 7, 8

13. Prys-Roberts C: Electrophysiology—The origin of the heart beat. In Prys-Roberts C (ed): The Circulation in Anaesthesia. Applied Physiology and Pharmacology. London, Blackwell Scientific, 1980, pp 37, 38–48

14. James TN: Anatomy of the A-V node of the dog. Anat Rec 148:15, 1964

15. Bachmann G: The inter-auricular time interval. Am J Physiol 41:309, 1916

16. Gross CM (ed): Grays Anatomy (ed 28): Philadelphia, Lea & Febiger, 1966, p 559

17. Lewis T: Mechanism and Graphic Registration of the Heart Beat (ed 3). London, Shaw and Sons, 1925

18. Scherf D: The mechanism of flutter and fibrillation. Am Heart J 71:273, 1966

19. Moe GK, Abildskov JA: Atrial fibrillation as a self-sustaining arrhythmia independent of focal discharge. Am Heart J 58:59–70, 1959

20. Rytland DA: The circus movement hypothesis and atrial flutter. Ann Intern Med 65:125, 1966

21. Chung EK: Parasystole. Prog Cardiovasc Dis 11:64, 1968

22. Massie E, Walsh TJ: Clinical Vectorcardiography and Electrocardiography. Chicago, Year Book, 1960

23. Scherf D, Choi KH, Bahadori A, et al: Parasystole. Am J Cardiol 12:527, 1963

24. Katz RL, Epstein RA: The interaction of anesthetic agents and adrenergic drugs to produce cardiac arrhythmias. Anesthesiology 29:763–784, 1968

25. Alper MH, Flack EW: Peripheral effects of anaesthetics. Ann Rev Pharmacol 9:273, 1969

26. Awalt CH, Frederickson EL: The contractile and cell membrane effects of halothane (Abstract). Anesthesiology 25:90, 1964

27. Hauswirth O, Schaer H: Effects of halothane on the sino-atrial node. J Pharmacol Exp Ther 158:36, 1967

28. Hauswirth O: Effects of halothane on single atrial ventricular and Purkinje fibers. Circ Res 24:745, 1969

29. Bosnjak ZJ, Campine JT: Effects of halothane, enflurane, and isoflurane on the SA node. Anesthesiology 58:314, 1983

30. Lynch C III, Vogel S, Sperelakis N: Halothane depression of myocardial slow-action potentials. Anesthesiology 55:360, 1981

31. Lynch C III: Differential depression of myocardial contractility by halothane and isoflurane in the guinea pig capillary muscle. Anesthesiology 64:620–631, 1986

32. Joas TA, Stevens WC: Comparison of the arrhythmic doses of epinephrine during forane, halothane, and fluroxene anesthesia in dogs. Anesthesiology 35:48, 1971

33. Johnston RR, Eger EI, Wilson C: A comparative interaction of epinephrine with enflurane, isoflurane, and halothane in man. Anesth Analg 55:709–712, 1976

34. Horrigan RW, Eger EI, Wilson C: Epinephrine-induced arrhythmias during enflurane anesthesia in man: A non-linear dose-response relationship and dose-dependent protection from lidocaine. Anesth Analg 57:547–550, 1978

35. Karl HW, Swedlow DB, Lee KW, et al: Epinephrine-halothane interactions in children. Anesthesiology 58:142–145, 1983

36. Sumikawa K, Ishizaka N, Suzaki M: Arrhythmogenic plasma level of epinephrine during halothane, enflurane, and pentobarbital anesthesia in the dog. Anesthesiology 58:322–325, 1983

37. Atlee JL, Malkinson CE: Potentiation by thiopental of halothane-epinephrine-induced arrhythmias in dogs. Anesthesiology 57:285–288, 1982

38. Miletich DJ, Albrecht RF, Seals C: Responses to

fasting and lipid infusion of epinephrine-induced arrhythmias during halothane anesthesia. Anesthesiology 48:245–248, 1978

39. Merin RG: New implications of fasting. Anesthesiology 48:236–237, 1978

40. Bernstein KJ, Gangat Y, Verosky M, et al: Halothane effect on beta-adrenergic receptors in canine myocardium. Anesth Analg 60:401–405, 1981

41. Koehntop DE, Liao JC, Van Bergen FH: Effects of pharmacologic alterations of adrenergic mechanisms by cocaine, tropolone, aminophylline, and ketamine on epinephrine-induced arrhythmias during halothane-nitrous oxide anesthesia. Anesthesiology 46:83–93, 1977

42. Atlee JL III, Rusy BF: Halothane depression of AV conduction studied by electrograms of the bundle of His in dogs. Anesthesiology 36:112–118, 1972

43. Kroll DA, Knight PR: Antifibrillatory effects of volatile anesthetics in acute occlusion/reperfusion arrhythmias. Anesthesiology 61:657–661, 1984

44. Davidsohn I, Henry JB: Todd Sanford Clinical Diagnosis by Laboratory Methods (ed 15). Philadelphia, WB Saunders, 1974, p 775

45. Levine HD: Electrolyte imbalance in the electrocardiogram. Mod Concepts Cardiovasc Dis 23:246, 1954

46. Pacifico AD, Digerness S, Kirklin JW: Acute alterations of body composition after open heart intracardiac operations. Circulation 41:331–341, 1970

47. Mandelbaum I, Morgan CR: Effect of extracorporeal circulation upon insulin. J Thorac Cardiovasc Surg 55:526–534, 1968

48. Surawicz B: Role of electrolytes and etiology and management of cardiac arrhythmias. Prog Cardiovasc Dis 8:364–386, 1966

49. Lepeschkin E: Modern Electrocardiography, vol 1. Baltimore, Williams & Wilkins, 1951

50. Drop LJ, Laver MB: Low plasma ionized calcium and response to calcium therapy in critically ill man. Anesthesiology 43:300–306, 1975

51. Gray R, Braunstein G, Krutzik S, et al: Homeostasis during coronary bypass surgery. Circulation 62(1):I57–I61, 1980

52. Das JB, Eraklis AN, Adams JG, et al: Changes in serum ionic calcium during cardiopulmonary bypass with hemodilution. J Thorac Cardiovasc Surg 62:449, 1971

53. Moffitt EA, Tarhan S, Goldsmith RS, et al: Patterns of total and ionized calcium and other electrolytes in plasma during and after cardiac surgery. J Thorac Cardiovasc Surg 65:751, 1973

54. Bronsky B, Dubin A, Waldstein SS, et al: Calcium in electrocardiogram. I. Electrocardiographic manifestations of hypoparathyroidism. Am J Cardiol 7:823, 1961

55. Burch GE, Giles TE: The importance of magnesium deficiency in cardiovascular disease. Am Heart J 94:649, 1977

56. Iseri LT, Freed J, Bures AR: Magnesium deficiency and cardiac disorders. Am J Med 58:837, 1975

57. Turlapty PDMV, Altura BM: Magnesium deficiency produces spasms of coronary arteries: Relationship to etiology of sudden death and ischemic heart disease. Science 208:198, 1980

58. Seller RH, Cangiano J, Kim KE, et al: Digitalis toxicity and hypomagnesemia. Am Heart J 79:57, 1970

59. Specter MJ, Schweizer E, Goldman RH: Studies on magnesium's mechanism of action in digitalis-induced arrhythmias. Circulation 52:1001–1005, 1975

60. Scheinmen MM, Sullivan RW, Hyatt KH: Magnesium metabolism in patients undergoing cardiopulmonary bypass. Circulation 39:235, 1969

61. Chernow B, Smith J, Rainey TG, et al: Hypomagnesemia: Implications for the critical care specialists. Crit Care Med 10:193–196, 1981

62. Singer I, Rotenberg D: Mechanisms of lithium action. N Engl J Med 289:254–260, 1973

63. Wilson JR, Kraus ES, Bailas MM, et al: Reversible sinus-node abnormality due to lithium carbonate therapy. N Engl J Med 294:1223–1224, 1976

64. Tangedahl TN, Gan GT: Myocardial irritability associated with lithium carbonate therapy. N Engl J Med 287:867–869, 1972

65. Azar I, Turndorf H: Paroxysmal left bundle branch block during nitrous oxide anesthesia in a patient on lithium carbonate: A case report. Anesth Analg 56:868–870, 1977

66. Spurr GB, Hutt BK, Horvath SM: Responses of dogs to hypothermia. Am J Physiol 179:139–145, 1954

67. Vandam LD, Burnap TK: Hypothermia. N Engl J Med 261:546–553, 595–603, 1959

68. Lange K, Weiner D, Gold MMA: Studies on mechanism of cardiac injury in experimental hypothermia. Ann Intern Med 31:989–1002, 1949

69. Osborn JJ: Experimental hypothermia. Respiratory and blood pH changes in relation to cardiac function. Am J Physiol 175:389, 1953

70. Emslie-Smith D, Sladden GE, Stirling GR: The significance of changes in the electrocardiogram in hypothermia. Br Heart J 21:343–351, 1959

71. Grosse-Brockhoff F, Schoedel W: Tierexperimentelle untersuchungen zur frage der therapie bei unterkuhlung. Arch Exp Pathol Pharmacol 201:417, 1943

72. Angelakos ET, Hagnauer AH: Pharmacological agents for the control of spontaneous ventricular fibrillation under progressive hypothermia. J Pharmacol Exp Ther 127:137–145, 1959

73. Lazzara R, El-Sherif N, Hope RR, et al: Ventricular arrhythmias and electrophysiological consequences of myocardial ischemia and infarction. Circ Res 42:740–749, 1978

74. Julian DG, Valentine TA, Miller GG: Disturbances of rate, rhythm, and conduction in acute myocardial

infarction: A prospective study of 100 consecutive unselected patients with the aid of electrocardiographic monitoring. Am J Med 37:915, 1964

75. DeSanctis RW, Block P, Hutter AM: Tachyarrhythmias in acute myocardial infarction. Circulation 45:681, 1972

76. Fisher FD, Tyroler HA: Relationship between ventricular premature contractions on routine electrocardiography and subsequent sudden death from coronary heart disease. Circulation 47:712, 1973

77. Vismara LA, Amsterdam EA, Mason DT: Relation of ventricular arrhythmias in the late hospital phase of acute myocardial infarction to sudden death after hospital discharge. Am J Med 59:6, 1975

78. El-Sherif N, Myerburg RJ, Scherlag BJ, et al: Electrocardiographic antecedents of primary ventricular fibrillation: Value of the R-on-T phenomenon in myocardial infarction. Br Heart J 38:415, 1976

79. deSoyza N, Bissett JK, Kane JJ, et al: Ventricular prematurity and its relationship to ventricular tachycardia in acute myocardial infarction in man. Circulation 50:529, 1974

80. Williams DO, Sherlag BJ, Hope RR, et al: The pathophysiology of malignant arrhythmias during acute myocardial ischemia. Circulation 50:1163, 1974

81. Vaughan Williams EM: Classification of antiarrhythmic drugs. In Sandoe E, Flensted-Jansene, Olesen KH (eds): Symposium on Cardiac Arrhythmias. Sodertalje, Sweden, AB Astra, 1970, pp 449–472

82. Millar JS, Vaughan Williams EM: Pacemaker selectivity. Influence on rabbit atria of ionic environment and of alinidine, a possible anion antagonist. Cardiovasc Res 15:335–350, 1981

83. Davis LD: Effect of changes in cycle length on diastolic depolarization produced by ouabain in canine Purkinje fibers. Circ Res 32:206–214, 1973

84. Ferrier GR, Saunders JH, Mendez C: A cellular mechanism for the generation of ventricular arrhythmias by acetylstrophanthidan. Circ Res 32:600–609, 1973

85. Rosen MR, Gelband H, Merker C, et al: Mechanisms of digitalis toxicity: Effects of ouabain on phase 4 of canine Purkinje fiber transmembrane potentials. Circ Res 47:681–689, 1973

86. Hoffman BF, Bigger JT Jr: Digitalis and allied cardiac glycosides. In Gilman AG, Goodman LS, Rall TW, et al (eds): The Pharmacological Basis of Therapeutics (ed 7). New York, McMillan, 1985, pp 724, 725

87. Rosen MR, Wit AL, Hoffman BF: Electrophysiology and pharmacology of cardiac arrhythmias. IV. Cardiac antiarrhythmic and toxic effects of digitalis. Am Heart J 89:391–399, 1975

88. Mudge GH, Lloyd BL, Greenblatt DJ, et al: Inotropic and toxic effects of a polar cardiac glycoside derivative in a dog. Circ Res 43:847–854, 1978

89. Gillis RA, Quest JA: The role of the central nervous system in the cardiovascular effects of digitalis. Pharmacol Rev 31:19–97, 1980

90. Rosen MR: Interactions of digitalis with the autonomic nervous system in relationship to cardiac arrhythmias. In Abboud F, Fozzard H, Gilmore J, et al (eds): Disturbances in Neurogenic Control of the Circulation. Bethesda, MD, American Physiological Society, 1981, pp 251–263

91. Smith TW, Braunwald E: Management of heart failure. In Braunwald E (ed): Heart Disease: A Textbook of Cardiovascular Medicine. Philadelphia, WB Saunders, 1980, p 524

88. Mudge GH, Lloyd BL, Greenblatt DJ, et al: Inotropic and toxic effects of a polar cardiac glycoside derivative in a dog. Cir Res 43:847–854, 1978

89. Gillis RA, Quest JA: The role of the central nervous system in the cardiovascular effects of digitalis. Pharmacol Rev 31:19–97, 1980

90. Rosen MR: Interactions of digitalis with the autonomic nervous system in relationship to cardiac arrhythmias. In Abboud F, Fozzard H, Gilmore J, et al (eds): Disturbances in Neurogenic Control of the Circulation. Bethesda, MD, American Physiological Society, 1981, pp 251–263

91. Smith TW, Braunwald E: The management of heart failure. In Braunwald E (ed): Heart Disease: A Textbook of Cardiovascular Medicine. Philadelphia, WB Saunders, 1980, p 524

92. Covino BG: Perioperative management of arrhythmias. In Kaplan JA (ed): Cardiac Anesthesia, Volume 2: Cardiovascular Pharmacology. Orlando, FL, Grune & Stratton, 1983, pp 397–412

93. Harrison DC, Winkle R, Sami M, et al: Comparative pharmacokinetics of new antiarrhythmic drugs. Am Heart J 100:1046–1054, 1980

94. Bassett AL, Hoffman BF: Antiarrhythmic drugs: Electrophysiological action. Ann Rev Pharmacol 11:143–170, 1971

95. Wittig J, Harrison LA, Wallace AG: Electrophysiological effects of lidocaine on distal Purkinje fibers of canine heart. Am Heart J 86:69–78, 1973

96. Vaughan Williams EM: A classification of antiarrhythmic actions reassessed after a decade of new drugs. J Clin Pharmacol 24:129–147, 1984

97. Birkhead JS, Vaughan Williams EM: Dual effect of disopyramide on atrial and atrioventricular conduction and refractory periods. Br Heart J 39:657–660, 1977

98. Strong JM, Parker M, Atkinson AJ: Identification of glycine xylidide in patients treated with intravenous lidocaine. Clin Pharmacol Ther 14:67–72, 1973

99. Hoffman BF, Rosen MR, Wit AL: Electrophysiology and pharmacology of cardiac arrhythmias. VII. Cardiac effects of quinidine and procainamide. Am Heart J 90:117, 1975

100. Kessler KM, Lowenthal DT, Warner H, et al: Quini-

dine elimination in patients with congestive heart failure or poor renal function. N Engl J Med 290:706–709, 1974

101. Bigger JT Jr, Hoffman BF: Antiarrhythmic drugs. *In* Gilman AG, Goodman LS, Gilman A (eds): The Pharmacological Basis of Therapeutics (ed 6). New York, Macmillan, 1980, pp 771, 781

102. Conn HL Jr, Luchi RJ: Some quantitative aspects of the binding of quinidine and related quinoline compounds by human serum albumin. J Clin Invest 40:509–516, 1961

103. Leahey EB Jr, Reiffel JA, Drusin RE, et al: Interaction between quinidine and digoxin. JAMA 240:533–534, 1978

104. Gerhardt RE, Knouss RF, Thyrum PT, et al: Quinidine excretion in aciduria and alkaluria. Ann Intern Med 71:927–933, 1969

105. Koster RW, Wellens HJJ: Quinidine-induced ventricular flutter and fibrillation without digitalis therapy. Am J Cardiol 38:519–523, 1976

106. Krone RJ, Miller JP, Kleiger RE, et al: The effectiveness of antiarrhythmic agents on early-cycle premature ventricular complexes. Circulation 63:664, 1981

107. Winkle RA, Glantz SA, Harrison DC: Pharmacologic therapy of ventricular arrhythmias. Am J Cardiol 36:629–650, 1975

108. Lima JJ, Goldfarb AL, Conti DR, et al: Safety and efficacy of procainamide infusions. Am J Cardiol 43:98–105, 1979

109. Gaffner C, Johnsson G, Sjogren J: Pharmacokinetics of procainamide intravenously and orally as conventional slow release tablets. Clin Pharmacol Ther 117:114, 1975

110. Collaste P, Karlsson E: Arrhythmia prophylaxis with procainamide: Plasma concentrations in relation to dose. Acta Med Scand 194:405, 1973

111. Reidenberg MM, Drayer DE, Levy M, et al: Polymorphic acetylation of procainamide in man. Clin Pharmacol Ther 17:722–730, 1975

112. Woosely RL, Roden DM: Importance of metabolites in antiarrhythmic therapy. Am J Cardiol 52:3C–7C, 1983

113. White RD: Cardiovascular pharmacology: Part I. *In* McIntyre KM, Lewis AJ (eds): Textbook of Advanced Cardiac Life Support. Dallas, American Heart Association, 1983, pp 104, 107

114. Strasberg B, Sclarovsky S, Erdberg A, et al: Procainamide-induced polymorphous ventricular tachycardia. Am J Cardiol 47:1309, 1981

115. Blomgren SE, Condemi JJ, Vaughn JH: Procainamide-induced lupus erythematosus: Clinical and laboratory observations. Am J Med 52:338, 1972

116. Roden DM, Reele SB, Higgins SB, et al: Antiarrhythmic efficacy, pharmacokinetics and safety of *N*-acetylprocainamide in human subjects: Compari-

son with procainamide. Am J Cardiol 46:463–468, 1980

117. Michelson EL, Spear JF, Moore EN: Effects of procainamide on strength-interval relations in normal and chronically infarcted canine myocardium. Am J Cardiol 47:1223, 1981

118. Wenger TL, Browning DL, Masterton CE, et al: Procainamide delivery to ischemic canine myocardium following rapid intravenous administration. Circ Res 46:789–795, 1983

119. Reid DS, Williams DO, Parashar SK: Disopyramide in the sick sinus syndrome—Safe or not? Br Heart J 39:348, 1977

120. Spurrell RAJ, Thorburn CW, Camm J, et al: Effects of disopyramide on electrophysiological properties of specialized conduction system in man and on accessory atrioventricular pathway in Wolff-Parkinson-White syndrome. Br Heart J 37:861, 1975

121. Podrid PG, Schoeneberger A, Lown B: Congestive heart failure caused by oral disopyramide. N Engl J Med 302:614, 1980

122. Koch-Weser J: Drug Therapy. Disopyramide. N Engl J Med 300:957, 1979

123. Zipes DP, Troup PJ: New antiarrhythmic agents: Amiodarone, aprinidine, disopyramide, ethmozin, mexiletine, tocainide, verapamil. Am J Cardiol 41:1005–1024, 1979

124. Chien YW, Lambert HJ, Karim A:: Comparative binding of disopyramide phosphate and quinidine sulfate to human plasma proteins. J Pharm Sci 63:1877–1879, 1974

125. Gillis RA, McClellan JR, Sauer TS, et al: Depression of cardiac sympathetic nerve activity by diphenylhydantoin. J Pharmacol Exp Ther 173:599, 1971

126. Evans DE, Gillis RS: Effect of diphenylhydantoin and lidocaine on cardiac arrhythmias induced by hypothalmic stimulation. J Pharmacol Exp Ther 191:506, 1974

127. Singh BN, Vaughan Williams EM: Explanation for the discrepancy in recorded cardiac electrophysiological actions of diphenylhydantoin and lidocaine. Br J Pharmacol 41:385, 1971

128. Bigger JT Jr, Weinberg DI, Kovalik ATW, et al: Effects of diphenylhydantoin on excitability and automaticity in the canine heart. Circ Res 26:1–15, 1970

129. Rosen MR, Danilo P Jr, Alonso MB, et al: Effects of therapeutic concentrations of diphenylhydantoin on transmembrane potentials of normal and depressed Purkinje fibers. J Pharmacol Exp Ther 197:594–604, 1976

130. Peon J, Ferrier GR, Moe GK: The relationship of excitability to conduction velocity in canine Purkinje tissue. Circ Res 43:125–135, 1978

131. Bigger JT Jr, Bassett AL, Hoffman BF: Electrophysiological effects of diphenylhydantoin on canine Purkinje fibers. Circ Res 22:221–236, 1968

132. Garson A, Kugler JD, Gillette PC, et al: Control of late postoperative ventricular arrhythmias with phenytoin in young patients. Am J Cardiol 46:290, 1980

133. Bigger JT Jr, Schmidt DH, Kutt H: Relationship between the plasma level of diphenylhydantoin sodium and its cardiac antiarrhythmic effects. Circulation 38:363–374, 1968

134. Kutt H, Winters W, Kokenge R, et al: Diphenylhydantoin metabolism, blood levels, and toxicity. Arch Neurol 11:642, 1964

135. Kutt H: Biochemical and genetic factors regulating dilantin metabolism in man. Ann NY Acad Sci 179:704–722, 1971

136. Lieberson AD, Shoumacher RR, Childress RH, et al: Effect of diphenylhydantoin on left ventricular function in patients with heart disease. Circulation 36:692, 1967

137. Konn RD, Kennedy JW, Blackmon JR: The hemodynamic effects of diphenylhydantoin. Am Heart J 73:500, 1967

138. Louis S, Kutt H, McDowell F: Cardiocirculatory changes caused by intravenous dilantin and its solvent. Am Heart J 74:523, 1967

139. Unger AH, Sklaroff HJ: Fatalities following intravenous use of sodium diphenylhydantoin for cardiac arrhythmias. JAMA 200:335, 1967

140. Southworth JL, McKusick VA, Peirce EC, et al: Ventricular fibrillation precipitated by cardiac catheterization. Complete recovery of the patient after 45 minutes. JAMA 143:717–720, 1950

141. Carden NL, Steinhaus JE: Lidocaine and cardiac resuscitation from ventricular fibrillation. Circ Res 4:680–683, 1956

142. Hitchcock P, Keown KK: Lidocaine and control of cardiac arrhythmias (Abstract). Fed Proc 17:378, 1958

143. Weiss WA: Intravenous use of lidocaine for ventricular arrhythmias. Anesth Analg 39:369–381, 1960

144. DeCliv-Lowe SG, Desmond J, North J: Intravenous lignocaine anaesthesia. Anaesthesia 13:138–146, 1958

145. Davis LD, Temte JV: Electrophysiological actions of lidocaine on canine ventricular muscle and Purkinje fibers. Circ Res 24:639–655, 1969

146. Bigger JT Jr, Reiffel JA: Sick sinus syndrome. Ann Rev Med 30:91–118, 1979

147. Gerstenblith G, Spear JF, Moore EN: Quantitative study of the effect of lidocaine on the threshold for ventricular fibrillation in the dog. Am J Cardiol 30:242–247, 1972

148. Arnsdorf MF, Bigger JT Jr: The effect of lidocaine on components of excitability in long mammalian cardiac Purkinje fibers. J Pharmacol Exp Ther 195:206–215, 1975

149. Singh BN, Vaughan Williams EM: Effect of altering potassium concentration on the action of lidocaine and diphenylhydantoin on rabbit atrial and ventricular muscle. Circ Res 29:286–295, 1971

150. Obayashi K, Hayakawa H, Mandell WJ: Interrelationships between external potassium concentration and lidocaine: Effects on canine Purkinje fiber. Am Heart J 89:221–226, 1975

151. Watanabe Y, Dreifus LS, Likoff W: Electrophysiological antagonism and synergism of potassium and antiarrhythmic agents. Am J Cardiol 12:702–710, 1963

152. Kupersmith J, Antman EM, Hoffman BF: In vivo electrophysiological effects of lidocaine in canine acute myocardial infarction. Circ Res 36:84–91, 1975

153. Wittig JH, Harrison LA, Wallace AG: Electrophysiological effects of lidocaine on distal Purkinje fibers of canine heart. Am Heart J 86:69–78, 1973

154. Bassett AL, Hoffman BF: Antiarrhythmic drugs: Electrophysiological actions. Ann Rev Pharmacol 11:143–170, 1971

155. El-Sherif N, Scherlag BJ, Lazzara R, et al: Re-entrant ventricular arrhythmias in the late myocardial infarction period. 4. Mechanism of action of lidocaine. Circulation 56:395, 1977

156. Davis RF, DeBoer LWV, Yasuda T, et al: Regional myocardial lidocaine concentration determines the antidysrhythmic effect in dogs after coronary artery occlusion. Anesthesiology 62:155–160, 1985

157. Zito RA, Caride VJ, Holford T, et al: Regional myocardial kinetics of lidocaine in experimental infarction: Modulation by regional blood flow. Am J Cardiol 47:265–270, 1981

158. Zito RA, Caride VJ, Holford T, et al: Regional myocardial lidocaine concentration following continuous intravenous infusion early and late after myocardial infarction. Am J Cardiol 50:497–502, 1982

159. Biehl D, Shnider SM, Levinson G, et al: Placental transfer of lidocaine: Effects of fetal acidosis. Anesthesiology 48:409–412, 1978

160. Eriksson E, Granberg PO: Studies on the renal excretion of Citanest® and Xylocaine®. Acta Anaesthesiol Scand [Suppl] 16:79, 1965

161. Yakaitis RW, Thomas JD, Mahaffey JE: Cardiovascular effects of lidocaine during acid-base imbalance. Anesth Analg 55:863–868, 1976

162. Lie KI, Wellens NJ, vanCapelle FJ: Lidocaine in the prevention of primary ventricular fibrillation. A double-blind, randomized study of 212 consecutive patients. N Engl J Med 291:1324–1326, 1974

163. deJong RH: Local Anesthetics (ed 2). Springfield, IL, Charles C. Thomas, 1977, p 216

164. Blumer J, Strong JM, Atkinson AJ: The convulsant potency of lidocaine and its o-dealkylated metabolites. J Pharmacol Exp Ther 186:31–36, 1973

165. Collinsworth KA, Kalman SM, Harrison DC: The clinical pharmacology of lidocaine as an antiarrhythmic drug. Circulation 50:1217–1230, 1974

166. Smith ER, Duce BR: The acute antiarrhythmic and toxic effects in mice and dogs of 2-ethylamino-2', 6'-acetoxylidine (L-86), a metabolite of lidocaine. J Pharmacol Exp Ther 179:580–585, 1971

167. Essman WB: Anticonvulsant properties of xylocaine in mice susceptible to audiogenic seizures. Arch Int Pharmacodyn Ther 164:376–386, 1966

168. Bernheard CG, Bohm E: Local anesthetics as anticonvulsants. A study on experimental and clinical epilepsy. Stockholm, Almqvist & Wiksel, 1965

169. Hood DD, Mecca RS: Failure to initiate electroconvulsive seizures in a patient pretreated with lidocaine. Anesthesiology 58:379–381, 1983

170. Campbell NPS, Zaidi SA, Agdgey AAJ, et al: Observations on hemodynamic effects of mexiletine. Br Heart J 41:182–186, 1979

171. Saunamaki KI: Hemodynamic effects of a new antiarrhythmic agent, mexiletine (KO1173), and ischaemic heart disease. Cardiovasc Res 9:788–792, 1975

172. Banim SO, DaSilva A, Stone D, et al: Observations of the hemodynamics of mexiletine. Postgrad Med J 53:74–76, 1977

173. Pozenel H: Hemodynamic studies on mexiletine a new antiarrhythmic agent. Postgrad Med J 53:78–80, 1977

174. Shaw TRD, Royds R: Effect of KO1173, a new antiarrhythmic drug, on contractile state of diseased left ventricle and on frequency of "stable" premature beats (Abstract). Br Heart J 35:558, 1973

175. Young MD, Hadidian Z, Horn HR, et al: Treatment of ventricular arrhythmias with oral tocainide. Am Heart J 100:1041–1045, 1980

176. Ikram H: Hemodynamic and electrophysiologic interactions between antiarrhythmic drugs and beta-blockers, with special reference to tocainide. Am Heart J 100:1076–1080, 1980

177. Kuhn L, Klicpera M, Kroiss A, et al: Antiarrhythmic and hemodynamic effects of mexiletine. Postgrad Med J 53:81–83, 1977

178. Winkle RA, Anderson JL, Peters F, et al: The hemodynamic effects of intravenous tocainide in patients with heart disease. Circulation 57:787–792, 1978

179. Nyquist O, Forssell G, Nordlander R, et al: Hemodynamic and antiarrhythmic effects of tocainide in patients with acute myocardial infarction. Am Heart J 100:1000–1005, 1980

180. Ryan WF, Karliner JS: Effects of tocainide on left ventricular performance at rest and during alterations in heart rate and systemic arterial pressure. Br Heart J 41:175–181, 1979

181. Abinader EG, Cooper M: Mexiletine use and control of chronic drug-resistant ventricular arrhythmias. JAMA 224:337–339, 1979

182. Dimarco JP, Garan H, Ruskin JN: Mexiletine for refractory ventricular arrhythmias: Results using serial electrophysiologic testing. Am J Cardiol 47:131–138, 1981

183. Podrid PJ, Lown B: Mexiletine for ventricular arrhythmias. Am J Cardiol 47:895–902, 1981

184. Horowitz JD, Amavekar SN, Morris PM, et al: Comparative trial of mexiletine and lignocaine in the treatment of early ventricular tachyarrhythmias after acute myocardial infarction. J Cardiovasc Pharmacol 3:409–419, 1981

185. Campbell RWF, Achuff SC, Pottage A, et al: Mexiletine in the prophylaxis of ventricular arrhythmias during acute myocardial infarction. J Cardiovasc Pharmacol 1:43–52, 1979

186. Bell JA, Thomas JM, Isaacson JR, et al: Prophylactic mexiletine in home coronary care. Br Heart J 48:285–290, 1982

187. Chamberlain DH, Jewitt DE, Julian DG, et al: Oral mexiletine in high-risk patients after myocardial infarction. Lancet 2:1324–1327, 1980

188. Winkle RA, Meffin PG, Fitzgerald JW, et al: Clinical efficacy and pharmacokinetics of a new orally effective antiarrhythmic, tocainide. Circulation 54:884–889, 1976

189. Engler R, Ryan W, LeWinter M, et al: Assessment of long-term antiarrhythmic therapy: Studies on the long-term efficacy and toxicity of tocainide. Am J Cardiol 43:612–618, 1979

190. Roden DM, Reele SB, Higgins SB, et al: Tocainide therapy for refractory ventricular arrhythmias. Am Heart J 100:15–22, 1980

191. Podrid PJ, Lown B: Tocainide for refractory systemic ventricular arrhythmias. Am J Cardiol 49:1279–1286, 1982

192. Rehnquist N: Comparison of tocainide with lidocaine in AMI. In Pottage A, Ryden L (eds): Workshop on Tocainide. Sweden, AB Hassle, 1981, pp 187–189

193. Campbell RWF, Bryson LG, Bailey BK, et al: Prophylactic administration of tocainide in acute myocardial infarction. In Pottage A, Ryden L (eds): Workshop on Tocainide. Sweden, AB Hassle, 1981, pp 201–204

194. Ryden L, Arnman K, Conradson TB, et al: Prophylaxis of ventricular tachyarrhythmias with intravenous and oral tocainide. In Harrison DC (ed): Cardiac Arrhythmias—A Decade of Progress. Boston, GK Hall, 1981, pp 227–247

195. Pottage A: Clinical profiles of new class I antiarrhythmic agents—tocainide, mexiletine, encainide, flecainide, and lorcainide. Am J Cardiol 52:24C–31C, 1983

196. Graffner C, Conradson TB, Hofvendahl S, et al: Pharmacokinetics of tocainide following intravenous and oral administration in healthy subjects and in patients with acute myocardial infarction. Clin Pharmacol Ther 27:64–71, 1980

197. Ronfeld RA, Wolshin EN, Block AJ: On the kinetics and dynamics of tocainide and its metabolites. Clin Pharmacol Ther 31:384–392, 1982

198. Oltmanns D: Tocainid-pharmakokinetik bei chronis-

cher lebererkrankung (Abstract). Z Cardiol 71:172, 1982

199. El Allaf B, Henrard L, Crochelet L, et al: Pharmacokinetics of mexiletine in renal insufficiency. Br J Pharmacol 14:431–435, 1982

200. Nitsch J, Steinbeck G, Luderitz B: Effect of kidney, liver, or heart insufficiency on plasma mexiletine levels. Internist 23:291–293, 1982

201. Campbell NPS, Kelly JG, Adgey AAJ, et al: The clinical pharmacology of mexiletine. Br J Clin Pharmacol 6:103–108, 1978

202. Wei JY, Bulkey BH, Schaeffer AH, et al: Mitral valve prolapse syndrome in recurrent ventricular tachyarrhythmias. Ann Intern Med 89:6, 1978

203. Zipes DP, Gaum WE, Foster PR, et al: Aprinidine for treatment of supraventricular tachycardias with particular application to Wolff-Parkinson-White syndrome. Am J Cardiol 40:586, 1977

204. Reiser J, Freeman AR, Greenspan K: Aprinidine-calcium-mediated antidysrhythmic effect (Abstract). Fed Proc 33:476, 1974

205. Delcroix C, Martin L, VanDurme JP, et al: Model for exchange kinetics of aprinidine in man after single and multiple doses. Acta Cardiol (Brux) (Suppl)18:251, 1974

206. vanLeuwen R, Meyboom RHB: Agranulocytosis and aprinidine. Lancet 2:1137, 1976

207. Gibson JK, Somani P, Bassett AL: Electrophysiologic effects of encainide (NJ9067) on canine Purkinje fibers. Eur J Pharmacol 52:161–169, 1978

208. Sami M, Mason JW, Peters F, et al: Clinical electrophysiologic effects of encainide, a newly developed antiarrhythmic agent. Am J Cardiol 44:526–532, 1979

209. Jackman WM, Zipes DP, Naccarelli GV, et al: Electrophysiology of oral encainide. Am J Cardiol 49:1270–1278, 1982

210. Tucker CR, Winkle RA, Peters FA, et al: Acute hemodynamic effects of intravenous encainide in patients with heart disease. Am Heart J 104:209–215, 1982

211. DiBianco R, Fletcher RD, Cohen AL, et al: Treatment of frequent ventricular arrhythmia with encainide: Assessment using serial ambulatory electrocardiograms, intracardiac physiologic studies, treadmill exercise tests, and radionuclide cineangiographic studies. Circulation 65:1134–1147, 1982

212. Kates RE, Harrison DC, Winkle RA: Metabolite accumulation during long-term oral encainide administration. Clin Pharmacol Ther 31:427–432, 1982

213. Olsson SB, Edvardsson N: Clinical electrophysiologic study of antiarrhythmic properties of flecainide: Acute intraventricular delayed conduction and prolonged repolarization in regular pace and premature beats using intracardiac monophasic action potentials with programmed stimulation. Am Heart J 102:864–871, 1981

214. Verdouw PD, Deckers JW, Conard GJ: Antiarrhythmic and hemodynamic actions of flecainide acetate (R-818) in the ischemic porcine heart. J Cardiovasc Pharmacol 1:473–486, 1979

215. Hodges M, Haugland JM, Granrud G, et al: Suppression of ventricular ectopic depolarization by flecainide acetate, a new antiarrhythmic agent. Circulation 65:879–885, 1982

216. Anderson JL, Stewart JR, Perry BA, et al: Oral flecainide for the treatment of ventricular arrhythmias. N Engl J Med 305:473–477, 1981

217. Duff HJ, Roden DM, Maffucci RJ, et al: Suppression of resistant ventricular arrhythmias by twice daily dosing with flecainide. Am J Cardiol 48:1133–1140, 1981

218. Lui HK, Lee G, Dietrich P, et al: Flecainide-induced QT prolongation and ventricular tachycardia. Am Heart J 103:567–569, 1982

219. Carmeliet E, Janssen PHA, Marsboom R, et al: Antiarrhythmic electrophysiologic and hemodynamic effects of lorcainide. Arch Int Pharmacodyn Ther 231:104–130, 1978

220. Echt DS, Mitchel LD, Kates RE, et al: Comparison of the electrophysiologic effects of intravenous and oral lorcainide in patients with recurrent ventricular tachycardia. Circulation 68:392–399, 1983

221. Barr MW, Farre J, Ross D, et al: Period electrophysiologic effects of lorcainide, a new antiarrhythmic drug. Br Heart J 45:292–298, 1981

222. Kasper W, Meinertz T, Kersting F, et al: Electrophysiological actions of lorcainide in patients with cardiac disease. J Cardiovasc Pharmacol 1:343–352, 1979

223. Almotrefi AA, Baker JBE: Antifibrillatory efficacy of encainide, lorcainide, and ORG6001 compared with lignocaine in isolated hearts of rabbits and guinea pigs. Br J Pharmacol 73:273–277, 1981

224. Keefe DL: Pharmacology of lorcainide. Am J Cardiol 54:18B–21B, 1984

225. Meinertz T, Kersting F, Kasper W, et al: Hemodynamic effects of a single intravenous dose of lorcainide in patients with heart disease. Eur J Pharmacol 18:461–465, 1980

226. Shita A, Bernard R, Mostinckx R, et al: Hemodynamic reactions after intravenous injection of lorcainide hydrochloride in acute myocardial infarction. Eur J Cardiol 12:237–242, 1981

227. Winkle RA, Keefe DL, Rodrigues I, et al: Pharmacodynamics of the initiation of antiarrhythmic therapy with lorcainide. Am J Cardiol 53:544–551, 1984

228. Jauhanchen E, Bechtol H, Kasper W, et al: Lorcainide kinetics. Clin Pharmacol Ther 26:187–205, 1979

229. Woestenborghs R, Michaels M, Haykants J: Simultaneous gas chromatographic determination of lorcainide hydrochloride and three of its principal metabolites in biological samples. J Chromatogr 164:169–176, 1979

230. Keefe DL, Kates RE, Winkle RA: Comparative electrophysiology of lorcainide in the dog. J Cardiovasc Pharmacol 6:808–815, 1984

231. Clotz U, Muller-Seydlitz P, Heimberg P: Pharmacokinetics of lorcainide in man: A new antiarrhythmic agent. Clin Pharmacokinet 3:407–418, 1978

232. Eyee YG, Kates RE: High-performance liquid chromatographic analysis of lorcainide and its active metabolite norlorcainide in human plasma. J Chromatogr 223:454–459, 1981

233. Kates RE, Keefe DL, Winkle RA: Lorcainide deposition kinetics in arrhythmia patients. Clin Pharmacol Ther 33:28–34, 1983

234. Klotz U, Fischer C, Muller-Seydlitz P, et al: Alterations in the disposition of differently cleared drugs in patients with cirrhosis. Clin Pharmacol Ther 26:221–227, 1979

235. Meinertz P, Kasper W, Kersting F, et al: Lorcainide kinetics and dynamics. Clin Pharmacol Ther 26:196–204, 1979

236. Ahlquist RP: A study of adrenotropic receptors. Am J Physiol 153:586–600, 1948

237. Lands AM, Arnold A, McAuliff JP, et al: Differentiation of receptor systems activated by sympathomimetic amines. Nature 214:597–598, 1967

238. Davis LT, Temte JV: Propranolol and the transmembrane potentials of ventricular muscle and Purkinje fibers of the dog. Circ Res 22:661–667, 1968

239. Woosley RL, Shand D, Cornhauser B, et al: Relation of plasma concentration and dose of propranolol to its effect on resistant ventricular arrhythmias. Clin Res 25:262A, 1967

240. Kupersmith J, Shiang H, Litwak RS, et al: Electrophysiological and antiarrhythmic effects of propranolol in canine acute myocardial ischemia. Circ Res 38:302–307, 1976

241. Evans GH, Wilkinson GR, Shand DG: The disposition of propranolol. IV. A dominant role for tissue uptake in the dose-dependent extraction of propranolol by the perfused rat liver. J Pharmacol Exp Ther 186:447–454, 1973

242. Evans GH, Nies AS, Shand DG: The disposition of propranolol. III. Decreased half-life and volume of distribution as a result of plasma binding in man, monkey, dog, and rat. J Pharmacol Exp Ther 186:114–122, 1973

243. Fitzgerald JD, O'Donnell SR: Pharmacology of four-hydroxypropranolol, a metabolite of propranolol. Br J Pharmacol 43:222–235, 1971

244. Shand DG: Drug therapy: Propranolol. N Engl J Med 293:280–284, 1975

245. Wood M, Shand DG, Wood AJJ: Propranolol binding in plasma during cardiopulmonary bypass. Anesthesiology 51:512–516, 1979

246. Miller RR, Olson HG, Amsterdam EA, et al: Propranolol-withdrawal rebound phenomenon: Exacerbation of coronary events after abrupt cessation of antianginal therapy. N Engl J Med 293:416–418, 1975

247. Shiroff RA, Mathis J, Zelis R, et al: Propranolol rebound—a retrospective study. Am J Cardiol 41:778–780, 1978

248. Lindenfeld J, Crawford MH, O'Rourke RA, et al: Adrenergic responsiveness after abrupt propranolol withdrawal in normal subjects and in patients with angina pectoris. Circulation 62:704–711, 1980

249. Ablad B, Carlsson E, Ek L: Pharmacological studies of two new cardioselective adrenergic beta-receptor antagonists. Life Sci 12:107–119, 1973

250. Lennard MS, Silas JH, Freestone, et al: Oxidation phenotype, a major determinant of metoprolol metabolism and response. N Engl J Med 307:1558–1560, 1982

251. Sonnenblick EH (ed): A symposium: Esmolol—An ultra-short-acting intravenous beta-blocker. Am J Cardiol 56:1F–62F, 1985

252. Gorczynski RJ, Shaffer JE, Lee RJ: Pharmacology of ASL-8052—A novel beta-adrenergic receptor antagonist with an ultra-short duration of action. J Cardiovasc Pharmacol 5:668–677, 1983

253. Gorczynski RJ: Basic pharmacology of esmolol. Am J Cardiol 56:3F–13F, 1985

254. Steck J, Sheppard D, Byrd RC, et al: Pulmonary effects of esmolol—an ultra short-acting beta adrenergeric blocking agent (Abstract). Clin Res 33:472A, 1985

255. Morganroth J, Horowitz LN, Anderson J, et al: Comparative efficacy and tolerance of esmolol to propranolol for control of supraventricular tachyarrhythmia. Am J Cardiol 56:33F–39F, 1985

256. Farmer JB, Kennedy I, Levy GT, et al: Pharmacology of AH5158: A drug which blocks both alpha- and beta-adrenoreceptors. Br J Pharmacol 45:660–675, 1972

257. Riley AJ: Some further evidence for partial agonist activity of labetalol. Br J Clin Pharmacol 9:517–518, 1980

258. Scott DB, Buckley FP, Drummond GB, et al: Cardiovascular effects of labetalol during halothane anesthesia. Br J Clin Pharmacol 3(suppl):817–821, 1976

259. Anderson JL: Antifibrillatory versus antiectopic therapy. Am J Cardiol 54:7A–13A, 1984

260. Boura ACA, Green AF: Actions of bretylium: Adrenergic neuron blocking and other effects. Br J Pharmacol 14:536–546, 1959

261. Chatterjee K, Mandel WJ, Vyden JK, et al: Cardiovascular effects of bretylium tosylate in acute myocardial infarction. JAMA 223:757–760, 1973

262. Anderson JL, Patterson E, Wagner JG, et al: Clinical pharmacokinetics of intravenous and oral bretylium tosylate in survivors of ventricular tachycardia or fibrillation: Clinical application of a new assay for bretylium. J Cardiovasc Pharmacol 3:485–499, 1981

263. Lucchesi BR: Rationale of therapy in the patient with acute myocardial infarction and life-threatening arrhythmias: A focus on bretylium. Am J Cardiol 54:14A–19A, 1984

264. Kniffen FJ, Lomas TE, Counsell RE, et al: The anti-arrhythmic and antifibrillatory actions of bretylium and its o-iodobenzyl trimethyl ammonium analog, UM-360. J Pharmacol Exp Ther 192:120–128, 1975

265. Cervoni Ellis CH, Mexwell RA: Antiarrhythmic action of bretylium in normal, reserpine-pretreated and chronically denervated dog hearts. Arch Int Pharmacodyn Ther 190:91–102, 1971

266. Mamm DH, Wang CM, El-Sayad S, et al: Effects of bretylium on rat cardiac muscle: The electrophysio-logical effects and its uptake and binding in normal and immunosympathectomized rat hearts. J Pharma-col Exp Ther 193:194–208, 1975

267. Tacker WA, Kiebauer MJ, Babbs CF, et al: The effect of newer antiarrhythmic drugs on defibrillation threshold. Crit Care Med 8:177–180, 1980

268. Haynes RE, Chinn TL, Copass MK, et al: Compari-son of bretylium tosylate and lidocaine in manage-ment of out-of-hospital ventricular fibrillation: A randomized clinical trial. Am J Cardiol 48:353–365, 1981

269. Nowak RM, Bodnar TJ, Droven S, et al: Bretylium tosylate as initial treatment for cardiopulmonary arrest: Randomized comparison with placebo. Ann Emerg Med 10:404–407, 1981

270. Terry G, Bellani CW, Higgins MR, et al: Bretylium tosylate in treatment of refractory ventricular ar-rhythmias complicating myocardial infarction. Heart 32:21–25, 1970

271. Bernstein JG, Koch-Weser J: The effectiveness of bretylium tosylate against ventricular arrhythmias. Circulation 45:1024–1034, 1972

272. Holder DA, Sniderman AD, Fraser G, et al: Experi-ence with bretylium tosylate by hospital cardiac arrest team. Circulation 55:541–544, 1977

273. Dhurandhar RW, Pickron J, Goldman AM: Brety-lium tosylate in the management of recurrent ventric-ular fibrillation complicating acute myocardial infarction. Heart Lung 9:265–270, 1980

274. McAlpin RN, Zellis EG, Kibowitz CF: Prevention of recurrent ventricular tachycardia with oral brety-lium tosylate. Ann Intern Med 72:909–912, 1970

275. Rosenbaum MB, Chiale PA, Halpern MS, et al: Clinical efficacy of amiodarone an antiarrhythmic agent. Am J Cardiol 38:934–944, 1976

276. Kaski JC, Girotti LA, Messuti H, et al: Long-term management of sustained, recurrent, symptomatic ventricular tachycardia with amiodarone. Circulation 64:273–279, 1981

277. Nademanee K, Hendrickson JA, Cannom DS, et al: Control of refractory life-threatening ventricular tachyarrhythmias by amiodarone. Am Heart J 101:759–768, 1982

278. Ward DE, Camm AJ, Spurrell RAJ: Clinical antiar-rhythmic effects of amiodarone in patients with resis-tant paroxysmal tachycardia. Br Heart J 44:91–95, 1980

279. Fogoros RN, Anderson KP, Winkle RA, et al: Amiodarone, clinical efficacy and toxicity in 96 patients with recurrent, drug-refractory arrhythmias. Circulation 68:88–94, 1983

280. Goupil N, Lenfant J: The effects of amiodarone on the sinus node activity of the rabbit heart. Eur J Pharmacol 39:23–31, 1976

281. Rosen MR, Wit AL: Electropharmacology of antiar-rhythmic drugs. Am Heart J 106:829–839, 1983

282. Mason JW, Hondeghem LM, Katzung BG: Amiodarone blocks inactivated cardiac sodium chan-nels. Pflugers Arch 396:79–81, 1983

283. Gloor HO, Urthaler F, James TN: The immediate electrophysiologic effects of amiodarone on the canine sinus node and the AV junctional region (Abstract). Am J Cardiol 49:981, 1982

284. Singh BN: Amiodarone: Historical development and pharmacologic profile. Am Heart J 106:788–797, 1983

285. Heger JJ, Prystowsky EN, Jackman WM, et al: Amiodarone: Clinical efficacy and electrophysiology during long-term therapy for recurrent ventricular tachycardia or fibrillation. N Engl J Med 305:539–545, 1981

286. Zipes DP, Prystowsky EN, Heger JJ: Amiodarone: Electrophysiologic actions, pharmacokinetics, and clinical effects. J Am Coll Cardiol 3:1059–1071, 1984

287. Singh BN, Nadenman EE: Amiodarone and thyroid function: Clinical implications during antiarrhythmic therapy. Am Heart J 106:857–868, 1983

288. Harriman RJ, Gomes JAC, Kang PS, et al: Effects of intravenous amiodarone in patients with inducible repetitive ventricular responses and ventricular tachycardia. Am Heart J 107:1109–1116, 1984

289. DeBoer LWV, Nosta JJ, Kloner RA, et al: Studies of amiodarone during experimental myocardial infarc-tion: Beneficial effects on hemodynamics and infarct size. Circulation 65:508–512, 1982

290. Haffajee CI, Love JC, Alpert JS, et al: Efficacy and safety profile of long-term amiodarone in the treat-ment of cardiac arrhythmias: Dosage experience. Am Heart J 106:935–943, 1983

291. Canada AT, Lasko LG, Haffajee CI: Disposition of amiodarone in patients with tachyarrhythmias. Curr Ther Res 30:968–974, 1981

292. Latini R, Tognoni G, Kates RE: Clinical effects of amiodarone. Clin Pharmacokinet 9:136–156, 1984

293. Andreasen F, Agerbaek H, Djerregaard P, et al: Phar-macokinetics of amiodarone after intravenous and oral administration. Eur J Clin Pharmacol 19:293–299, 1981

294. Mostow ND, Rakita L, Vrobel TR, et al: Amiodarone: Intravenous loading for rapid compres-sion of complex ventricular arrhythmias. J Am Coll Cardiol 4:97–104, 1984

295. Kerin NZ, Blevins RD, Frumin H, et al: Intravenous

and oral loading versus oral loading alone with amiodarone for chronic refractory ventricular arrhythmias. Am J Cardiol 55:89–91, 1985

296. Harris L, McKeena WJ, Rowland E, et al: Side effects and possible contraindications of amiodarone use. Am Heart J 106:916–921, 1983

297. Rikita L, Sobol SM, Mostow N, et al: Amiodarone pulmonary toxicity. Am Heart J 106:906–914, 1983

298. Marchlinski FE, Gansler S, Waxman HL, et al: Amiodarone pulmonary toxicity. Ann Intern Med 97:839–845, 1982

299. Kudenchuk PJ, Pierson BJ, Greene HL, et al: Prospective evaluation of amiodarone pulmonary toxicity. Chest 86:541–548, 1984

300. Veltri EP, Reid PR: Amiodarone pulmonary toxicity: Early changes and pulmonary function tests during amiodarone rechallenge. J Am Coll Cardiol 6:802–805, 1985

301. Marcus FI, Fontaine GH, Frank R, et al: Clinical pharmacology and therapeutic applications of the antiarrhythmic drug amiodarone. Am Heart J 101:480–493, 1981

302. Berger A, Binichett C, Nicod P, et al: Effect of amiodarone on serum triiodothyronine, reverse triiodothyronine, thyroxin and thyrotropin. A drug influencing peripheral metabolism of thyroid hormones. J Clin Invest 58:255–259, 1976

303. Kerin NZ, Blevins RD, Benaderet D, et al: Relation of serum reverse T3 to amiodarone antiarrhythmic efficacy and toxicity. Am J Cardiol 57:128–130, 1986

304. Buchser E, Chiolero R, Martin P, et al: Amiodarone-induced hemodynamic complications during anesthesia. Anaesthesia 38:1008–1009, 1983

305. Gallagher JD, Lieberman RW, Meranze J, et al: Amiodarone-induced complications during coronary artery surgery. Anesthesiology 55:186–188, 1981

306. Braunwald E: Mechanism of action of calcium-channel-blocking agents. N Engl J Med 307:1618–1627, 1982

307. Katz AM, Messineo FC, Herbette L: Ion channels in membranes. Circulation 65(Suppl 1):I2–I10, 1982

308. Triggle BJ, Swamy BC: Pharmacology of agents that affect calcium agonists and antagonists. Chest 78:174–179, 1980

309. Reves JG, Kissin I, Lell WA, et al: Calcium entry blockers: Uses and implications for anesthesiologists. Anesthesiology 57:504–518, 1982

310. VanBreemen C, Aaronson P, Loutzenheiser R: Sodium-calcium interactions in mammalian smooth muscle. Pharmacol Rev 30:167–208, 1978

311. Katz AM, Messinel FC: Lipids and membrane function: Implications in arrhythmias. Hosp Pract 16:49, 1981

312. Gettes LS: Possible role of ionic changes in the appearance of arrhythmias. Pharmacol Ther B2:787, 1976

313. Triggle DJ: Calcium antagonists: Basic chemical and pharmacological aspects. *In* Weiss GB (ed): New Perspectives on Calcium Antagonists. Bethesda, MD, American Physiological Society, 1981, pp 1–18

314. Fleckenstein A: Pharmacology of calcium in myocardium, cardiac pacemakers and vascular smooth muscle. Ann Rev Pharmacol Toxicol 17:149–166, 1977

315. Henry P: Comparative pharmacology of calcium antagonists: Mephtamine, verapamil and topiza. Am J Cardiol 46:1047–1058, 1980

316. Kazada F, Jarthoff B, Meyer H, et al: Pharmacology of a new calcium antagonist compound, isobutyl methyl 1,4-dihydro-2,6-dimethyl-4-(2-nitrofentyl)-3,5-pyridinedicarb oxylate) nisoldipine, k5552). Arzneimitteforsch 30:2144–2162, 1980

317. Triggle DJ: Biochemical pharmacology of calcium blockers. *In* Flaim SF, Xellis R (eds): Calcium Blockers: Mechanisms of Action and Clinical Applications. Baltimore, Urban and Swartzenberg, 1981

318. Satoh K, Yanagisawa T, Taira N: Coronary vasodilator and cardiac effects of optical isomers of verapamil in the dog. J Cardiovasc Pharmacol 2:309–318, 1980

319. Roy PR, Spurrell IAJ, Sowton GE: The effect of verapamil on the conduction system in man. Postgrad Med J 50:270, 1974

320. Schlepper M, Weppner HG, Merle H: Hemodynamic effects of supraventricular tachycardias and their alterations by electrically and verapamil-induced termination. Cardiovasc Res 12:28–33, 1978

321. Kopman EA: Intravenous verapamil to relieve pulmonary congestion in patients with mitral valve disease. Anesthesiology 58:374–376, 1983

322. Kapur PA, Flacke WE, Olewine SK: Comparison of effects of isoflurane versus enflurane on cardiovascular and catecholamine responses to verapamil in dogs. Anesth Analg 61:193–194, 1982

323. Kates RA, Kaplan JA, Hug CC, et al: Hemodynamic interactions of verapamil and isoflurane in dogs. Anesth Analg 61:194–195, 1982

324. Singh BN, Nademanee K, Feld G: Calcium blockers in the treatment of cardiac arrhythmias. *In* Flaim SF, Zelis R (eds): Calcium Blockers: Mechanisms of Actions and Clinical Applications. Baltimore, Urban and Swartzenberg, 1982, p 258

325. Mangiardi LM, Hariman RJ, McAllister RG, et al: Electrophysiologic and hemodynamic effects of verapamil: Correlation with plasma drug concentrations. Circulation 57:366–372, 1978

326. Smogyi A, Albreacht M, Kleims G, et al: Pharmacokinetics, bioavailability, and ECG response of verapamil in patients with liver cirrhosis. Br J Clin Pharmacol 12:51–60, 1981

327. Kates RE, Keefe DLD, Schwart J, et al: Verapamil disposition kinetics in chronic atrial fibrillation. Clin Pharmacol Ther 30:44–51, 1981

328. Henry CD: Comparative pharmacology of calcium antagonists: Nifedipine, verapamil and diltiazem. Am J Cardiol 46:1047–1058, 1980

329. Brichard G, Zimmerman PD: Verapamil in cardiac dysrhythmias during anesthesia. Br J Anaesth 42:1005–1012, 1970

330. Lawson NW, Kraynack BJ, Gintautas J: Neuromus-

cular and electrocardiographic responses to verapamil in dogs. Anesth Analg 62:50–54, 1983

331. Kraynack BJ, Lawson NW, Gintautas J: Neuromuscular blocking action of verapamil in cats. Can Anaesth Soc J 30:242–247, 1983

332. Keefe DL, Miura D, Somberg JC: Supraventricular tachyarrhythmias: Their evaluations and treatment. Am Heart J 111:1150–1161, 1986

333. Somberg JC, Miura D, Keefe DL: The treatment of ventricular rhythm disturbances. Am Heart J 111:1162–1176, 1986

Robert A. Kates, M.D.

13

Antianginal Drug Therapy

A comprehensive understanding of the clinical pharmacology of antianginal drugs requires a knowledge of the pathophysiology of angina pectoris. Angina pectoris is a clinical symptom first described in 1772 by Dr. William Heberden as a strangling sensation brought on by walking and relieved by rest.[1] The afferent neuronal limb of anginal pain is comprised of unmyelinated sympathetic nerve fibers within the myocardium that are incorporated into the cardiac sympathetic plexis, enter the spinal cord between the eighth cervical and fifth thoracic ganglia, and travel via the thalamus to the cerebral cortex.[2] The actual stimulus of these afferent nerve fibers is unknown but may involve a change in extracellular pH, potassium concentration, or oxygen tension due to myocardial ischemia or the focal release of bradykinin, histamine, or serotonin.[3,4] Referred pain is frequently perceived in the distribution of somatic afferent fibers of the arms and mandible, which enter the same spinal cord segments as the cardiac sympathetic fibers[5] (see Chapter 15).

Ischemia occurs when coronary blood flow is insufficient for delivery of adequate myocardial oxidative substrates and removal of metabolic wastes. The coronary vascular system normally autoregulates by altering arteriolar vascular tone to provide adequate blood flow for a spectrum of meta-bolic demands from rest to exercise loads requiring four times the resting flow rate.[6] Insufficient resting blood flow or reductions in coronary vascular reserve (maximum flow capacity) usually arise when coronary occlusive disease increases the vascular resistance in epicardial coronary arteries. High vascular resistance can be produced by "fixed" atherosclerotic stenoses, vasospasm (Prinzmetal's or variant angina), or a combination of functional epicardial vasoconstriction (at the site of atherosclerotic disease) and atherosclerotic stenosis.[7] There is recent evidence that vasoconstriction can also develop in small intramyocardial arteries, which may be the etiology of "variable threshold angina" in patients who have no angiographic evidence of epicardial coronary artery spasm.[8,9] A 50 percent diameter reduction limits coronary reserve so that myocardial ischemia occurs during exercise (exercise-induced angina).[6] Diameter reductions greater than 80–85 percent can prevent adequate flow at rest (unstable and rest angina).[6] Fixed stenoses of less than 80 percent can produce ischemia at rest if concurrent vasomotion at the site of atherosclerotic disease further reduces the luminal diameter (unstable angina)[10,11] (Fig. 13-1). Myocardial ischemia can also develop from platelet adhesion and thrombus formation on the diseased coronary endothelium. If the thrombus spontane-

CARDIAC ANESTHESIA, SECOND EDITION
ISBN 0-8089-1848-6

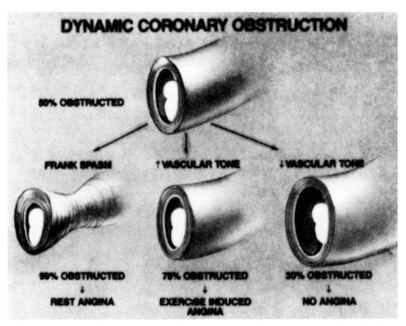

Fig. 13-1. Illustration of how dynamic coronary vascular tone can determine whether a "fixed" atherosclerotic lesion will produce rest-induced, exercise-induced or no angina. (From Epstein SE, et al: Hemodynamic principles in the control of coronary blood flow. Am J Cardiol 56:4E–10E, 1985, with permission.)

ously lyses, this can produce unstable angina symptoms, but if lysis does not occur, an acute myocardial infarction will result. Partial epicardial stenosis most frequently causes subendocardial ischemia, resulting in ST-segment depression on the electrocardiogram (ECG). Variant angina, producing total epicardial vascular obstruction, causes transmural ischemia with ST-segment elevation on the ECG.

In addition to coronary vascular pathology, hemodynamic factors that decrease coronary blood flow and increase myocardial oxygen consumption can also precipitate myocardial ischemia. Since flow to the left ventricle predominantly occurs during diastole, tachycardia, which reduces diastolic time, will reduce coronary blood flow. A decrease in coronary perfusion pressure (aortic diastolic pressure minus left ventricular end-diastolic pressure) due to decreased aortic diastolic pressure or increased left ventricular end-diastolic pressure (LVEDP) will decrease coronary blood flow. An increase in LVEDP will decrease blood flow by increasing extrinsic compression of intramyocardial arterial vessels, predominantly in the subendocardium. An increase in myocardial oxygen demand (increased heart rate, preload, afterload, or contractility) can also produce myocardial ischemia in patients with

decreased myocardial vascular reserve. The relative importance of the hemodynamic factors influencing myocardial ischemia was evaluated in a canine model of critical coronary stenosis.[12] It was found that increasing afterload evoked the mildest degree of ischemia; more pronounced ischemia was produced by increasing preload, and the most serious ischemia was induced by tachycardia (see Chapters 1 and 15).

Redistribution of intramyocardial blood flow can also cause ischemia by a "coronary steal" phenomenon (Fig. 13-2).[6] When two arteriolar resistance beds receive blood from the same moderately stenotic epicardial vessel, the arterioles of the collateral-dependent bed may require full dilation by autoregulation to prevent ischemia (flow to this area is pressure dependent), while arterioles supplied directly from the moderately stenotic epicardial vessel may require only minimal dilatation for baseline metabolic requirements. An arteriolar dilator stimulus, such as exercise, will dilate the minimally dilated arterioles and increase blood flow through the stenotic epicardial vessel. Since the pressure gradient across a stenosis is directly proportional to the flow, the perfusion pressure to the collaterally supplied vessel decreases, resulting in ischemia (Fig. 13-2A). Similarly, an "endocardial steal" can occur from a

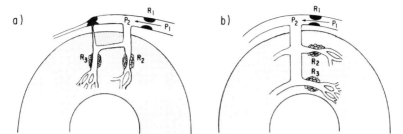

Fig. 13-2. (a) Coronary vascular arrangement that can produce a "coronary steal" due to increased myocardial work or arteriolar dilating drugs. Dilation of R_2 arterioles will increase flow through epicardial vessel (R_1). This increased flow will decrease the distal coronary arterial pressure (P_2), producing ischemia in the R_3 region, which is already maximally dilated. (b) By the same principle, dilation of epicardial resistance vessels (R_2) will decrease perfusion pressure in the subendocardium (R_3), producing subendocardial ischemia. (Modified from Epstein SE, et al: Hemodynamic principles in the control of coronary blood flow. Am J Cardiol 56:4E–10E, 1985, with permission.)

stenotic epicardial vessel that feeds both the subepicardium and subendocardium (Fig. 13-2B). Since myocardial oxygen demand is higher in the subendocardium, these arterioles may be maximally dilated while the epicardial vessels are minimally dilated. An arteriolar dilator stimulus may increase flow to the subepicardium at the expense of the subendocardium.[4] The endocardial:epicardial flow ratio will fall, and subendocardial ischemia will occur. Drugs that decrease myocardial oxygen demand (thereby preserving arteriolar tone in the less jeopardized regions) will decrease steal patterns of blood flow, while exercise or potent arteriolar dilators, such as sodium nitroprusside, will "steal" flow away from jeopardized myocardium[6] (see Chapters 1 and 15).

The therapeutic effects of antianginal drugs appear to be primarily due to hemodynamic effects that decrease myocardial oxygen demand and improve coronary blood flow. Nitrates and calcium channel blockers, however, also directly dilate coronary arteries, which can improve myocardial perfusion by redistribution of intramyocardial flow, decreased epicardial vascular tone, or prevention of coronary spasm. The three classes of antianginal drugs discussed in this chapter are the organic nitrates, beta-adrenergic receptor blocking drugs, and calcium channel blocking drugs. Modern antianginal drug therapy began with nitroglycerin in the 1870s to which the beta-adrenergic receptor blocking drugs were added in the 1950s and the calcium channel blocking drugs in the 1970s. Each class of compounds complements the other forms of antianginal therapy so that modern antianginal drug therapy is frequently comprised of a combination of drugs from each of these classes of compounds.

ORGANIC NITRATES

Historical Background

Prior to the discovery of the antianginal effects of organic nitrates, the relief of anginal symptoms by amyl nitrite was described by Lord Brunton, who wrote in 1857, "On pouring from five to ten drops of the nitrite on a cloth and giving it to the patient to inhale, the physiological action took place in from thirty to sixty seconds; and simultaneously with the flushing of the face the pain completely disappeared."[13] In 1846, Sobrero synthesized nitroglycerin (NTG) and discovered that a small quantity placed on the tongue elicited a severe headache.[14] The first widespread application of NTG was as a component of dynamite, invented by Alfred B. Nobel, who later went on to endow the Nobel Prize awards.[14] NTG's antianginal properties were originally described in 1879 by Dr. William Murrell after he administered NTG to patients with angina pectoris because of "the similarity existing between its general action and that of nitrite of amyl."[15] During the 20th century, new analogues of NTG were synthesized, and different methods for systemic drug absorption were developed so that organic nitrates can now provide acute as well as chronic antianginal drug therapy. In 1968, Viljoen first administered NTG intramuscularly during coronary artery bypass surgery (CABS),[16] and eight years later Kaplan et al demonstrated the effectiveness of intraoperative intravenous (IV) NTG.[17] This study placed NTG within the pharmaceutical armamentarium of the anesthesiologist.

Vascular Smooth Muscle Cell

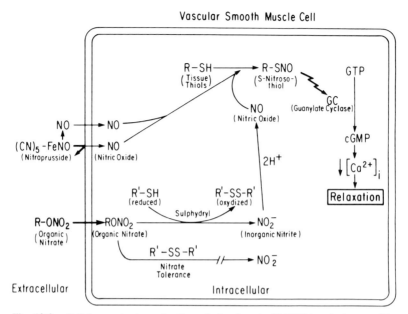

Fig. 13-3. Cellular mechanism of action of nitroglycerin (R-ONO₂) and nitroprusside ((CN)₅-FeNO). Different pathways lead to a decrease in "available" intracellular calcium via activation of guanylate cyclase. The proposed mechanism of nitrate tolerance is illustrated by depletion of reduced sulphydryl groups (R-SH). (Modified from Ignarro, et al: Mechanism of vascular smooth muscle relaxation by organic nitrates, nitrites, nitroprusside and nitric oxide: Evidence for the involvement of S-nitrosothiols as active intermediates. J Pharmacol Exp Ther 218:739–749, 1981, with permission.)

Mechanism of Action

Several cardiovascular compounds, including organic nitrates, sodium nitroprusside, and calcium channel blockers, possess vasodilatory properties. Their pharmacodynamic effects (vasodilation) are similar, and considerable evidence implicates a final common pathway involving a decrease in myoplasmic calcium availability. However, each class of vasodilator compounds has unique molecular mechanisms prior to convergence into the common pathway involving myoplasmic calcium levels.[18,19]

Unlike calcium channel blockers and beta-adrenergic blockers, whose site of action is located on the cell membrane, organic nitrates must be absorbed intracellularly in order to interact with a specific intracellular nitrate receptor[19] (Fig. 13-3). Reaction with the sulphydryl moiety on the nitrate receptor is necessary for denitration and formation of inorganic nitrite (NO₂⁻), which subsequently reacts with hydrogen ions to form nitric oxide (NO).[20] Sodium nitroprusside (SNP) differs from nitrates in that it releases nitric oxide spontaneously, circumventing the necessity for sulphydryl molecules.[19] Nitric oxide interacts with tissue thiols to form S-nitroso-thiols, which acti-

vate guanylate cyclase catalyzing the formation of cyclic guanosine monophosphate (cGMP). Extensive pharmacologic evidence now strongly indicates that cGMP is the essential mediator for vascular smooth muscle relaxation and that organic nitrates produce vasodilation by increasing the intracellular content of cGMP.[21,22] The link between cGMP and cellular calcium metabolism is not yet fully elucidated; however, several studies indicate that organic nitrates do interfere with cellular calcium flux.[18] Unlike the calcium channel blockers, which inhibit calcium influx across the cell membrane, nitrates appear to inhibit calcium mobilization from intracellular stores and also possibly enhance calcium efflux from vascular smooth muscle cells.[23,24] The reduction in free intracellular calcium impairs the interaction between actin and myosin that produces smooth muscle relaxation.

Cardiovascular Effects of Organic Nitrates

Vasodilation, predominantly in the vascular beds of the venous circulation, is the major pharmacodynamic effect of the organic nitrates (Fig.

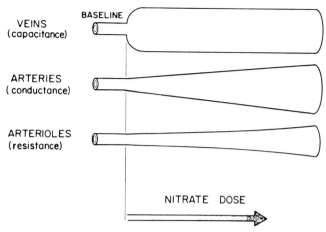

Fig. 13-4. Relative potency of increasing nitroglycerin dosage on different vascular beds. (From Abrams J: Hemodynamic effects of nitroglycerin and long-acting nitrates. Am Heart J 110:216–224, 1985, with permission.)

13-4).[14,25-28] Tissue sensitivity to the dilating effects of NTG is greatest in smooth muscle of venous beds; higher nitrate doses are required to dilate systemic arterial vessels.[14,25,27,28] Pharmacokinetic evidence also indicates that the high nitrate sensitivity of venous smooth muscle is enhanced by higher blood levels and greater tissue uptake on the venous side compared with the arterial side of the circulation.[29,30] Dilation of arteriolar resistance vessels occurs only at relatively high doses of nitrates, not usually reached during chronic nitrate therapy, although easily achieved by IV NTG.[25,31] Therefore, chronic antianginal nitrate therapy usually does not affect systemic vascular resistance (SVR), mean arterial pressure (MAP), or diastolic arterial pressure.[19] The systolic component of arterial blood pressure may decrease during nitrate therapy due to an increase in aortic compliance.[19,32]

The vascular effects of nitrates profoundly influence cardiac performance, myocardial oxygen demand, and coronary blood flow. The increase in venous capacitance lowers left and right ventricular filling pressures by reducing venous return to the heart.[33] Radionuclide scintillation measurements indicate that sublingual NTG administration to patients with coronary atherosclerotic heart disease (CAD) decreases pulmonary blood volume.[34] This decrease in left ventricular preload indirectly reduces ventricular volume during systole, which in turn reduces systolic wall tension or afterload as well as the myocardial work load.[33-35] The nitrate-induced decrease in preload and systolic wall tension will variably affect cardiac output, depending on the

patient's underlying cardiovascular status (Fig. 13-5).[36] Patients in congestive heart failure (CHF) usually respond with an increase in cardiac output (CO) due to the reduction in systolic wall tension or afterload.[36] Also, CHF is frequently associated with mitral regurgitation due to dilatation of the mitral valve apparatus. A reduction in left ventricular volume by NTG has been shown to reduce the functional regurgitant orifice of the mitral valve, enhancing forward blood flow.[37] The improvement in cardiac performance often reduces the high baseline sympathetic tone, and heart rate decreases. In contrast, patients with normal or low ventricular filling pressures may experience a decrease in cardiac output due to inadequate preload after nitrate-induced venodilation.[36] The subsequent decrease in arterial blood pressure elicits a reflex increase in sympathetic tone, which increases heart rate and contractility.[33,35] Amelioration of myocardial ischemia can also improve cardiac performance by reducing ischemic dysfunction.[37-40]

Although drug-induced changes in preload and systolic wall tension can profoundly alter cardiac performance, experimental evidence indicates that NTG has no direct effects on myocardial contractility.[38] Nitroglycerin may improve myocardial contractility in patients with CAD; however, this appears to be due to a reduction in myocardial ischemia (Fig. 13-5).[39] Studies have demonstrated that NTG increases ejection fraction during exercise in patients with CAD but not in normal subjects.[37,39,40] Numerous studies have also shown improved regional contractile function in ischemic myocardium due to

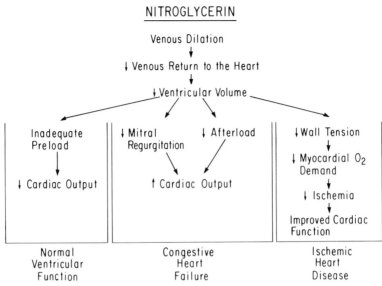

Fig. 13-5. The nitrate-induced decrease in ventricular volume and systolic wall tension (afterload) will variably affect cardiac output depending on the patient's underlying cardiovascular status.

improved blood flow and decreased ischemia.[41,42] Just as NTG improves left ventricular performance, it also has antiarrhythmic properties in patients with CAD. Nitroglycerin decreases the frequency of premature ventricular contractions during acute myocardial infarction and unstable angina.[43,44] Since nitrates have no direct electrophysiologic effects, these effects are ascribed to an amelioration of myocardial ischemia.

Effects on Myocardial Blood Flow

Organic nitrates influence myocardial blood flow indirectly via hemodynamic changes and directly by coronary arterial dilation (Fig. 13-6). Nitrate-induced hemodynamic changes increase coronary perfusion pressure by lowering LVEDP more

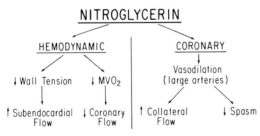

Fig. 13-6. Nitroglycerin influences myocardial blood flow indirectly by hemodynamic changes and by direct effects on coronary blood vessels.

than aortic diastolic pressure. The decrease in LVEDP reduces extrinsic tissue compression of coronary vessels in the subendocardium, thereby improving subendocardial blood flow. Hemodynamic changes can also *decrease* coronary blood flow via autoregulation. Nitrate-induced reductions in preload and wall tension decrease myocardial oxygen demand, which causes an autoregulatory decrease in coronary blood flow. This has been demonstrated in humans at rest, during exercise, and during pacing-induced tachycardia.[45,46]

Major differences in the vasodilating effects of nitrates have been demonstrated between epicardial and resistance (arteriolar) coronary arterial vessels.[11,33] Studies on isolated coronary arteries demonstrate that, unlike adenosine (a potent arteriolar dilator), therapeutic doses of NTG block the constriction of vascular smooth muscle of large coronary arteries but not coronary arterioles.[47] In fact, dose-dependent studies in conscious dogs demonstrate systemic venodilation and dilation of large coronary arteries at low-dose NTG, and systemic and coronary arteriolar dilation only at a much higher dose.[25] The effects of nitrates on coronary vascular tone in chronically instrumented canine studies demonstrate a biphasic effect on blood flow. Intravenous administration of high NTG doses (8 and 32 μg/kg) causes direct coronary arteriolar vasodilation, overriding coronary autoregulation as evidenced by an increase in coronary blood flow and coronary sinus oxygen

Table 13-1

Clinical Pharmacokinetics of the Organic Nitrates

Drug	Route	Dosage	Onset of Action (min)	Duration of Action (hr)
Isosorbide dinitrate	Sublingual	2.5–10 mg q 2–4 hr	5	1–3
	Oral	10–60 mg q 4–6 hr	30	4–6
Nitroglycerin	Sublingual	0.1–0.6 mg q 1–3 hr	1.5–2	0.5–1
	Ointment	7.5–30 mg q 4–6 hr	15–30	3–6
Pentaerythritoltetranitrate	Oral	20–60 mg q 6 hr	30	4–7

Modified from Kaplan JA: Nitrates. *In* Kaplan JA (ed): Cardiac Anesthesia, vol 2. Cardiovascular Pharmacology. Orlando, FL, Grune & Stratton, 1983, pp 151–180.

saturation.[33] After discontinuation of the NTG infusion, the fall in blood nitrate levels is accompanied by a decrease in coronary blood flow below baseline levels, while coronary sinus oxygen saturation returns to baseline. This biphasic response is interpreted as a direct coronary arteriolar dilating effect at high nitrate doses, followed by a coronary autoregulation-induced decrease in coronary flow at lower nitrate levels when the hemodynamic effects of NTG predominate. Clinical studies also demonstrate that NTG selectively dilates epicardial coronary arteries in humans.[48] Small IV doses of NTG (75–150 μg), which did not affect aortic pressure or heart rate, have been shown angiographically to increase the diameter of the left anterior descending and circumflex coronary arteries as well as collaterally filled vessels.[48,49] Smaller epicardial arteries (0.3–1.0 mm) appear to show the greatest increase in diameter from NTG. Recent work in prostaglandin pharmacology has demonstrated that part of the action of NTG on coronary vasodilation might involve its effects on myocardial prostaglandin metabolism. Although controversial, therapeutic levels of NTG have been shown to stimulate prostacyclin, a potent coronary arterial dilator, and these dilator effects have been experimentally ablated by prostaglandin synthesis inhibitors.[50]

Pharmacokinetics of the Organic Nitrates

Three nitrate compounds are clinically available in the United States: isosorbide dinitrate (Isordil; ISDN), glyceryl trinitrate (nitroglycerin), and pentaerythritol tetranitrate (Peritrate), which are comprised of two, three, and four nitrate groups, respectively (Table 13-1). The pharmaceutical industry has also developed a spectrum of drug delivery techniques utilizing enteric delivery via sublingual, masticated, and swallowed routes; cutaneous delivery via ointments and polymer gels; and IV delivery. Although most nitrates are well absorbed from the gastrointestinal tract, extensive first-pass hepatic metabolism (denitration and glucuronidation) has stirred controversy over the actual systemic bioavailability and clinical efficacy of oral nitrates. It has now been extensively demonstrated, however, that enterally administered nitrates are efficacious for chronic antianginal drug therapy due to relatively large enteric doses (overwhelming the first-pass hepatic metabolism) as well as the pharmacologic activity of some of the metabolites.

NITROGLYCERIN

Nitroglycerin is fully absorbed from the stomach, but hepatic metabolism to relatively inactive metabolites yields only a 2–10 percent absolute bioavailability.[14] Its high lipid solubility results in a large apparent volume of distribution, 3–4 l/kg, with highest drug tissue levels measured in liver (the organ of metabolism) and vascular smooth muscle tissue (the target organ).[30] Rapid hepatic metabolism produces a short plasma half-life of 2 minutes and 4.4 minutes after intravenous bolus and sublingual administration, respectively.[51] However, the duration of effect increases with CHF and liver dysfunction.[52] The hemodynamic effects of NTG have been found to correlate closely with the plasma drug levels; plasma levels of 1–2 ng/ml produce venodilation, and drug levels over 3 ng/ml produce both venous and arterial vasodilation.[53]

Drug delivery systems for NTG have been designed to obviate the problems of first-pass hepatic metabolism and the short plasma half-life. Sublingual delivery into the systemic venous system results in an 80 percent bioavailability; however, the half-life is very short and the duration of effect is only $1/2$ to 1 hour.[19] Transdermal drug delivery with ointments of 2 percent nitroglycerin maintain therapeutic blood levels for 4 hours, and recently developed polymer gels can produce constant blood levels for up to 24 hours.[54]

The development of IV NTG administration techniques is a milestone for acute care of patients with CAD who might require rapid drug titration over a wide spectrum of plasma nitrate levels. Since NTG is absorbed into standard polyvinylchloride tubing, extensive research was necessary to develop a delivery system that would deliver constant and accurate doses of NTG.[55] Commercially available IV delivery systems that do not absorb NTG can now be used for quick and accurate titration to therapeutic end points.

ISOSORBIDE DINITRATE

Orally administered ISDN was the focus of controversy over the efficacy of orally administered, long-acting nitrates.[56] It was claimed in the 1970s that, although well absorbed from the stomach, complete first-pass hepatic elimination resulted in no therapeutic bioavailability.[14] However, subsequent studies demonstrated that considerable amounts of unchanged drug do reach the systemic circulation (20 percent), and although denitrated metabolites have less potency, high blood levels of the metabolites that have longer half-lives than ISDN contribute to pharmacodynamic activity.[57] Peak blood levels are reached 15 minutes after sublingual and 30 minutes after oral administration.[19,57] The half-life of ISDN is 30 minutes with a slow terminal elimination phase, so that the pharmacodynamic effect can be maintained for 4–6 hours after oral administration.[19,57]

PENTAERYTHRITOL TETRANITRATE

Pentaerythritol tetranitrate is slowly and incompletely absorbed from the gastrointestinal tract, with peak plasma concentrations reached in 4–6 hours after oral administration.[58,59] The metabolite of the tetranitrate, pentaerythritol trinitrate, is more active than the parent compound, and, therefore, the tetranitrate can be considered the precursor of the active moiety, pentaerythritol trinitrate.[19,58,59] The trinitrate has a long elimination half-life (11.4 hours), and drug effects last longer than 6 hours. This long duration of action is probably due to enterohepatic recirculation or reconversion to pharmacologically active free nitrates in peripheral tissues.[59]

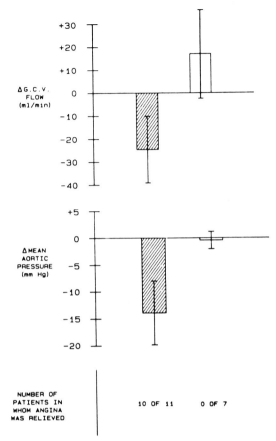

Fig. 13-7. The effect of nitroglycerin on myocardial blood flow (great cardiac vein [G.C.V.]) in patients with left anterior descending coronary artery disease. Response to systemic (sublingual or intravenous, hatch bars) and intracoronary (open bars) NTG is shown. Antianginal effects occurred only with systemic nitroglycerin, accompanied by a reduction in G.C.V. flow. This suggests that the antianginal effects were due to a reduction in oxygen demand—not an increase in supply. (From Fuchs RM, et al: Am J Cardiol 51:19–23, 1983, with permission.)

Therapeutic Uses of Organic Nitrates

ANTIANGINAL THERAPY

Mechanism of action. Nitroglycerin exerts its antianginal effects by inducing advantageous hemodynamic and direct coronary vascular effects. Numerous studies indicate that both pharmacologic effects are important. The importance of the hemodynamically induced reduction in myocardial oxygen demand is exemplified by clinical studies that demonstrate that although intracoronary NTG administra-

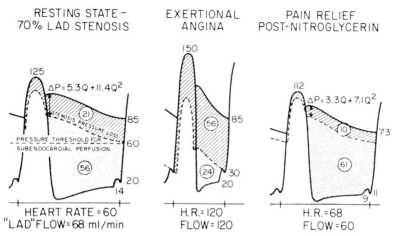

Fig. 13-8. Hemodynamic response to exercise and sublingual nitroglycerin in a hypothetical patient with 70 percent left anterior descending coronary artery (LAD) stenosis is illustrated with aortic, left ventricular, and poststenotic coronary pressures. The crosshatched area is the pressure lost (Δ P) for the specific blood flow (Q) through the stenosis. The stippled area between the poststenotic and left ventricular diastolic pressure is the coronary perfusion pressure. Increased flow, as with exercise, increases the Δ P. Subendocardial ischemia occurs when the threshold for adequate perfusion is crossed as with exertional angina. Nitroglycerin improves the coronary perfusion pressure compared with the resting state by (1) coronary dilation, which reduces the stenosis pressure loss, and (2) decreased preload, which increases the coronary perfusion pressure (from 56 to 61 mm Hg) despite a 12 mm Hg fall in aortic pressure (HR, heart rate). (Modified from Brown BG, et al: Mechanisms of NTG Action. Circulation 64(6):1089–1097, 1981.)

tion increases coronary blood flow, it is not as effective as IV NTG in relieving pacemaker-induced myocardial ischemia (Fig. 13-7).[60,61] After an IV bolus of NTG, patients experience a brief increase in coronary blood flow followed by a persistent autoregulated decrease in flow which accompanies the antianginal effects at rest and during exercise, supporting the hypothesis that the antianginal effects of the nitrates are predominantly due to a decrease in myocardial oxygen demand, not an increase in coronary blood flow.[45,46] Although these data of global blood flow do not rule out intramyocardial redistribution of blood flow to ischemic myocardial tissue, which has been documented, other studies demonstrate that concurrent with the antianginal effects of IV NTG, blood flow to the ischemic regions may actually decrease.[60] Furthermore, in an experimental animal model, NTG reduced metabolic acidosis in ischemic myocardial tissue without increasing blood flow, also probably due to a hemodynamically induced decrease in oxygen consumption.[62]

In contrast, the importance of the direct coronary vascular effects of NTG has been demonstrated experimentally by improved subendocardial perfusion, collateral blood flow, and dilation of epicardial

arteries perfusing ischemic myocardial tissue after *intracoronary* NTG.[48,63–65] Intracoronary NTG doses, which are devoid of systemic effects, increase blood flow to ischemic tissue, reduce ST-segment elevation, and improve ischemic systolic function and diastolic compliance.[48,66] Radioisotope and angiography studies in patients with CAD indicate that IV NTG is a vasodilator of epicardial (both normal and atherosclerotic) and collateral coronary arteries.[48,67,68] Nitroglycerin has been shown to increase blood flow to ischemic regions of myocardium supplied by collateral vessels, while SNP (in doses that produce similar systemic hemodynamic effects) decreases myocardial flow to ischemic regions.[69] Nitroprusside dilates resistance arteries, which can produce a "coronary steal" from ischemic to normal myocardium, while NTG dilates large coronary arteries and collateral vessels, which supply ischemic myocardial tissue.[69] Furthermore, intraoperative and postoperative studies following CABG indicate that NTG increases coronary blood flow to myocardial tissue supplied by coronary collateral vessels and severely stenosed epicardial vessels.[70,71]

Clearly, the antianginal properties of NTG are multifactorial (Fig. 13-8). Reductions in preload and

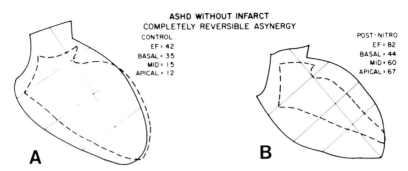

Fig. 13-9. (A) The control ventriculogram shows a reduced ejection fraction and significant asynergy. (B) Nitroglycerin increases the ejection fraction and abolishes the asynergy. (From Reddy SP: Reversibility of left ventricular asynergy by nitroglycerin in coronary artery disease. Am Heart J 90:479–486, 1975, with permission.)

systolic wall tension reduce myocardial oxygen demand and increase subendocardial blood flow, while coronary arterial dilation increases oxygen delivery and flow redistribution to ischemic tissue. Corwin and Reiffel summarized three clinical situations for which specific antianginal effects theoretically predominate.[72] Patients with partial coronary artery obstruction primarily benefit from the decrease in oxygen consumption at rest and during exercise (hemodynamic effects). When a coronary artery is totally occluded, dilation of collateral vessels and redistribution of blood flow improves regional perfusion (coronary vascular effects). Patients with vasospastic angina benefit by vascular smooth muscle relaxation from organic nitrates (coronary vascular effects).

Exertional angina. Nitrate therapy relieves episodes of acute ischemia and prophylactically enhances exercise capacity.[73,74] Of all the clinically used antianginal drugs, only sublingual, inhaled, or IV NTG or inhaled amyl nitrite have a sufficiently rapid onset to be useful for acute anginal attacks.[73] Maximal antianginal relief occurs within 3 minutes, and effectiveness is maintained for about 1 hour.[73] Isosorbide dinitrate is the most popular long-acting nitrate for prophylactic enhancement of exercise tolerance. Oral ISDN administration exerts beneficial hemodynamic effects (lower ventricular filling pressures), increases exercise tolerance, and reduces ST depression for 3–5 hours.[19]

Unstable angina pectoris and variant angina. Unstable angina pectoris occurs at rest or during exercise and is clinically significant because of its disabling nature and the possibility of progression to acute myocardial infarction.[75] Nitrates are the

cornerstone of therapy with maximum improvement demonstrated when IV NTG is titrated to reduce arterial pressure by approximately 10 percent or to a systolic pressure of 100–110 mm Hg.[2] Relief of chest pain and ST-segment depression is accompanied by an improvement in regional and global ejection fraction (Fig. 13-9).[76] Intravenous NTG is effective in patients refractory to sublingual NTG, and a therapeutic effect can be maintained for prolonged periods of time.[77] A retrospective study of 45 patients with unstable angina pectoris demonstrated immediate pain relief in 22, relief by titration of NTG in 18, and no relief in 3 patients. Doses ranged from 5 to 267 μg/min with a mean optimal therapeutic dose of 54 μg/min.[77]

Variant angina commonly occurs at rest, exercise tolerance is good, and the angina is associated with ST-segment elevation. Standard therapy for variant angina includes NTG and long-acting nitrate preparations.[78-80] Several clinical comparisons have demonstrated that chronic therapy with ISDN is comparable with the calcium channel blockers for prophylactic efficacy in patients with variant angina;[81,82] however, combined nitrate and calcium blocker therapy may provide added benefit over either drug alone.[83] Coronary artery spasm also occurs intraoperatively,[83] postoperatively after myocardial revascularization,[84] and in the cardiac catheterization laboratory secondary to ergonovine provocation or intracoronary catheter stimulation.[85] Intravenous or intracoronary NTG may be necessary to effectively reverse the spasm and correct the ECG signs of ischemia or the ischemia-induced dysrhythmias. Intracoronary NTG doses of 25–100 μg relieved spasm that occurred spontaneously or after ergonovine provocation in the catheterization laboratory.[85] Buxton et al and Cohen et al found that after

CABG, large intracoronary doses of NTG were needed to relax the spasm, and they recommended using intracoronary doses of 0.1–1.0 mg when patients are refractory to IV NTG.[84,86]

Acute myocardial infarction. Intravenous NTG was at one time contraindicated for the treatment of acute myocardial infarction because of the possibility of hypotension and reflex tachycardia.[87] However, animal studies clearly show a reduction in the extent of ischemic damage, and clinical studies have demonstrated the safety and efficacy of IV NTG during acute myocardial infarction. Experimental studies demonstrate increased collateral blood flow to ischemic regions and decreased infarction size.[88] This beneficial effect is dose specific, however; higher doses of NTG, which reduce coronary perfusion pressure, produce no effect or even a detrimental effect on the degree of ischemic damage.[89]

Clinical studies have extensively documented that IV NTG administration during acute myocardial infarction improves hemodynamic conditions and reduces infarct size as well as the frequency of ventricular ectopic beats.[43,90–96] Maximum benefit probably occurs when acute myocardial infarction is accompanied by CHF; however, as long as hypotension is avoided, it appears that patients without heart failure also benefit.[91] Compared to SNP, IV NTG is safer and more advantageous for ischemic myocardial tissue when used to treat CHF or hypertensive complications of acute myocardial infarction.[92] Nitroglycerin infusions in doses averaging 0.5 μg/kg/min predominantly decreased preload with only minimal changes in arterial blood pressure or heart rate. This was associated with a consistent decrease in ST-segment elevation.[93] When titrated to a 10 percent reduction in MAP, NTG produced a decrease in preload and SVR and an increase in CO accompanied by a decrease in infarction size as measured by cardioselective isoenzymes of creatine kinase.[90] A similar protocol demonstrated that the subgroup of patients with inferior myocardial infarcts attained the most protective effect from NTG.[94] It is unclear why NTG infusions produce greater beneficial effects during inferior infarctions than anterior infarctions; however, it is suggested that this might be due to a greater frequency of coronary spasm in the right than left coronary artery or a more favorable effect of NTG on right ventricular loading conditions and perfusion.[94] *Intracoronary* administration of NTG has also been shown to relieve coronary artery spasm during acute myocardial infarction.[95] The time from onset of ischemic pain to institution of NTG therapy

appears to be important, since a greater incidence in clinical improvement was noted when NTG treatment was initiated within 10 hours.[96] These clinical studies indicate the IV NTG titration to produce a slight (10 percent) reduction in MAP should improve salvage of myocardial tissue during acute myocardial infarction.

PERIOPERATIVE NITROGLYCERIN THERAPY

Intravenous NTG is now recognized as an integral component of the anesthetic management of cardiac surgical patients. The perioperative indications for IV NTG include treatment of myocardial ischemia, CHF, systemic and pulmonary arterial hypertension, and coronary arterial spasm. The usual intraoperative indications are as follows:[*]

1. Hypertension greater than 20 percent above control values
2. Pulmonary capillary wedge pressure greater than 18–20 mm Hg
3. AC and V waves greater than 20 mm Hg
4. ST changes greater than 1 mm
5. Acute right ventricular or left ventricular dysfunction
6. Coronary artery spasm

At the conclusion of cardiopulmonary bypass, IV NTG may be especially useful under the following circumstances:[*]

1. Elevated pulmonary capillary wedge pressure
2. Elevated pulmonary or systemic vascular resistance
3. Infusion of oxygenator reservoir volume
4. Transfusion of blood products
5. Incomplete revascularization
6. Ischemia (ST-segment changes in leads II or V_5)
7. Ischemia-induced ventricular dysrhythmias
8. Intraoperative myocardial infarction
9. Coronary artery spasm (ST elevation, dysrhythmias)

Preoperative nitrate therapy. Most authors agree that chronic nitrate therapy with oral and transcutaneous nitrate preparations should be continued as scheduled until the time of surgery. Decreases in CO and increases in SVR have been documented when nitrol ointment patches are abruptly discontinued.[19] It is also thought that withdrawal may lead to increased

*Modified from Kaplan JA. Nitrates. *In* Kaplan JA (ed): Cardiac Anesthesia: Cardiovascular Pharmacology. Orlando, FL, Grune & Stratton, 1983, pp 151–180.

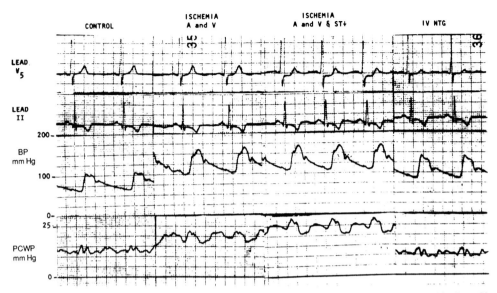

Fig. 13-10. Nitroglycerin relieved postintubation intraoperative myocardial ischemia as evidenced by large V waves in the pulmonary capillary wedge pressure (PCWP) tracing and then by ST-segment depression. (From Kaplan JA, Wells PH: Early diagnosis of myocardial ischemia using the pulmonary arterial catheter. Anesth Analg 60(11):789–793, 1981, with permission.)

sensitivity of the coronary and systemic vasculature to vasoconstrictor stimuli.[19] Nitrol ointment can provide continuous intraoperative therapeutic blood levels and can be easily continued postoperatively by the transdermal route. Careful attention to intravascular volume is important since hypovolemia can be accentuated by the venodilating effects of nitrate therapy.

Intraoperative hemodynamic effects. The intraoperative effects of NTG are similar to its reported hemodynamic properties in awake humans—predominantly venodilation. However, since *intravenous* nitroglycerin is now administered in the perioperative period, high plasma levels are easily achieved within the dose range of 1–3 µg/kg/ min, and systemic arteriolar dilation with decreases in SVR and blood pressure often occur.[97] For equal reductions in blood pressure, however, a larger reduction in pulmonary capillary wedge pressure (PCWP) occurs with NTG than SNP. Since preload may be greatly reduced at these doses of NTG, CO frequently decreases, except in patients with left ventricular failure in whom the decrease in afterload predominates and CO may increase. Heart rate does not increase except at doses that are accompanied by a decrease in systemic arterial blood pressure, yet this effect may be modified by patients who are concurrently receiving beta-adrenergic receptor blockers.

The predominant venodilating effect of NTG versus the arteriolar dilating effect of SNP has also been demonstrated during cardiopulmonary bypass at 30°C. At equal doses, (1.5–2.0 µg/kg/min), SNP had a greater effect on SVR, while NTG caused a greater reduction in the venous reservoir volume (indicating an increase in total body venous capacitance).[28]

Intraoperative ischemia. Intraoperative administration of NTG improves the myocardial oxygen balance and reduces ischemic ST-segment changes.[98] Compared with SNP, blood pressure reduction with NTG causes less of a reduction in coronary perfusion pressure and a greater improvement in ST-segment depression.[99] During halothane anesthesia for hip replacement surgery, blood pressure reduction to a systolic pressure of 75 mm Hg was accompanied by ischemic ECG changes in 38 percent of patients in the SNP group but no patients in the NTG group.[99] This apparent difference in myocardial perfusion could be partially due to the significantly higher mean and diastolic blood pressures in the NTG group compared with the SNP group despite the similar systolic pressures. The development of prominent V waves in the PCWP waveform can precede ischemic ST-segment changes and may be an early indicator of myocardial ischemia (Fig. 13-10). Prompt administration of NTG has been reported to reduce V waves and to preclude the progression to ischemic ST-segment changes.[100]

The hemodynamic and myocardial metabolic effects of NTG have been evaluated during halothane anesthesia for CABG.[97] High doses of IV NTG (1–3 μg/kg/min) decreased MAP, SVR, and left ventricular filling pressure; heart rate and cardiac index frequently did not change. Concurrently, myocardial oxygen consumption decreased and coronary sinus oxygen content increased, as measured from a coronary sinus catheter. Although NTG increased global myocardial oxygen availability, this study did not assess regional myocardial perfusion; however, regional ischemia was not detected by ECG monitoring. The dose of NTG appears to be important for prophylactic ischemic protection. Nitroglycerin, 0.5 μg/kg/min, was found not to be superior to placebo for prevention of ischemic ST changes during fentanyl anesthesia for cardiac surgery.[101] A recent study comparing two doses of IV NTG (0.5 and 1.0 μg/kg/min) during noncardiac surgery in patients with CAD demonstrated that the higher dose was necessary to prevent ST-segment depression, suggesting that a dose of less than 1.0 μg/kg/min is not effective for prophylactic treatment of myocardial ischemia.[102] Importantly, during the higher dose NTG therapy, intravenous fluids (619 ± 174 ml) were administered to prevent a reflex increase in heart rate. Although IV NTG administration must be titrated according to hemodynamic effects, this reported effective antianginal dose (1.0 μg/kg/min) is in agreement with several previous studies and probably represents clinically important therapeutic dosing information.

Iatrogenic myocardial ischemia is a consequence of aortic cross-clamping. Adequate delivery of cardioplegia minimizes ischemic damage; however, delivery distal to coronary stenosis is sometimes difficult. Although controversial, the addition of NTG to cardioplegic solutions has been shown to improve myocardial protection and reduce coronary vascular resistance during cardioplegic delivery.[103]

Perioperative antihypertensive therapy. Perioperative hypertension occurs in 33–61 percent of patients undergoing CABG surgery.[104] Intravenous nitroglycerin, 1–3 μg/kg/min, effectively reduces perioperative hypertension by decreasing SVR and preload.[105,106] Intravenous ISDN also reduces blood pressure in the perioperative period of cardiac surgery, but not as effectively as NTG.[106] Studies indicate that NTG is as effective as SNP in controlling hypertension before and after cardiopulmonary bypass. Whereas CO usually increases with SNP, it

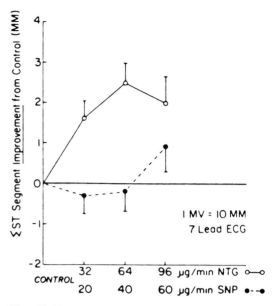

Fig. 13-11. Improvement from control ST-segment depression is shown for both nitroglycerin and nitroprusside. Nitroglycerin significantly improved the ST segments at all doses, whereas the two smaller doses of nitroprusside did not change the ST-segment depression. (From Kaplan JA: Vasodilator therapy during coronary artery surgery. J Thorac Cardiovasc Surg 77:301–308, 1979, with permission.)

frequently does not change or decreases with NTG due to large reductions in preload. Although studies indicate equal antihypertensive efficacy, there appear to be some patients who require the more potent arteriolar dilator, SNP, for adequate blood pressure control.[107] In addition, during cardiopulmonary bypass, NTG was relatively ineffective for blood pressure control compared with SNP.[108] This can be partially explained by recent information that demonstrates that NTG is absorbed by the cardiopulmonary bypass apparatus, so that patients may not be receiving the expected dose.[109] Antihypertensive therapy with NTG appears to improve the myocardial oxygen balance better than SNP. Coronary sinus blood sampling demonstrated that for equal reductions in MAP, myocardial lactate extraction increased with NTG and decreased with SNP.[110,111] Compared with SNP, NTG was shown to produce greater improvement in ischemic ST changes (Fig. 13-11).[112] These studies indicate that when an improvement in cardiac output is of primary importance, SNP might be the preferred antihypertensive, while NTG is the antihypertensive of choice when myocardial ischemia is suspected.

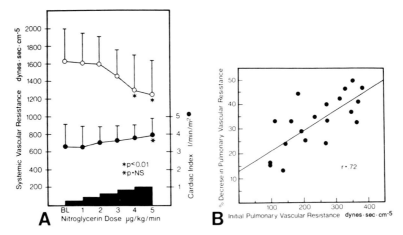

Fig. 13-12. (A) The dose-dependent effect of nitroglycerin on systemic and pulmonary vascular resistance (PVR) in pediatric patients for congenital heart surgery. (B) Patients with the highest baseline PVR had the greatest response. (From Ilbawi MN, et al: Circulation 72(suppl II):II101–II107, 1985, with permission.)

Pulmonary effects. Nitroglycerin has been shown to reduce pulmonary vascular resistance (PVR) effectively during adult cardiac surgery[108] and to reverse reactive pulmonary hypertension following pediatric congenital heart surgery (Fig. 13-12).[113] The nitroglycerin-induced decrease in pulmonary artery systolic pressure is accompanied by an improvement in right ventricular function.[114] Compared with SNP, for an equal reduction in systemic arterial blood pressure, PVR was reduced to a greater extent with NTG in a canine model of pulmonary hypertension.[115] As with all vasodilators, a decrease in pulmonary arteriolar resistance can prevent hypoxic pulmonary vasoconstriction, thereby reducing ventilation:perfusion ratios in atelectatic lung segments. A reduction in MAP to 65 mm Hg by NTG in postoperative CABG patients was accompanied by an increase in intrapulmonary shunting from 9.3 to 16.5 percent and a fall in arterial oxygen tension.[116] Chronic mitral valve disease is often associated with a gradient between PCWP and left atrial pressure due to reversible pulmonary vasoconstriction.[117] This gradient, which can continue in the postoperative period, can be reduced by NTG, which is thought to produce this effect by pulmonary venodilation.[117] Nitroglycerin also relaxes bronchial smooth muscle in large airways of patients without bronchospastic disease during fentanyl-diazepam anesthesia for CABG surgery.[117] However, its effect on patients with reactive airway disease is controversial, with some studies demonstrating an in-

crease and others no change in pulmonary function tests.

Intraoperative left ventricular failure. Nitroglycerin can be useful for the treatment of intraoperative left ventricular failure. The decrease in SVR combined with the decrease in systolic ventricular volume frequently increases cardiac output. Also, during CABG surgery, left ventricular dysfunction is commonly ischemia induced, and, in this setting, the amelioration of myocardial ischemia may increase ventricular diastolic compliance and improve ventricular systolic function. If the effects of NTG alone do not sufficiently maintain adequate cardiac function, an inotrope is sometimes required. Dopamine as well as dobutamine combined with NTG augments CO in patients with severe congestive heart failure.[118,119]

Coronary spasm. Coronary artery spasm is a complication of CABG surgery and can be associated with ST-segment elevation, severe myocardial dysfunction, and ventricular dysrhythmias. Its etiology is probably multifactorial, including underlying vasospastic disease or withdrawal of chronic vasodilator therapy as well as large temperature shifts, electrolyte changes, and high catecholamine levels after cardiopulmonary bypass. Intracoronary NTG, 200–1000 μg, has been reported to cause immediate relaxation of the affected coronary artery and resolution of the symptoms.[86] In the acute situation, the effects of IV NTG may be augmented by administration of sublingual nifedipine.[86]

Adverse Effects of Organic Nitrate Therapy

Long-term nitrate therapy can be complicated by nitrate tolerance and nitrate dependence. Nitrate tolerance is thought to be due to repeated nitrate-induced oxidation of intracellular sulphydryl groups, which are necessary for the conversion of the nitrate molecule into the active vasodilator (Fig. 13-3).[120,121] The lack of reduced sulphydryl groups, which produces tolerance, can be quickly reversed by a disulphide-reducing agent.[20] Animal studies in vivo and in vitro demonstrate that nitrate tolerance to vasodilation is related to the duration of exposure, dosing interval, and nitrate dose.[120] Several clinical studies have also demonstrated that repeated doses of ISDN result in a blunted blood pressure response despite maintenance of ISDN plasma levels.[121] Nitrate cross-tolerance has also been demonstrated by the fact that nitroglycerin-induced changes in blood pressure and venous capacitance were greater before than after 4 weeks of ISDN therapy.[122] Further studies are necessary to determine if patients receiving preoperative IV NTG infusions become tolerant to intraoperative NTG therapy.

Drug dependence is defined by the appearance of physical symptoms following drug withdrawal. Nitrate dependence first became evident among NTG ammunition workers exposed to industrial amounts of nitrates who developed chest pain 2–3 days after removal from the work environment.[123] Animal studies of nitrate dependence have demonstrated lack of coronary vascular responsiveness to intravenous ergonovine initially; however, 40 hours after withdrawal from 6 weeks of chronic NTG therapy, ergonovine readily produced coronary spasm.[124] This suggests that withdrawal from nitrates may lead to rebound vasoconstriction and increased arterial responsiveness of vasoconstrictor stimuli.[19] Compelling clinical evidence of nitrate dependence does not yet exist; however, abrupt cessation of nitrate therapy should probably be avoided in the perioperative period.

Induction of methemoglobinemia is another concern with nitrate administration. Nitrite, the metabolite of organic nitrates, converts oxyhemoglobin to methemoglobin, which interferes with oxygen delivery because of the inability of methemoglobin to transport oxygen and by a shift to the left in the oxyhemoglobin dissociation curve.[19] Development of methemoglobinemia in the perioperative period is rare; however, it has been reported from nitrate overdose and excessive intravenous doses.[125,126] Treatment of severe cases involves administration of 100 percent oxygen, 100 mg of methylene blue, and blood exchange transfusions.

Three adverse drug interactions have been reported with organic nitrates. Ethacrynic acid, which oxidizes sulphydryl groups, has been shown to produce a state of refractoriness to vasodilation from nitrates. However, a recent animal study demonstrated that this effect of ethacrynic acid may be primarily seen in vitro and not in vivo.[127] Indomethacin, which inhibits prostaglandin E, has been shown in animals to reduce the vasodilator potency of nitrates.[128] This is in accordance with other data, suggesting that vasodilation from nitrates may be mediated by prostaglandins.[50] Of particular interest to anesthesiologists is a potential interaction between IV NTG and pancuronium bromide. Although the mechanism is uncertain, NTG has been found to double the intensity and duration of pancuronium-induced neuromuscular blockade in cats.[129]

BETA-ADRENERGIC RECEPTOR BLOCKERS

Mechanism of Action

A comprehensive knowledge of beta-adrenergic receptor blocking drugs necessitates an understanding of basic pharmacologic principles of receptor pharmacology and competitive drug inhibition. The receptor for the beta-blockers is the beta-adrenergic receptor, which is composed of membrane proteins located on the outer surface of cell membranes.[130] These receptors are stimulated by adrenergic agonists, such as neurotransmitters (norepinephrine and dopamine), or hormonal mediators (epinephrine). Beta-agonist binding stimulates an enzyme, adenyl cyclase, to increase cellular levels of cyclic adenosine monophosphate (cAMP) (Fig. 13-13).[130] Cyclic AMP, the "second messenger," initiates functional modifications of cellular enzymes, which produce the characteristic beta-adrenergic physiologic response.[130] Since the generation of cAMP is proportional to the concentration of agonist–receptor complexes, beta-adrenergic sympathetic activity is proportional to the concentration of receptors occupied by agonist compounds.

The degree of receptor occupation is related to the concentration of adrenergic agonists at receptor sites plus the *affinity* of agonists for the receptor.[131] The higher the affinity, the greater proportion of receptors occupied per concentration of compounds at the receptor. The magnitude of the elicited

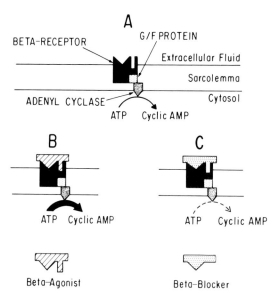

Fig. 13-13. Schematic of molecular mechanism of beta-blocking drugs. (A) The beta-receptor on the external surface of the sarcolemma is coupled to adenyl cyclase on the inner surface of the sarcolemma by the G/F protein. (B) Binding of an agonist modifies cellular function by enhancing cAMP production. (C) Beta-blockers also bind to the receptor, but (unless they possess intrinsic sympathomimetic activity) do not increase the rate of cAMP production. Occupation of the receptor by the beta-blocker prevents beta agonist binding and activation of adenyl cyclase. (From Hager WD, et al: *In* β-Blockers: The Extended Family. 1984, pp 205, with permission.)

response depends on the concentration of compound–receptor complexes as well as the agonist's *intrinsic activity,* which is the efficacy of a compound for stimulating a response (in this case, adenyl cyclase activation) or "the capacity to stimulate for a given occupancy."[132] For beta-adrenergic receptors, in the relative intrinsic activity of the agonists in isolated perfused rabbit hearts, isoproterenol is greater than epinephrine, which is greater than norepinephrine.[133] A beta-adrenergic agonist is a compound that possesses affinity and intrinsic activity. A pure beta-adrenergic receptor blocker (or antagonist) has affinity but lacks intrinsic activity (Fig. 13-14). Many clinically available beta-blocking drugs possess some degree of intrinsic sympathomimetic activity and are not pure antagonists.[134]

Beta-adrenergic receptor blocking drugs are competitive antagonists of beta-adrenergic agonists. The degree of receptor occupation by the antagonist is determined by the relative concentrations of the blocker and agonist as well as the specific receptor affinity of each of these compounds. Since the beta-blocking drugs are *competitive* antagonists, a sufficient increase in the agonist concentration will overcome any degree of blockade. The key pharmacologic feature of competitive antagonism is a parallel rightward displacement of the agonist dose–response curve without a reduction in the maximum elicited response (Fig. 13-15).[135]

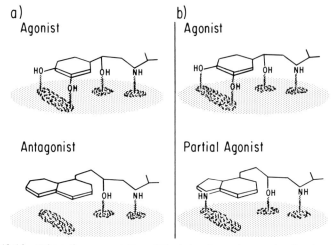

Fig. 13-14. Schematic representation of the beta-adrenergic receptor showing (a) the molecular attachment points for an agonist (isoproterenol) and an antagonist (propranolol) lacking sympathomimetic activity, versus (b) an agonist and a partial agonist (pindolol) with intrinsic sympathomimetic activity. (From Clark BJ: Beta-adrenoceptor-blocking agents: Are pharmacologic differences relevant? Am Heart J 104:334–345, 1982, with permission.)

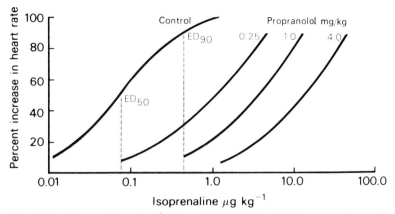

Fig. 13-15. Characteristics of competitive inhibition by beta-blocking drugs. Increasing doses of propranolol cause a parallel rightward displacement in the isoproterenol (Isoprenaline) dose–response curve without a reduction in the maximum elicited response by high doses of isoproterenol. (From Prys-Roberts C: *In* Prys-Roberts C (ed): Pharmacokinetics of Anaesthesia. Oxford, Blackwell Scientific, 1984, p 295, with permission.

Beta-adrenergic receptors were first identified in 1948 by Ahlquist[136] and were subsequently subdivided into beta$_1$- and beta$_2$-adrenergic receptors by Lands et al in 1967.[133] Beta$_1$-receptor stimulation primarily involves cardiac function, producing positive chronotropic and inotropic effects and increasing the electrical excitability of myocardial tissue (Table 13-2).[137] Noncardiac beta$_1$-receptors stimulate renin secretion in the kidney and aqueous humor production in the eye.[137] The primary actions of beta$_2$-receptor stimulation are noncardiac, involving arteriolar vasodilation (predominantly in skeletal muscle tissue), bronchodilation, and metabolic effects (stimulation of insulin secretion, glucogenolysis, glyconeogenesis, and lipolysis).[137] Beta$_2$-receptors also affect extrarenal potassium homeostasis.[138] Stimulation of beta$_2$-receptors redistributes potassium from the extracellular to intracellular space.

Recent evidence indicates the presence of cardiac beta$_2$-adrenergic receptors in humans.[139] This subpopulation of cardiac beta-receptors is responsible for a portion of the isoproterenol-induced inotropic response of isolated strips of human atrial and ventricular myocardium.[139] In fact, radioligand studies have demonstrated a substantial proportion of beta$_2$-receptors in human right ventricular tissue.[139] Cardiac beta$_2$-receptor stimulation also affects the chronotropic response to isoproterenol in humans as evidenced by the fact that atenolol and metoprolol, which are beta$_1$-selective, are less potent than propranolol (beta$_1$ and beta$_2$) in blunting the heart rate response to isoproterenol.[140] Postsynaptic beta$_2$-receptor sites and presynaptic beta$_2$-receptors that

Table 13-2
Differential Effects of Beta Stimulation

Beta$_1$ Effects	Beta$_2$ Effects
Cardiac	Smooth muscle
Increased chronotropy	Peripheral vasodilation
	Bronchodilation
Increased inotropy	Uterine relaxation
Increased excitability	Cardiac*
Increased plasma renin	Increased chronotropy
Increased aqueous	Increased inotropy
humor	Metabolic
	Stimulation of insulin secretion
	Stimulation of glycogenolysis
	Stimulation of gluconeogenesis
	Stimulation of lipolysis
	Potassium homeostasis
	Extracellular to intracellular potassium redistribution
	Skeletal muscle tremor

*Recent evidence of cardiac beta$_2$-receptors.[139,140]
Modified from Slogoff S: Beta-Adrenergic Blockers. *In* Kaplan JA (ed): Cardiac Anesthesia: Cardiovascular Pharmacology. Orlando, FL, Grune & Stratton, 1983, pp 181–208.

exert a positive feedback on norepinephrine release have been postulated. The clinical significance of cardiac beta$_2$-receptors in cardiac surgical patients is not yet understood; however, these potential effects need to be appreciated when comparing the pharmacodynamic effects of beta$_1$-selective with nonselective beta-blocking drugs.

Classification of Beta-Blockers

Beta-blocking drugs presently available for clinical systemic use in the United States include acebutolol, atenolol, esmolol, labetalol, metoprolol, nadolol, pindolol, propranolol, and timolol. Esmolol should be available shortly. These drugs have a number of associated properties and characteristics that can be used to subdivide this class of compounds, including cardioselectivity, intrinsic sympathomimetic activity (ISA), membrane-stabilizing activity (MSA), and concomitant alpha-adrenergic blocking properties (Table 13-3) (see Chapter 12).

CARDIOSELECTIVITY

The beta-adrenergic receptor blockers can be subdivided into compounds that nonselectively block both beta$_1$- and beta$_2$-receptors (labetalol, nadolol, pindolol, propranolol, and timolol) and those that possess a greater blocking potency for beta$_1$- than beta$_2$-receptor subtypes (acebutolol, atenolol, esmolol, and metoprolol). Since beta$_1$-receptors represent the predominant beta-adrenergic innervation in the heart, beta$_1$-selective blockers are commonly referred to as cardioselective although, as has been mentioned above, beta$_2$-receptors have now been identified in cardiac tissue. It is important to realize that these drugs are "cardioselective" and not cardiospecific, meaning that they have a relative increased potency for beta$_1$-receptors but do not totally lack effects on beta$_2$-receptors.[137]

INTRINSIC SYMPATHOMIMETIC ACTIVITY

The beta-blocking drugs can also be classified into compounds that possess or do not possess intrinsic sympathomimetic activity.[141] Beta-blocking drugs with ISA are acebutolol, esmolol, labetalol, and pindolol. Beta-blockers with ISA not only block receptor occupancy by agonist compounds, but also produce a degree of stimulation of the beta-receptor (Fig. 13-14).[141] In order for beta-blocking drugs to be clinically useful, however, the ISA properties must be considerably less than the intrinsic activity of agonist compounds. In fact, the first isolated beta-

Table 13-3

Associated Pharmacologic Properties of the Beta-Blocking Drugs

Drug	Relative Beta$_1$ Selectivity	Intrinsic Sympathomimetic Activity	Membrane-Stabilizing Activity
Acebutolol	+	+ +	+
Atenolol	+ +	0	0
Esmolol	+ +	+	+
Labetalol*	0	? + B$_2$	+
Metoprolol	+ +	0	0
Nadolol	0	0	0
Pindolol	0	+ +	0
Propranolol	0	0	+ +
Timolol	0	0	0

*Labetalol has additional alpha-adrenergic blocking activity.

blocker, dichloro-isoproterenol, was not therapeutically useful largely because of prominent ISA.[142]

Beta-blocking drugs with ISA possess significant hemodynamic differences from beta-blockers without ISA.[141] Human studies in vitro demonstrate a direct vasodilating effect of pindolol on both arteries and veins.[142] Resting heart rate, cardiac output, and peripheral blood flow are maintained due to ISA in the face of low levels of endogenous catecholamines (Fig. 13-16).[143] During moderate exercise, however, the beta-blocking effect predominates and heart rate is reduced to a similar degree as with beta-blockers without ISA. It should also be noted that this difference between drugs with and without ISA may only be evident at maximum blocking doses.[141]

MEMBRANE-STABILIZING ACTIVITY

Acebutolol, esmolol, labetalol, and propranolol possess membrane-stabilizing properties in vitro; however, in clinically relevant doses, beta-blockers do not exhibit any MSA.[137] Membrane-stabilizing activity has been demonstrated not to be a therapeutic property, since the D(+) isomer of propranolol, which has the MSA but lacks the beta-blocking effects of racemic (clinically used) propranolol, lacks antianginal, antihypertensive, and antiarrhythmic properties.[137] The only therapeutic modality in which this property may have possible therapeutic effects is when propranolol is used as a component of cardioplegia solutions in which high concentrations are

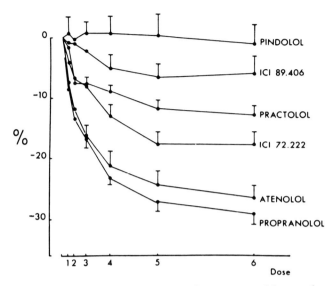

Fig. 13-16. Beta-blocker dose–response curves for percentage of decrease from resting cardiac output after pindolol and ICI 89.406 (high degree of ISA), practolol and ICI 72.222 (lesser degree of ISA), and propranolol and atenolol (no ISA). Beta-blocking drugs with ISA produce less of a reduction in heart rate and cardiac output during periods of low levels of endogenous catecholamines, such as at rest. (From Taylor SH: Intrinsic sympathomimetic activity: Clinical fact or fiction? Am J Cardiol 52:16D–26D, 1983, with permission.)

delivered directly into the coronary circulation.[144] In these cardioplegic doses, the MSA may contribute to cardioplegic protection.

NONSELECTIVE BETA-BLOCKADE PLUS ALPHA-ADRENERGIC BLOCKING PROPERTIES

Labetalol, a relatively new beta-blocking drug, is the only clinically available beta-blocker that possesses concomitant alpha-adrenergic blocking properties.[145,146] The beta-blocking properties are about one-third as potent as propranolol, and the alpha-blocking properties are one-tenth as potent as phentolamine.[147] The alpha-blocking component of labetalol produces distinct hemodynamic effects. Unlike most beta-blockers, cardiac output is not reduced with labetalol, probably due to a reduction in SVR from alpha-adrenergic blockade.[145] This also results in a potent antihypertensive effect from labetalol.[146]

Cardiovascular Effects of Beta-Blocking Drugs

The cardiovascular effects of beta-blocking drugs are directly due to inhibition of beta-receptor stimulation by catecholamines. The greater the degree of sympathetic activity (or stimulation), the more prominent will be the effect of the beta-blockers;[148] minimal effects are seen at rest. The reduction in resting heart rate from beta-blockers without ISA is due to blockade of low levels of sympathetic activity producing a prevalence of vagal (parasympathetic) tone.[137] At rest, the ISA of certain beta-blockers, such as pindolol, balances the beta-blockade of the low levels of endogenous catecholamines, and minimal changes in heart rate occur; however, during exercise with increasing sympathetic activity, the beta-blocking effect of pindolol predominates.[141] The effect of beta-blockers on CO usually parallels the negative chronotropic effect, so that drugs possessing ISA cause less of a reduction in CO at rest than beta-blockers without ISA (Fig. 13-16).

Most beta-blocking drugs increase SVR by two mechanisms: directly by blockade of $beta_2$-adrenergic–mediated vasodilation and indirectly by reflex alpha-adrenergic–mediated vasoconstriction responding to a decrease in blood pressure.[141] Theoretically, SVR should be elevated to the greatest extent by nonselective beta-adrenergic receptor blockers, while cardioselective beta-blockers with ISA should have the least effect. However, a review of several clinical studies involving 410 patients revealed no significant difference in the peripheral arterial effects between acute administration of cardioselective (atenolol and metoprolol) and nonselective beta-blockers (propranolol and timolol); SVR increased acutely and then returned to baseline during chronic drug administration.[149] Beta-blockers possessing ISA do have the least effect on SVR except for labetalol, which produces a considerable decrease in SVR due to its alpha-adrenergic blocking properties.[141,145]

The effect of beta-blockers on vital organ blood flow has been extensively evaluated. The reduction in CO from beta-blocker therapy is accompanied by a fall in peripheral blood flow including renal plasma flow;[150] however, other studies have shown no effect on renal blood flow.[151] The reduction in peripheral perfusion does not affect cerebral perfusion, which remains unchanged.[152] The decrease in heart rate with a resultant increase in the diastolic perfusion time allows for a substantial increase in coronary blood flow.[137] However, the reductions in cardiac sympathetic tone, heart rate, and blood pressure reduce myocardial oxygen requirements, which often results in an autoregulatory-induced decrease in coronary blood flow.[137] Cardioselectivity does not impart different coronary vascular effects than those of nonselective beta-blockers.[153]

Noncardiac Pharmacodynamics

BRONCHIAL SMOOTH MUSCLE

Although patients without pulmonary pathology do not usually manifest a change in pulmonary function from beta-blockade, patients suffering from bronchospastic disease who are dependent on beta-sympathetic tone to maintain adequate airway patency are sensitive to beta-blockade and demonstrate an increase in airway resistance as evidenced by a decrease in FEV_1.[154,155] Severe bronchoconstriction can be provoked by the administration of beta-blockers to asthmatics. The beta-adrenergic receptor blockers have also been shown to produce a small increase in airway obstruction in patients with chronic obstructive pulmonary disease and may reduce the respiratory response to carbon dioxide.[156] Cardioselective beta-blockers appear to have some advantages in patients with bronchospastic disease. For a given negative chronotropic effect, atenolol produces less of a reduction in FEV_1 and less inhibition of isoproterenol-induced bronchodilation in asthmatic patients than does propranolol.[157] However, it

must be appreciated that cardioselective beta-blocking drugs only show modest selectivity in the lungs.[137] Another clinical study demonstrated that atenolol and metoprolol both decreased FEV_1 in asthmatics.[155] Beta-blockers with ISA (pindolol) may have fewer detrimental effects on patients with bronchospastic disease, causing less of a reduction in peak airway flow rate and FEV_1, than propranolol (Table 13-4).[141]

GLUCOSE METABOLISM

The $beta_2$-adrenergic system affects glucose metabolism by stimulating insulin secretion, glycogenolysis, and gluconeogenesis.[137] Beta-blockade does not affect resting glucose or insulin levels in nondiabetics; however, the hyperglycemic response to serum catecholamines is inhibited,[158] and insulin release in response to a glucose load and increased beta-stimulation (exogenous isoproterenol) is ablated.[159] Beta-blocking drugs can have adverse effects in diabetics by reducing insulin secretion and reducing the recovery rate from insulin-induced hypoglycemia, since this is dependent on catecholamine stimulation of glycogenolysis.[137,160] Beta-blocking drugs also mask the symptomatology of hypoglycemia—tachycardia, palpitations, and tremors.[137,160] The cardiovascular effects of hypoglycemic-induced epinephrine secretion, a rise in systolic and a fall in diastolic pressure, are converted to rises in systolic and diastolic pressures due to blockade of the $beta_2$-mediated vasodilation.[161] Beta-blockers can also influence glucose homeostasis in the perioperative period. A recent report of severe hypoglycemia following tympanoplasty in a nondiabetic, hypertensive child treated with propranolol demonstrated that propranolol can enhance the susceptibility of children to hypoglycemia.[162] Perioperative hypoglycemia is especially dangerous because premedication and anesthetics can mask the subjective symptoms of hypoglycemia.

LIPID METABOLISM

High levels of catecholamines increase tissue lipolysis and plasma levels of free fatty acids, which enhances myocardial free fatty acid uptake and utilization.[137,141] In this setting, beta-blockers, which reduce lipolysis and decrease plasma free fatty acid levels, shift myocardial metabolism from the utilization of fatty acids to carbohydrates.[163] Since glucose metabolism consumes less oxygen than fatty acid metabolism for equal amounts of energy production, this metabolic effect of beta-blockers may be protective during myocardial ischemia.[137,163]

Table 13-4

Spirometric Comparison of Pindolol and Propranolol in Nine
Patients With Bronchospastic Disease

	Control	Propranolol	Propranolol Withdrawal	Pindolol
FEV$_1$/VC	55%	↓13.2%	↑14.1%	↓3.0%
		$p < 0.01$	$p < 0.01$	NS

Propranolol produced significant bronchoconstriction while pindolol (with intrinsic sympathomimetic activity) did not. $p < 0.01$ or NS from control.

FEV$_1$ = Forced expiratory volume at 1 second; VC = vital capacity.

From Frishman W., Davis R., Strom J., et al: Clinical pharmacology of the new beta-adrenergic blocking drugs. Part 5. Pindolol (LB-46) therapy for supraventricular arrhythmia: A viable alternative to propranolol in patients with bronchospasm. Am Heart J 98:393–398, 1979, with permission.

HEMATOLOGIC EFFECTS

Beta-blockers produce functional changes in hemoglobin that can augment their antianginal effects. Oxygen delivery to tissues may be improved by a shift to the right in the oxyhemoglobin dissociation curve, which has been demonstrated in vitro as well as in vivo.[164] The P$_{50}$ in anginal patients was 31.7 ± 0.1 mm Hg during propranolol administration, and 28.2 ± 0.9 mm Hg after discontinuation of the drug.[164]

Pharmacokinetics of Beta-Blocking Drugs

An appreciation of the pharmacokinetic properties of beta-blocking drugs is useful for understanding their bioavailability, duration of action, and the effects of tissue dysfunction on drug metabolism and elimination. Most beta-blockers can be divided into lipophilic and hydrophilic compounds. This division has pharmacologic merit because the degree of lipophilicity affects multiple pharmacokinetic properties of these drugs (Table 13-5).

LIPOPHILIC BETA-BLOCKING DRUGS

Lipophilic compounds include labetalol, metoprolol, propranolol, and timolol. (Pindolol has moderate lipid solubility characteristics.) Lipophilicity imparts excellent absorption from the gastrointestinal tract; however, these drugs then undergo extensive first-pass hepatic metabolism resulting in only a fraction of the drug reaching the systemic circulation.[137] First-pass hepatic metabolism is highly variable, producing high individual differences in plasma concentrations despite similar oral doses.[153] The first-pass hepatic extraction can become saturated with high oral doses, which can increase the bioavailability of propranolol from 30 to 50 percent.[165] Liver metabolism is mainly via hepatocyte detoxification mechanisms utilizing glucuronide conjugation and oxidative deamination.[137] Hepatic metabolism is dependent on normal hepatic cellular function and hepatic blood flow so that cirrhosis and congestive heart failure prolong the plasma half-life.[153,166] Beta-blocking drugs (such as propranolol) which reduce hepatic blood flow will decrease their own rate of drug metabolism.[156] The water-soluble metabolic products of hepatic metabolism are excreted by the kidney, but since the liver is the principal organ of drug elimination for lipophilic beta-blockers, drug effect is not greatly prolonged in patients with renal failure. However, an active metabolite of propranolol can accumulate and exert hemodynamic effects during severe renal failure.[167] Lipid solubility also imparts a large apparent volume of distribution because of uptake into peripheral tissues. A drug concentration effect of propranolol in lung, liver, and heart tissue has been confirmed in animal studies.[137] This may explain a longer duration of cardiac effects of propranolol than would be expected from plasma drug levels.

Lipophilic compounds can be highly bound to plasma proteins. This has pharmacodynamic significance because it is only the free, unbound drug that distributes out of the plasma to the sites of action and produces the biologic effects.[168] Plasma protein binding accounts for 83–95 percent of the total plasma concentrations of propranolol.[169,170] Alterations in the amount of plasma proteins by disease states as well as drug competition for available protein bind-

Table 13-5
Pharmacokinetic Properties of Beta-Blocking Drugs

	Lipid Solubility Log Partition Coefficient (Octanol:Water)	Absorption (% Ingested)	Bioavailability (% Ingested)	Elimination Half-Life (hr)	Mechanism of Drug Elimination	Beta$_1$-Blockade Potency Ratio (Propranolol = 1.0)
Propranolol	3.65	90	30	4-6	Hepatic	1.0
Labetalol	3.13	100	30	3-5	Hepatic	0.3
Metoprolol	2.15	95	50	3-4	Hepatic	1.0
Timolol	2.10	90	50	4-5	Hepatic	6.0
Pindolol	1.75	90	75	3-4	Hepatic/renal	6.0
Nadolol	0.71	30	30	14-24	Renal	1.0
Acebutolol	0.55	100	100	3-4	Renal/hepatic	0.3
Atenolol	0.23	50	40	6-9	Renal	1.0

Difference between percentage of absorption and percentage of bioavailability primarily reflects first-pass hepatic metabolism.
Modified from Slogoff, S: Beta-Adrenergic Blockers. In Kaplan JA (ed): Cardiac Anesthesia: Cardiovascular Pharmacology. Orlando, FL, Grune & Stratton, 1983, p 193.

ing sites can affect pharmacokinetic activity of pro-pranolol.[168] Heparin increases plasma levels of nonesterified free fatty acids, which compete with propranolol for albumin binding sites.[169] Hepariniza-tion, as well as cardiopulmonary bypass (which decreases plasma protein concentrations), has been found to significantly decrease plasma protein bind-ing of propranolol.[169,170] These heparin-induced changes in protein binding of propranolol result in more biologically active propranolol and can possi-bly explain the hemodynamic effects associated with heparin administration for cardiopulmonary bypass.

HYDROPHILIC BETA-BLOCKING DRUGS

The hydrophilic beta-blocking drugs include acebutolol, atenolol, and nadolol.[171,172] Their low lipid solubility decreases the rapidity of gastrointesti-nal absorption; however, this does not appear to be clinically relevant. These drugs do not undergo sig-nificant hepatic metabolism so that bioavailability following oral administration is not affected by first-pass hepatic elimination.[137] Atenolol and nadolol, which are among the most hydrophilic beta-blocking drugs, are eliminated almost entirely by renal excre-tion.[172] Total body clearance of these drugs is depen-dent upon the glomerular filtration rate. The normal glomerular filtration rate is 0.1–0.15 l/min; the total body clearance of atenolol and nadolol is 0.1 and 0.18 l/min, respectively.[172] The higher clearance of nadolol is probably due to additional excretion via the biliary tract.[137] In contrast, the lipophilic drugs, which are extensively extracted from the blood dur-ing passage through the liver, have a total body clear-ance that is in the same range as the hepatic blood flow (1.0–2.0 l/min).[172] The decreased total body clearance of the water-soluble compounds imparts a relatively long elimination half-life, enabling ateno-lol and nadolol to be effective with once-daily oral dosing. The half-life of these drugs is inversely pro-portional to the creatinine clearance and can be greatly prolonged in patients with renal insuffi-ciency;[137,172] however, liver dysfunction does not affect their elimination half-life.

Acebutolol is a hydrophilic beta-blocker that undergoes significant hepatic metabolism as well as renal excretion.[171] It has a total body clearance of 0.62 l/min, reflecting extrarenal as well as renal excretion.[171] The major route for metabolism is by hydrolysis, producing diacetolol, which has car-dioselective beta-blocking properties similar to ace-butolol. Since renal elimination is important, the plasma half-lives of acebutolol and diacetolol are increased in parallel with the degree of renal insuffi-ciency.[171]

Pindolol, which is moderately lipid soluble, is eliminated 50 percent via hepatic metabolism and 40 percent via renal excretion of unchanged drug.[173] The total plasma drug clearance is midway between the clearance rates of renal and hepatically eliminated drugs (0.4 l/min). Patients with renal insufficiency demonstrate a compensatory increase in hepatic metabolism of pindolol, and more than a 50 percent reduction in dose is seldom necessary.[173]

New Beta-Adrenergic Receptor Blocking Drugs

ESMOLOL

Esmolol is a newly developed beta-blocking drug which is effective for the treatment of supraven-tricular tachyarrhythmias as well as intraoperative hypertension and tachycardia due to surgical stress. It is cardioselective and possesses minimal ISA and MSA.[174] Like other beta-blockers, its clinical phar-macodynamic properties are due to beta-adrenergic receptor blockade; no significant receptor-indepen-dent effects have been identified. The distinctive property of esmolol is due to its pharmacokinetics;[174] an ultrashort duration of action enables intravenous titration of beta-blockade and rapid withdrawal of drug effect. After cessation of intravenous adminis-tration, a rapid decrease in blood levels occurs, pre-dominantly due to rapid metabolism during transport through the vascular bed (Fig. 13-17). In fact, the total body clearance of esmolol in dogs is 350 ml/kg/min, which is greater than the cardiac output.[174] Metabolism of esmolol is due to hydrolysis of the methyl ester in the molecule by blood esterases located in the cytosol of red blood cells. The metabo-lites are methanol and an acid metabolite that pos-sesses minimal beta-blocking properties.[174-176] The esterase enzyme in red blood cells is not inhibited by physostigmine, and although in anesthetized dogs large doses of esmolol do not modify the magnitude and duration of the effect of succinylcholine, an inhibitory effect of esmolol on human plasma cholin-esterase activity has been demonstrated in vitro.[174,175]

Esmolol pharmacokinetics have been exten-sively studied in humans. It has an extremely rapid distribution half-life of 2 minutes and an elimination half-life of 9 minutes. Because of its ultrashort kinetic properties, steady-state levels of esmolol can be rapidly achieved within 5 minutes with loading dose infusion techniques, and recovery from beta-blockade is complete 10–20 minutes after termina-tion of infusion.[176] Esmolol infusions in humans in the range of 25–300 μg/kg/min produce linear dose-

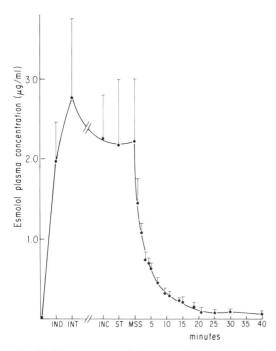

Fig. 13-17. Plasma esmolol concentrations from a continuous esmolol infusion begun prior to induction (IND) and intubation (INT) and continued through incision (INC), sternotomy (ST), and maximal sternal spread (MSS) for cardiac surgery. Termination of the infusion after MSS resulted in an extremely rapid decay in plasma levels, relecting short alpha- and beta-elimination half-lives of 1.3 and 9.8 minutes, respectively. (From deBruijn NP, et al: (abstr) Proc SCA, Montreal, 1986, with permission.)

related hemodynamic effects.[177] Clinical studies demonstrate dose-dependent decreases in heart rate and cardiac index at rest and during exercise, as well as inhibition of isoproterenol-induced increases in heart rate and blood pressure.[177] The cardiovascular effects of esmolol at rest and during exercise were found to be similar to propranolol except that resting SVR and exercise systemic blood pressure were lower with esmolol.[174,178] Characteristic of the beta-blocking drugs, the electrophysiologic effects of esmolol are due to blockade of adrenergic tone at the SA and AV nodes, producing a decrease in sinus node rate and AV conduction and an increase in AV refractoriness. The electrophysiologic effects on SA node function, AV nodal conduction, and A-H interval are comparable with those of other beta-blocking drugs. In the clinical setting, there was no electrophysiologic effect on the His–Purkinje or ventricular tissue[179] (see Chapter 12).

Esmolol is comparable in safety and efficacy with propranolol for the treatment of supraventricular tachyarrhythmias.[180] A therapeutic reduction in heart rate was achieved in 70 percent of patients, although conversion to normal sinus rhythm occurred in only 15 percent. The pharmacokinetic properties of esmolol, however, make it ideally suited for short-term dysrhythmia therapy as may be necessary with intraoperative dysrhythmias and for acute drug testing in the clinical electrophysiology laboratory. The most frequent adverse reaction during treatment of supraventricular tachycardia was hypotension during esmolol rates of 150 μg/kg/min, which resolved in 20–90 minutes after discontinuation of the drug.

Esmolol may also be useful for treating myocardial ischemia and infarction. Experimental ischemia models demonstrate that esmolol reduces myocardial infarction size and improves recovery of regional myocardial function after reversible ischemia.[181] The long duration of action of the currently available beta-blocking drugs limits their use in certain subgroups of acute myocardial infarction patients because of the risk of adverse effects. These high-risk patients include those with left ventricular dysfunction, cardiac conduction problems, borderline-to-low blood pressure, and bronchospastic disease. Esmolol can be administered with careful monitoring, and if adverse effects develop, the drug dose can be reduced or terminated, and the adverse effect will rapidly dissipate. The safety and efficacy of esmolol have been demonstrated in patients with acute myocardial infarction accompanied by hypertension. Doses as high as 300 μg/kg/min for up to 420 minutes decreased heart rate and blood pressure. Thirty minutes after discontinuing the infusion, the parameters returned to baseline and chronic therapy was then instituted with conventional oral beta-blocking drugs.[181]

The relative cardioselective effects of esmolol have been demonstrated in asthmatic patients. Esmolol produces a slight, clinically insignificant increase in specific airway resistance and sensitivity to drug-induced bronchoconstriction.[182] No adverse effects were seen in 60 patients with chronic obstructive pulmonary disease when esmolol was used to treat supraventricular tachyarrhythmias.[177]

LABETALOL

Labetalol is a relatively new beta-blocking drug that combines selective, competitive, reversible alpha$_1$-adrenergic blockade with nonselective, beta-blocking activity.[145,146] It is indicated for the treatment of systemic arterial hypertension. In humans, the ratios of alpha- to beta-blockade have been estimated to be 1:3 and 1:7 after oral and intravenous administration, respectively. Intrinsic sympathetic activity has been identified at beta$_2$-adrenergic receptors but not at beta$_1$-receptors. Membrane-stabilizing properties have been demonstrated in animals at doses higher than required for complete alpha- and beta-blockade.

The unique pharmacology of labetalol originates from the effect of concomitant alpha- and beta-blockade, which induces a reduction in SVR without significant changes in heart rate or CO at rest.[145,146] Vasodilation is the mechanism of blood pressure reduction with labetalol in contrast to most beta-blockers, which reduce blood pressure by decreases in heart rate and CO.[145,146] At high levels of exercise, there may be some reduction in CO, but in patients with ischemic heart disease this was smaller than with propranolol.[145,146] Labetalol appears to block the exercise-induced increase in blood pressure more than the increase in heart rate.[183] In studies with normotensive angina patients, it has less antianginal effectiveness than propranolol.[146,183] Bronchoconstriction from labetalol is a consideration since it is a nonselective beta-blocking drug; however, beta$_2$-ISA provides some protection since the degree of bronchoconstriction appears to be less than with propranolol.[184] The pharmacokinetic properties of labetalol are similar to those of propranolol, and the metabolism is predominantly through conjugation to glucuronide metabolites in the liver with extensive first-pass metabolism. The elimination half-life after intravenous administration is 5.5 hours, and the total body clearance is 2.0 l/min.[137,145,146]

Therapeutic Uses of Beta-Blocking Drugs

EXERTIONAL ANGINA

Beta-blocking drugs are effective in exertional or unstable angina when an increase in endogenous catecholamine levels is expected and when a decrease in baseline sympathetic support of cardiac function can be tolerated without cardiac decompensation.[137] They have been shown to decrease the frequency of angina attacks and NTG requirements and increase exercise tolerance.[137] However, in angina associated with coronary spasm, beta-blockers are not effective and may actually be harmful due to unopposed alpha-adrenergic influences on the coronary vasculature.[185] By simultaneous blockade of alpha- and beta-receptors in the coronary vasculature, labetalol might incur less risk of coronary spasm than other beta-blockers.[186]

The principal mechanism for the antianginal effects of the beta-blockers is due to a reduction in myocardial oxygen consumption via antagonism of sympathetic effects on cardiac function (Fig. 13-18).[137] The reduction in heart rate will also improve coronary blood flow. The reduction in

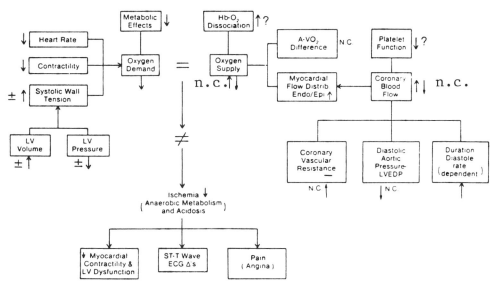

Fig. 13-18. Effects of beta-blockers on the balance between myocardial oxygen demand and oxygen supply. (Modified from Frishman WH: β-adrenergic blocking drugs in ischemic heart disease. *In* Clinical Pharmacology of the β-Adrenoceptor Blocking Drugs. East Norwalk, CT, Appleton-Century-Crofts, 1984, pp 257–272.)

myocardial oxygen consumption by beta-blockers is, however, limited by a potential increase in left ventricular volume due to the reduction in sympathetically supported myocardial contractility. This is especially true in patients with left ventricular dysfunction. Patients with the largest end-diastolic volumes before propranolol experience the greatest increase in ventricular volume after propranolol administration.[187] Beta-blockers with ISA, such as pindolol, produce less of an increase in left ventricular volume and might, therefore, be advantageous as antianginal agents in patients with compromised ventricular function. However, while beta-blockade decreases contractility in normal myocardial tissue, the reduction in oxygen demand can reduce regional myocardial ischemia and thereby improve regional function in ischemic myocardial tissue.[62] The antianginal effects of beta-blockers do not appear to be due to myocardial tolerance of greater cardiac workloads, but rather to a reduction in the rate of increase in heart rate–blood pressure product (myocardial oxygen demand) during increasing levels of exercise.[188,189] Interestingly, when beta-blocked patients with ischemic heart disease are exercised, chest pain occurs at a lower rate–pressure product than before administration of beta-blockers. This is presumably due to increased left ventricular volume and wall tension after beta-blockade.[189]

ACUTE MYOCARDIAL INFARCTION

Several randomized double-blind studies have demonstrated that beta-blocking drugs reduce the incidence of sudden death within the first 1–3 years after acute myocardial infarction.[190-192] The major causes of death after acute myocardial infarction are recurrent infarction, dysrhythmias, and left ventricular dysfunction.[193] Beta-blockers reduce the incidence of postinfarction ventricular dysrhythmias and increase the threshold of ventricular fibrillation probably by blocking the dysrhythmogenic effect of excess catecholamines, which accompany acute myocardial infarction and are a consequence of the amelioration of ischemia.[190,194]

Experimental evidence also suggests that if reinfarction is not averted, the subsequent infarct size will be reduced. Animal studies indicate that beta-blockers can salvage ischemic myocardial tissue; however, the time between drug administration and onset of infarction is critical.[195] Propranolol administered before infarction caused a 53 percent reduction in infarct size versus a 28 percent reduction when propranolol was given 3 hours after infarction and had no effect on infarct size when given 6 hours after

coronary ligation.[195] A randomized trial of 400 patients demonstrated that atenolol administration within 12 hours of chest pain caused a 30 percent reduction in enzymatically estimated infarct size.[190] "Threatened" infarction may also be prevented by beta-blockade.[194] The efficacy of the different beta-blockers appears to be due to beta-blocking action and is not related to cardioselectivity or membrane-stabilizing effects. It has been suggested that beta-blockers with ISA, such as pindolol and oxprenolol (available in Europe), might have fewer beneficial effects after acute myocardial infarction.[194] In fact, The European Infarction Study with oxprenolol had to be prematurely terminated because of an increased mortality in the oxprenolol group.[196] Singh and Venkatesh outlined a subset of acute myocardial infarction patients who would most likely benefit from beta-blocker therapy: (1) patients with threatened infarction; (2) patients who develop ischemia in the postinfarction period, especially with major ST segment elevation; and (3) postinfarction patients with hypertension.[194]

SYSTEMIC ARTERIAL HYPERTENSION

The antihypertensive properties of beta-blockers were accidently discovered in 1964 by Prichard while treating a patient with angina pectoris.[197] Presently, all clinically available beta-blocking drugs in the United States are indicated for the treatment of mild-to-moderate hypertension.[198,199] Equipotent doses of nonselective, cardioselective, and beta-blockers with ISA are equally effective. Labetalol is most effective due to its combined beta- and alpha-adrenergic–blocking properties; it is also the only beta-blocker that is effective for the treatment of severe hypertensive emergencies.[145,146]

The primary antihypertensive hemodynamic effect of beta-blockers (except labetalol) is a reduction in cardiac output.[130,198] Proposed antihypertensive effects for beta-blockers include:*

1. Hemodynamic effects, including reduction in cardiac output and vasodilation (labetalol)
2. Decreased renin release from kidney
3. Decreased plasma aldosterone
4. Neural actions, including inhibition of central beta-receptors in the brain to reduce central adrenergic outflow, inhibition of peripheral presyn-

---

*Modified from Frolich ED: Pharmacologic and physiologic considerations of adrenoceptor blockade. Am J Med Oct:9–14, 1983.

aptic beta-receptors to reduce alpha- and beta-adrenergic stimulation, and reset arterial baroreceptors

5. Effects on prostaglandin metabolism

Beta-blockers reduce blood pressure by decreasing CO; SVR increases acutely and then returns to normal during chronic drug therapy.[198] Beta-blocking drugs with ISA produce less of a reduction in CO.[143] Labetalol is the only beta-blocking drug that reduces blood pressure by a reduction in SVR; CO does not change or may actually increase in hypertensive patients.[145] A number of studies indicate that modulation of renal renin release is one of the antihypertensive mechanisms of the beta-blockers.[130,198] All beta-blockers have recently been shown to reduce basal and stimulated plasma renin levels. Although renin levels are decreased in all beta-blocked patients, however, urinary aldosterone levels only decrease in hypertensive responders, suggesting that an important antihypertensive effect is a reduction in aldosterone release through the renin-angiotensin pathway.[198] There is also evidence that the hypotensive effect may be due to blockade of prejunctional beta-adrenergic receptors, which inhibits efferent sympathetic stimulation of both beta- and alpha-adrenergic receptors in vascular smooth muscle.[198] Beta-blockers that enter the central nervous system (propranolol) have been shown to promote a release of norepinephrine in the brain which stimulates *central* alpha-receptors, leading to a decrease in peripheral sympathetic tone.[130,198] Other mechanisms that are less well proven are the effects of beta-blockers on baroreceptor sensitivity and prostaglandin release.[198]

Since all beta-blocking drugs are effective in equipotent doses, selection of the most appropriate one is usually determined by the associated pharmacologic effects. In patients with high resting heart rates, beta-blockers without ISA may be most useful; in patients with chronic obstructive pulmonary disease, cardioselective agents may be most appropriate; patients with borderline congestive heart failure may experience a therapeutic advantage from a beta-blocker with ISA or labetalol with both beta- and alpha-adrenergic blocking properties. Adequate blood pressure control often requires concomitant therapy with a diuretic or vasodilator. These therapeutic combinations are clinically advantageous because beta-blockers prevent reflex tachycardia from vasodilators and attenuate thiazide-induced hypokalemia.[198]

Table 13-6
Antiarrhythmic Mechanisms for Beta-Blockers*

1. Beta-blockade
   Electrophysiologic properties
      Nodal tissue: depresses conduction velocity and automaticity, and increases refractory period
      Ventricular tissue: depresses excitability
   Prevention of ischemia
      Decreases automaticity and inhibits reentry mechanisms
      Blockade of excess catecholamines
2. Membrane stabilizing effects
   Quindine-like properties not significant in clinical doses
3. Other associated properties (cardioselectivity, intrinsic sympathomimetic activity, alpha-blocking properties) do not appear to contribute to antiarrhythmic effectiveness

*Modified from Frishman, et al: Physiologic and metabolic effects. *In* Clinical Pharmacology of the β-Adrenoceptor Blocking Drugs. East Norwalk, CT, Appleton-Century-Crofts, 1984, pp 27–50.

CARDIAC DYSRHYTHMIAS

The beta-blocking drugs have little direct antirrhythmic effects, and although membrane-stabilizing and quinidine-like actions have been demonstrated experimentally, they are only evident in doses much higher than would be achieved clinically (Table 13-6).[137] The electrophysiologic and antiarrhythmic properties of the beta-blockers are due to blockade of the beta-adrenergic receptors on SA and AV nodal tissue, which decreases the slope of phase 0 and phase 4 depolarization, reducing conduction velocity and automaticity, respectively, and increases the refractory period in AV nodal tissue.[137] These properties are therapeutic for sinus tachycardias and dysrhythmias that involve AV nodal tissue, such as paroxysmal supraventricular tachycardias, in which the AV node participates in the reentry circuit.[130] The decreased AV conduction velocity and increased AV refractory period are also useful in slowing the ventricular rate during atrial fibrillation and flutter.[130] The antiarrhythmic properties that reduce ventricular dysrhythmias during myocardial ischemia result from an amelioration in the severity of ischemia and a blockade of the electrophysiologic effects of excess catecholamines[190,193,194] (See Chapter 12).

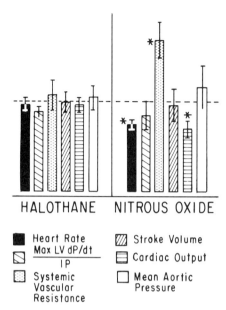

HALOTHANE   NITROUS OXIDE

■ Heart Rate   ▨ Stroke Volume
▧ Max LV dP/dt / IP   ▤ Cardiac Output
▨ Systemic Vascular Resistance   ☐ Mean Aortic Pressure

Fig. 13-19. The effect of propranolol, 0.2 mg/kg, in dogs anesthetized with a baseline halothane anesthetic (dashed line) or nitrous oxide anesthetic. Higher baseline sympathetic tone during nitrous oxide anesthesia resulted in a more pronounced effect from beta-blockade. Asterisks denote p < 0.05, significant change after propranolol. (Modified from Foex P, Prys-Roberts C: J Anaesth 46:397–404, 1974.)

PERIOPERATIVE USES OF BETA-BLOCKING DRUGS

Hemodynamic interactions with anesthetic drugs. Since the pharmacologic properties of the beta-blockers are due to receptor blockade of sympathetic stimulation, anesthetic techniques and intraoperative stimuli that induce high levels of sympathetic activity are conditions in which beta-blocking drugs have the most prominent cardiovascular effects.[135] Propranolol administration to animals during catecholamine-inducing anesthetic techniques, such as cyclopropane and nitrous oxide-based anesthesia, results in large reductions in heart rate and cardiac output and an increase in SVR due to unopposed alpha-adrenergic receptor stimulation (Fig. 13-19).[200] During experimentally induced intraoperative stress such as hypercarbia, which stimulates endogenous catecholamines, propranolol produced the same effect.[201] In contrast, 1-MAC doses of the inhalational anesthetics, halothane and isoflurane, which do not augment sympathetic tone, react less dramatically with beta-blocking drugs (Fig. 13-19).[201-203] Propranolol has a simple additive

myocardial depressant effect with these potent inhalational anesthetic drugs.[135] Propanolol administration during high-dose enflurane or enflurane plus hypovolemia has been reported to produce profound myocardial depression in dogs; however, recent information has demonstrated that propranolol or metoprolol does not substantially depress cardiac function during enflurane anesthesia.[204-206] Several recent animal and clinical studies have examined the interaction between esmolol and anesthetics. During 1-MAC enflurane anesthesia in dogs, esmolol, 300 μg/kg/min, completely blocked the isoproterenol-induced increase in heart rate; also, although left ventricular contractility was decreased, hemodynamic stability was preserved.[207] However, in this animal study, esmolol administration in higher doses (1000 and 3000 μg/kg/min) caused cardiovascular collapse and death, suggesting a relatively narrow range of safety during enflurane anesthesia.[207] Another study, which compared esmolol in awake dogs with enflurane- or halothane-anesthetized dogs, confirmed the greater hemodynamic depression by esmolol during inhalational anesthesia than in awake animals; however, there was no hemodynamic distinction between halothane or enflurane.[208]

Preoperative beta-blocker therapy. Patients presenting for CABG surgery are commonly receiving beta-blocking drugs for treatment of hypertension as well as ischemic heart disease. Controversial therapeutic recommendations in the 1970s resulted in preoperative discontinuation of chronic beta-blocker therapy because of a suspected dangerous interaction between beta-blocking drugs and anesthetics.[209] Subsequent studies reversed this recommendation and demonstrated that (1) beta-blocker withdrawal can result in perioperative hypertension, myocardial ischemia, myocardial infarction, and dangerous tachyarrhythmias; and (2) continuation of beta-blocker therapy until surgery did not increase the incidence of bradycardia, hypotension, intraoperative complications, or death.[210-213] Discontinuation of propranolol 10–48 hours preoperatively was associated with a greater rise in blood pressure and a higher incidence of postoperative dysrhythmias than when propranolol was administered on the morning of surgery and continued immediately postoperatively (Fig. 13-20).[214] A recent study of withdrawal versus maintenance of preoperative metoprolol prior to CABG surgery with neuroleptanesthesia demonstrated more preoperative and intraoperative myocardial ischemia when metoprolol was discontinued.[215] Continuation of propranolol or metoprolol until car-

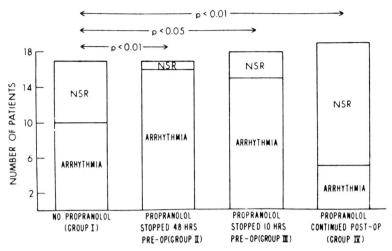

Fig. 13-20. The incidence of postoperative supraventricular arrhythmias versus normal sinus rhythm (NSR) after coronary artery bypass graft surgery in the different propranolol treatment groups. There was a significant increase in the frequency of arrhythmias in group II patients (propranolol discontinued 48 hours preoperatively) and group III patients (propranolol discontinued 10 hours preoperatively) compared with group I patients (no propranolol). Group IV patients (propranolol maintained preoperatively and postoperatively) had a significantly lower incidence of arrhythmias compared with group I patients. (From Frishman, et al: β-adrenoceptor blockade and coronary artery surgery. *In* Clinical Pharmacology of the β-Adrenoceptor Blocking Drugs. East Norwalk, CT, Appleton-Century-Crofts, 1984, pp 367–392, with permission.)

diac surgery resulted in stable hemodynamic performance during morphine, fentanyl, and sufentanil anesthesia.[215,216] Chronic preoperative propranolol therapy produced a plasma concentration-dependent attenuation in intraoperative stress-induced increases in heart rate and, to a lesser degree, arterial pressure and cardiac index (Fig. 13-21).[216]

A beta-blocker withdrawal syndrome consisting of tachyarrhythmias, hypertension, and myocardial ischemia was identified during several clinical trials of medical patients receiving beta-blocking drugs alternating with placebo.[217] A possible mechanism for this withdrawal phenomenon is a beta-blockade–induced increase in beta-adrenergic receptor density. This was demonstrated experimentally by a 43 percent increase in the beta-receptor density (measured in human lymphocytes) that developed within 5 days of propranolol administration and required 4–7 days after propranolol withdrawal to return to baseline.[218] An increase in responsiveness to isoproterenol has also been shown after discontinuation of propranolol administration to healthy volunteers.[219]

Intraoperative beta-blocker therapy. Beta-blocking drugs can be administered intraoperatively to attenuate the hemodynamic response to intraopera-

tive stress. Propranolol, metoprolol, labetalol, and esmolol are available as intravenous preparations. Propranolol will diminish the heart rate and blood pressure response to rapid-sequence endotracheal intubation.[220] The optimal time interval between propranolol (0.01 mg/kg IV) and intubation has been shown to be 5 minutes.[220] Interestingly, this does not correlate with plasma propranolol levels, suggesting a disparity between myocardial tissue levels and plasma drug levels because of rapid uptake by cardiac tissue. A labetalol infusion (0.5 mg/kg bolus followed by 0.1 mg/kg/min) begun preoperatively and continued into the operative period for cardiac surgery was found to attenuate the hemodynamic response to endotracheal intubation, but did not produce hemodynamic effects during low levels of stimulation, 5 minutes before or 5 minutes after intubation (Fig. 13-22).[221]

The unique pharmacokinetic properties of esmolol make it an extremely useful beta-blocking drug in the perioperative period.[222] The ability to rapidly titrate the desired degree of beta-blockade, maintain stable levels of blockade during the infusion, and terminate its hemodynamic effect by discontinuing the drug infusion allows for ideal treatment of intense but brief periods of stressful stimuli (Fig. 13-17 and

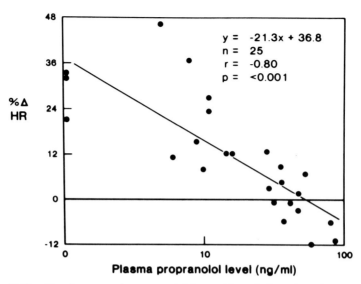

Fig. 13-21. Chronic preoperative propranolol therapy blunts the hemodynamic response to intraoperative stress as evidenced by a propranolol plasma concentration-dependent attenuation of heart rate response to maximal sternal spread. (From Sill JC, et al: Influence of propranolol plasma levels on hemodynamics during coronary artery bypass surgery. Anesthesiology 60:455–463, 1984, with permission.)

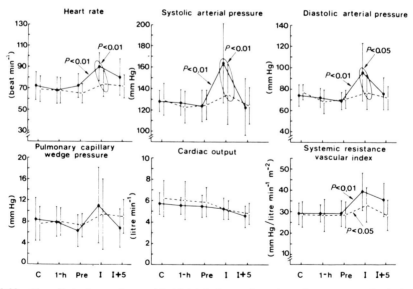

Fig. 13-22. The effect of a continuous labetalol infusion on hemodynamic response to intubation during cardiac surgery. Measurements are taken before labetalol (C), 1 hour after beginning infusion (1-h), prior to intubation (Pre), just after intubation (I), and 5 minutes after intubation (I + 5) in the placebo group (solid line) and labetalol group (dashed line). Labetalol blocked the immediate response to intubation by blocking heart rate and peripheral vasoconstriction. (Modified from Fischler M, et al: Circulatory responses to thiopentone and tracheal intubation in patients with coronary artery disease. Br J Anaesth 57:493–496, 1985.)

Control

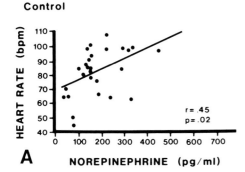

A

Esmolol

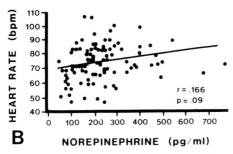

B

Fig. 13-23. Postintubation heart rate (HR) and norepinephrine (NE) levels in patients during coronary artery bypass graft surgery. There is a weak but significant association between HR and NE in untreated patients (A) but no association in patients receiving beta₁-blockade with esmolol (B). This demonstrates beta-blockade of the adrenergic response to intubation. (From Reves JG, et al: Perioperative use of esmolol. Am J Cardiol 56(11):57F–60F, 1985, with permission.)

13-23). Furthermore, since myocardial function can become severely depressed after aortic cross-clamping, esmolol obviates the inherent risk of administering long-acting beta-blocking drugs before cardiopulmonary bypass.

Three multicenter clinical studies have demonstrated that esmolol is safe during narcotic-based anesthesia and that it effectively blocks the tachycardia and hypertension during induction of anesthesia and tracheal intubation for CABG surgery, carotid endarterectomy, and other noncardiac surgical procedures. The hemodynamic effects of esmolol appear to depend on the patient's cardiovascular status, underlying sympathetic tone, concurrent anesthesia, and vasoactive drug therapy.[222] In patients who were not beta-blocked during diazepam–nitrous oxide anesthesia, esmolol infusions at doses greater than

100 μg/kg/min decreased heart rate and mean blood pressure after intubation; cardiac index and SVR did not change.[223] Esmolol also blocked the heart rate and blood pressure response to intubation during a thiopental, nitrous oxide, enflurane anesthetic for noncardiac surgery.[224] In healthy noncardiac patients, esmolol blocked the rise in heart rate and blood pressure that occurred during a ketamine induction.[225] During a stress-free interval of high-dose fentanyl anesthesia for cardiac surgery, esmolol produced no measured hemodynamic effects, demonstrating the need for stress-induced sympathetic activity in order to manifest a substantial hemodynamic effect.[226] In chronically beta-blocked patients during diazepam–enflurane anesthesia, esmolol and control groups both demonstrated minimal heart rate response to intubation indicating that esmolol is less effective in well beta-blocked patients.[227] Recently, Dagnino and Prys-Roberts demonstrated a technique for assessing the degree of beta-receptor blockade in humans during "balanced" anesthesia using intraoperative isoproterenol dose–response curves (Fig. 13-24).[228] During anesthesia, as in awake patients, preoperative cardioselective and nonselective beta-blocker therapy shifted the dose–response curve to the right. This can be a useful tool for evaluating intraoperative beta-blocker therapy.

The electrophysiologic effects of beta-blocking drugs during anesthesia have recently been evaluated. Prolongation of the Q-T interval (corrected for heart rate), which is related to duration of the action potential, has been shown to occur after succinylcholine administration and endotracheal intubation.[229] This is presumably due to increased sympathetic tone and can be dysrhythmogenic. Intravenous metoprolol, 30–40 μg/kg, decreases the Q-T interval after succinylcholine administration and intubation and reduces the incidence of ventricular dysrhythmias.[230] This antiarrhythmic effect can have therapeutic importance, especially in patients with baseline ventricular dysrhythmias or prolonged Q-T interval syndromes. Propranolol was also shown to reestablish SA nodal dominance during an accelerated AV junctional rhythm in a patient anesthetized with enflurane.[231]

The combined alpha- and beta-blocking properties of labetalol make it a potentially useful drug for intraoperative blood pressure control. Intravenous labetalol has been evaluated as a component of controlled hypotension during a halothane anesthetic.[232,233] Labetalol, 25 mg IV, during 1% halothane in patients without cardiovascular disease, caused a significant decrease in heart rate, blood

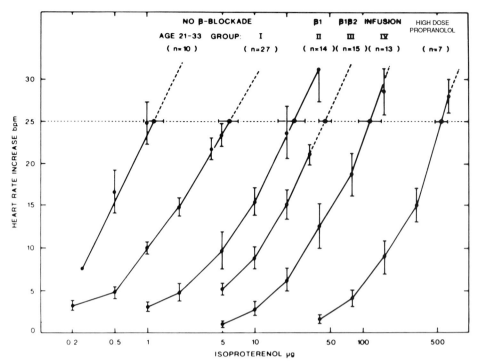

Fig. 13-24. Intraoperative isoproterenol dose–response curves used to evaluate the degree of beta-blockade in four groups of anesthetized patients: group I (no beta-blockers), group II (cardioselective beta-blockers), group III (non-cardioselective beta-blockers), and group IV (labetalol infusion). Also plotted are a group of awake controls and a group of high-dose propranolol patients from a previous study. All curves are significantly different from each other ($p < 0.01$) except between groups II and III ($p < 0.1$). (From Dagnino, et al: Anesth Analg 64:305–311, 1985, with permission.)

pressure, and SVR. Cardiac index and stroke volume were modestly reduced; however, increasing inspired halothane concentrations to 3% caused a substantial decrease in blood pressure and cardiac index and an increase in central venous pressure.[232,233] It was concluded that, provided deep levels of halothane are avoided, labetalol is a satisfactory agent for inducing hypotensive anesthesia.[232,233] Another similar study of labetalol, 30–50 mg IV, during halothane anesthesia demonstrated that the chronotropic effect persists into the postoperative period despite dissipation of the vasodilation.[232]

Postoperative indications. Propranolol therapy in the postoperative period has been shown to reduce the incidence of supraventricular tachyarrhythmias when restarted within 24 hours of CABG surgery.[234] Recently, a bolus-infusion technique for maintaining steady-state therapeutic propranolol levels after cardiac surgery has been reported.[235] Propranolol, 3 mg IV in divided doses, followed by 0.7 μg/kg/min, produced stable levels of 30–50 ng/ml and a right-

ward shift of the isoproterenol dose–response curve which was similar at 0.5 and 2 hours after beginning the infusion.[235]

Esmolol and labetalol have also been shown to be useful postoperative antihypertensive agents. Esmolol has been demonstrated to be as efficacious as SNP in patients with mild-to-moderate hypertension after cardiac surgery (Fig. 13-25).[236] During an esmolol infusion, blood pressure was reduced by a heart rate–induced decrease in cardiac output, and SVR was unchanged. In contrast, SNP reduced blood pressure by decreasing SVR. Labetalol has also been evaluated for treating postoperative hypertension following heart surgery.[237] However, unlike its effects in nonsurgical hypertensive patients in whom the antihypertensive effect of labetalol is due to a decrease in SVR, in postoperative cardiac surgical patients the antihypertensive effect is due to a decrease in cardiac index, while SVR does not change. It is suggested that postoperative cardiac surgical patients may be more sensitive to the beta-blocking effects of labetalol, so that this drug should

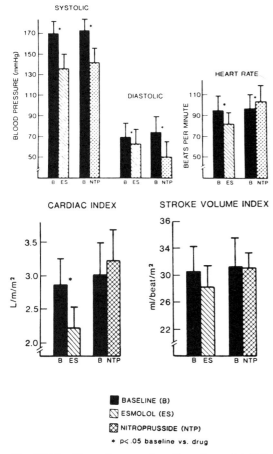

Fig. 13-25. The antihypertensive effect of esmolol (ES) compared with nitroprusside (NTP) in postoperative cardiac surgical patients. Both drugs are effective at reducing blood pressure while maintaining stroke volume. However, cardiac output is maintained by an increase in heart rate after NTP but decreases along with heart rate after ES. (Modified from Gray RJ, et al: Use of esmolol in hypertension after cadiac surgery. Am J Cardiol 56:49F–56F, 1985.)

be given with caution to patients with evidence of impaired left ventricular function.

Adverse Effects of Beta-Blocker Therapy

The adverse effects of the beta-blockers are a direct extension of their pharmacologic properties.[199] Because most of the complications are predictable, they can be minimized by avoiding beta-blockers in specific subsets of patients.

Beta-blockers can precipitate heart failure in patients who are dependent on high sympathetic tone or rapid heart rates for adequate cardiac output.[199] Patients with sinus node dysfunction can develop sinus arrest and slow idiopathic rhythms, so institution of pacing capabilities is recommended prior to pharmacologic beta-blockade in this group of patients.[199] In patients with AV node disease, beta-blockers can precipitate second-degree and third-degree heart block; however, this is rare.[199] Clinical trials indicate that beta-blockers with ISA, such as pindolol or the combined beta- and alpha-blocker labetalol, may be less likely to precipitate heart failure or heart block.[137,199]

Adverse noncardiac reactions are primarily due to the effects of beta$_2$-blockade. Bronchospasm is a primary concern, and although this is more likely to occur in patients with obstructive airway disease, it has also been reported in subjects without known lung disease.[137,199] Less of a reduction in FEV$_1$ and a greater brochodilator response to beta$_2$-agonists have been demonstrated with "cardioselective" compared with nonselective beta-blocking drugs. However, all beta-blockers should be avoided in patients requiring theophylline preparations or beta$_2$-agonists to maintain adequate bronchiolar potency.[137,155,157,199] An increase in claudication symptoms in patients with peripheral vascular disease receiving beta-blocking drugs has been reported and is probably due to a combination of beta$_1$-blockade (reduced CO) and beta$_2$-blockade (increased SVR).[137,141,199] Symptoms occur less often with pindolol, probably due to beta$_2$-agonist effects on vascular tone.[141] Adverse metabolic effects of beta-blockers involve carbohydrate and lipid metabolism. Beta-blocker therapy in diabetics may prolong the duration and mask the symptoms of hypoglycemia.[137,158,160,199] Propranolol may also inhibit insulin release in response to hyperglycemia.[137,158,199] The serum lipid profile is altered by beta-blockers as evidenced by increasing blood levels of high-density lipoprotein and triglycerides.[137] Beta-blocking drugs also decrease free fatty acid availability for skeletal muscle metabolism, which might be responsible for early exercise fatigue.[137,141] A slight increase in serum potassium may develop after beta-blockade largely due to inhibition of beta-adrenergic receptor stimulation of the skeletal muscle sodium–potassium pump; however, a fall in serum aldosterone may also be involved.[199] Nonselective beta-blocker therapy has been shown to increase serum potassium concentrations during CABG surgery.[138] This increase in serum potassium can be accentuated during stress or concomitant alpha-agonist administration.[238]

CALCIUM CHANNEL BLOCKING DRUGS

The calcium channel blocking drugs are the most recent class of compounds to join the therapeutic armamentarium of antianginal drugs. The concept of calcium antagonism as a principal mechanism of action of cardiac drugs was originated in 1964 by A. Fleckenstein who reported that verapamil "mimicked the myocardial contractile effects of simple calcium withdrawal"; ventricular contractile force is diminished without a major change in the electrical action potential.[239] Subsequent investigations demonstrated that not only were the myocardial contractile properties depressed but so were a spectrum of cardiovascular functions that require transmembrane calcium influx, specifically vascular smooth muscle contraction, and SA and AV node automaticity and conduction. After these pharmacologic properties were demonstrated with nifedipine and D600 (a methoxy-verapamil derivative), Fleckenstein designated these drugs as members of a new family of mechanistically related compounds, which he termed *calcium antagonists*.[239] Diltiazem was added to this group following its synthesis in 1975 by Nakagima in Japan.[239] The proper nomenclature of this category of drugs remains controversial; they are referred to as *calcium antagonists, calcium channel blockers, calcium-entry blockers,* and *slow-channel blockers.* This chapter uses the *Index Medicus 1986* terminology: *calcium channel blockers* or *calcium channel blocking drugs.*

Cardiovascular Calcium Physiology

Calcium plays a critical role in the regulation of cardiovascular electrophysiologic and contractile function. Initiation of cardiac and vascular contraction depends on an adequate concentration of myoplasmic calcium in the vicinity of the actin and myosin contractile elements. Although the source of this myoplasmic calcium is from the intracellular calcium storage sites (sarcoplasmic reticulum, mitochondria, transverse tubular system, and the inner surface of cell membrane), the activation of intracellular calcium release requires an influx of calcium from the extracellular fluid.[240] The influx of extracellular calcium is regulated by the calcium channels.

The calcium channels have been described as proteinaceous pores embedded within the lipid-bilayer matrix of the cardiac cell membrane (sarcoplasma).[241,242] Little is known of the molecular structure of these channels; however, certain physiologic characteristics have been elucidated and sche-

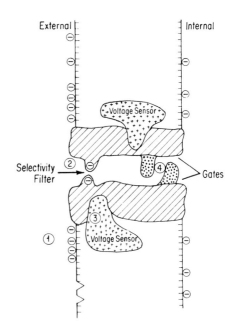

Fig. 13-26. Schematic representation of a calcium channel depicted as a proteinaceous membrane pore. A selectivity filter (2) confers ion selectivity by specific molecular dimension and charge density characteristics. Voltage sensor components (3) link membrane depolarization with channel opening and closing via the gating mechanism (4). Negatively charged sites (1) on the external surface serve as calcium (cation) binding sites. (Modified from Triggle DJ: Biochemical pharmacology of calcium blockers. *In* Flaim SF, Zelis R (eds): Calcium Blockers: Mechanisms of Action and Clinical Applications. Baltimore, Urban and Schwarzenberg, 1982, pp 121–134.)

maticized (Fig. 13-26). The calcium channel has a negatively charged site of specific dimension and charge density which functions as a "selectivity filter" producing relative specificity of the channel for calcium ions. The channel also has "voltage-sensor components" by which the electrical potential of the cell membrane influences the opening and closing of the channel through orientation of the gating mechanism. The gating mechanism also has a time-dependent characteristic that closes the calcium channel within the range of 30–300 msec.[243] The calcium channel has been termed a "slow channel" because its kinetic properties are slow relative to the "fast" sodium channel.[244] Binding of catecholamines to beta-adrenergic receptors in cardiac tissue increases the magnitude of the calcium influx by recruiting additional numbers of active calcium channels during depolarization.[245] Although calcium entry through these channels is not an energy-dependent process,

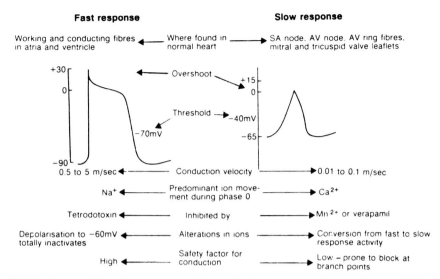

Fig. 13-27. Characteristics of fast response (sodium) and slow response (calcium) action potentials in cardiac muscle. (From Singh BN, et al: Calcium antagonists: Clinical use in the treatment of arrhythmias. Drugs 25:125–153, 1983, with permission.)

energy is required for maintenance of the channels. Myocardial ischemia and the subsequent depletion of cellular ATP results in a large influx of extracellular calcium through dysfunctional calcium channels, producing pathologic cellular calcium overload and organelle destruction.[246]

Electrical depolarization is the major stimulus for initiation of the inward calcium current in cardiac tissue. Two electrophysiologically distinct groups of cardiac tissues are represented by (1) fast-response action potentials in atrial, ventricular, and Purkinje tissue and (2) slow-response action potentials in SA and AV nodal tissue (Fig. 13-27). Depolarization of atrial, ventricular, and Purkinje tissue from their resting membrane potential of −90 mv is induced by activation of fast sodium channels and rapid sodium influx, which produces the characteristic brisk upstroke (phase 0) in the action potential.[247] As the membrane potential increases above −50 mv, the calcium channels open with relatively slow kinetic properties producing the prolonged plateau phase of the action potential.[243] The sodium channels are refractory in SA and AV nodal tissue due to a relatively high resting membrane potential of −60 mv, and membrane depolarization occurs by activation of the calcium channels as the resting membrane potential increases above −50 mv.[243,244] The inward calcium current produces a slower upstroke (phase 0) in the nodal action potential, and therefore, slower conduction velocity than in ventricular tissue. Myocar-

dial ischemia can increase the resting membrane potential in ventricular tissue. Thus, the action potential and electrophysiologic properties resemble nodal tissue with automaticity characteristics and reduced conduction velocity, which can produce dangerous ventricular dysrhythmias due to automatic foci and reentry mechanisms.[244]

The influx of extracellular calcium during depolarization stimulates a large release of intracellular calcium stores, primarily from the sarcoplasmic reticulum, which sufficiently increases the concentration of calcium in the vicinity of myofibrils to produce contraction (Fig. 13-28).[240] The magnitude of the trans-sarcoplasmic calcium influx regulates the intensity of contraction by modulating the amount of calcium mobilized from the intracellular calcium stores.[240] Activation and intensity of myofibrillar contraction is dependent on calcium concentration, beginning when the myoplasmic calcium concentration increases from 10^{-7} to 10^{-6} M and generating maximal mechanical activity at 10^{-5} M.[248] Attachment of calcium to a specific binding site on troponin releases the inhibitory effect of the troponin–tropomyosin complex from the actin filaments, thus enabling cross-bridge formation between actin and myosin. The relaxation cycle occurs by withdrawal of calcium from the myoplasm into the sarcoplasmic reticulum, which is an energy-dependent process utilizing ATP.

Braunwald has described six other mechanisms

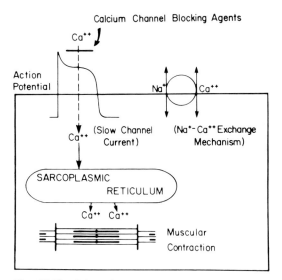

Fig. 13-28. Schematic representation of calcium influx during the plateau phase of ventricular depolarization and "calcium-triggered" calcium release from sarcoplasmic reticulum initiating muscular contraction. Calcium channel blocking drugs block Ca^{++} influx during the plateau phase of the action potential. The Na^+-Ca^{++} exchange mechanism also regulates cellular Ca^{++} levels. (Modified from Antman EM, et al: Calcium channel blocking agents in the treatment of cardiovascular disorders Part I: Basic and clinical electrophysiologic effects. Ann Intern Med 93:875–885, 1980.)

that, in addition to the calcium channels, control myoplasmic calcium concentrations:[241] (1) sodium–calcium exchange pump on the sarcolemma which pumps calcium out of the cell and is driven by the influx of sodium down its concentration gradient (Fig. 13-28); the positive inotropic effect of digitalis originates from inhibition of the sodium–potassium pump which decreases the transcellular sodium gradient; this decrease in the sodium gradient reduces the activity of the sodium–calcium pump, resulting in a greater concentration of intracellular calcium and a positive inotropic effect; (2) the sarcolemma possesses a calcium ATPase that extrudes calcium from the cell by an energy-requiring process; (3) a calcium-stimulated magnesium ATPase pumps calcium into the lumen of the sarcoplasmic reticulum, which terminates mechanical contraction; (4) calcium can also be taken up and released by the mitochondria and inner surface of the sarcolemma; (5) a variety of ionophores can transport calcium directly across the sarcolemma, down its concentration gradient; and (6) myoplasmic calcium concentrations can be buffered by binding to intracellular proteins such as troponin and calmodulin.

Calcium also regulates vascular smooth muscle contraction; however, less is known about the calcium cycle in vascular tissue than in cardiac tissue. Potential-dependent calcium channels (PDCs) and

STIMULUS-CONTRACTION COUPLING EVENTS IN VASCULAR SMOOTH MUSCLE

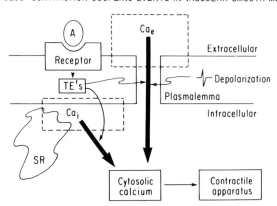

Fig. 13-29. Schematic representation of alpha-agonist (A)–stimulated receptor-operated Ca^{2+} channels (ROCs), which primarily increase cytosolic Ca^{2+} by releasing Ca_i from the sarcoplasmic reticulum (SR). Stimulation of ROC also increases extracellular Ca^{2+} (Ca_e) influx. Transduction events (TEs) represent the link between receptor stimulation and calcium mobilization. Membrane depolarization causes Ca_e influx via potential-dependent Ca^{2+} channels. (Modified from Ratz PH, et al: Species and blood vessel specificity in the use of calcium for contraction. *In* Flaim SF, Zelis R (ed): Calcium Blockers: Mechanisms of Action and Clinical Applications. Baltimore, Urban and Schwarzenberg, 1982, pp 77–98.)

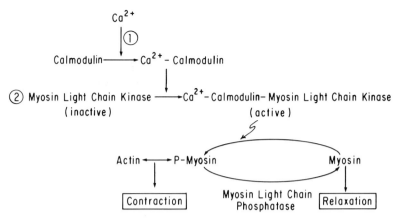

Fig. 13-30. The activation sequence of mechanical contraction in vascular smooth muscle. The calcium (Ca^{++}) calmodulin complex (1) activates myosin light chain kinase (2), which catalyzes the phosphorylation of myosin (P-myosin). Cross-bridge formation between P-myosin and actin produces mechanical contraction. (From Andersson KE, et al: On the mechanism of action of calcium antagonists. Acta Med Scand [Suppl] 681:11–24, 1984, with permission.)

receptor-operated calcium channels (ROCs) have been described that represent electromechanical and pharmacomechanical coupling, respectively (Fig. 13-29).[241] When stimulated by membrane depolarization, PDCs initiate vasoconstriction via an influx of extracellular calcium. Stimulated by alpha-adrenergic agonists, ROCs primarily increase myoplasmic calcium concentrations by a direct release of intracellular calcium stores (from the sarcoplasmic reticulum) and only to a minor extent by an influx of extracellular calcium.[249] The relative importance of extracellular calcium influx from ROC stimulation varies among different vascular beds. This may be a major factor in determining the response of the vessel to calcium channel blocking drugs, since the calcium channel blockers affect the influx of extracellular calcium but do not affect the release of intracellular calcium except in concentrations well above the clinical range.[241,249] Canine epicardial coronary artery constriction in response to norepinephrine, which is due to an influx of extracellular calcium, can be effectively blocked by calcium channel blocking drugs.[249] In contrast, rabbit vertebral artery constriction in response to norepinephrine, which is due to a direct release of intracellular calcium, is difficult to antagonize with calcium blockers.[249]

The intracellular regulatory protein of vascular smooth muscle contraction is not troponin (which is not present in vascular smooth muscle), but calmodulin, a calcium-binding protein (Fig. 13-30).[250] An increase in intracellular calcium concentration pro-duces increasing levels of the calcium–calmodulin complex. Calcium–calmodulin–dependent phosphorylation of the light chain of myosin is the regulatory step for initiating actin–myosin interactions in vascular smooth muscle. Vascular relaxation is produced by myosin light chain phosphatase, which dephosphorylates the myosin light chain, decoupling actin and myosin. The decrease in myoplasmic calcium is accomplished by activation of pumps, such as sodium–potassium ATPase, calcium ATPase, or the sodium–calcium exchange system.[251]

Cellular Mechanism of Action of Calcium Channel Blocking Drugs

Calcium channel-blocking drugs are structurally dissimilar compounds that are grouped due to their influence on transmembrane calcium conductivity. According to Fleckenstein, five pharmacologic prerequisites determine drug placement into this class of compounds;[239] calcium channel blocking drugs should produce (1) a selective decrease of calcium-dependent myocardial contractile energy expenditure without a major effect on the sodium-dependent ventricular action potential; (2) a dose-dependent inhibition of SA node automaticity and AV node conduction; (3) a reduction in vascular smooth muscle contractility, particularly in coronary and systemic arterial vessels; (4) an antianginal effect; and (5) a direct protective effect against ischemic myocardial damage.[239] All three of the calcium channel blocking drugs presently available in the United States (verapamil, nifedipine, and diltiazem) satisfy these five pharmacologic properties. In contrast to the binding of beta-blocking drugs to a uniform cellular receptor, however, the structural variability of the calcium channel blockers is consistent with different modes and sites of action.[251] The heterogeneity of calcium channel blocker binding sites in cardiac tissue has been evaluated using nimodipine (a nifedipine derivative) as a membrane receptor marker. Specific binding of nimodipine to the sarcolemma was found to be competitively inhibited by nifedipine, partially inhibited by verapamil, and stimulated by diltiazem, suggesting distinct, albeit related, sites of action.[252] Electrophysiologic studies demonstrate that verapamil alters the kinetics of the calcium channels by slowing the activation and inactivation kinetics of the gating mechanism of the calcium channel.[241,252] The potency of verapamil and, to a lesser extent, diltiazem, is frequency dependent, such that the more rapid the cardiac cycling the more potent will be the effect of these drugs on transmembrane calcium influx.[241,252] Diltiazem and verapamil also appear to preferentially block inactivated calcium channels. In contrast, nifedipine blocks calcium channels independent of activation state or frequency of depolarization.[241,252]

The ability of the calcium channel blocking drugs to inhibit calcium influx into vascular smooth muscle has been well documented. Although still controversial, recent evidence indicates that calcium channel blocking drugs preferentially inhibit postsynaptic alpha$_2$-adrenergic stimulation of vascular smooth muscle.[253,254] The potency of the vasodilating effects of the calcium channel blockers in various vascular beds depends on the extent to which transmembrane calcium influx (versus mobilization of intracellular calcium stores) is the result of ROC stimulation.[249,255] Vascular smooth muscle in the arteriolar beds is more sensitive than in the venous beds to the effects of calcium channel blockers, and the arteries in the coronary circulation appear to be the most sensitive.[249]

Cardiovascular Effects of Calcium Channel Blocking Drugs

ELECTROPHYSIOLOGIC EFFECTS

Since SA and AV nodal cells depend on calcium influx for depolarization, it is not surprising that verapamil, nifedipine, and diltiazem inhibit the elec-

Table 13-7

Comparative Cardiovascular Effects of the Calcium Channel Blocking Drugs

	Diltiazem	Nifedipine	Verapamil
Heart rate	↓	reflex ↑	↑ or ↓
AV nodal conduction rate	↓	− or reflex ↑	↓↓
LV contractility	−	− or reflex ↑	↑ or ↓
Peripheral vasodilation	+	+ + +	+ +
Coronary vasodilation	+ + +	+ + +	+ +

Modified from Ram CVS: Southwestern internal medicine conference: Calcium antagonists in the treatment of hypertension. Am J Med Sci 290(3):118–133, 1985.

trophysiologic properties of these tissues. In isolated tissue preparations, all calcium channel blocking drugs decrease the rate of spontaneous diastolic depolarization and increase the membrane threshold potential, which effectively decreases the rate of spontaneous firing of nodal tissue (negative chronotropy). The rate of rise and overshoot of the nodal action potential are also decreased, which slows conduction velocity (negative dromotropy).[239,256,257] High concentrations of calcium channel-blocking drugs will actually cause a standstill of impulse generation from SA and AV nodal tissue.[239,256]

Despite similar direct electrophysiologic effects in isolated tissues, important distinctions exist among these compounds when administered to intact animals and humans (Table 13-7). A drug-induced reduction in systemic blood pressure can increase sympathetic and decrease parasympathetic tone to the heart, which counteracts direct negative chronotropic and dromotropic effects. Therefore, the relative potencies of the electrophysiologic versus the peripheral vascular effects of the calcium channel blocking drugs are important. An extensive review of the literature by Mitchell et al has comprehensively compared the electrophysiologic effects of verapamil, nifedipine, and diltiazem in humans.[257]

Diltiazem produces the most potent negative chronotropic effect, with an approximate 10 percent reduction in heart rate. Nifedipine and, to a lesser extent, verapamil result in a reflex increase in heart rate. These reflex increases in heart rate are seen more commonly with acute administration. Chronic administration of nifedipine does not affect heart rate, while diltiazem and verapamil produce either no change or a slight reduction.[257] However, verapamil, like diltiazem, can produce a large reduction in heart rate including sinus arrest in patients with SA node disease.

Both verapamil and diltiazem slow antegrade and retrograde conduction through the AV node by approximately 15–25 percent during fixed-rate pacing.[257] Despite equal depression of conduction, however, verapamil increases AV nodal refractoriness more than diltiazem. This property has been used to explain the greater incidence of first-degree and second-degree AV block with verapamil. In contrast, nifedipine facilitates AV nodal conduction by 14 percent during fixed-rate pacing and reduces the AV nodal refractory period. This has been ascribed to increased autonomic tone by a reduction in blood pressure from nifedipine.[239,256,257]

The calcium channel blocking drugs do not produce a clinically significant effect on conduction velocity or refractoriness of normal atrial, ventricular, or Purkinje tissue.[257] Although they tend to shorten the plateau phase of the action potential, this is not reflected in clinical electrophysiologic characteristics. However, membrane depolarization in ischemic ventricular tissue may be dependent on slow calcium influx, and measurable electro-physiologic effects can be demonstrated from the calcium channel-blocking drugs, ie, decreases in automaticity and conduction velocity and an increase in refractoriness.[243]

HEMODYNAMIC EFFECTS

Calcium channel-blocking drugs influence cardiovascular hemodynamics through direct effects on myocardial contractility, SA and AV nodal conduction, and vascular smooth muscle tone. Isolated heart tissue preparations and specific animal models that maintain a constant contraction rate, preload, and afterload demonstrate that all calcium channel blockers directly depress myocardial contractility in a dose-dependent fashion.[239,256,257] This is believed to be due to a reduction in available intracellular calcium necessary to release the inhibition of troponin–tropomyosin from actin and myosin.[241,258] However, since vasodilatation also alters cardiac performance (by affecting afterload and reflex autonomic tone), evaluation of the direct negative inotropic effects of these drugs becomes complex in the intact organism. The importance of sympathetic responses to calcium channel blocker–induced vasodilation is demonstrated in pentobarbital-anesthetized animal preparations in which diltiazem, nifedipine, and verapamil do not cause myocardial depression until institution of beta-blockade with propranolol.[259,260]

The net hemodynamic effects of calcium channel blockers in intact animals and humans depend on the drugs' relative potency for each distinct cardiovascular function (Table 13-7). In the whole-animal preparation, nifedipine induces vasodilation at lower dosage than is necessasry to produce negative chronotropic, dromotropic, and inotropic effects.[261] In the therapeutic dose range, the resultant vasodilation produces a reduction in afterload and a reflex sympathetic discharge, which overrides any direct negative chronotropic, dromotropic, and inotropic actions.[261] The resultant hemodynamic profile is similar to a pure vasodilator; cardiac output, heart rate, and AV nodal conduction rate usually increase. In contrast, verapamil and diltiazem have a similar potency on AV nodal conduction and vasodilation.[260,261] The negative dromotropic effect of verapamil is more potent than that of diltiazem; however, in a dose range that produces electrophysiologic effects (increase in P-R interval), vasodilation occurs, and only minimal changes in contractility are evident with either drug.[258,259] As the dosage increases, more pronounced systemic vasodilatation may occur, but the reflex-induced increase in sympathetic tone is not sufficient to offset the negative dromotropic effect.[258] When given in equipotent coronary vasodilating doses in dogs, verapamil and diltiazem cause a prolongation of AV conduction time, whereas nifedipine decreases AV nodal conduction time.[257] The negative inotropic effects are more prominent with verapamil than diltiazem, and myocardial depression may develop when verapamil is given to patients with baseline cardiac dysfunction.[260]

Pharmacokinetics of the Calcium Channel Blocking Drugs

VERAPAMIL

Verapamil is rapidly and extensively absorbed from the gastrointestinal tract, undergoes extensive first-pass hepatic metabolism (85 percent of the absorbed drug), and is highly protein bound in human plasma (Table 13-8). Plasma levels of the demethylated and dealkylated metabolites of verapamil may be twice as high as those of the parent drug, and one, nor-verapamil, contributes about 15 percent of the hemodynamic effects of the drug.[261] From a single oral dose, measurable effects on AV conduction time are evident within 30 minutes, and

Table 13-8
Pharmacokinetic Features of Calcium Channel Blocking Drugs

Drug	Available Form	Average Elimination Half-life (hr)	Metabolism Metabolite Activity, and Excretion	Dosage
Diltiazem	30- and 60-mg tablets	4–5	Hepatic metabolism; metabolites partially active; 70 percent gastrointestinal excretion	Initial: 30 mg four times daily; maximum: 240 mg/day (possibly higher)
Nifedipine	10-mg capsules	3–4 (wide individual variation)	Hepatic metabolism; inactive metabolites; 80 percent renal excretion	Initial: 10 mg three or four times daily; maximum: 120–180 mg/day
Verapamil	Injectable solution	3–7	Hepatic metabolism; active metabolites; 70 percent renal excretion	IV: bolus of 0.075–0.15 mg/kg (average in adults: 5–10 mg): maintenance infusion of 0.005 mg/kg/min;
	80- and 120-mg tablets			oral: initial: 80 mg three or four times daily; maximum: 480 mg/day

Modified from Ram CVS: Southwestern internal medicine conference: Calcium antagonists in the treatment of hypertension. Am J Med Sci 290(3):118–133, 1985.

peak blood levels occur in 1–2 hours.[262] When administered by rapid intravenous injection, verapamil serum levels fall in a biexponential pattern with a distribution half-life of 3.5 minutes and an elimination half-life of 110.5 minutes.[263] After intravenous injection, the peak vasodilatory effects occur by 5 minutes and return to baseline by 30 minutes; but the antiarrhythmic effects, also appearing in 5 minutes, may remain 6 hours later, suggesting preferential binding of verapamil to the AV nodal tissue.[262] It has been suggested that racemic verapamil undergoes stereospecific presystemic hepatic metabolism with preferential clearance of the more active (−) isomer. This explains the requirement for two to three times higher plasma verapamil levels after oral than after intravenous drug administration in order to produce an equivalent prolongation in the P-R interval. Because of the unrestricted high-efficiency hepatic extraction, verapamil kinetics exhibit flow-dependent hepatic metabolism, so that drugs that reduce liver blood flow (eg, halothane) will prolong the elimination half-life.[263] Verapamil has also been shown to increase plasma digoxin levels by about 60

percent during chronic administration of both drugs, leading to the recommendation to reduce digoxin doses.[264]

For the treatment of supraventricular dysrhythmias, the recommended dose is a single bolus injection of 5–10 mg (0.075–0.15 mg/kg) over 1–3 minutes while monitoring the electrocardiogram and blood pressure.[261,262,265] A second dose may be safely repeated in 30 minutes, and, if continuous blood levels are desired, an infusion of 0.005 mg/kg/min may be necessary. The dose should be reduced in patients with myocardial dysfunction. The initial dose for oral therapy is 40–80 mg every 8 hours, which may be increased over 2–3 days to the usual daily dose of 240–360 mg, with a maximum dose of 480 mg daily.

NIFEDIPINE

Nifedipine, like verapamil, is almost completely absorbed from the gastrointestinal tract, undergoes first-pass hepatic metabolism (40 percent of absorbed drug), and is strongly protein bound (91–99 percent) (Table 13-8).[266] Approximately 80 percent of the hepatic metabolites, which are inactive, are excreted by the kidneys, and 20 percent are excreted via the gastrointestinal tract. When administered orally, nifedipine appears in the plasma in 20 minutes with peak concentrations occurring in 1–2 hours. When administered via the sublingual route, it is rapidly absorbed through the buccal mucosa and has an onset of action of 5–10 minutes.[266] A single intravenous bolus of nifedipine, 0.5–1.0 mg, produces vasodilation almost immediately, and the effects dissipate in approximately 10 minutes.[266] Bolus administration results in a redistribution half-life of 13 minutes and an elimination half-life of 1.3 hours. After oral administration, a third phase with a half-life of about 8 hours prolongs the duration of effect.[266] Nifedipine is highly unstable when exposed to light, and, although this has hampered pharmacokinetic studies in the past and complicates intravenous drug handling and administration, it does not appear to affect kinetic properties. However, the effect of light transmission to the blood via cardiopulmonary bypass apparatus has not yet been evaluated.

The usual starting dose is 10 mg orally or sublingually three times a day. The dose is then increased until desired results are achieved or until unwanted side effects, usually hypotension, are encountered. The maximum oral dose recommended is 120 mg daily.[266] In certain patients, the drug must be administered every 4 hours or symptoms will recur between doses. Intravenous nifedipine can be administered as a bolus of 10–20 μg/kg and maintained as an infusion of 1–3 μg/kg/min.

DILTIAZEM

Orally administered diltiazem is rapidly and extensively absorbed (95 percent); however, due to efficient first-pass hepatic metabolism, the absolute bioavailability is 40 percent (Table 13-8).[267] Elimination occurs primarily via the liver, with only 0.4 percent excreted unchanged by the kidneys. After oral administration, diltiazem first appears in the blood in 15 minutes, and peak concentrations occur after 60–90 minutes.[267] Onset of action is within 30 minutes after oral administration, and it has an elimination half-life of 4–5 hours. The major metabolite, desacetyldiltiazem, has 25–50 percent of the pharmacodynamic activity of diltiazem, but low blood levels of this metabolite during chronic therapy result in minimal hemodynamic effects.[267] A significant relationship has been demonstrated between plasma concentration and antianginal efficacy.[268] Patients with poor therapeutic response had blood levels of less than 100 ng/ml, while responders had levels between 100 and 200 ng/ml.[268] The usual oral dose

of diltiazem is 30–60 mg every 8 hours; however, when necessary, the dosage has been increased to 120 mg 3 times daily.

Therapeutic Uses of Calcium Channel Blocking Drugs

EXERTIONAL ANGINA

Numerous clinical trials have demonstrated that diltiazem, nifedipine, and verapamil reduce the frequency of angina attacks, nitroglycerin usage, and ischemic ECG changes in patients with exertional angina.[269-271] These antianginal properties of the calcium channel blocking drugs have been ascribed to three basic effects: (1) a decrease in myocardial oxygen demand; (2) an improvement in myocardial blood flow by direct coronary vasodilation; and (3) a cardioprotective effect during transient myocardial ischemia (see acute myocardial infarction below).[272,273] Although still controversial, the antianginal effects are usually ascribed more to a decrease in myocardial oxygen demand than an increase in myocardial oxygen supply (Fig. 13-31). In fact, calcium channel blocking drugs often produce a decrease in coronary sinus blood flow, as well as in oxygen consumption at rest and during atrial pacing.[274] These measurements of global myocardial blood flow, however, do not preclude an increase in regional blood flow, which has been demonstrated in jeopardized regions of myocardium.[275]

A decrease in systolic ventricular wall tension (afterload) is the major mechanism by which the calcium channel blockers reduce myocardial oxygen demand.[261] Unlike nitrates, which reduce ventricular wall tension by venodilating or reducing preload, the calcium channel blockers reduce afterload by arterial dilation.[276] Chronic use of the calcium channel blocking drugs does not produce a substantial decrease in heart rate; in fact, it may occasionally increase with nifedipine.[257] Although individual patients occasionally experience a beneficial reduction in heart rate with high doses of diltiazem or verapamil,[257] this does not appear to be their major antianginal mechanism. Calcium channel blockers directly depress contractility in isolated tissue; however, the increase in reflex sympathetic tone due to vasodilation usually offsets any direct negative inotropic effect. Ischemic heart disease can also produce abnormalities in ventricular diastolic function with an impairment in myocardial relaxation, which can decrease subendocardial perfusion. An improvement in diastolic relaxation has been demonstrated with

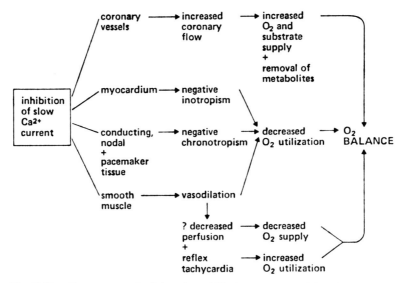

Fig. 13-31. Consequences of calcium channel blockers on myocardial O_2 balance. Due to reflex responses, negative chronotropism and inotropism may not be important. (From Nayler WG, Dillon JS, Daly MJ: Cellular sites of action of calcium antagonists and β-adrenoceptor blockers. *In* Prospectives in Cardiovascular Research, Vol 9. Calcium Antagonists and Cardiovascular Disease. 1984, pp 181–191, with permission.)

verapamil and nifedipine, which may reflect reduced subendocardial ischemia, alterations in left ventricular loading conditions, or primary myocardial effects on cellular calcium flux.[277]

Calcium channel blockers can have adverse hemodynamic effects in anginal patients. Excessive vasodilation, especially with nifedipine, can produce hypotension and reflex tachycardia.[276,277] Verapamil administration to patients with baseline left ventricular dysfunction can severely reduce contractility and compromise myocardial perfusion pressure due to left ventricular distension and systemic hypotension.[260]

All calcium channel blocking drugs are also potent coronary arterial dilators and can improve oxygen delivery to ischemic myocardial tissue. The calcium channel blockers have been shown to block epicardial coronary vasoconstriction, especially in areas of fixed stenosis, in response to alpha-adrenergic stimulation.[48] An improvement in collateral blood flow to ischemic myocardium has been demonstrated,[278] and it has been claimed that these drugs may accelerate the formation of new collateral vessels.[275,279] Preliminary data also suggest that calcium channel blockers can increase the generation of prostacyclin in the coronary circulation.[280] The vasodilatory and antiplatelet effects of prostacyclin may contribute to the antianginal properties of the calcium channel blocking drugs.

VARIANT ANGINA AND UNSTABLE ANGINA PECTORIS

Coronary spasm is the principal cause of myocardial ischemia in patients with variant angina.[7] The underlying mechanism for the increased coronary vasomotion with variant angina is controversial; however, thromboxane A_2 and platelet-releasing factors, as well as decreased production of or sensitivity to the vasodilator prostacyclin, have been implicated. An enhanced responsiveness to alpha-adrenergic stimulation by epicardial coronary vessels may also be important.[11,48,276] It has also been postulated that the primary abnormality may be due to increased sarcolemma calcium stores, which could result in a greater rise in intracellular calcium on stimulation of vascular smooth muscle.[281]

Conventional therapy for ischemic heart disease with nitrates and beta-blockers is not necessarily optimal for the treatment of coronary vasospastic disease, which may exist alone (variant angina) or as a component of unstable angina. Although sublingual or IV NTG is efficacious in preventing or relieving coronary spasm, the prophylactic use of long-acting nitrates is not as reliable.[282] Propranolol, beneficial for treating ischemia due to increased oxygen demand, may potentiate coronary spasm by blocking beta-adrenergic receptors and allowing for alpha-adrenergic neurogenic dominance of the coronary

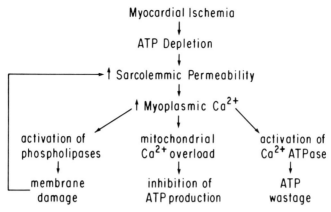

Fig. 13-32. ATP depletion from myocardial ischemia results in a massive Ca^{++} influx, which further augments ischemic tissue injury.

vessels.[185] The potent coronary vasodilating properties of the calcium channel blockers suggest their efficacy for the treatment of variant and unstable angina.[48] Diltiazem, nifedipine, and verapamil all relieve anginal symptoms in patients with unstable angina.[283] In a well-controlled, randomized, double-blind study, the addition of nifedipine to a regime of nitrates and propranolol decreased anginal symptoms and improved outcome.[284] Calcium channel blockers are extremely effective and often superior to nitrates for prophylactic therapy of coronary spasm.[285] They reduce the frequency of variant angina attacks, the need for sublingual NTG, and the occurrence of ST-segment changes.[283] Dangerous ventricular dysrhythmias associated with variant angina also respond to calcium channel blocker therapy.[285] There are few studies that compare the effectiveness of the three clinically available calcium channel blockers for the treatment of variant angina. Nifedipine and verapamil produce similar relief from symptoms and reduction in ST-segment changes.[286] One study suggests less efficacy from verapamil than nifedipine or diltiazem; however, the drugs were not compared in the same patients.[287]

ACUTE MYOCARDIAL INFARCTION

During the evolution of an acute myocardial infarction, sarcolemmic permeability increases, allowing a massive influx in extracellular calcium (Fig. 13-32).[246] Cellular ATP stores are rapidly depleted because mitochondrial calcium uptake impairs mitochondrial energy production, and enhanced activity of calcium-activated ATPases accelerates ATP utilization.[246] The influx of extracellular calcium also activates intracellular phospholipases, leading to severe sarcolemmal injury and irreversible structural damage.[246] Since initial calcium entry during ischemia is via the calcium channels, the calcium channel blockers may be protective.[273,283] Experimental evidence demonstrates a protective effect of calcium channel blockers during brief periods of ischemia; however, they are less effective during prolonged ischemia, which produces generalized destruction of the sarcolemma and cellular organelles. When given to animals before or soon after onset or ischemia, nifedipine reduces the extent of irreversible myocardial injury; verapamil reduces ischemic contracture, mitochondrial calcium overload, and infarction size; and diltiazem reduces reperfusion injury.[273,283]

Initial clinical trials with calcium channel blocker administration shortly after onset of acute myocardial infarction have not demonstrated substantial beneficial effects. Two large clinical studies (337 patients) of nifedipine administration within 5–12 hours of onset of infarction symptoms failed to demonstrate cardiac enzyme evidence of myocardial salvage.[284,285] Verapamil administered within 8 hours and continued for 2 days postinfarction, however, reduced enzyme estimation of infarct size.[283] Further studies need to investigate the potential ability of specific calcium channel blocking drugs for improving pharmacologic salvage in conjunction with emergency reperfusion procedures utilizing thrombolytic drugs and percutaneous transluminal coronary angioplasty.

CARDIAC ANTIARRHYTHMICS

The antiarrhythmic properties of calcium channel blocking drugs can be correlated with their electrophysiologic effects.[257,265] The predominant effect of verapamil and diltiazem is slowing conduction

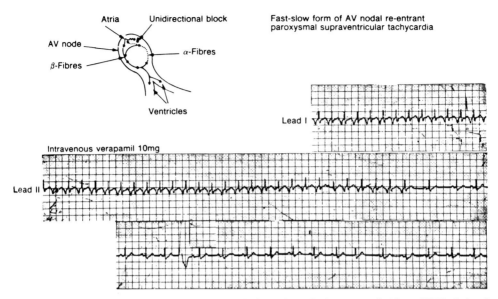

Fig. 13-33. An example of conversion of supraventricular tachycardia by verapamil, 10 mg IV Blockade of alpha fibers converts unidirectional block to bidirectional block, terminating the reentry circuit. (Modified from Singh BN: Calcium antagonists: Clinical use in the treatment of arrhythmias. Drugs 25:125–153, 1983.)

through the AV node with prolongation of the refractory period.[257] Automaticity of the SA node is usually not affected in intact animals and humans.[257] Verapamil and diltiazem terminate paroxysmal supraventricular tachycardia (SVT) and slow the ventricular response to atrial fibrillation and flutter.[265] Chronic oral therapy provides prophylactic therapy for SVT and controls ventricular response to atrial fibrillation and flutter[265] (See Chapter 12).

Most paroxysmal SVT occurs as a result of intranodal reentrant mechanisms. The AV node develops functional longitudinal dissociation of conduction pathways, one having a longer conduction time than the other.[265] When the faster pathway develops anterograde block, conduction occurs only down the slow fibers, and the fast pathway is stimulated in a retrograde fashion, which then cycles back down the slow pathway to create the reentry mechanism of SVT. There is now increasing agreement that intravenous verapamil, 10–15 mg, is the drug of choice for terminating SVT with narrow QRS complex (Fig. 13-33).[265] Recent clinical trials also demonstrate that intravenous diltiazem (the intravenous form is not presently available for clinical use) is also effective; however, its efficacy has not been compared with that of verapamil. It has been reported by Singh et al that the success rate of verapamil can be improved to almost 100 percent by simultaneous carotid massage or the addition of intravenous edrophonium, 5–10 mg, immediately after verapamil administration.[265] Preexcitation syndromes, like Wolff-Parkinson-White, are most responsive to verapamil if the antegrade pathway involves the AV node. However, if atrial fibrillation or flutter complicates preexcitation syndromes, the negative dromotropic effects of calcium channel blockers on the AV node may facilitate anterograde traffic through an accessory pathway, which can precipitate ventricular tachycardia and fibrillation.[265]

SYSTEMIC ARTERIAL HYPERTENSION

Chronic systemic arterial hypertension is usually due to an augmentation in systemic vascular resistance. Like other vasodilators, the calcium channel blockers decrease arterial blood pressure by relaxing arteriolar smooth muscle (Fig. 13-34).[288] The forearm resistance vessels have been found to be more sensitive in hypertensive patients than normotensives to the dilating effect of verapamil.[288,289] This may be due to enhanced activity of the potential-dependent calcium channels in hypertensives, which is believed to be one of the basic functional disorders in essential hypertension.[289] Blockade of these augmented potential-dependent channels and inhibition of postsynaptic alpha$_2$-adrenergic receptor–mediated vasoconstriction by the calcium channel blocking drugs are two proposed mechanisms of their antihypertensive effects.[253,254,286] Clinical trials have demonstrated

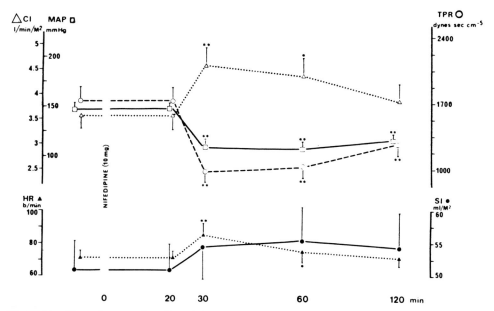

Fig. 13-34. The antihypertensive effect of nifedipine is demonstrated from 17 patients with essential hypertension. Blood pressure (MAP) reduction is produced by a decrease in total peripheral resistance (TPR). Cardiac index (CI) and heart rate (HR) increase while stroke index (SI) does not significantly change (single and double asterisks denote significant differences from pre-nifedipine at p < 0.05 and p < 0.01, respectively). (From Guazzi MD: Use of the calcium channel blocking agents in the treatment of systemic arterial hypertension. *In* Stone PH, Antman EM (eds): Calcium Channel Blocking Agents in the Treatment of Cardiovascular Disorders. New York, Futura Publishing Company, 1983, pp 377–401, with permission.)

that diltiazem, nifedipine, and verapamil are all effective in decreasing blood pressure when used as sole antihypertensive agents.[267,286] Their antihypertensive effects are also additive with beta-blocking drugs, alpha-methyldopa, and thiazide diuretics.[267,286] Sublingual nifedipine (10–20 mg) has also been found to be effective in malignant hypertensive crisis.[288]

OTHER POTENTIAL CLINICAL INDICATIONS

Pulmonary hypertension may be exacerbated by varying degrees of reversible pulmonary arteriolar constriction.[290] Clinical studies indicate clinical improvement from calcium channel blocking drugs.[290] Nifedipine decreases pulmonary arterial pressure and pulmonary vascular resistance in patients with chronic obstructive lung disease.[290] The magnitude of the reduction in pulmonary arterial pressures correlates with the severity of baseline hypoxemia.[289] A number of studies have also demonstrated favorable results in patients with primary pulmonary hypertension.[290] If pulmonary hypertension has already compromised the right ventricle, however, a further decompensation in right ventricular

function may develop after nifedipine despite a decrease in pulmonary vascular resistance. The long-term effectiveness and safety of calcium channel blockers for treating pulmonary hypertension remains to be established, particularly with regard to the effects on right ventricular function.[290]

Calcium channel blocking drugs may exert a favorable effect on bronchospastic lung disease since many of the pathophysiologic events are calcium-dependent processes.[291] Nifedipine and verapamil attenuate bronchoconstriction due to exercise, histamine, and antigens.[291] Bronchodilation may be due to a direct effect on bronchial smooth muscle as well as an inhibition of calcium-dependent mediator release from activated mast cells.[291] Unfortunately, the protective effects in patients with exercise-induced asthma appear to be modest.[291] Although presently available calcium channel blockers are not highly effective for treating bronchospastic lung disease, new calcium channel blockers may be developed with more specific effects on bronchial smooth muscle and mast cells. Their lack of *adverse* pulmonary effects, however, makes calcium channel blockers (as opposed to beta-blockers) excellent antianginal drugs for coronary artery patients with bronchospastic lung disease.

Recent information reveals that, like myocardial ischemia, *cerebral* ischemia is heralded by an influx of extracellular calcium, which is associated with a precipitous decrease in intracellular levels of ATP.[292,293] Cerebral vasospasm, a contributing factor to neuronal damage, often accentuates cerebral ischemia by preventing adequate reperfusion. Calcium channel blockers may provide therapeutic benefits during cerebral injury by preventing postischemic cerebral vasospasm and reducing ischemic cellular injury.[293] Nimodipine, a nifedipine analogue, prevents spasm of cerebral arteries in rabbits.[293] In patients with acute ischemic strokes, intravenous nimodipine was associated with a dose-dependent increase in blood flow to the ischemic hemisphere.[292] Nimodipine, administered after a 17-minute episode of complete cerebral ischemia, improved the neurologic outcome in monkeys.[294] Although prompt restoration of cerebral perfusion pressure is of paramount importance for minimizing ischemic cerebral damage, new analogues of calcium channel blockers may prove useful for minimizing brain damage resulting from severe hemodynamic instability during cardiac surgery.

PERIOPERATIVE USES OF THE CALCIUM CHANNEL BLOCKING DRUGS

Hemodynamic interactions with anesthetic drugs. Since the calcium channel blocking drugs rely on reflex responses of the autonomic nervous system to establish their net pharmacodynamic profile, the interaction between these drugs and anesthetic agents must be appreciated from an understanding of direct drug effects, as well as of the effect of general anesthesia on reflex autonomic response. Additionally, the halogenated inhalational anesthetic drugs have pharmacologic properties similar to the calcium channel blocking drugs. Halothane decreases the rate of firing of SA nodal tissue and prolongs AV nodal conduction,[295,296] which could enhance the negative chronotropic and dromotropic properties of verapamil and diltiazem. Direct myocardial depression from halogenated inhalational anesthetics may be due to the same mechanism of action as the calcium channel blockers, ie, an inhibition of trans-sarcolemmal calcium influx;[297,298] however, there is also evidence of effects on intracellular calcium flux at the sarcoplasmic reticulum and the actinomyosin ATPase system.[299,300] These effects on myocardial calcium flux may augment the negative

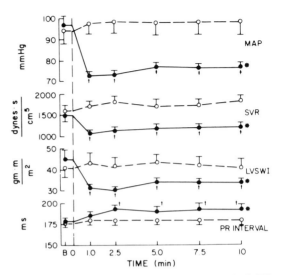

Fig. 13-35. Cardiovascular effects of verapamil, 0.075 mg/kg (solid lines), versus placebo (broken lines) during narcotic-based anesthesia for coronary artery bypass surgery in patients with normal baseline cardiac function. Blood pressure (MAP) reduction is produced by a decrease in systemic vascular resistance (SVR), while cardiac output did not change (not shown). The P-R interval increased but no patient progressed beyond a first-degree AV block. LVSWI = left ventricular stroke work index. (t = p < 0.005 from baseline; * = p < 0.05 between groups over time). (From Kates RA, et al: Cardiovascular responses to verapamil during coronary artery bypass graft surgery. Anesth Analg 62:821–826, 1983, with permission.)

inotropic effects of the calcium channel blockers. Halothane, like calcium channel blocking drugs, also directly relaxes vascular smooth muscle, although the mechanisms may differ. While calcium channel blockers are less effective in attenuating the norepinephrine-stimulated receptor-operated calcium channels on vascular smooth muscle, halothane effectively blocks norepinephrine-induced contraction of vascular smooth muscle.[301] Furthermore, attenuation of carotid baroreceptor function by inhalational anesthetics can blunt the increased reflex sympathetic tone that normally accompanies a decrease in blood pressure from the calcium channel blocking drugs.[302]

Intravenous verapamil, 5 mg, has been administered to patients with normal cardiac conduction and myocardial function during a narcotic-based anesthetic technique for CABG surgery (Fig. 13-35).[303] The major hemodynamic effect of verapamil prior to cardiopulmonary bypass was peripheral vasodilation and a moderate reduction in blood pressure; CO and

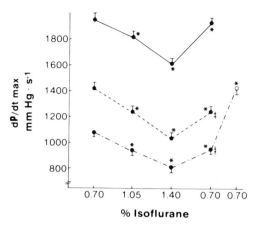

Fig. 13-36. In this canine right-heart bypass preparation, the dose-dependent myocardial depression (left ventricular dP/dt max) by isoflurane alone is shown (solid line; $p < 0.001$). This myocardial depression is enhanced in a dose-dependent manner by low-dose (broken line) and high-dose (broken line with dots) verapamil ($p < 0.05$). Calcium chloride (o) partially reversed the inhibition of isoflurane plus verapamil. (From Kates RA, et al: Hemodynamic interactions of verapamil and isoflurane. Anesthesiology 59(2):132–138, 1983, with permission.)

PCWP did not change.[303] Although the P-R interval increased, first-degree AV block did not occur, and all patients tolerated the remainder of surgery without problems.[303] From this study and multiple clinical experiences, it appears that verapamil can be safely administered intraoperatively to patients with normal cardiac function during a narcotic anesthetic.[304] Drug interaction studies between verapamil and halogenated inhalational anesthetics yield more cautious conclusions. A canine right-heart bypass preparation was used to evaluate the direct myocardial effects of verapamil during an isoflurane anesthetic (Fig. 13-36). In this preparation, heart rate and rhythm, preload, and mean arterial pressure were held constant. The depression in left ventricular function produced by isoflurane was augmented in a dose-dependent fashion by verapamil. A reduction in isoflurane levels or administration of calcium chloride partially reversed the combined myocardial depression of isoflurane and verapamil. In the intact animal, verapamil was evaluated during nitrous oxide, halothane, isoflurane, and enflurane anesthetics.[305–308] Although conflicting data exist, these studies demonstrate that verapamil administration to dogs and swine can produce dose-dependent myocardial depression during halothane anesthesia, as evidenced by a decrease in CO and left ventricular pressure

development (dP/dt) and an increase in PCWP.[306,308] In contrast, during nitrous oxide analgesia in swine, verapamil produced an increase in CO and a decrease in SVR.[306] Verapamil administration during inhalational anesthetics may decrease blood pressure by reducing CO, not SVR. This might be partially explained as a hypotensive-stimulated increase in plasma catecholamines that antagonizes the vasodilation but not the myocardial depression from verapamil. In a canine study, verapamil appears to be less well tolerated during enflurane than during isoflurane or halothane anesthesia (Fig. 13-37).[307] Cardiac dysfunction in the enflurane group was also associated with a high incidence of AV conduction disturbances.[307] In contrast to these animal studies, verapamil has been administered during CABG surgery to patients anesthetized with halothane, and it produced a transient decrease in blood pressure and SVR while CO was maintained.[309] In this study, a decrease in coronary perfusion pressure demonstrated that the vasodilation might cause myocardial ischemia.[309]

Although nifedipine does not depress the heart in vivo, it does have direct myocardial depressant properties in vitro. The direct cardiac effects of halothane plus nifedipine in the isolated rat heart produced additive negative inotropic effects.[310] However, in intact animals anesthetized with fentanyl, nifedipine produced a hemodynamic profile similar to sodium nitroprusside, ie, vasodilation and an increase or no change in heart rate and cardiac output.[311] Increasing the depth of halothane anesthesia from 1 MAC to 2 MAC decreases the reflex-induced increase in heart rate after nifedipine, indicating that higher concentrations of halothane attenuate autonomic reflex responses (Fig. 13-38).[312] The importance of autonomic reflexes was further demonstrated by abolishment of the nifedipine-induced increase in heart rate during halothane anesthesia by pretreatment with propranolol.[313] Nifedipine has been administered intraoperatively during narcotic and inhalational anesthetic (halothane and isoflurane) techniques; with each technique, nifedipine decreased blood pressure by vasodilation and cardiac output was maintained.[314,315] Intravenous nifedipine (7.5 μg/kg) administered to halothane-anesthetized patients with normal global left ventricular function, prior to surgical incision for CABG surgery, produced a slight decrease in left ventricular dP/dt and MAP; however, the mild myocardial depression was offset by a decrease in SVR resulting in no change or an increase in CO.[316] In beta-blocked patients, heart rate does not change, or increases slightly, but in patients who

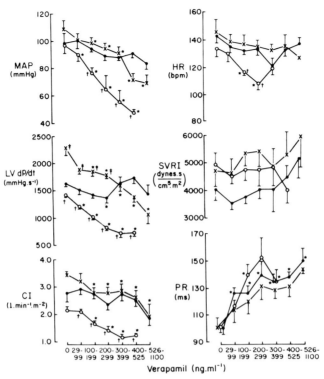

Fig. 13-37. Comparison of the hemodynamic effects of increasing verapamil levels during 1-MAC enflurane (open circles), halothane (filled circles), and isoflurane (crosses) anesthesia in dogs. During enflurane anesthesia, verapamil produced a significantly greater reduction in mean arterial pressure (MAP), left ventricular (LV) dP/dt, cardiac index (CI), and heart rate (HR) compared with the other two groups (+, p < 0.05 enflurane compared with both halothane and isoflurane). (From Kapur PA, et al: Comparison of cardiovascular responses to verapamil during enflurane, isoflurane, or halothane anesthesia in the dog. Anesthesiology 61:156–160, 1984, with permission.)

were not beta-blocked, the reflex increases in heart rate can be substantial. An excessive decrease in blood pressure accompanied by a reflex increase in heart rate can produce myocardial ischemia in patients with CAD.

The interaction between diltiazem and inhalational anesthetics has been evaluated in isolated tissue and intact animal studies. The maximum force of contraction of isolated guinea pig atria was depressed to a greater extent by the combination of diltiazem plus isoflurane than by either drug alone.[317] Isoflurane-anesthetized dogs receiving diltiazem infusions to produce clinically relevant blood levels (157 ± 13 ng/mg) experienced a prolongation in the P-R interval and a slight decrease in left ventricular dP/dt, but no significant changes in heart rate, blood pressure, or cardiac output.[318] Increasing diltiazem blood levels (250–400 ng/ml) resulted in a progression of the negative dromotropic effects to second-

degree heart block in some animals. Similar diltiazem blood levels caused a prolongation in the P-R interval and second-degree heart block but no reduction in dP/dt or CO in dogs receiving fentanyl (100 μg/kg/hr).[319] Although clinical evaluations of the hemodynamic interaction between diltiazem and anesthetic agents are lacking, these animal studies indicate that if diltiazem becomes available for intravenous administration, it may produce minimal hemodynamic effects during general anesthesia provided that safe drug dosages are used and the patient does not have SA or AV nodal dysfunction. In summary, since the pharmacodynamic properties of the calcium channel blocking drugs are dependent on direct tissue effects plus reflex responses to vasodilation, the resultant hemodynamic profiles during anesthesia depend on the direct cardiovascular effects of the anesthetic plus its effect on baroreceptor reflexes (Fig. 13-39).

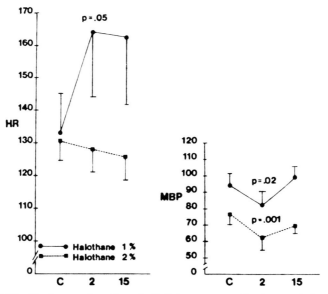

Fig. 13-38. The hypotensive effect of nifedipine causes a reflex increase in heart rate during 1 percent halothane in dogs. However, 2 percent halothane prevented the reflex increase in heart rate despite a similar reduction in blood pressure from nifedipine. (Modified from Tosone SR, et al: Hemodynamic responses to nifedipine in dogs anesthetized with halothane. Anesth Analg 62:903–908, 1983.)

Preoperative calcium channel blocker therapy. As with the beta-blocking drugs, several studies have evaluated the safety and hemodynamic consequences of maintenance of calcium channel blocker therapy until surgery. It was initially recommended to withdraw patients from nifedipine prior to cardiac surgery because of suspected severe hypotension during fentanyl induction.[320] However, a subsequent study demonstrated no difference between patients who did and did not receive preoperative nifedipine.[321] A prospective randomized trial with nifedipine withdrawal for 24 hours versus nifedipine

administration until the time of surgery demonstrated a greater need for vasodilators after cardiopulmonary bypass in the nifedipine-withdrawal group compared with the group maintained on nifedipine until surgery (58 percent versus 14 percent, respectively).[322] This may be due to maintenance of vasodilation or a possible rebound vasoconstrictor state in the patients who were withdrawn from nifedipine 24 hours preoperatively. Isolated human coronary arteries have demonstrated a state of hyperresponsiveness to constrictor stimuli following nifedipine withdrawal.[323] Withdrawal of diltiazem therapy in the preoperative

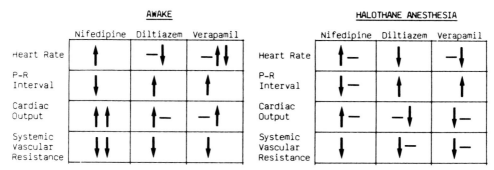

Fig. 13-39. Theoretical hemodynamic profiles of the calcium channel blocking drugs in awake subjects versus during halothane anesthesia. Effect on variables are designated as follows: ↑, increase; ↓, decrease, —, no change. When multiple symbols are present, the initial designated effect is most likely to occur.

period has been associated with possible coronary spasm after coronary revascularization.[324] A prospective randomized study evaluated the effects of preoperative diltiazem therapy on hemodynamic performance during CABG surgery in fentanyl-anesthetized patients.[325] Systemic vascular resistance during cardiopulmonary bypass was lower in patients receiving diltiazem until surgery compared with patients who had diltiazem withheld 12 hours before surgery, but the lower blood pressure was responsive to phenylephrine. There were no other hemodynamic differences between the groups. These studies indicate that calcium channel blockers can be safely continued preoperatively. Beneficial effects on myocardial oxygenation, protection against myocardial ischemic injury, and possible prevention of postcardiopulmonary bypass coronary spasm are all possible advantages of maintenance of calcium channel blocker therapy until surgery.

Intraoperative antiarrhythmic uses. Intravenous verapamil has been successfully used for the treatment of intraoperative SVT; however, its potential pharmacologic interactions with various anesthetic drugs must be appreciated. Evidence also indicates that halothane-induced ventricular dysrhythmias may be caused by reentry ventricular circuits, especially in the presence of elevated catecholamine levels. Verapamil and diltiazem both protect against epinephrine-induced ventricular dysrhythmias in halothane-anesthetized dogs, as well as in halothane-anesthetized dogs receiving aminophylline infusions.[306,326,327] Alpha-adrenergic stimulation and an increase in MAP have been implicated as possible mechanisms of epinephrine-induced ventricular dysrhythmias. The antiarrhythmic effects of verapamil and diltiazem might involve these two dysrhythmogenic mechanisms, since calcium channel blockers decrease arterial blood pressure and block the vasoconstricting effects of postsynaptic alpha-adrenergic stimulation.[253,254] Diltiazem decreased the incidence of spontaneous ventricular dysrhythmias during narcotic as well as inhalational anesthetics.[327] Verapamil has also been shown to terminate refractory ventricular fibrillation following removal of the aortic cross-clamp during cardiopulmonary bypass.[328]

Intraoperative antihypertensive uses. The antihypertensive effects of intravenous nifedipine have been evaluated during cardiac surgery. An intravenous bolus of nifedipine, 400 μg, administered to hypertensive fentanyl-anesthetized patients prior to

cardiopulmonary bypass, controlled blood pressure within 1 minute with a 36 percent decrease in SVR, while CO and heart rate increased 14 percent and 12 percent, respectively.[315] Hemodynamic effects returned to baseline within 10 minutes. Nifedipine infusion (2–5 μg/kg/min) was found to be as effective as SNP for treating hypertension during fentanyl-nitrous oxide anesthesia for cardiac surgery (Fig. 13-40).[329] Both drugs reduced blood pressure to baseline values within 3 minutes by decreasing SVR. In contrast to SNP, nifedipine significantly increased stroke volume index (23 percent). This difference in stroke volume may be due to a reduction in PCWP (left ventricular underloading) with SNP and to no change in the nifedipine group. Its antihypertensive effectiveness, preservation of cardiac function, and potential beneficial effects on ischemic myocardial tissue might make intravenous nifedipine an important antihypertensive for patients with CAD. Intravenous nifedipine is presently in clinical trials and may be released for clinical use in the near future. As with other vasodilators, such as NTG and SNP, a reduction in hypoxic pulmonary vasoconstriction, which can increase pulmonary shunting, must be considered, especially in patients with pre-existing lung disease.[330]

Intraoperative myocardial preservation. All three clinically available calcium channel–blocking drugs have been evaluated as myocardial protective agents prior to ischemia and as adjuncts to cold potassium cardioplegia during aortic cross-clamping for cardiac surgery.[331] The theoretical benefits of incorporating calcium channel blockers in standard cardioplegic solutions may be due to (1) preservation of ATP during ischemia by a reduction in energy utilization; (2) protection against mitochrondrial dysfunction from calcium overload; (3) coronary vasodilation, which may improve cardioplegic delivery; and (4) a decreased incidence of reperfusion dysrhythmias.

Animal studies show that the combination of nifedipine and potassium cardioplegia reduces postischemic myocardial edema and improves diastolic relaxation and systolic contractile function.[332] A recent clinical study incorporating nifedipine into cardioplegic solutions during cardiac surgery demonstrated an improvement in left ventricular stroke work index after bypass and a significant reduction in low cardiac output death.[333] Nifedipine, administered at the end of bypass, has also been shown to correct diastolic dysfunction (severe noncompliance) and to allow termination of cardiopulmonary bypass

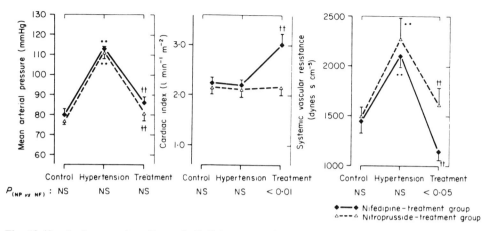

Fig. 13-40. Antihypertensive effects of nifedipine versus nitroprusside during cardiac surgery. Both drugs effectively reduced blood pressure; however, cardiac output was higher in the nifedipine group despite similar heart rates (not shown). The difference in cardiac output between the treatment groups may be due to a 38 percent decrease in left ventricular filling pressure in the nitroprusside group but no change in the nifedipine group (not shown). The symbols are as follows: *, $p < 0.05$, and **, $p < 0.01$, between control and hypertension; and +, $p < 0.05$, and ++, $p < 0.01$, between hypertension and treatment periods. (From Hess W, et al: Nifedipine versus nitroprusside for controlling hypertensive episodes during coronary artery bypass surgery. Eur Heart J 5:140–145, 1984, with permission.)

after aortic valve replacement in a patient with hypertrophic cardiomyopathy.[334] Numerous animal trials have demonstrated that verapamil preserves cellular ATP stores, mitochondrial function, and cardiac performance after global ischemia.[335,336] However, the clinical efficacy of verapamil as an additive to cold potassium cardioplegia is highly controversial. In high-risk cardiac surgical patients, verapamil was associated with improved postischemic cardiac function; however, a recent evaluation of verapamil cardioplegia in patients with normal global left ventricular function undergoing CABG surgery demonstrated no benefit and an increased incidence of transient AV nodal block and inotropic requirements.[337] The additon of diltiazem to cardioplegia solutions in animals improved preservation of left ventricular function and intracellular levels of creatine phosphate, but an impairment in ATP production was noted after reperfusion.[338]

Intraoperative myocardial ischemia and coronary artery spasm. Intraoperative myocardial ischemia refractory to NTG has been reported to respond to intravenous verapamil, 7.5 mg (Fig. 13-41).[339,340] These cases may represent coronary spasm during CABG surgery. Coronary artery spasm occurring immediately after CABG surgery has been effectively treated by intravenous and intracoronary NTG followed by nifedipine, 30 mg, via nasograstric

tube; however, in some cases, I.V. NTG might prove ineffective and systemic calcium channel blockers might be required.[341,342]

Adverse Effects of Calcium Channel Blocker Therapy

These potent cardiovascular drugs can produce a spectrum of adverse cardiovascular effects, which are usually due to (1) an extension of their pharmacologic properties; (2) an interaction with concomitant drug therapy; or (3) an underlying disease process (Table 13-9).

A review of 262 studies encompassing 8072 patients receiving verapamil has revealed a 9 percent incidence of adverse effects, with severe reactions requiring discontinuation of the drug in 1 percent of patients.[262] Oral verapamil is well tolerated and has a very low incidence of gastric intolerance or constipation (gastrointestinal motility is calcium dependent). Intravenous administration occasionally produces hypotension and disturbances in AV node conduction. Serious adverse hemodynamic effects such as severe hypotension, bradycardia, and, rarely, ventricular asystole have occurred from drug overdose or pre-existing ventricular dysfunction, conduction disturbances, or severe hypertrophic cardiomyopathies.[343]

Because of its potent negative dromotropic

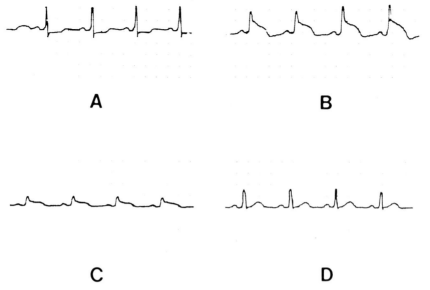

Fig. 13-41. Treatment of nitroglycerin-refractory myocardial ischemia with verapamil: (A) preinduction, (B) after intravenous nitroglycerin during apparent coronary artery spasm, (C) after verapamil, 2.5 mg IV; and (D) after verapamil, 7.5 mg IV, total dose. (From Nussmeier N, et al: Verapamil treatment of intraoperative coronary artery spasm. Anesthesiology 62:539–541, 1985, with permission.)

effects, verapamil should be used cautiously with beta-adrenergic–blocking drugs and digitalis preparations. Asystole attributed to intravenous verapamil has been reported in two patients pretreated with digitalis and practolol (a beta-blocker available in Europe).[344] Hypotension and myocardial depression can also occur due to the combined negative inotropic effects of verapamil and beta-blockers.[262] Cau-

tion also should be used when verapamil is administered with other antiarrhythmics. Patients receiving verapamil and disopyramide, an antiarrhythmic with myocardial depressant properties, have developed profound hypotension.[345] Adverse reactions due to the negative inotropic effect of verapamil are usually amenable to therapy with calcium chloride or other inotropic drugs, such as epinephrine

Table 13-9
Side Effects of Antianginal Drugs

	Hypotension, Flushing, and Headache	Left Ventricular Dysfunction	Decreased Heart Rate and Atrioventricular Block*	Gastrointestinal Symptoms	Bronchoconstriction†
Beta-blockers	0	+ +	+ + +	+	+ + +
Nitrates	+ + +	0	0	0	0
Diltiazem	+	+	+	0	0
Nifedipine	+ + +	0	0	0	0
Verapamil	+	+	+ +	+ +	0

Key: 0, absent; +, mild; + +, moderate; + + +, sometimes severe.
*In patients with sick-sinus syndrome or conduction system disease.
†In patients with obstructive lung disease.
From Braunwald E: Mechanism of action of calcium channel blocking agents. N Engl J Med 307:1618, 1982, with permission.

or isoproterenol.[346] Bradycardias or high-degree AV block do not respond well to calcium and may require isoproterenol or temporary cardiac pacing.[346]

A review of 5008 patients receiving chronic nifedipine therapy revealed that side effects, usually related to the drug's potent vasodilatory action, occurred quite frequently, with a rate of 17 percent.[347] Headache occurred in 5.9 percent of patients, a sensation of heat and facial flush in 5.1 percent, dizziness in 2.7 percent, and hypotension, palpitations, or peripheral edema in 1.6 percent. Adverse gastrointestinal problems, including nausea and vomiting, were noted in 5.2 percent. In only a low percentage of patients (4.7 percent), adverse reactions caused discontinuance of therapy. Since its major side effect is hypotension, the drug should be used with caution in patients who are concurrently receiving other vasodilators.

In a review of diltiazem therapy in 7884 patients, adverse effects appeared to be infrequent (3.9 percent).[267,281] Cardiovascular side effects, facial flushing, and bradycardia occurred in 1 percent of patients, gastrointestinal disturbances in 1 percent, and dizziness and headache in 0.4 percent. A hypersensitivity drug rash developed in 1.3 percent of patients. Diltiazem should be given carefully to patients with disturbances in cardiac conduction. AV block has been reported when the drug is administered concurrently with beta-blockade or digitalis toxicity although this is rare.[267]

Recent evidence suggests that calcium channel blockers may potentiate the effects of neuromuscular blocking drugs. The direct effects of calcium channel blockers on neuromuscular function are quite controversial. Although Kraynack et al have demonstrated a dose-related depression of skeletal muscle twitch to indirect stimulation in various animal species, others have shown no effects or even facilitation of neuromuscular transmission by the calcium channel blocking drugs.[348-351] Some animal studies, however, indicate that verapamil potentiates pancuronium. Verapamil, in clinically relevant doses, enhanced the twitch depression produced by succinylcholine and pancuronium in rabbits.[350] It is suggested that verapamil may affect ion conductance at the postsynaptic acetylcholine-activated channels on the muscle fiber.[350] It is also possible that verapamil, which has local anesthetic potency, might possess a presynaptic depressant effect on nerve conduction.[262] A case report has described a patient receiving chronic verapamil therapy who had a prolonged neuromuscular blockade following pancuronium (2 mg) and tubocurarine (5 mg), which was resistant to neostigmine,

but promptly responded to edrophonium, 0.5 mg/kg.[352] Another case was reported of acute respiratory failure due to muscle weakness following intravenous verapamil in a patient with Duchenne's muscular dystrophy.[353] These clinical case reports and animal studies suggest that verapamil may reduce skeletal muscle reserve in the perioperative period when administered to patients with neuromuscular disease or in conjunction with neuromuscular blockers.

Although verapamil has been recommended as adjunctive therapy for malignant hyperthermia, recent evidence indicates that calcium channel blockers are probably not effective for treating malignant hyperthermia and that potentially dangerous drug interactions may develop between verapamil and dantrolene.[354,355] In the isolated guinea pig heart, verapamil and dantrolene produced additive myocardial depression.[356] In chloralose-anesthetized swine, the combined administration of both drugs was associated with marked hyperkalemia and cardiovascular collapse.[357] These experimental studies suggest that verapamil should not be administered to malignant hyperthermia patients treated with dantrolene.

COMBINATION ANTIANGINAL THERAPY

Each class of antianginal drugs—nitrates, betablockers, and calcium channel blockers—has distinct mechanisms of action that improve the myocardial oxygen balance (Table 13-10). Their pharmacologic profiles include distinct hemodynamic properties, as well as detrimental effects (Tables 13-9 and 13-10). Combinations of these compounds have pharmacologic appeal because the effects of one drug can be used to counterbalance the detrimental effects and complement the beneficial properties of another drug.[272,276]

The physiologic reflex responses of nitrates and nifedipine, tachycardia and increased inotropy, are clearly detrimental in patients with ischemic heart disease. The negative chronotropic and inotropic activity of the beta-blockers effectively counteracts these reflex responses (Fig. 13-42). The beneficial hemodynamic effects of the nitrates and calcium channel blockers also appear to be complementary. Nitrates reduce preload, which decreases ventricular wall tension (radius times pressure) by a reduction in ventricular volume (radius); while calcium channel blockers are primarily arterial dilators, which decrease systolic wall tension by decreasing systolic ventricular pressure and frequently increasing ejec-

Table 13-10

Comparative Effects of Nitrates, Beta-Blockers, and Calcium Channel
Blockers on Determinants of Myocardial Oxygen Uptake and Coronary Blood Flow

	Nitrates	Beta-Blockers	Calcium Channel Blockers		
			Diltiazem	*Verapamil*	*Nifedipine*
Myocardial oxygen uptake					
Contractility	NC ↑	⬇	NC	NC ↓	NC ↑
Heart rate	↑	⬇	NC ↓	↓↑	↑
LV wall tension					
Volume	⬇	↑	?	NC ↑	↓
Systolic pressure	↓	↓	↓	↓	↓
Diastolic pressure	⬇	↑	NC	NC ↑	NC
Coronary blood flow					
Aortic pressure	NC ↓	↓	↓	↓	↓
Coronary resistance	⬇	↑	⬇	⬇	⬇
Epicardial artery size	⬆	↓	↑↑	↑↑	↑↑

Small arrow, minor effect; two small arrows, moderate effect; large arrow, major effect; NC, no change;
NC↑, no change or increase; NC↓, no change or decrease; ↑↓, increase or decrease.
Source: Modified from Conti; Perspectives in Cardiovascular Research, vol 9. 1984.

tion fraction due to a decrease in SVR (Table 13-11). The combination of decreased preload and afterload produces a major reduction in myocardial oxygen consumption. The myocardial depressant effects of beta-blockers, which produce an increase in left ventricular volume, are potentially detrimental in patients with left ventricular dysfunction.[187] This can be offset by combination therapy with nitrates or calcium channel blockers due to their effects on preload and SVR, respectively.[358] Patients with mild conduction abnormalities may also tolerate the combination of nifedipine and beta-blockers better than beta-

blockers alone.[276] Direct vascular effects are also complementary in that NTG is a more potent epicardial coronary arterial dilator, while calcium channel blockers strongly inhibit epicardial coronary arterial constriction (coronary spasm) in response to alpha-adrenergic stimuli and serotonergic coronary receptor stimulation (Table 13-12).[48]

Recent clinical reports have demonstrated the beneficial effects of combination antianginal drug therapy. Several well-designed clinical trials have shown that the addition of nifedipine to patients receiving nitrates and beta-blocking drugs results in

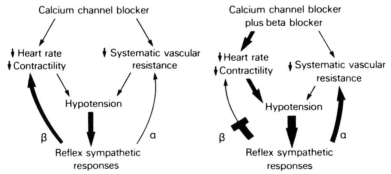

Fig. 13-42. Direct hemodynamic effects (downward arrows) and reflex responses (upward arrows) from calcium channel blockers alone (A) and in combination with beta-blockers (B). (From Leon MB: Combination therapy with calcium channel blockers and beta-blockers for chronic stable angina pectoris. Am J Cardiol 55:69B–80B, 1985, with permission.)

Table 13-11

Comparative Drug Effects on Global and Regional Left Ventricular
Function During Exercise (Versus Control) in Patients With Ischemic Heart Disease

	Global LV Function								Regional LV Function		
	HR	SBP	DBP	PAPD	CI	TVR	EF	EDVI	NL	ISCH	SCAR
Nitroglycerin	(↑)	—	(↓)	↓	—	—	(↑)	(↓)	—	↑	—
Nifedipine	↑	↓	↓	↓	↑	↓	(↑)	—	—	↑	—
Metoprolol	↓	↓	—	↑	(↓)	↑	—	—	↓	(↑)	—

Significant group differences are represented by different symbols: arrows indicate changes versus control; arrows in parentheses indicate changes that are significant by single comparison but not by multiple group comparison. Abbreviations: LV, left ventricular; HR, heart rate; SBP, systolic blood pressure; DBP, diastolic blood pressure; PAPD, pulmonary artery diastolic pressure; CI, cardiac index; TVR, total vascular resistance; EF, ejection fraction; EDVI, end-diastolic volume index; NL, normal segment; ISCH, ischemic segment; SCAR, scar segment; ↑, increase; ↓, decrease; —, no significant change versus control.

From Pfisterer M, et al: Comparative effects of nitroglycerin, nifedipine and metoprolol on regional left ventricular function in patients with one-vessel coronary disease. Circulation 67:291, 1983, with permission.

Table 13-12

Effects of Nitrates Versus Calcium Channel Blockers in
Vascular Smooth Muscle Relaxation

	Nitrites and Nitrates	Ca^{++} Blockers
Large extramural coronary arteries	+ + + +	+ + +
Coronary arterioles	Only in high doses with intracoronary, not sublingual, administration	With low doses s.l., orally, and IV
Venous system	+ + + +	None
Eccentric stenoses	Short (1 hr)	Long (3–4 hr)
Coronary spasm	+ +	+ + + +
Mechanism	Intracellular sequestration of Ca^{++}; induction of cGMP	Inhibition of Ca^{++} influx into the cell; no effect on Ca^{++} efflux

Key: strong effect, + + + +; moderate effect, + + +; mild effect, + +.

Modified from Lichtlen PR, Engel H-J, Rafflenbeul W: Calcium entry blockers, especially nifedipine, in angina of effort: Possible mechanisms and clinical implications. In Opie LH (ed): Perspectives in Cardiovascular Research, vol 9. 1984, pp 221–236.

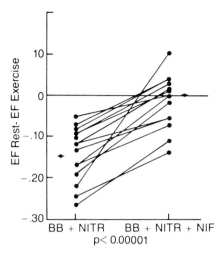

Fig. 13-43. The decrease in global ejection fraction (EF) from rest to exercise is an index of inducible or reversible myocardial ischemia. The addition of nifedipine (NIF) to maximal angina therapy with beta-blockers (BB) plus nitrates (NITR) produced a significant reduction in exercise-induced ischemia (EF Rest − EF Exercise). (From Nesto RW, et al: Addition of nifedipine to maximal beta-blocker-nitrate therapy: Effects on exercise capacity and global left ventricular performance at rest and during exercise. Am J Cardiol 55:3E–8E, 1985, with permission.)

improved relief of anginal symptoms and improved left ventricular function at rest and during exercise (Fig. 13-43).[261,284,359,360] Since patients presenting for CABG surgery frequently receive maximum medical therapy including nitrates, beta-blockers, and calcium channel blocking drugs, the cardiovascular effects of combined antianginal drug therapy as well as the pharmacology of the individual drugs must be appreciated by the anesthesiologist.

REFERENCES

1. Heberden W: Some account of a disorder of the breast. Med Trans Coll Phys (Lond) 2:59, 1772
2. Cohn P, Braunwald E: Chronic ischemic heart disease. *In* Braunwald E (ed): Heart Disease: A Textbook of Cardiovascular Medicine. Philadelphia, WB Saunders, 1984, pp 1334–1393
3. Levine HJ: Difficult problems in the diagnosis of chest pain. Am Heart J 100:108, 1980
4. Del Banco PL, Del Bene E, Sicuteri F: Heart Pain. *In* Bonica JJ (ed): Advances in Neurology, vol 4. New York, Raven Press, 1974, pp 375–381
5. Mountcastle VB: Pain and temperature sensibilities. *In* Bonica JJ (ed): Medical Physiology (ed 13). St. Louis, CV Mosby, 1974
6. Epstein SE, Cannon RO, Talbot TL: Hemodynamic principles in the control of coronary blood flow. Am J Cardiol 56:4E–10E, 1985
7. Conti CR: Large vessel coronary vasospasm: Diagnosis, natural history and treatment. Am J Cardiol 55:41B–49B, 1985
8. Cannon RO, Watson RM, Rosing DR, et al: Angina caused by reduced vasodilator reserve of the small coronary arteries. J Am Coll Cardiol 1:1359–1373, 1983
9. Cannon RO, Leon MB, Watson RM, et al: Chest pain and "normal coronary arteries"—Role of small coronary arteries. Am J Cardiol 55:50B–60B, 1985
10. Epstein SE, Talbot TL: Dynamic coronary tone in precipitation, exacerbation and relief of angina pectoris. Am J Cardiol 48:797–803, 1981
11. Vatner SF: Regulation of coronary resistance vessels and large coronary arteries. Am J Cardiol 56:16E–22E, 1985
12. Szekeres L, Udvary E: Haemodynamic factors influencing myocardial ischaemia in a canine model of coronary artery stenosis: The effects of nitroglycerin: Br J Pharmacol 79:337–345, 1983
13. Brunton TL: Use of nitrite of amyl in angina pectoris. Lancet 2:97–98, 561–564, 1857
14. Needleman P: Biotransformation of organic nitrates. *In* Needleman P (ed): Organic Nitrates. Berlin, Heidelberg, New York, Springer 1975, pp 57–95
15. Murrell W: Nitroglycerin as a remedy for angina pectoris. Lancet 1:80–81, 1879
16. Viljoen JF: Anaesthesia for internal mammary implant surgery. Anaesthesia 23:515–520, 1968
17. Kaplan JA, Dunbar RW, Jones EL: Nitroglycerin infusion during coronary artery surgery. Anesthesiology 45:11–21. 1976
18. Fleckenstein A, Nakayama K, Fleckenstein-Grun G,

et al: Interactions of vasoactive ions and drugs with Ca-dependent excitation-contraction coupling of vascular smooth muscle. *In* Carafoli E, Clementi F, Drabikowski W, et al. (eds): Calcium Transport in Contraction and Secretion. Amsterdam, Oxford, New York, Elsevier-North-Holland, 1975, pp 555–566

19. Abshagen U: Organic nitrates. *In* Abshagen U (ed): Clinical Pharmacology of Antianginal Drugs, vol 76. Berlin, Heidelberg, New York, Tokyo, Springer-Verlag, 1985, pp 287–364

20. Needleman P, Jarschik B, Johnson EM: Sulfhydril requirement for relaxation of vascular smooth muscle. J Pharmacol Exp Ther 187:324–331, 1973

21. Axelsson KI, Wikberg JES, Andersson RGG: Relationship between nitroglycerin, cyclic GMP, and relaxation of vascular smooth muscle. Life Sci 24:1779–1786, 1979

22. Katsuki S, Arnold WP, Murad F: Effects of sodium nitroprusside, nitroglycerin and sodium azide on levels of cyclic nucleotide. J Cyclic Nucleotide Res 3:239–247, 1977

23. Zsoter TT, Henein NF, Willchinsky C: The effect of sodium nitroprusside on the uptake and efflux of calcium from rabbit and rat vessels. Eur J Pharmacol 45:7–12, 1977

24. Karashima T: Actions of nitroglycerin on smooth muscles of the guinea pig and rat portal veins. Br J Pharmacol 69:489–497, 1980

25. Bassenge E, Holtz J, Kinadeter H, et al: Threshold dosages of nitroglycerin for coronary artery dilatation, afterload reduction and venous pooling in conscious dogs. *In* Lichtlen PR, Engel HJ, Schrey A, et al (eds): Nitrates III. Berlin, Heidelberg, New York, Springer, 1981, p 238

26. Stiefel A, Kreye VAW: On the haemodynamic differences between sodium nitroprusside, nitroglycerin, and isosorbide nitrate: Comparison of their vasorelaxant effects in vitro and of their inactivation in vivo. Naunyn Schmiedebergs Arch Pharmacol 325:270–274, 1984

27. Imhof PR, Ott B, Frankhauser P, et al: Difference in nitroglycerin dose-response in the venous and arterial beds. Eur J Clin Pharmacol 31:193–199, 1981

28. Gerson H, Allen FB, Seitzer JL, et al: Arterial and venous dilation by nitroprusside and nitroglycerin— Is there a difference? Anesth Analg 61:256–260, 1982

29. Brymer JF, Stetson PL, Walton JA, et al: Correlation of hemodynamic effects and plasma levels of nitroglycerin. Clin Res 27:229A, 1979

30. Fung HL, Sutton SC, Kamiya A: Blood vessel uptake and metabolism of organic nitrates in the rat. J Pharmacol Exp Ther 228:334–341, 1984

31. Staurer BE, Scherpe A: Ventricular function and coronary hemodynamics after intravenous nitroglycerin in coronary artery disease. Am Heart J 95(2):210–219, 1978

32. Westling H, Jansson L, Jonson B, et al: Vasoactive drugs and elastic properties of human arteries in vivo, with special reference to the action of nitroglycerin. Eur Heart J 5:609–616, 1984

33. Vatner SF, Pagani M, Rutherford JD, et al: Effects of nitroglycerin on cardiac function and regional blood flow distribution in conscious dogs. Am J Physiol 234:244–252, 1978

34. Slutsky R, Mancini GBJ, Costello D, et al: Radionuclide analysis of pulmonary blood volume: The response to spontaneous angina pectoris and sublingual nitroglycerin in patients with coronary artery disease. Am Heart J 105:243–248, 1983

35. Greenberg H, Dwyer EM Jr, Jameson AG, et al: Effects of nitroglycerin on the major determinants of myocardial oxygen consumption: An angiographic and hemodynamic assessment. Am J Cardiol 36:426–432, 1975

36. Bussmann WD, Lohner J, Kaltenbach M: Orally administered isosorbide dinitrate in patients with and without left ventricular failure due to acute myocardial infarction. Am J Cardiol 39:91–96, 1977

37. Packer M: Mechanisms of nitrate action in patients with severe left ventricular failure: Conceptual problems with the theory of venosequestration. Am Heart J 110(1):259–264, 1985

38. Gmeiner R: Effect of nitroglycerin on the mechanical and metabolic performance of the isolated aerobic and hypoxic rat heart. Eur J Cardiol 2:47–54, 1974

39. Hayashi H, Kobayashi A, Yamashita T, et al: Effects of nitroglycerin on left ventricular function in patients with ischemic heart disease. Jpn Heart J 26(2): 209–217, 1985

40. Harris PJ, Roubin GS, Sadick NN, et al: The effect of high-dose intravenous nitroglycerin on cardiovascular hemodynamic features and left ventricular function at rest and during exercise in patients with exertional angina. Am J Cardiol 52:113A–118A, 1983

41. McAnulty JH, Hattenhauer MT, Rosch J, et al: Improvement in left ventricular wall motion following nitroglycerin. Circulation 51:140–145, 1975

42. Dumeshil JG, Ritman EL, Davis GD, et al: Regional left ventricular wall dynamics before and after sublingual administration of nitroglycerin. Am J Cardiol 36:419–425, 1975

43. Bussman WD, Neumann K, Kaltenbach M: Effects of intravenous nitroglycerin on ventricular ectopic beats in acute myocardial infarction. Am Heart J 107:940–944, 1984

44. Gagnon RM, Lemire J, Beaudet R: Intravenous use of nitroglycerin to control severe ventricular arrhythmias in unstable angina. Can Med Assoc J 123:1131–1133, 1980

45. Kupper W, Bleifeld W: Effect of nitrates on myocardial blood flow, myocardial lactate extraction and hemodynamics during angina pectoris. *In* Rudolph W, Schrey A (eds): Nitrate II. Munich Vienna, Baltimore, Urban and Schwarzenberg, 1980, p 86

46. Lichtlen P, Halter J, Gattiker K: The effect of isosorbide dinitrate on coronary blood flow, coronary resistance and left ventricular dynamics under exercise in patients with coronary artery disease. Basic Res Cardiol 69:402–421, 1974

47. Harder DR, Belardinelli L, Sperelakis N, et al: Differential effects of adenosine and nitroglycerin on the action potentials of large and small coronary arteries. Circ Res 44:176–182, 1979

48. Brown BG: Response of normal and diseased epicardial coronary arteries to vasoactive drugs: Quantitative arteriographic studies. Am J Cardiol 56:23E–29E, 1985

49. Feldman RL, Pepine CJ, Curry RC, et al: Coronary arterial responses to graded doses of nitroglycerin. Am J Cardiol 43:91–97, 1979

50. Trimarco B, Cuocolo A, VanDorne D, et al: Late phase of nitroglycerin-induced coronary vasodilatation blunted by inhibition of prostaglandin synthesis. Circulation 71(4):840–848, 1985

51. Armstrong PW, Armstrong JA, Marks GS: Blood levels after sublingual nitroglycerin. Circulation 59:585–588, 1979

52. Porchet H, Bircher J. Noninvasive assessment of portosystemic shunting: Evaluation of a method to investigate systemic availability of oral glyceryl trinitrate by digital plethysmography. Gastroenterology 82:629–637, 1982

53. Armstrong PW, Armstrong JA, Marks GS: Pharmacokinetic-hemodynamic studies of intravenous nitroglycerin in congestive cardiac failure. Circulation 62:160–166, 1980

54. Muller P, Imhof PR, Burkart F, et al: Human pharmacological studies of a new transdermal system containing nitroglycerin. Eur J Clin Pharmacol 22:473–480, 1982

55. Baaske DM, Amann AH, Wagenknecht DM, et al: Nitroglycerin compatibility with intravenous fluid filters, containers, and administration sets. Am J Hosp Pharm 37:201–205, 1980

56. Carr CJ: History of the synthesis and pharmacology of isosorbide dinitrate. Am Heart J 110(1):197–201, 1985

57. Chausseaud LF, Down WH, Grundy RK: Concentrations of the vasodilator isosorbide dinitrate and its metabolites in the blood of human subjects. Eur J Clin Pharmacol 8:157–160, 1975

58. Davidson IWF, Miller HS Jr, DiCarlo FJ: Pharmacodynamics and biotransformation of pentaerythritol tetranitrate in man. J Pharm Sci 60:274–277, 1971

59. DiCarlo FJ, Crew MC, Brusco LS, et al: Metabolism of pentaerythritol trinitrate. Clin Pharmacol Ther 22:309–315, 1977

60. Fuchs RM, Brinker JA, Gusman PA, et al: Regional coronary blood flow during relief of pacing-induced angina by nitroglycerin: Implications for mechanism of action. Am J Cardiol 51:19–22, 1983

61. Amende I, Simon R, Hood WP, et al: Direct and indirect effects of nitroglycerin on systolic and diastolic left ventricular function. In Lichten PR, Engle HJ, Schrey A, et al. (eds): Nitrate III. Berlin, Heidelberg, New York, Springer, 1981, pp 126–133

62. Shibano T, Abiko Y: Effects of nitroglycerin, dipyridamole and propranolol on myocardial pH and PO_2 during regional ischemia in the dog heart. Arch Int Pharmacodyn 264:274–289, 1983

63. Kedem J, Talafih K, Weiss HR: Improvement in regional myocardial O_2 supply and O_2 consumption by nitroglycerin during ischemia. Eur J Pharmacol 112:47–55, 1985

64. Sakamoto S, Yokoyama M, Fukuzaki S: Dilatation of coronary stenosis as the salutary effect of nitroglycerin in relief of myocardial ischemia in the dog. J Cardiovasc Pharmacol 7:562–568, 1985

65. Gorman MW, Sparks HV: Nitroglycerin causes vasodilation within ischemic myocardium. Cardiovasc Res 14:515–521, 1980

66. Liu P, Houle S, Burns RJ, et al: Effect of intracoronary nitroglycerin on myocardial blood flow and distribution in pacing-induced angina pectoris. Am J Cardiol 55:1270–1276, 1985

67. Brown BG, Bolson EL, Petersen RB, et al: The mechanisms of nitroglycerin action: Stenosis vasodilation as a major component of the drug response. Circulation 64:1089–1097, 1981

68. Feldman RL, Joyal M, Conti CR, et al: Effect of nitroglycerin on coronary collateral flow and pressure during acute coronary occlusion. Am J Cardiol 54:958–963, 1984

69. Mann T, Cohn PF, Holman BL, et al: Effect of nitroprusside on regional myocardial blood flow in coronary artery disease. Results in 25 patients and comparison with nitroglycerin. Circulation 57:732–738, 1978

70. Klein RC, Grehl TM, Stengert KB, et al: Evaluation of the effects of systemic nitroglycerin on perfusion of ischemic myocardium in coronary heart disease assessed intraoperatively by antegrade blood flow through intact saphenous vein bypass grafts. Am Heart J 101(3):292–299, 1985

71. Simon R, Amende I, Lichtlen PR: Effects of nitroglycerin on blood velocity and flow in coronary arteries and bypass grafts in man. In Lichtlen PR, Engel HJ, Schrey A, et al: (eds): Nitrates III. Berlin, Heidelberg, New York, Springer, 1981, pp 202–208

72. Corwin S, Reiffel JA: Nitrate therapy for angina pectoris: Current concepts about mechanism of action and evaluation of currently available preparations. Arch Intern Med 145:538–543, 1985

73. Reichek N: Role of nitroglycerin in effort angina. Am J Med 74:33–39, 1983

74. Kaski JC, Plaza LR, Meran DO, et al: Improved coronary supply: Prevailing mechanism of action of nitrates in chronic stable angina. Am Heart J 110:238–245, 1985

75. Hurst JW, King SB, Walter PF, et al: The clinical

recognition and management of coronary atherosclerotic heart disease. *In* Hurst JW, Logue RB, Rackley CE, et al. (eds): The Heart (ed 6). New York, McGraw-Hill, 1986, pp 882–1008

76. Sharma B, Hodges M, Asinger RW, et al: Left ventricular function during spontaneous angina pectoris: Effect of sublingual nitroglycerin. Am J Cardiol 46:34–41, 1980

77. Mikolich JR, Nicoloff NB, Robinson PH, et al: Relief of refractory angina with continuous intravenous infusion of nitroglycerin. Chest 77:375–379, 1980

78. Gensini GG: Arteriographic demonstration of the release of coronary artery spasm by isosorbide dinitrate: A twenty-five-year retrospective study. Am Heart J 110:201–203, 1985

79. Curry RC Jr: Prinzmetal angina: Provocative test and current treatment. JAMA 240:677–679, 1978

80. Hillis LD, Braunwald E: Coronary artery spasm. N Engl J Med 299:695–702, 1978

81. Hill JA, Feldman RL, Pepine CJ, et al: Randomized double-blind comparison of nifedipine and isosorbide dinitrate in patients with coronary arterial spasm. Am J Cardiol 49:431–438, 1982

82. Ginsburg R, Lamb IH, Schroeder JS, et al: Randomized double-blind comparison of nifedipine and isosorbide dinitrate therapy in variant angina pectoris due to coronary artery spasm. Am Heart J 103:44–48, 1982

83. Pichard AD, Ambrose J, Mindich B, et al: Coronary artery spasm and perioperative cardiac arrest. J Thorac Cardiovasc Surg 80:249–254, 1980

84. Buxton AE, Goldberg S, Harken A, et al: Coronary artery spasm immediately after myocardial revascularization. N Engl J Med 304:1249–1253, 1981

85. Pepine CJ, Feldman RL, Conti CR: Action of intracoronary nitroglycerin in refractory coronary artery spasm. Circulation 65:411–414, 1982

86. Cohen DJ, Roley RW, Ryan JM: Intraoperative coronary artery spasm successfully treated with nitroglycerin and nifedipine. Ann Thorac Surg 36(1):97–100, 1983

87. Ihlen H, Myhre E, Smith H: Potential deleterious haemodynamic effects of glyceryl trinitrate on myocardial ischaemia in man. Br Heart J 52:510–515, 1984

88. Jugdutt BL, Becker LC, Hutchins GM, et al: Effects of intravenous nitroglycerin on collateral blood flow and infarct size in the conscious dog. Circulation 63:17–28, 1981

89. Fukuyama T, Schechtman KB, Roberts R: The effects of intravenous nitroglycerin on hemodynamics, coronary blood flow and morphologically and enzymatically estimated infarct size in conscious dogs. Circulation 62:1227–1238, 1980

90. Bussman WD, Passek D, Seidel W, et al: Reduction of CK and CK-MB indexes of infarct size by intravenous nitroglycerin. Circulation 63:615–622, 1981

91. Borer JS, Redwood DR, Levitt B, et al: Reduction in myocardial ischemia with nitroglycerin or nitroglycerin plus phenylephrine administered during acute myocardial infarction. N Engl J Med 293:1008–1012, 1975

92. Flaherty JT: Comparison of intravenous nitroglycerin and sodium nitroprusside in acute myocardial infarction. Am J Med 74:53–60, 1983

93. Flaherty JT, Come PC, Baird MG, et al: Effects of intravenous nitroglycerin on left ventricular function and ST-segment changes in acute myocardial infarction. Br Heart J 38:612–621, 1976

94. Jaffe AS, Geltman EM, Tiefenbrunn AJ, et al: Reduction of infarct size in patients with inferior infarction with intravenous glyceryl trinitrate: A randomised study. Br Heart J 49:452–460, 1983

95. Oliva PB, Breckenridge JC: Arteriographic evidence of coronary arterial spasm in acute myocardial infarction. Circulation 56:366–374, 1977

96. Flaherty JT, Becker LC, Bulkley BH, et al: A randomised prospective trial of intravenous nitroglycerin in patients with acute myocardial infarction. Circulation 68(3):576–588, 1983

97. Sethna DN, Moffitt EA, Bussell JA, et al: Intravenous nitroglycerin and myocardial metabolism during anesthesia in patients undergoing myocardial revascularization. Anesth Analg 61:828–833, 1982

98. Kaye SE, Diami W, Gattiker R: Intravenous nitroglycerin during surgery for coronary artery disease. Anaesth Intens Care 9:247–254, 1981

99. Fahmy NR: Nitroglycerin as a hypotensive drug during general anesthesia. Anesthesiology 49:17–20, 1978

100. Kaplan JA, Wells PH: Early diagnosis of myocardial ischemia using the pulmonary arterial catheter. Anesth Analg 60:789–793, 1981

101. Thomson IR, Mutch AC, Culligan JD: Failure of intravenous nitroglycerin to prevent intraoperative myocardial ischemia during fentanyl-pancuronium anesthesia. Anesthesiology 61:385–393, 1984

102. Coriat P, Daloz M, Bousseau D, et al: Prevention of intraoperative myocardial ischemia during noncardiac surgery with intravenous nitroglycerin. Anesthesiology 61:193–196, 1984

103. McKeown PP, McClelland JS, Bone DK, et al: Nitroglycerin as an adjunct to hypothermic hyperkalemic cardioplegia. Circulation 68(suppl II):II107–II111, 1983

104. Estafanous FG, Tarazi RC: Systemic arterial hypertension associated with cardiac surgery. Am J Cardiol 46:685–694, 1980

105. Tobias MA: Comparison of nitroprusside and nitroglycerin for controlling hypertension during coronary artery surgery. Br J Anaesth 53:891–896, 1981

106. Thys DM, Sivak G, Kaplan JA: The role of isosorbide dinitrate in the treatment of perioperative hypertension. Am Heart J 110:273–276, 1985

107. Guggiari M, Dagreau F, Lienhart A, et al: Use of

nitroglyercin to produce controlled decreases in mean arterial pressure to less than 50 mm Hg. Br J Anaesth 57:142–147, 1985

108. Townsend GE, Wynands JE, Walley DG, et al: A profile of intravenous nitroglycerin use in cardiopulmonary bypass surgery. Can Anaesth Soc J 30(2):142–147, 1983

109. Dasta JF, Jacobi J, Wu LS, et al: Loss of nitroglycerin to cardiopulmonary bypass apparatus. Crit Care Med 11(1):50–52, 1983

110. Fremes SE, Weisel RD, Mickle DAG, et al: A comparison of nitroglycerin and nitroprusside: I. Treatment of postoperative hypertension. Ann Thorac Surg 39(1):53–59, 1985

111. Ihlwn H: Different effects of nitroglycerin and nitroprusside on myocardial blood flow and metabolism. Scand J Clin Lab Invest [Suppl] 173:75–79, 1984

112. Kaplan JA, Jones EL: Vasodilator therapy during coronary artery surgery: Comparison of nitroglycerin and nitroprusside. J Thorac Cardiovasc Surg 77:301–309, 1979

113. Damen J, Hitchcock JF: Reactive pulmonary hypertension after a switch operation. Br Heart J 53:223–225, 1985

114. Konstam MA, Salem DN, Isner JM, et al: Vasodilator effect on right ventricular function in congestive heart failure and pulmonary hypertension: End-systolic pressure-volume relation. Am J Cardiol 54:132–136, 1984

115. Pearl RG, Rosenthal MH, Ashton JPA: Pulmonary vasodilator effects of nitroglycerin and sodium nitroprusside in canine oleic acid-induced pulmonary hypertension. (in press)

116. Anjou-Lindskog E, Broman L, Broman M, et al: Effects of nitroglycerin on central haemodynamics and VA/Q distribution during ventilation with F_IO_2 = 1.0 in patients after coronary bypass surgery. Acta Anaesthesiol Scand 28:27–33, 1984

117. Halperin JL, Brooks KM, Rothlauf EB, et al: Effect of nitroglycerin on the pulmonary venous gradient in patients after mitral valve replacement. J Am Coll Cardiol 5(1):34–39, 1985

118. Awan NA, Evenson MK, Needham KE, et al: Effect of combined nitroglycerin and dobutamine infusions in left ventricular dysfunction. Am Heart J 106(1):35–40, 1983

119. Loeb HS, Ostrenga JP, Gual W, et al: Beneficial effects of dopamine combined with intravenous nitroglycerin on hemodynamics in patients with severe left ventricular failure. Circulation 68(4):813–820, 1984

120. Sponer G, Strein K, Dietmann K, et al: Investigations about the development of tolerance to organic nitrates in conscious dogs. Arzneimittelforsch Drug Res 34(II)1510–1516, 1984

121. Leier CV: Nitrate tolerance. Am Heart J 110:224–232, 1985

122. Manyari DE, Smith ER, Spragg J: Isosorbide dinitrate and glyceryl trinitrate: Demonstration of cross

tolerance in the capacitance vessels. Am J Cardiol 55:927–931, 1985

123. Hogstedt C, Andersson K: A cohort study on mortality among dynamite workers. J Occup Med 21:553–556, 1979

124. Reeves WC, Cook L, Wood MA, et al: Coronary artery spasm after abrupt withdrawal of nitroglycerin in rabbits. Am J Cardiol 55:1066–1069, 1985

125. Zurick AM, Wagner RH, Starr NJ, et al: Intravenous nitroglycerin, methemoglobinemia, and respiratory distress in a postoperative cardiac surgical patient. Anesthesiology 61:464–466, 1984

126. Kaplan KJ, Taber M, Teagarden JR, et al: Association of methemoglobinemia and intravenous nitroglycerin administration. Am J Cardiol 55:181–183, 1985

127. Moffat JA, Abdollah H, Rollwage D, et al: Ethacrynic acid: Acute hemodynamic effects and influence on the in vivo and in vitro response to nitroglycerin in the dog. J Cardiovasc Pharmacol 7:637–642, 1985

128. Morcillo E, Reid PR, Dubin N, et al: Myocardial prostaglandin E release by nitroglycerin and modification by indomethacin. Am J Cardiol 45:53–57, 1980

129. Glisson SN, Sanchez MM, El-Etr A, et al: Nitroglycerin and neuromuscular blockade produced by gallamine, succinylcholine, D-tubocurarine, and pancuronium. Anesth Analg 59:117–122, 1980

130. Hager WD, Messineo FC, Katz AM: β-Blockers: The extended family. Adv Intern Med 30:201–229, 1984

131. Goth A: Basic mechanisms of drug action. In Medical Pharmacology. St. Louis, CV Mosby, 1974, pp 7–14

132. Nelson E: Physicochemical and pharmaceutic properties of drugs that influence the results of clinical trials. Clin Pharmacol Ther 3:673, 1962

133. Lands AM, Arnold A, McAuliff JP, et al: Differentiation of receptor systems activated by sympathomimetic amines. Nature 214:597–598, 1967

134. Taylor SH, Silke B, Lee PS, et al: Haemodynamic dose-response effects of intravenous beta-blocking drugs with different ancillary properties in patients with coronary heart disease. Eur Heart J 3:564–569, 1982

135. Prys-Roberts C: Adrenergic mechanisms, agonist and antagonist drugs. In Prys-Roberts C (ed): The Circulation in Anaesthesia: Applied Phyiology and Pharmacology. Oxford, Blackwell, 1980, p 375

136. Ahlquist RP: A study of adrenotropic receptors. Am J Physiol 153:586–600, 1948

137. Prichard BNC: β-Adrenoceptor blocking agents. In Abshagen U (ed): Clinical Pharmacology of Antianginal Drugs, Vol 76. Berlin, Heidelberg, New York, Tokyo, Springer-Verlag, 1985, pp 385–458

138. Lundborg P: The effect of adrenergic blockade on potassium concentrations in different conditions. Acta Med Scand [Suppl] 672:121–125, 1983

139. Ask JA, Stene-Larsen G, Helle KB, et al: Functional

β_1 and β_2-adrenoceptors in the human myocardium. Acta Physiol Scand 123:81–88, 1985

140. Brown JE, McLeod AA, Shand DG: Evidence for cardiac β_2-adrenoceptors in man. Clin Pharmacol Ther 33(4):424–428, 1983

141. Taylor SH: Intrinsic sympathomimetic activity: Clinical fact or fiction? Am J Cardiol 52:16D–26D, 1983

142. Thulesium O, Gjores JE, Berlin E: Vasodilating properties of beta-adrenoceptor blockers with intrinsic sympathetic activity. Br J Clin Pharmacol 13:229S–230S, 1982

143. Velasco M, Vizcarrondo H, Rubina-Quintana A, et al: A comparative study between pindolol and nadolol on systemic and cardiac hemodynamics in hypertensive patients. Curr Ther Res 32:663–668, 1982

144. Magee PG, Gardner TJ, Flaherty JT: Improved myocardial protection with propranolol during induced ischemia. Circulation 62(1):49–56, 1980

145. Lund-Johansen P: Pharmacology of combined α-β-blockade. (II) Haemodynamic effects of labetalol. Drugs 28(suppl 2):35–50, 1984

146. Prichard BNC: Combined α- and β-receptor inhibition in the treatment of hypertension. Drugs 28(suppl 2):51–68, 1984

147. Weiner N: Drugs that inhibit adrenergic nerves and block adrenergic receptors. In Gilman AC, Goodman LS, Gilman A (eds): The Pharmacological Basis of Therapeutics. New York, MacMillan, 1980, pp 176–210

148. McDevitt DG: The assessment of β-adrenoceptor blocking drugs in man. Br J Clin Pharmacol 4:413–425, 1977

149. Manin T, Veld AJ, Schalekamp MADH: How intrinsic sympathomimetic activity modulates the haemodynamic responses to β-adrenoceptor antagonists. A clue to the nature of their antihypertensive mechanism. Br J Clin Pharmacol 13(suppl 2):245S–257S, 1982

150. Bauer JH, Brooks CS: The long-term effect of propranolol therapy on renal function. Am J Med 66:405–410, 1979

151. Pasternack A, Porsti P, Poyhonen L: Effects of pindolol and propranolol on renal function of patients with hypertension. Br J Clin Pharmacol 13(suppl 2):241S–244S, 1982

152. Griffith DNW, James IM, Newbury PA, et al: The effect of β-adrenergic receptor blocking drugs on cerebral blood flow. Br J Clin Pharmacol 7:491–494, 1979

153. Stephens J, Hayward R: Effects of selective and non-selective beta-adrenergic blockade on coronary dynamics in man assessed by rapid atrial pacing. Br Heart J 40:856–863, 1978

154. Gribbin HR, MacKay AD, Baldwin CJ, et al: Bronchial and cardiac β-adrenoceptor blockade—A comparison of atenolol, acebutolol and labetalol. Br J Clin Pharmacol 12:61–65, 1981

155. Greefhorst APM, van Herwaarden CLA: Comparative study of the ventilatory effects of three beta$_1$-selective blocking agents in asthmatic patients. Eur J Clin Pharmacol 20:417–421, 1981

156. Chester FH, Shwartz HJ, Fleming GM: Adverse effects of propranolol on airway function in non-asthmatic chronic obstructive lung disease. Chest 79:540–544, 1981

157. Ellis ME, Sahay JN, Chatterjee SS, et al: Cardioselectivity of atenolol in asthmatic patients. Eur J Clin Pharmacol 21:173–176, 1981

158. Potter DE: Effects of adrenergic activators and inhibitors of the endocrine system. In Szekeres L (ed): Adrenergic Activators and Inhibitors. Berlin, Heidelberg, New York, Springer, 1981, pp 161–211

159. Reeves RL, Sen JB, Summit NJ: The effect of metoprolol and propranolol on pancreatic insulin release. Clin Pharmacol Ther 31:262–263, 1982

160. Barnett AH, Leslie D, Watkins PJ: Can insulin-treated diabetics be given beta-adrenergic blocking drugs? Br Med J 1:976–978, 1980

161. Prichard BNC, Ross EJ: Use of propranolol in conjunction with alpha-receptor blocking drugs in phaeochromocytoma. Am J Cardiol 18:394–398, 1966

162. Zeligs MA, Lockhart CH: Perioperative hypoglycemia in a child treated with propranolol. Anesth Analg 62:1035–1037, 1983

163. Opie LH, Thomas M: Propranolol and experimental myocardial infarction: Substrate effects. Postgrad Med J 52(suppl):124–133, 1976

164. Schrumpf JD, Sheps DS, Wolfson S, et al: Altered hemoglobin-oxygen affinity with long-term propranolol therapy in patients with coronary artery disease. Am J Cardiol 40:76–82, 1977

165. Nies AS, Shand DG: Clinical pharmacology of propranolol. Circulation 52:6–15, 1975

166. Sotaniemi EA, Pelkonen O, Arranto AJ, et al: Effect of liver function on beta-blocker kinetics. Drugs 25:113–120, 1983

167. Thompson FD, Joekes AM, Foulkes DM: Pharmacodynamics of propranolol in renal failure. Br Med J 2:434–436, 1972

168. Greenblatt DJ, Sellers EM, Koch-Weser J: Importance of protein binding for the interpretation of serum or plasma drug concentrations. J Clin Pharmacol 22:259–263, 1982

169. Wood M, Shand DG, Wood AJJ: Propranolol binding in plasma during cardiopulmonary bypass. Anesthesiology 51:512–516, 1979

170. Kates RA, Bai SA, Reves JG, et al: Anesthetic and operative effect on plasma protein binding of propranolol and verapamil during cardiac surgery. Anesthesiology 63:A21, 1985

171. Singh BN, Thoden WR, Ward A: Acebutolol: A review of its pharmacological properties and therapeutic efficacy in hypertension, angina pectoris and arrhythmia. Drugs 29:531–569, 1985

172. Regardh C-G: Pharmacokinetics of β-adrenoceptor antagonists. In Poppers PJ, VanDijk B, vanElzakker AHM (eds): β-Blockade and Anaesthesia. Netherlands, Astra Pharm BV, 1980, pp 29–45.

173. Ohnhaus EE, Nuesch E, Meier J, et al: Pharmacokinetics of unlabelled and 14-C labelled pindolol in uraemia. Eur J Clin Pharmacol 7:25–29, 1974

174. Gorczynski RJ, Shaffer JE, Lee RJ: Pharmacology of ASL-8052, a novel beta-adrenergic receptor antagonist with an ultra-short duration of action. J Cardiovasc Pharmacol 5:668–677, 1980

175. Barabas E, Kirkpatrick T, Zsigmond EK: Inhibitory effect of esmolol on human plasma cholinesterase *in vitro*. Anesthesiology 61:A308, 1984

176. Sum CY, Yacobi A, Kartzinel R, et al: Kinetics of esmolol, an ultra-short acting beta-blocker, and its major metabolite. Clin Pharmacol Ther 34:427–434, 1984

177. Lowenthal DT, Porter S, Saris SD, et al: Clinical pharmacology, pharmacodynamics and interactions with esmolol. Am J Cardiol 56:14F–18F, 1985

178. Iskandrian AS, Hakki A, Laddu A. Effects of esmolol on cardiac function: Evaluation by noninvasive techniques. Am J Cardiol 56:27F–32F, 1985

179. Greenspan AM, Speilman SR, Horowitz LN, et al: Electrophysiology of esmolol. Am J Cardiol 56:19F–26F, 1985

180. Morganroth J, Horowitz LN, Anderson J, et al: Comparative efficacy and tolerance of esmolol to propranolol for control of supraventricular tachyarrhythmia. Am J Cardiol 56:33F–39F, 1985

181. Kloner RA, Kirshebaum J, Lange R, et al: Experimental and clinical observations on the efficacy of esmolol in myocardial ischemia. Am J Cardiol 56:40F–48F, 1985

182. Steck J, Sheppard D, Byrd RC, et al: Pulmonary effects of esmolol—An ultra short-acting beta-adrenergic blocking agent. Clin Res 33:472A, 1985

183. Halprin S, Frishman W, Kirschner M, et al: Clinical pharmacology of the new beta-adrenergic blocking drugs. Part II. Effects of oral labetalol in patients with both angina pectoris and hypertension: A preliminary experience. Am Heart J 99:388–396, 1980

184. Larsson K: Influence of labetalol, propranolol and practolol in patients with asthma. Eur J Respir Dis 63:221–230, 1982

185. Williams DO: Effects of antianginal agents on the coronary circulation. Am Heart J 101:473–479, 1981

186. Taylor SH: α- and β-blockade in angina pectoris. Drugs 28(suppl 2):69–87, 1984

187. Crawford MH, LeWinter MM, O'Rourke RA, et al: Combined propranolol and digoxin therapy in angina pectoris. Ann Intern Med 83:449–455, 1975

188. Boudoulas H, Lewis RP, Rittgers SE, et al: Increased diastolic time: A possible important factor in the beneficial effect of propranolol in patients with coronary artery disease. J Cardiovasc Pharmacol 1:503–513, 1979

189. Robinson BF: The mode of action of beta-antagonists in angina pectoris. Postgrad Med J 47:41–43, 1971

190. Johns VJ: Beta-blocking drugs for arrhythmias, hypertension, and ischemic heart disease. Am J Surg 147:725–730, 1984

191. The Norwegian Multicenter Study Group: Timolol-induced reduction in mortality and reinfarction in patients surviving acute myocardial infarction. N Engl J Med 304:801–807, 1981

192. β-Blocker Heart Attack Trial Research Group: A randomized trial of propranolol in patients with acute myocardial infarction. 1. Mortality results. JAMA 247:1707, 1982

193. Lichstein E: Why do beta-receptor blockers decrease mortality after myocardial infarction? J Am Coll Cardiol 6(5):973–975, 1985

194. Singh BN, Venkatesh N: Prevention of myocardial reinfarction and of sudden death in survivors of acute myocardial infarction: Role of prophylactic β-adrenoceptor blockade. Am Heart J 107(1):189–200, 1984

195. Miura M, Thomas R, Ganz W, et al: The effect of delay in propranolol administration on reduction of myocardial infarct size after experimental coronary artery occlusion in dogs. Circulation 59:1148–1157, 1979

196. The European Infarction Study Group: European Infarction Study (EIS). A secondary prevention study with slow release oxprenolol after myocardial infarction: Morbidity and mortality. Eur Heart J 5:189–202, 1984

197. Prichard BNC: Hypotensive action of pronethalol. Br Med J 1:1227–1228, 1964

198. Thadani U: Beta-blockers in hypertension. Am J Cardiol 52:10D–15D, 1983

199. Gerber JG, Nies AS: Beta-adrenergic blocking drugs. Ann Rev Med 36:145–164, 1985

200. Craythorne NWB, Huffington PE: Effects of propranolol in the cardiovascular response to cyclopropane and halothane. Anesthesiology 27:580, 1966

201. Foex P, Prys-Roberts C: Interactions of beta-receptor blockade and PCO_2 levels in the anaesthetized dog. Br J Anaesth 46:397–404, 1974

202. Horan BF, Prys-Robert C, Roberts JG, et al: Haemodynamic responses to isoflurane anaesthesia and hypovolaemia in the dog, and their modification by propranolol. Br J Anaesth 49:1179–1187, 1977

203. Roberts JG, Foex P, Clarke TNS, et al: Hemodynamic interactions of high-dose propranolol pretreatment and anaesthesia in the dog. I: Halothane dose-response studies. Br J Anaesth 48:315, 1976

204. Henriksson BA, Biber B, Haggendal J, et al: Cardiovascular effects of enflurane and asphyxia during long-term beta$_1$-adrenoceptor blockade. Acta Anaesthesiol Scand 29:363–370, 1985

205. Horan BF, Prys-Robert C, Hamilton WK, et al: Haemodynamic responses to enflurane anaesthesia and hypovolaemia in the dog, and their modification by propranolol. Br J Anaesth 49:1189–1197, 1977

206. Zimpfer M, Gilly H, Krosl P, et al: Importance of

myocardial loading conditions in determining the effects of enflurane on left ventricular function in the intact and isolated canine heart. Anesthesiology 58:159–169, 1983

207. Reves J, Kissin I, Fournier S: Effects of esmolol, a short-acting beta-blocker in enflurane-anesthetized dogs. Anesthesiology 61:A17, 1984

208. Gatt S, Hurley R, Fox J, et al: Evaluation of acute cardiovascular effects of esmolol in the dog—Awake and anesthetized with halothane and enflurane. Anesthesiology 61:A17, 1984

209. Viljoen JF, Estafanous G, Kellner GA: Propranolol and cardiac surgery. J Thorac Cardiovasc Surg 64:826–830, 1972

210. Heikkila H, Jalonen J, Laaksonen V, et al: Metoprolol medication and coronary artery bypass grafting operation. Acta Anaesthesiol Scand 28:677–682, 1984

211. Foex P: Beta-blockade in anaesthesia. J Clin Hosp Pharm 8:183–190, 1983

212. Stanley TH, deLange S, Boxcoe MJ, et al: The influence of chronic preoperative propranolol therapy on cardiovascular dynamics and narcotic requirements during operation in patients with coronary artery disease. Can Anaesth Soc J 29(4):319–324, 1982

213. Whelton PK, Flaherty JT, MacAllister NP, et al: Hypertension following coronary artery bypass surgery: Role of preoperative propranolol therapy. Hypertension 2:291–298, 1980

214. Kadish A, Oka Y, Becker R, et al: Propranolol withdrawal: Cause of post-coronary bypass arrhythmias and hypertension. Circulation 60:104, 1979

215. Ponten J, Haggendal J, Milocco I, et al: Long-term metoprolol therapy and neuroleptanesthesia in coronary artery surgery: Withdrawal versus maintenance of β_1-adrenoreceptor blockade. Anesth Analg 62:380–390, 1983

216. Still JC, Nugent M, Moyer TP, et al: Influence of propranolol plasma levels on hemodynamics during coronary artery bypass surgery. Anesthesiology 60:455–463, 1984

217. Miller RR, Olson HG, Amsterdam EA, et al: Propranolol-withdrawal-rebound phenomenon. Exacerbation of coronary events after abrupt cessation of anti-anginal therapy. N Engl J Med 293:416–418, 1975

218. Aarons RD, Nies AS, Gal J, et al: Elevation of β-adrenergic receptor density in human lymphocytes after propranolol administration. J Clin Invest 65:949–957, 1980

219. Boudoulas H, Lewis RP, Kates RE, et al: Hypersensitivity to adrenergic stimulation after propranolol withdrawal in normal subjects. Ann Intern Med 87:433–436, 1977

220. Safwat AM, Fung DL, Bilton DC: The use of propranolol in rapid sequence anaesthetic induction: Optimal time interval for pretreatment. Can Anaesth Soc J 31(6):638–641, 1984

221. Fischler M, DuBois C, Broadty D, et al: Circulatory responses to thiopentone and tracheal intubation in patients with coronary artery disease. Br J Anaesth 57:493–496, 1985

222. Reves J, Flezzani P: Perioperative use of esmolol. Am J Cardiol 56:57F–62F, 1985

223. Menkhaus P, Reves J, Kissin I, et al: Cardiovascular effects of esmolol in anesthetized humans. Anesth Analg 64:327–334, 1985

224. Korenaga GM, Kirkpatrick A, Lord JG, et al: Effect of esmolol on tachycardia induced by endotracheal intubation (Abstract). Anesth Analg 64:238, 1985

225. Gold M, Brown M, Selem J: The effect of esmolol on hemodynamics after ketamine induction and intubation. Anesthesiology 61:A19, 1984

226. Girard D, Shulman BJ, Thys DM, et al: The safety and efficacy of esmolol during myocardial revascularization. Anesthesiology 65:157–165, 1986

227. deBruijn NP, Reves JG, Croughwell N, et al: Pharmacokinetics and pharmacodynamics of esmolol in beta-blocked patients undergoing CABG (Abstract). Proc SCA, Montreal, 1986

228. Dagnino J, Prys-Roberts C: Assessment of β-adrenoceptor blockade during anesthesia in Humans. Anesth Analg 64:305–311, 1985

229. Saarnivaara L, Lindgren L: Prolongation of the QT interval during induction of anaesthesia. Acta Anaesthesiol Scand 27:126–130, 1983

230. Saarnivaara L, Lindgren L, Hynynen M: Effects of practolol and metoprolol on QT interval, heart rate and arterial pressure during induction of anaesthesia. Acta Anaesthesiol Scand 28:644–648, 1984

231. Brewlow MJ, Evers AS, Lebowitz P: Successful treatment of accelerated junctional rhythm with propranolol: Possible role of sympathetic stimulation in the genesis of this rhythm disturbance. Anesthesiology 62:180–182, 1985

232. Cope DHP, Crawford MC: Labetalol in controlled hypotension. Br J Anaesth 51:359–365, 1979

233. Scott DB, Buckley FP, Littlewood DG, et al: Circulatory effects of labetalol during halothane anaesthesia. Anaesthesia 33:145–156, 1978

234. Oka Y, Frishman W, Becker RM, et al: Clinical pharmacology of the new beta-adrenergic blocking drugs, Part 10. Beta-adrenoceptor blockade and coronary artery surgery. Am Heart J 99:255–269, 1980

235. McDonald DH, Hug CC, Kaplan JA: Continuous propranolol infusion: Isoproterenol response. Anesthesiology 57:A69, 1982

236. Gray RJ, Bateman TM, Czer LSC, et al: Use of esmolol in hypertension after cardiac surgery. Am J Cardiol 56:49F–56F, 1985

237. Meretoja DA, Allonen H, Arola M, et al: Combined alpha- and beta-blockade with labetalol in post-open heart surgery hypertension. Chest 78(6):810–815, 1980

238. Williams ME, Rosa RM, Silva P, et al: Impairment

of extrarenal potassium disposal by α-adrenergic stimulation. New Engl J Med 311(3):145–148, 1984

239. Fleckenstein A: History of calcium antagonists. Circ Res 52(suppl I):3–16, 1983

240. Fabiato A: Calcium-induced release of calcium from the cardiac sarcoplasmic reticulum. Am J Physiol 245:C1–C14, 1983

241. Braunwald E: Mechanism of action of calcium channel blocking agents. N Engl J Med 307(26):1615–1627, 1982

242. Schwartz A: Cellular action of calcium channel blocking drugs. Ann Rev Med 35:325–339, 1984

243. Reuter H: The dependence of the slow inward current in Purkinje fibers on the extracellular calcium concentration. J Physiol (Lond) 192:479–492, 1967

244. Gettes LS: Possible role of ionic changes in the appearance of arrhythmias. Pharmacol Ther 2(4):787–810, 1976

245. Mitchell MR, Powell T, Terrar DA, et al: Characteristics of the second inward current in cells isolated from rat ventricular muscle. Proc R Soc Lond [Biol] 219:447–469, 1983

246. Reimer KA, Jennings RB, Tatum AH: Pathobiology of acute myocardial ischemia: Metabolic, functional and ultrastructural studies. Am J Cardiol 52:72A–81A, 1983

247. Fozzard HA, Hiraoka M: The positive dynamic current and its inactivation properties in cardiac Purkinje fibers. J Physiol (Lond) 234:569–586, 1973

248. Solaro RJ: The role of calcium in the concentration of the heart. In Flaim SF, Zelis R (eds): Calcium Blockers: Mechanisms of Action and Clinical Applications. Baltimore, Munich, Urban and Schwarzenberg, 1980, pp 21–36

249. Ratz PH, Flaim SF: Species and blood vessel specificity in the use of calcium for contraction. In Flaim SF, Zelis R (eds): Calcium Blockers: Mechanisms of Action and Clinical Applications. Baltimore, Munich, Urban and Schwarzenberg, 1982, pp 77–98

250. Silver PJ, Stull JT: The role of calcium in the contraction of vascular smooth muscle. In Flaim SF, Zelis R (eds): Calcium Blockers: Mechanisms of Action and Clinical Applications. Baltimore, Munich, Urban and Schwarzenberg, 1980, pp 37–51

251. vanHoutte PM: Calcium entry blockers, vascular smooth muscle and systemic hypertension. Am J Cardiol 55:17B–23B, 1985

252. Millard RW: Chronotropic, inotropic and vasodilator actions of diltiazem, nifedipine, and verapamil. A comparative study of physiological responses and membrane receptor activity. Circ Res 52(part II):I29–39, 1983

253. Pedrinelli R, Tarazi RC: Interference of calcium entry blockade in vivo with pressor responses to α-adrenergic stimulation: Effects of two unrelated blockers on responses to both exogenous and endogenously released norepinephrine. Circulation 69(6):1171–1176, 1984

254. Timmermans PBMWM, van Meel JCA, van Zwieten PA: Calcium antagonists and α-receptors. Eur Heart J 4(suppl):11–17, 1983

255. Godfraind T, Miller RC: Specificity of action of Ca^{++} entry blockers: A comparison of their actions in rat arteries and in human coronary arteries. Circ Res 25(suppl I):81–91, 1983

256. Henry PD: Comparative cardiac pharmacology of calcium blockers. In Flaim SF, Zelis R (eds): Calcium Blockers: Mechanisms of Action and Clinical Applications. Baltimore, Munich, Urban and Schwarzenberg, 1980, pp 135–153

257. Mitchell LB, Schroeder JS, Mason JW: Comparative clinical electrophysiologic effects of diltiazem, verapamil and nifedipine: A review. Am J Cardiol 49:629–635, 1982

258. Zsoter TT, Church JG: Calcium antagonists: Pharmacodynamic effects and mechanism of action. Drugs 25:93–112, 1983

259. Nakaya H, Schwartz A, Millard RW: Reflex chronotropic and inotropic effects of calcium channel blocking agents in conscious dogs. Circ Res 52:302–311, 1983

260. Chew CYC, Hecht HS, Colett JT, et al: Influence of severity of ventricular dysfunction on hemodynamic responses to intravenously administered verapamil in ischemic heart disease. Am J Cardiol 47:917–922, 1981

261. Hugenholtz PG. Calcium antagonists. In Abshagen U (ed): Clinical Pharmacology of Antianginal Drugs. Berlin, Heidelberg, New York, Tokyo, 1985, pp 459–538

262. Singh BN, Ellrodt G, Peter CT: Verapamil: A review of its pharmacological properties and therapeutic use. Drugs 15:169–197, 1978

263. Merin RG, Chelly J, Abernethy D, et al: Inhalational anesthetics (IAs) alter the pharmacokinetics of verapamil. Anesthesiology 63:A205, 1985

264. Klein HO, Kaplinsky E: Verapamil and digoxin: Their respective effects on atrial fibrillation and their interaction. Am J Cardiol 50:894–902, 1982

265. Singh BN, Nademanee K, Bady SH: Calcium antagonists: Clinical use in the treatment of arrhythmias. Drugs 25:125–153, 1983

266. Raemsch KD, Sommer J: Pharmacokinetics and metabolism of nifedipine. Hypertension 5(suppl II):II18–II24, 1983

267. Chaffman, Brogden RN: Diltiazem: A review of its pharmacological properties and therapeutic efficacy. Drugs 29:387–454, 1985

268. Morselli PL, Rovel V, Mitchard M, et al: Pharmacokinetics and metabolism of diltiazem in man (observations on healthy volunteers and angina pectoris patients). In Bing RJ (ed): New Drug Therapy With a Calcium Antagonist. Amsterdam, Princeton, Exerpta Medica, 1979, pp 152–168

269. Frishman WH, Klein NA, Strom JA, et al: Superiority of verapamil to propranolol in stable angina pectoris: A double-blind, randomized crossover trial. Circulation 65(suppl 1):I51–I59, 1982

270. Mueller HS, Chahine RA: Interim report of multi-center double-blind, placebo-controlled studies of nifedipine in chronic stable angina. Am J Med 71:645–655, 1981

271. Strauss WE, McIntyre KM, Parisi AF, et al: Safety and efficacy of diltiazem hydrochloride for the treatment of stable angina pectoris: Report of a cooperative clinical trial. Am J Cardiol 49:560–566, 1982

272. Leon MB, Rosing DR, Bonow RO, et al: Combination therapy with calcium channel blockers and beta-blockers for chronic stable angina pectoris. Am J Cardiol 55:69B–80B, 1985

273. Reimer KA, Jennings RB: Effects of calcium channel blockers on myocardial preservation during experimental acute myocardial infarction. Am J Cardiol 55:107B–115B, 1985

274. Ferlinz J, Turbow ME: Antianginal and myocardial metabolic properties of verapamil in coronary artery disease. Am J Cardiol 46:1019–1026, 1980

275. Engel HJ, Lichtlen PR: Beneficial enhancement of coronary blood flow by nifedipine. Comparison with nitroglycerin and beta-blocking agents. Am J Med 71:658–666, 1981

276. Conti RC: Recommendations for combination antianginal therapy. Cardiovasc Med: 11(part 1) 21–26, 1986

277. Bonow RO: Effects of calcium channel blocking agents on left ventricular diastolic function in hypertrophic cardiomyopathy and in coronary artery disease. Am J Cardiol 55:172B–178B, 1985

278. Henry PD, Schuchleib R, Clark RE, et al: Effect of nifedipine on myocardial ischemia: Analysis of collateral flow, pulsatile heart and regional muscle shortening. Am J Cardiol 44:817–824, 1979

279. Schmier J: Formation of collaterals in association with calcium antagonists. In Lichtlen PR (ed): Coronary Angiography and Angina Pectoris. Stuttgart, Georg Thieme, 1976, pp 334–342

280. Mehta JL: Influence of calcium-channel blockers on platelet function and arachidonic acid metabolism. Am J Cardiol 55:158B–164B, 1985

281. Flaim S, Zelis R: Clinical use of calcium entry blockers. Fed Proc 40:2887–2889, 1981

282. Gunther S, Muller JE, Mudge GH, et al: Therapy of coronary vasoconstriction in patients with coronary artery disease. Am J Cardiol 47:157–162, 1981

283. Winniford MD, Willerson JT, Hillis LD: Calcium antagonists for acute ischemic heart disease. Am J Cardiol 55:116B–124B, 1985

284. Gerstenblith G: Nifedipine in unstable angina: A double-blind randomized trial. New Engl J Med 306:885–889, 1982

285. Ellrodt G, Chew CYC, Singh BN: Therapeutic implications of slow-channel blockade in cardio-circulatory disorders. Circulation 62:669–679, 1980

286. Winniford MD, Johnson SM, Mauritson DR, et al: Verapamil therapy for Prinzmetal's variant angina: Comparison with placebo and nifedipine. Am J Cardiol 50:913–918, 1982

287. Kimura E, Kishida H: Treatment of variant angina with drugs: A survey of 11 cardiology institutes in Japan. Circulation 63:844–848, 1982

288. Huysmans FM, Slulter HE, Thien T, et al: Acute treatment of hypertensive crisis with nifedipine. Br J Clin Pharmacol 16:725–727, 1983

289. Robinson BF, Dobbs RJ, Bayley S: Response of forearm resistance vessels to verapamil and sodium nitroprusside in normotensive and hypertensive men: Evidence for a functional abnormality of vascular smooth muscle in primary hypertension. Clin Sci 63:33–42, 1982

290. Rubin LJ: Calcium channel blockers in primary pulmonary hypertension. Chest 88(4):257S–260S, 1985

291. Fanta CH: Calcium channel blockers in prophylaxis and treatment of asthma. Am J Cardiol 55:202B–209B, 1985

292. Gelmers HJ: Calcium channel blockers: Effects on cerebral blood flow and potential uses for acute stroke. Am J Cardiol 55(3):144B–148B, 1985

293. Weir B: Calcium antagonists, cerebral ischemia and vasospasm. Can J Neurol Sci 11(2):239–246, 1984

294. Steen PA, Gisvold SE, Milde JH, et al: Nimodipine improves outcome when given after complete cerebral ischemia in primates. Anesthesiology 62:406–414, 1985

295. Bosnjak ZJ, Kampine JP: Effects of halothane, enflurane, and isoflurane on the SA node. Anesthesiology 58:314–321, 1983

296. Atlee JL III, Alexander SC: Halothane effects on conductivity of the AV node and Purkinje system in the dog. Anesth Analg 56:378–386, 1977

297. Bosnjak ZJ, Kampine JP: The effects of halothane on transmembrane potentials, Ca^{++} transients and papillary muscle tension. Anesth Analg 63:A191, 1984

298. Lynch C III, Vogel S, Sperelakis N: Halothane depression of myocardial slow action potentials. Anesthesiology 55:360–368, 1981

299. Su JY, Kerrick WGL: Effects of halothane Ca^{++}-activated tension development in mechanically disrupted rabbit myocardial fibers. Pflugers Arch 375:111–117, 1978

300. Merin RG, Kumazawa T, Honig CR: Reversible interaction between halothane and Ca^{++} on cardiac actomyosin adenosine triphosphatase: Mechanism and significance. J Pharmacol Exp Ther 190:1–14, 1974

301. Price ML, Price HL: Effects of general anesthetics on contractile responses of rabbit aortic strips. Anesthesiology 23:16–20, 1962

302. Seagard JL, Hopp FA, Donegan JH, et al: Halothane and the carotid sinus reflex: Evidence for multiple sites of action. Anesthesiology 57:191–202, 1982

303. Kates RA, Kaplan JA: Cardiovascular responses to verapamil during coronary artery bypass graft surgery. Anesth Analg 62:821–826, 1983

304. Zimpfer M, Fitzal S, Tonczar L: Verapamil as a hypotensive agent during neuroleptanaesthesia. Br J Anaesth 53:885–889, 1981

305. Norfleet EA, Heath KR, Kopp VJ, et al: Verapamil—Different cardiovascular responses during N₂O analgesia and halothane anesthesia. Anesthesiology 57:A75, 1982

306. Kapur PA, Flacke WE: Epinephrine-induced arrhythmias and cardiovascular function after verapamil during halothane anesthesia in the dog. Anesthesiology 55:218–225, 1981

307. Kapur PA, Bloor BC, Flacke WE, et al: Comparison of cardiovascular responses to verapamil during enflurane, isoflurane, or halothane anesthesia in the dog. Anesthesiology 61:156–160, 1984

308. Kates RA, Zaggy AP, Norfleet EA, et al: Comparative cardiovascular effects of verapamil, nifedipine, and diltiazem during halothane anesthesia in swine. Anesthesiology 61:10–18, 1984

309. Schulte-Sasse U, Hess W, Markschies-Hornung A, et al: Combined effects of halothane anesthesia and verapamil on systemic hemodynamics and left ventricular myocardial contractility in patients with ischemic heart disease. Anesth Analg 63:791–798, 1984

310. Marshall AG, Kissin I, Reves JG, et al: Interaction between negative inotropic effects of halothane and nifedipine in the isolated rat heart. J Cardiovasc Pharmacol 5:592–597, 1983

311. Griffin RM, Dimich I, Jurado R, et al: Cardiovascular effects of nifedipine infusions during fentanyl anesthesia. Anesthesiology 61:A10, 1984

312. Tosone SR, Reves JG, Kissin I, et al: Hemodynamic responses to nifedipine in dogs anesthetized with halothane. Anesth Analg 62:903–908, 1983

313. Springman SR, Redon D, Rusy BF: The effect of nifedipine on the circulation during morphine-N₂O analgesia and halothane anesthesia. Anesth Analg 62:284–285, 1983

314. Spiss CK, Zadrobilek E, Weindlmayr-Goettel M, et al: Nifedipine induced hypotension in man: Hemodynamic response during isoflurane and halothane anesthesia. Anesthesiology 63:A93, 1985

315. Rogers A, Curling PE, Cooper S, et al: Intravenous nifedipine for treatment of intraoperative hypertension. Anesthesiology 63:A24, 1985

316. Schulte-Sasse U, Hess W, Markschies-Hornung A, et al: Cardiovascular interactions of halothane anesthesia and nifedipine in patients subjected to elective coronary artery bypass surgery. Thorac Cardiovasc Surg 31:261–265, 1983

317. Broadbent MP, Swan PC, Jones RM: Interactions between diltiazem and isoflurane: An in vitro investigation in isolated guinea pig atria. Br J Anaesth 57:1018–1021, 1985

318. Kapur PA, Tippit SE: Correlation of cardiovascular effects with plasma levels of diltiazem during isoflurane anesthesia. Anesthesiology 61:A12, 1984

319. Griffin RM, Dimich I, Pratilas V, et al: Cardiovascular effects of diltiazem infusion during fentanyl anesthesia. Anesth Analg 64:223, 1985

320. Freis ES, Lappas DG: Chronic administration of calcium entry blockers and the cardiovascular responses to high doses of fentanyl in man. Anesthesiology 57:A295, 1982

321. Roach GW, Moldenhauer CC, Hug CC, et al: Hemodynamic responses to fentanyl or diazepam-fentanyl anesthesia in patients on chronic nifedipine therapy. Anesthesiology 61:A374, 1984

322. Casson WR, Jones RM, Parsons RS: Nifedipine and cardiopulmonary bypass. Anaesthesia 39:1197–1201, 1984

323. Nelson DO, Graham CA, Frederiksen JW, et al: Alteration of contractile activity of human vascular smooth muscle following acute withdrawal of calcium channel blocker. Circulation 68(suppl III):III323, 1983

324. Engelman RM, Hadji-Rousou I, Breyer RH, et al: Rebound vasospasm after coronary revascularization in association with calcium antagonist withdrawal. Ann Thorac Surg 37(6):469–472, 1984

325. Larach DR, Hensley FA, Pae LR, et al: A randomized study of diltiazem withdrawal prior to coronary artery bypass surgery. Anesthesiology 63:A23, 1985

326. Lina AA, Leon-Ruiz EN, Fouts KE, et al: Influence of verapamil and aminophylline on epinephrine dysrhythmias under halothane anesthesia. Anesthesiology 63:A84, 1985

327. Iwatsuki N, Katoh M, Ono K, et al: Antiarrhythmic effect of diltiazem during halothane anesthesia in dogs and in humans. Anesth Analg 64:964–970, 1985

328. Kapur PA, Norel E, Dajee H, et al: Verapamil treatment of intractable ventricular arrhythmias after cardiopulmonary bypass. Anesth Analg 63:460–463, 1984

329. Hess W, Schulte-Sasse U, Tarnow J: Nifedipine versus nitroprusside for controlling hypertensive episodes during coronary artery bypass surgery. Eur Heart J 5:140–145, 1984

330. Zadrobilek E, Spiss CK, Redl G, et al: Nifedipine-induced hypotension in man: Intrapulmonary shunting during isoflurane and halothane anesthesia. Anesthesiology 63:A521, 1985

331. Guyton RA, Dorsey LM, Kates RA, et al: Enhancement of cardioplegic myocardial protection with calcium entry blockers. J Med Assoc Ga73:707–711, 1984

332. Magovern GJ, Dixon CM, Burkholder JA: Improved myocardial protection with nifedipine and potassium-based cardioplegia. J Thorac Cardiovasc Surg 82:239–244, 1981

333. Clark RD, Magovern GJ, Christlief IY, et al: Nifedipine cardioplegia experience: Results of a 3-year cooperative clinical study. Ann Thorac Surg 36:654–662, 1983

334. Lee TH, DiSesa VJ, Cohn LH, et al: Correction of intraoperative diastolic myocardial dysfunction with nifedipine. Clin Cardiol 6:549–552, 1983

335. Bersohn MM, Shine KI: Verapamil protection of ischemic isolated rabbit heart: Dependence on pretreatment. Am Coll Cardiol 15:659–671, 1983

336. Yamamoto F, Manning AS, Baimbridge MV, et al: Cardioplegia and slow calcium channel blocker studies with verapamil. J Thorac Cardiovasc Surg 86:252–261, 1983

337. Guffin AV, Kates RA, Holbrook GW, et al: Verapamil and myocardial preservation in patients undergoing coronary artery bypass surgery. Ann Thorac Surg 41:587–591, 1986

338. Barner HB, Jellinek M, Standeven JW, et al: Cold blood-diltiazem cardioplegia. Ann Thorac Surg 33(1):55–63, 1982

339. Humphrey LS, Blanck TJJ: Intraoperative use of verapamil for nitroglycerin-refractory myocardial ischemia. Anesth Analg 64:68–71, 1985

340. Nussmeier NA, Slogoff S: Verapamil treatment of intraoperative coronary artery spasm. Anesthesiology 62:539–541, 1985

341. Buston AE, Goldberg S, Harken A, et al: Coronary artery spasm immediately after myocardial revascularization. N Engl J Med 304:1249–1253, 1981

342. Lewis BH, Muller JE, Rutherford J, et al: Nifedipine for coronary artery spasm after revascularization. N Engl J Med 306:992–993, 1982

343. Stone PH, Antmans EM, Muller JE, et al: Calcium channel blocking agents in the treatment of cardiovascular disorders. Part II: Hemodynamic effects and clinical applications. Ann Intern Med 93:886–904, 1980

344. Cullhed I, Karlsson L: The effect of verapamil on the regularization of auricular fibrillation. *In* Cantor, Aulendorf (eds): Symposium on Arrhythmias: Isoptin. Gotenburg, Sweden, 1972, pp 27–28

345. Ross D, Vohra J, Sloman JG: Disopyramide in myocardial infarction. Lancet 1:330, 1978

346. Harriman RJ, Mangiardi LM, McAllister RD Jr, et al: Reversal of the cardiovascular effects of verapamil by calcium and sodium: Differences between electrophysiologic and hemodynamic responses. Circulation 59:797–804, 1979

347. Ebner F, Dunschede HB: Haemodynamic, therapeutic mechanism of action and clinical findings of adalat use based on worldwide clinical trials. *In* Jatene AD, Lichten PR (eds): The Third International Adalat Symposium. Amsterdam, Excerpta Medica, 1976, pp 283–300

348. Kraynack BL, Lawson NW, Gintautas J: Neuromuscular blocking action of verapamil in cats. Can Anaesth Soc J 30(3):242–247, 1983

349. Kraynack BJ, Lawson NW, Gintautas J, et al: Effects of verapamil on indirect muscle twitch responses. Anesth Analg 62:827–830, 1983

350. Durant NN, Nguyen N, Katz RL: Potentiation of neuromuscular blockade by verapamil. Anesthesiology 60:298–303, 1984

351. Sata T, Ono H: Facilitation of neuromuscular transmission by calcium antagonists, diltiazem, nifedipine and verapamil in the dog. Arch Int Pharmacodyn 249:235–246, 1981

352. Jones RM, Cashman JN, Casson WR, et al: Verapamil potentiation of neuromuscular blockade: Failure of reversal with neostigmine but prompt reversal with edrophonium. Anesth Analg 64:1021–1025, 1985

353. Zalman F, Perloff JK, Durant NN, et al: Acute respiratory failure following intravenous verapamil in Duchenne's muscular dystrophy. Am Heart J 105(3):510–511, 1983

354. Zukaitis MG, Hoech GP, Williams CH, et al: Verapamil attenuation of malignant hyperthermia syndrome in susceptible pigs. Anesthesiology 57:A228, 1982

355. Bikhazi GB, Thomas KC, Foldes FF: Effects of verapamil and EDTA on mammalian muscle in vitro. Anesthesiology 51:S275, 1979

356. Roewer N, Rumberger E, Bode H, et al: Electrophysiological and mechanical interactions of verapamil and dantrolene on isolated heart muscle. Anesthesiology 63:A274, 1985

357. Saltzman LS, Kates RA, Corke BC, et al: Hyperkalemia and cardiovascular collapse after verapamil and dantrolene administration in swine. Anesth Analg 63:473–478, 1984

358. Vetrovec GW, Parker VE: Acute electrophysiologic, hemodynamic and left ventricular effects of nifedipine and beta-blocker interactions: Maintenance of global and regional left ventricular wall motion. Am J Cardiol 55:21E–26E, 1985

359. Muller JE: Nifedipine and conventional therapy for unstable angina pectoris: A randomized double-blind comparison. Circulation 69:728, 1984

360. Nesto RW, White HD, Ganz P, et al: Addition of nifedipine to maximal beta-blocker-nitrate therapy: Effects on exercise capacity and global left ventricular performance at rest and during exercise. Am J Cardiol 55:3E–8E, 1985

Carol L. Lake, M.D.

14

Chronic Treatment of Heart Failure

Heart failure is the pathophysiologic state in which an abnormality of myocardial function prevents pumping of blood at a rate sufficient to meet the metabolic requirements during exercise. Congestive heart failure (CHF) is a syndrome characterized by pulmonary or systemic congestion accompanied by a low cardiac output (CO). However, not all patients with heart failure have elevated venous pressures; while, conversely, severe pulmonary or systemic congestion can occur in humans with normal hearts. Thus, either myocardial or congestive failure can be seen. Heart failure is usually classified using the New York Heart Association classification as listed below.*

Class I—No limitation. Ordinary physical activity does not cause symptoms.
Class II—Slight limitation of physical activity. Ordinary physical activity will result in symptoms.
Class III—Marked limitation of physical activity. Less than ordinary activity leads to symptoms.
Class IV—Inability to carry on any activity without symptoms. Symptoms are present at rest.

*Modified from Criteria Committee of the New York Heart Association.

ETIOLOGY AND CLINICAL RECOGNITION

Heart failure may be caused by either cardiac or noncardiac causes. These causes include work overload states, such as the pressure overload of valvular stenosis or hypertension, or the volume overload of valvular regurgitation; high output states (arteriovenous fistulas, thyrotoxicosis); oxygen deprivation (either hypoxia or ischemia); restricted diastolic filling from pericardial disease, hypertrophic cardiomyopathy, or mitral stenosis; and myocardiopathies (viral, idiopathic, or metabolic) in which there is a primary disturbance of contractility. These and other causes of heart failure are listed below.

Cardiac work overload (pressure, volume)
Dysrhythmias
Infarction or ischemia
Physical or emotional stress
Systemic infections
Pulmonary embolism
High-output states (hyperthyroidism)
Endocarditis or myocarditis
Discontinuation or reduction of therapy

It is relatively easy to recognize the overt symptoms of CHF, including elevated central venous pressure (CVP), pulmonary rales, peripheral edema, small peripheral pulses, cardiac enlargement, or an S_3 gallop. Normally, the jugular veins are visible no more than 2 cm above the sternal angle with the patient in a 45° upright position. In heart failure, the actual CVP can be estimated by adding 5 cm to the vertical distance of the venous pulsations.

One of the earliest symptoms of CHF is dyspnea on exertion. Although central circulatory pressures may be normal at rest, exercise abnormally increases left ventricular end-diastolic pressure (LVEDP) in patients with CHF. Comparable increases in pulmonary venous and capillary pressures produce dyspnea. Pulmonary vascular engorgement decreases pulmonary compliance and increases the transpulmonary airway gradient to increase the work of breathing. Dyspnea results primarily from pulmonary capillary hypertension, although decreased CO may also be responsible. Cough, often nocturnal, dry and nonproductive, occurs early in CHF. Dyspnea also occurs at rest when the LVEDP is chronically elevated.

At a later stage than dyspnea comes orthopnea, the sensation of dyspnea or labored breathing while recumbent. Recumbency not only decreases ventilatory reserve by elevation of the diaphragm, but also increases venous return. Venous return is also increased by increased reabsorption of fluid from dependent areas. Paroxysmal nocturnal dyspnea, dyspnea occurring after 3–4 hours of recumbent sleep, results from a similar mechanism, but represents a more advanced stage of heart failure.

Rales develop when the transudation of fluid from the capillaries into interstitial and interalveolar spaces exceeds the capacity of pulmonary lymphatics to remove it. Dependent portions of the lung are the first affected, but all areas may become involved. Bronchospasm and bronchial wall edema result in generalized wheezing and rhonchi. Fluid transudation into the pleural spaces causes right or bilateral pleural effusions.

Chest radiographs demonstrate cardiomegaly and increased pulmonary vascular markings, most prominent at the lung apices, since blood flow is redistributed there when pulmonary vascular resistance (PVR) increases at the bases in CHF. Lymphatic congestion results from pulmonary vascular engorgement and presents as Kerley B lines, horizontal lines extending 1–2 cm from the lateral chest wall into the lung fields.

Peripheral edema is due to an expansion of the interstitial fluid volume. Capillary fluid dynamics, lymph flow, interstitial fluid pressure, and interstitial compartment compliance are the factors which regulate interstitial fluid volume.[1] In heart failure, the primary factors responsible for edema are the increased venous capillary pressure and the decreased CO with consequent renal fluid retention.[1] Peripheral edema occurs in dependent portions of the body, such as the legs and feet of ambulatory patients and the lumbosacral area of recumbent patients.

Other signs and symptoms of CHF which may be present are hepatomegaly, hydropericardium, and cyanosis. The span of the liver is increased and extends well below the right costal margin. Echocardiography frequently identifies pericardial fluid, although usually insufficient to produce tamponade. With a low cardiac output, flow through capillary beds is reduced, increasing the extraction of oxygen from hemoglobin. The increased amount of reduced hemoglobin in capillary beds causes cyanosis of skin and mucous membranes. Excessive sweating, due to increased adrenergic activity, also occurs. Nocturia, because of the increased CO at rest, results from stimulated diuresis. S_3 and S_4 gallops are heard on auscultation. The electrocardiogram is nonspecific in CHF, and cardiac catheterization is rarely necessary to establish the diagnosis. It is more difficult to recognize subtle changes of cardiac dysfunction. Exercise testing is a noninvasive means to determine aerobic capacity or maximal oxygen uptake, anaerobic threshold, the severity of failure, and cardiovascular reserve.[2] An exercise test using a bicycle ergometer or treadmill will demonstrate an abnormal cardiovascular response to stress. Heart failure is characterized in these circumstances by an exaggerated increase in cardiac filling pressure and an attenuated increase in CO. Both can be measured either invasively using a pulmonary artery catheter and thermodilution cardiac outputs, or noninvasively by impedance cardiography and observation of the jugular venous pulse.

In normal individuals, right upper quadrant abdominal compression does not affect jugular venous pressure or causes only a transient increase. With CHF, there is a prompt increase in jugular venous pressure that remains elevated as long as abdominal compression is maintained. Two phenomena are probably responsible for a positive hepatojugular reflux: (1) The rising diaphragm which tamponades the heart and prevents ventricular filling; and (2) mobilization of blood from abdominal viscera augmenting venous return to a heart which cannot respond to increased venous return.[3]

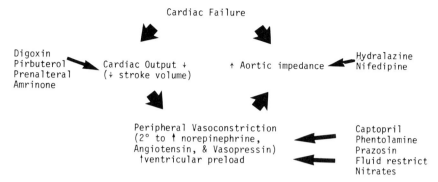

Fig. 14-1. The vicious cycle of cardiac failure. The compensatory mechanisms of vasoconstriction and fluid retention actually worsen ventricular performance. The points where therapeutic intervention can break or modify the cycle are demonstrated.

PATHOPHYSIOLOGY

Although impaired myocardial performance is usually present in patients with CHF, complex multisystem involvement initiates a positive feedback among the heart, peripheral circulation, and other vital organ systems, resulting in the clinical syndrome (Fig. 14-1). These feedback mechanisms involve aortic impedance, ventricular preload, sodium retention, peripheral edema, neurohumoral responses from the renin-angiotensin, vasopressin-antidiuretic hormone (ADH), or sympathetic nervous systems, as well as myocardial hypertrophy and ischemia[4] (Table 14-1). All of these mechanisms are systemic responses to the inadequate pump.

Impaired Myocardial Performance

PRIMARY MYOCARDIAL DISEASE

Myocardial failure is characterized by decreases in the force and speed of muscle contraction. Both the velocity of shortening and the maximum rate of force development are decreased in heart failure. However, the elasticity of the heart, measured in terms of the series elastic properties, are unchanged and there is little or no change in passive length-tension relations of isolated failing heart muscles[5] (Table 14-2).

Right-heart failure commonly accompanies left-heart failure. Chronic pulmonary venous hypertension increases PVR and right ventricular afterload. During exercise, pulmonary artery pressure, right ventricular, and right atrial pressures increase secondary to the increase in left ventricular filling and pulmonary venous pressures.

ROLE OF AORTIC IMPEDANCE

Normal aortic impedance includes both a compliance component from the large arteries and a resistive component from the smaller arteries and arterioles. Ventricular afterload includes not only aortic impedance, but also the contribution from ventricular volume and wall thickness, as well as the

Table 14-1

Pathophysiology of Heart Failure

Hemodynamic alterations
  Decreased myocardial contractility
  Increased preload
  Increased afterload
  Increased heart rate
Neurohumoral responses
  Sympathetic activation
  Increased renin-angiotensin-aldosterone system
    activity
  Increased vasopressin levels

Table 14-2

Mechanical Alterations in Heart Failure

Decreased force of contraction
Decreased speed (velocity) of contraction
Decreased maximum rate of force development
Little or no change in passive length-tension
  relations
Unchanged series elastic properties

Source: Adapted from Parmley WW: Pathophysiology of congestive heart failure. Am J Cardiol 55:9A–14A, 1985.

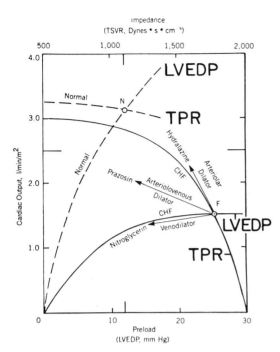

Fig. 14-2. The output of the normal heart (dotted lines) is regulated primarily by the left ventricular end-diastolic pressure (LVEDP) and very little by total peripheral resistance (TPR or TSVR). The failing heart (solid lines), however, is quite sensitive to alterations in afterload. Thus, the benefits of arterial vasodilation (hydralazine) are significant. Venodilators (nitroglycerin) decrease preload, but fail to improve cardiac output. Mixed arteriovenous dilators (prazosin) increase cardiac output and decrease preload. (From Mason DT: Treatment of acute and chronic congestive heart failure by vasodilator-afterload reduction. Arch Intern Med 140:1577–1581, 1980, with permission.)

viscous and inertial properties of the blood. Together, these factors comprise the wall stress or force per unit area faced by the ventricle and vary during ventricular ejection. Normally the left ventricle is principally regulated by changes in preload rather than afterload. The failing heart becomes very sensitive to alterations of afterload because it cannot compensate by augmentation of contractile force or by the Frank-Starling mechanism[6] (Fig. 14-2). Impedance is significantly increased in patients with heart failure.[7]

ROLE OF PRELOAD

A large end-diastolic ventricular volume results from impaired left ventricular emptying. The diastolic compliance of the ventricle may also be decreased in failure. Other alterations in CHF that

increase preload are decreased venous compliance due to increased sympathetic activity, increased intravascular volume, and sodium retention.

Neurohumoral Responses

SYMPATHETIC NERVOUS SYSTEM RESPONSE

Activation of the sympathetic nervous system is suggested by the elevated plasma norepinephrine often seen in patients with CHF.[8] Tachycardia, diaphoresis, and peripheral vasoconstriction also implicate the sympathetic nervous system. Coronary sinus norepinephrine is also increased.[9] As CHF progresses, the myocardial catecholamine stores are depleted, because sympathetic nerve endings in the heart fail to synthesize, store, and release catecholamines. However, myocardial dopamine content may be increased.[10] Augmentation of cardiac contractility in response to local release of catecholamines is lost, although normal myocardial responsiveness is maintained. It is not, however, the loss of myocardial catecholamines per se that *causes* heart failure.[11]

In addition, there is a blunted peripheral response to catecholamines, possibly as a consequence of "down regulation" of the alpha-adrenergic receptors exposed to chronically elevated plasma norepinephrine levels in CHF.[12] This finding has been noted in patients with CHF given infusions of up to 2.5 μg/min of norepinephrine without hemodynamic response.

RENIN-ANGIOTENSIN-ALDOSTERONE SYSTEM RESPONSE

Renin, a proteolytic enzyme produced in the granular juxtaglomerular cells of the kidney, initiates the formation of angiotensin I from angiotensinogen, a tetradecapeptide alpha-globulin synthesized in the liver.[13] Angiotensin I, which is biologically inactive, is cleaved by the carboxypeptidase, angiotensin converting enzyme (ACE), in the lung and other tissues to the vasoactive angiotensin II (ANG II).[13] ANG II and angiotensin III, formed by hydrolyis of ANG II, stimulate aldosterone secretion. Angiotensin III is also vasoactive, though less so than ANG II. The half-life in the circulation of renin is between 4 and 15 minutes, but that of ANG II is only 30 seconds. Renin release is governed by the macula densa, an intrarenal "stretch-type" receptor, renal sympathetic nerves, and circulating potassium, vasopressin, ANG II, and epinephrine.[14,15]

Plasma renin activity (PRA) is elevated in some, but not all, patients with CHF.[16] There appear to be two extremes, patients with markedly elevated and markedly suppressed PRA. Sodium intake is pivotal in this response with increased PRA in sodium depletion.[17] Because the macula densa is sensitive to stretch, there is an inverse relationship between renal perfusion and renin secretion.[15] Decreased stretch, such as occurs with decreased CO and CHF, increases secretion of renin. High-renin heart failure is characterized by a low serum sodium,[18] although diuretic therapy affects this response.[19] Hyperaldosteronism also results from decreased hepatic metabolism of aldosterone in heart failure.

Several factors may stimulate renin release in CHF: decreased renal blood pressure and flow ("baroreceptor theory"), increased sympathetic activity by cardiac mechanoreceptors ("sympathetic nervous system theory"), and decreased macula densa sodium or intracellular ionized calcium ("macula densa theory").[4] In normal individuals, low-pressure mechanoreceptors in the right atrium respond to sudden resumption of upright posture and decreased venous return by stimulation of renin release. This does not occur in patients with heart failure.[20] Total body sodium, and thus decreased sodium delivery to the distal tubule, stimulates renin release.[21] Which of these factors is responsible for renin release in CHF is uncertain.

Angiotensin II is a potent vasoconstrictor that inappropriately increases vascular tone, permitting further impedance of forward flow and reduction of cardiac output. Angiotensin II also directly stimulates aldosterone release from the adrenal gland to retain fluid and sodium.[17] Aldosterone release stimulates renal potassium release. Angiotensin II plays a major role in mediating renal blood flow in patients with CHF.

VASOPRESSIN-ADH SYSTEM RESPONSE

Plasma arginine vasopressin levels are elevated in patients with CHF, potentiating the peripheral vasoconstriction induced by ANG II and norepinephrine to maintain arterial pressure.[22] The elevated vasopressin level, coupled with the increased sodium content in blood vessels, increases plasma volume,

vascular stiffness, and systemic vascular resistance.[23,24] There is little correlation between either norepinephrine or PRA and arginine vasopressin, indicating that different mechanisms are probably responsible for their control.[22]

Myocardial Energetics in Failure

BIOCHEMICAL CHANGES IN THE FAILING MYOCARDIUM

The function of contractile proteins is defective in CHF. Although there is considerable controversy resulting from difficulties in defining the correct time to measure biochemical parameters, it appears that myocardial mitochondrial function is abnormal during CHF, but may be normal when the compensated hypertrophic phase is studied.[25] The myofibrillar ATPase activity and high-energy phosphate stores are decreased in hypertrophy and heart failure, which is responsible for the depressed mechanical performance of these hearts.[26] The actomyosin ATPase activity is related to the velocity of shortening in CHF. The myosin isozymes are altered with a shift from fast to slow isozymes[5] (Table 14-3).

ENERGY PRODUCTION AND UTILIZATION

The processes of energy production, such as substrate uptake, intermediary metabolism, and oxidative phosphorylation were noted to be normal in older studies of the failing heart.[5,27] The concentrations of both creatine phosphate and adenosine triphosphate (ATP) were maintained. However, more recent studies suggest the possibility of depletion of high-energy phosphates in CHF,[5] or that the ATP might be depleted in some small vital compartment responsible for muscle contraction, but this has not been documented. Changes in other energy-linked functions, such as calcium transport in the sarcoplasmic reticulum or mitochondria, may be affected in CHF before energy production or utilization themselves.

EXCITATION-CONTRACTION COUPLING

Calcium ion is particularly important in myocardial contractility and in the initiation of myocardial contraction. During diastole, extracellular calcium is concentrated in the region of the sarcolemma, while intracellular calcium is sequestered in the sarcoplasmic reticulum. When the cell membrane is excited, there is rapid entry of extracellular calcium into the cell. As depolarization spreads via the sarcotubular system, intracellular calcium is released to activate

Table 14-3
Biochemical Changes in CHF

Decreased myofibrillar ATPase activity
Decreased myocardial synthesis and storage of NE
? Decreased ATP and CP
Decreased sarcoplasmic reticulum function
Increased myocardial collagen content

the contractile proteins. For myocardial relaxation to occur, the intracellular calcium must be taken up by the sarcoplasmic reticulum and calcium must efflux from the cell. In heart failure, a decrease in the function of the sarcoplasmic reticulum with a decreased rate of uptake of calcium and decreased calcium stores have been reported, but the total uptake of calcium by the sarcoplasmic reticulum may be normal.[28]

Role of the Kidney in Congestive Heart Failure

Blood flow to the renal cortex is abut 3–5 ml/gm/min, which is considerably in excess of that required for metabolism. Blood perfusing the capillaries of the glomerulus is ultrafiltered, the first step in urine formation. The glomerular hydrostatic pressure, essentially the systemic arterial pressure modified by afferent and efferent capillary tone, is the main driving force for filtration. This hydrostatic pressure offsets the plasma oncotic and intratubular pressures which would retard filtration. An increased blood flow relative to metabolic needs and the low renal vascular resistance demonstrate the importance of normal cardiovascular function to the kidney.

Either decreased systemic arterial pressure or increased renal vascular resistance, particularly at the afferent arteriole (due to increased sympathetic activity, exogenous catecholamines, or ANG II) can reduce glomerular capillary pressure and filtration. Renal plasma flow is decreased in CHF, but the precise mechanism is complex and poorly understood.[29] Other intrarenal hemodynamic factors than glomerular perfusion can also affect renal function. Peritubular capillary hydrostatic and oncotic pressures determine the net absorption of sodium from the plasma ultrafiltrate. The increased filtration fraction seen in CHF increases peritubular capillary oncotic pressure and sodium reabsorption.[30]

Hyponatremia is often seen in patients with CHF. Proximal tubular reabsorption of sodium is enhanced, but in the ascending limb of Henle's loop sodium reabsorption is reduced. The countercurrent system of the renal medulla depends upon the hypertonic inner medulla created by sodium chloride in the loop of Henle. If insufficient sodium is delivered to the loop because of increased proximal tubular reabsorption, the ability of the kidney to concentrate and dilute urine is reduced, contributing to the hyponatremia of heart failure. Thus, therapy in CHF must aim to increase renal blood flow and to relieve renal vasoconstriction.

Compensatory Mechanisms

The compensatory mechanisms for CHF include increased preload (Frank-Starling mechanism), myocardial contractility, and myocardial hypertrophy. A decreased venous pressure (preload) or resistance to ejection (afterload) can also prevent the decline in cardiac function when the heart moves onto the descending limb of Starling's curve (Fig. 14-2). Other responses to a low CO are the redistribution of CO to vital organs such as the brain and myocardium, slowing of the circulation time, and decreased oxyhemoglobin affinity. The oxyhemoglobin dissociation curve is shifted rightward secondary to increased 2, 3 diphosphoglycerate (2,3DPG) levels to enhance the availability of oxygen to the tissues.[31] The slow circulation time also facilitates oxygen delivery to the tissues. Redistribution of CO is particularly noticeable during exercise when reduction of flow to the mesenteric and renal vascular beds is prominent.[32]

FRANK-STARLING MECHANISM

Starling observed that "the mechanical energy set free on passage from the resting to the contracted state is a function of the length of the muscle fibers." Thus, the relationship between stroke volume and end-diastolic volume can be used to evaluate changes in ventricular function (Fig. 14-2). In CHF, an increased preload or end-diastolic volume sustains stroke volume. The presence of a descending limb on Starling's curve remains debatable.

MYOCARDIAL HYPERTROPHY AND OTHER MECHANICAL ALTERATIONS

The pressure- and volume-overloaded left ventricle responds by increasing muscle mass to attempt to maintain its performance. Protein synthesis and myocardial hypertrophy, thus, would at first glance appear to be desirable responses. However, the hypertrophy eventually further impairs performance as a result of the change in compliance of the ventricle with its thickened wall. Systolic function may also be impaired due to ingrowth of collagen during the hypertrophic process. An increase in ventricular end-diastolic pressure may decrease coronary perfusion pressure, particularly in the subendocardium, giving rise to myocardial ischemia which further impairs myocardial function.

Increasing the heart rate will increase the force of contraction through operation of the strength-interval relationship. However, this effect is less prominent in intact hearts than in the depressed heart.

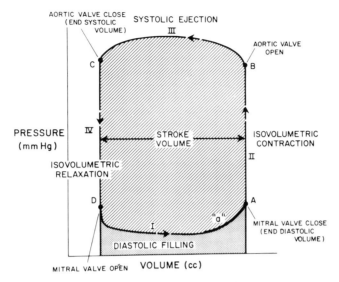

Fig. 14-3. Ventricular filling is passive during early and midventricular diastole. (I) The atrial kick (a) from atrial contraction completes left ventricular filling (the LVEDP and left ventricular end-diastolic volume). Isovolumetric contraction occurs (II), increasing intraventricular pressure with little change in volume. The aortic valve opens when intraventricular pressure exceeds aortic pressure and rapid ventricular ejection occurs (III) until intraventricular pressures decrease below aortic pressure. Ventricular relaxation is initially isovolumetric (IV) until LV pressure decreases below left atrial pressure and the mitral valve opens. (From Barash PB, Kopriva CJ: Cardiac pump function and how to monitor it. *In* Thomas S (ed): Manual of Cardiac Anesthesia. New York, Churchill Livingstone, 1984, p 1–34, with permission.)

Tachycardia can, nonetheless, improve ventricular function by increasing contractility, although the duration of diastolic filling is reduced.

PERIPHERAL CIRCULATORY RESPONSES

Inappropriate vasoconstriction in both the arterial and venous circulations results from the increased sympathetic nervous system activity. These alterations which maintain arterial blood pressure may actually further worsen cardiac function.

THERAPY

The cardiac output is determined by the product of stroke volume and heart rate, while stroke volume is dependent upon preload, afterload, and myocardial contractility. Arterial blood pressure is the product of systemic vascular resistance (SVR) and CO. Analysis of ventricular pump function may be performed by measurement of ventricular pressure-volume relationships over the entire cardiac cycle (Fig. 14-3).

Therefore, therapy for CHF is rationally determined by alterations of these parameters (Fig. 14-4).

The first principle of treatment of CHF is to identify and, if possible, correct the cause. This may include valve replacement, myocardial revascularization, or other surgical procedures. If the cause is noncorrectable, the goal of therapy is to reduce the work of the heart, reduce SVR, decrease ventricular preload, and enhance myocardial contractility. Thus, measures such as sodium restriction by diet and diuretic therapy will decrease ventricular size. Sodium restriction to 1000 mg/day also decreases extracellular water and intravascular blood volume.

Myocardial work is decreased by decreasing oxygen demand. Myocardial oxygen consumption depends upon heart rate and ventricular chamber volume. Tachycardia is avoided by control of physical and mental activity (ie, rest), or normalization of cardiac rhythm if atrial fibrillation or another supraventricular tachycardia is present. Likewise, bradyarrhythmias are avoided by pacemaker insertion or modification of drug regimens causing sinus node dysfunction.

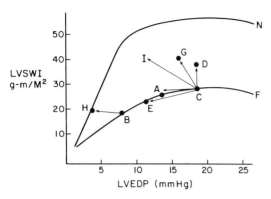

Fig. 14-4. It is preferable to use left ventricular stroke work index (LVSWI) ([Mean blood pressure (MAP)-mean pulmonary wedge pressure (PWP)] × SVI × 0.0136) rather than SV or CO on the Y axis of a Starling curve since LVSWI includes: (1) measurement of both systolic and diastolic performance (MAP and PWP); (2) major variables altering cardiac performance such as heart (SVI), preload (PWP) and afterload (MAP); (3) LVSWI defines the area within the pressure volume loop in (Fig. 14-3). N = normal heart—Starling Curve; F = failing heart—Starling curve; D = digoxin therapy in failing heart; G = failing heart (C) treated with arteriolar dilator in pt with ↑LVEDP; H = failing heart (B) treated with arteriolar dilator in pt with low LVEDP; A = diuretic therapy in failing heart; E = failing heart treated with venodilator; C = position on Starling curve of a failing heart; I = failing heart treated with both arterial and venodilators or combined with a positive inotropic drug.

Afterload reduction with vasodilator drugs reverses the excessive SVR seen in patients with CHF. Improved regional blood flow after vasodilator therapy may relieve the metabolic acidosis caused by the low CO of CHF. Although venodilator therapy does little to improve stroke output, the ventricular chamber size and pressure, ventricular wall stress, and myocardial oxygen consumption decrease in response to the increased venous capacitance. If ventricular pressures are low, venodilators can worsen stroke output by moving the heart down the ascending limb of Starling's curve. Inotropic drugs increase myocardial contractility and decrease ventricular filling pressure.

Patients with advanced CHF and hypoperfusion at rest require invasive monitoring (pulmonary and intra-arterial catheters) and therapy with intravenous agents. The therapeutic modalities discussed in this chapter may be efficacious in such patients, but the discussion will primarily focus on chronic ambulatory patient management without invasive monitors.

All pharmacologic interventions should be monitored by daily determinations of body weight, frequent physical examination, and analysis of serum electrolytes every 6–12 weeks in outpatients. More frequent determinations will be necessary in the acute stages or in patients requiring hospitalization. Mild CHF usually requires only a digitalis glycoside; moderate failure, digitalis and a diuretic. Severe failure is managed with digitalis, diuretics, positive inotropic and vasodilator drugs.

Digitalis

MECHANISM OF ACTION

Digitalis binds with the enzyme sodium-potassium ATPase, which generates the energy for extrusion of sodium from the cell during phase 4 of the resting membrane potential. Thus, intracellular sodium gradually accumulates and intracellular potassium is lost.[33] The elevated intracellular sodium increases the availability of calcium to the contractile protein system.[33,34] Digitalis exerts its positive inotropic effects independent of catecholamine liberation.

CARDIOVASCULAR EFFECTS

Digitalis augments both force and velocity of contraction in failing hearts, and, in the nonfailing heart, increases contractility without raising cardiac output.[35,36] Ventricular end-diastolic volume and end-diastolic pressure are decreased as demonstrated on the modified Starling curve (Fig. 14-4). Heart size decreases which, in turn, decreases myocardial wall tension, myocardial oxygen consumption, and angina. Although digitalis increases systolic arterial pressure, pulse pressure, and peripheral resistance in normal patients by a direct constrictor effect on arterial and venous smooth muscle,[33,34,37] it decreases SVR and venomotor tone in patients with heart failure.[33,38] Despite its weak inotropic effect, digitalis remains the primary drug for chronic cardiac failure. Vasodilator therapy may supplement, but has not replaced, digoxin therapy.[39] Digoxin is particularly useful if atrial fibrillation is coexistent with failure.

ELECTROPHYSIOLOGIC EFFECTS

Digitalis increases phase 4 depolarization and causes the resting potential to become less negative.[34,36] The duration of the action potential is shortened. Conduction through the atrioventricular (A-V) node and Purkinje tissue is delayed.[33] Vagal activity is usually increased in the presence of digitalis; thus the atrial refractory period is shortened and the refractory period of the A-V node prolonged.[33,34,37] The ventricular refractory period and automaticity in Purkinje cells is also enhanced[33] (Chapter 12).

PHARMACOKINETICS

The onset of action with digoxin occurs within 15 to 30 minutes after intravenous administration, with a peak effect in $1^1/_2$–5 hours. The beta half-life is 36 hours. Even with the improved bioavailability resulting from current dissolution standards for digoxin tablets, the bioavailability of the drug in tablet form is less than 85 percent.[4] The gelatin capsule preparation increases the bioavailability to 90–95 percent, necessitating a reduction in dose from that of tablets, but enhancing its usefulness in patients with malabsorption.[40] The volume of distribution is large, 5–8 liters/kg, and it is extensively bound to heart and skeletal muscle. Elimination is primarily by glomerular filtration and tubular secretion with about 30 percent of digoxin being excreted unchanged in urine.[41]

The therapeutic level of digoxin is 0.5–2 ng/ml,[42] with toxicity at plasma concentrations of digoxin of 2.5 ng/ml or greater.[34] Samples for digoxin levels should be obtained 5–6 hours after oral doses, 2–4 hours after intravenous doses, and 8–10 hours after intramuscular doses to be reliable indicators of myocardial digoxin levels. Digoxin doses should be reduced in patients with renal insufficiency,[42] since renal metabolism is the principal method for elimination, although some hepatic metabolism occurs.

PREPARATIONS

The most frequently prescribed digitalis glycoside for either oral or intravenous use is digoxin. For rapid digitalization of the undigitalized patient in heart failure, an oral dose of 0.0075 mg/kg is given in three divided doses every 6 hours. Maintenance doses are 0.125–0.5 mg daily. Alternatively, doses of 0.125–0.5 mg daily given for 7 days will slowly digitalize the patient. If intravenous therapy is needed, 0.5 to 0.75 mg IV of digoxin is given, followed in 60 minutes or, preferably, in 2–3 hours, by additional 0.125–0.250-mg increments as needed up to 2 mg. The effect is maximal within 1–3 hours, and digitalization is complete within 12 hours with intravenous dosing. Maintenance doses are needed in 12–24 hours. Digoxin can be given intramuscularly as well, although injection is accompanied by pain at the injection site, delayed absorption, and lower serum concentrations.[43] Digoxin is relatively contra-

indicated in patients with hypoxia, sinus node dysfunction, hypokalemia, hypercalcemia, and hypertrophic cardiomyopathy. Doses must also be carefully individualized in patients with renal dysfunction.

INTOXICATION

Although digitalis intoxication can occur in any patient receiving the drug, the elderly[44] and those with hypothyroidism[45] are particularly prone. Digitalis toxicity is enhanced by the presence of hypoxia, electrolyte imbalance such as hypomagnesemia, hypercalcemia, hypokalemia, or the concurrent administration of drugs such as propranolol, reserpine, diuretics, amiodarone,[46,47] verapamil,[48,49] or quinidine.[50]

The cardiac symptoms of digitalis toxicity arise from two mechanisms[51]: (1) enhanced automaticity, and (2) atrioventricular block. The increased automaticity is seen in intracellular electrophysiologic preparations as after-depolarizations, after-potentials, or triggered activity, which result from oscillating release of calcium ions from the sarcoplasmic reticulum.[52] The dysrhythmias in digitalis intoxication include nonparoxysmal junctional tachycardia, atrioventricular junctional escape rhythm, ventricular bigeminy or trigeminy, and ventricular ectopic beats, either alone or with ventricular tachycardia.[53] Atrial flutter, atrial fibrillation, and wide-complex ventricular tachycardia are very rare in digitalis toxicity. Digitalis toxicity in patients with atrial fibrillation is characterized by a slow, but irregular ventricular response, or a regularization of fibrillation due to a nodal Wenckebach pattern. Patients with toxicity often demonstrate worsening CHF.

Extracardiac symptoms of toxicity originate in the gastrointestinal and nervous systems, including anorexia, nausea, vomiting, diarrhea, abdominal pain,[33] headache, drowsiness, disorientation, confusion, dizziness, syncope, paresthesias, neuralgias, delirium, and convulsions. The gastrointestinal symptoms are probably a result of medullary chemoreceptor stimulation,[54] rather than direct gastrointestinal irritation, as digoxin can be detected in the cerebrospinal fluid. Digoxin also appears to accumulate in peripheral nervous tissue such as sympathetic ganglia.[55] Blurred or yellow vision, white halos around dark objects, diplopia, scotomas, and optic neuritis are less common symptoms.

The first step in the treatment of toxicity is discontinuation of digitalis, which is sufficient in mild cases. Potassium, which binds loosely to the myocardium and delays subsequent digitalis binding, should be given if serum concentrations are low. However, digitalis is firmly bound, and potassium has little effect on glycoside already attached to the heart. Diuretics causing potassium loss and infusions of carbohydrates that cause intracellular movement of potassium should be avoided. Potassium is contraindicated when high degrees of AV block are present.

For serious digitalis-induced dysrhythmias lidocaine, procainamide, phenytoin, propranolol, or DC shock may be required. DC countershock may be required for drug-resistant ventricular tachycardia or fibrillation accompanied by shock, although ventricular dysrhythmias resulting from DC shocks may be fatal. The frequency of ventricular dysrhythmias after electroconversion of supraventricular dysrhythmias can be reduced by using the lowest amount of energy that will convert the dysrhythmias, coupled with lidocaine to suppress PVCs.[56]

INTERACTIONS WITH OTHER DRUGS

Concomitant administration of quinidine,[46,50] amiodarone,[46,47] nifedipine, and verapamil[48,49] increases serum digoxin concentrations. In the case of quinidine, both renal and nonrenal clearance are affected, with inhibition of tubular secretion the most likely renal mechanism.[54] Serum digoxin is unaffected by disopyramide, lidocaine, aprindine, mexilitene, and propranolol. Anesthetic agents which increase tolerance to digitalis in experimental animals include diethyl ether, methoxyflurane, enflurane, isoflurane, ketamine, and Innovar (Janssen Pharmaceutica, Piscataway; NJ).[57]

Diuretics

The glomerular filtrate is an ultrafiltrate of plasma presented to the proximal tubule for sodium reabsorption. Hydrogen ion and organic acid secretion also occur in the proximal tubule. About 70 percent of sodium reabsorption occurs in the proximal tubule. The reabsorption of sodium is an active, energy-requiring process in which sodium accompanied by chloride is transported out of the tubular fluid, and hydrogen ion is secreted into the tubular fluid. In the ascending limb of Henle's loop, chloride is actively transported and sodium passively follows. Because the ascending limb is impervious to water, the tubular fluid is dilute. Of the sodium presented to the ascending limb, 55–60 percent is reabsorbed. In the distal convoluted tubule, another 5–10 percent of the sodium is reabsorbed. Reabsorption in the distal convoluted tubule and collecting duct depends on ADH. If ADH is present, tubular water is extracted. If absent, no water is reabsorbed. Aldosterone regu-

lates the sodium reabsorption in exchange for hydrogen and potassium in the distal convoluted tubule and collecting duct. Only 3 percent of the sodium is reabsorbed here (Fig. 14-5).

Although diuretics have no direct effect on the intrinsic myocardial activity of the failing heart, they often reverse the physiological imbalance produced by hypoperfusion of the kidney. In CHF, renal hypoperfusion stimulates the kidney to retain water and sodium by activation of the renin-angiotensin-aldosterone system, increased proximal tubular sodium reabsorption due to an increased filtration fraction, and redistribution of renal blood from the cortex to the salt-conserving medulla. Water and sodium retention expand extracellular volume to increase preload. Diuretics inhibit solute reabsorption in the renal tubule, enhancing the elimination of water and sodium. Ethacrynic acid and furosemide redistribute renal blood flow toward the renal cortex with less salt conservation. Their effects on the Starling curve are seen in Fig. 14-4. Cardiac output is often decreased by diuresis, but congestion is relieved. Diuretic therapy must be carefully monitored since effective circulating blood volume is actually reduced in CHF, and further decreases in blood volume can be detrimental. In fact, as diuresis is stimulated, regulatory processes counterbalance their effect and limit the response. Examples of these regulatory processes are: (1) decreased blood volume decreases CO, renal blood flow, and glomerular filtration (filtration fraction is increased since renal blood flow is decreased more than glomerular filtration); (2) increased filtration fraction elevates peritubular oncotic pressure, enhancing sodium reabsorption proximal to the loop of Henle; and, (3) gradual increase in plasma aldosterone occurs after 5–6 days due to activation of the renin-angiotensin system. Prolonged diuretic therapy depleting total body sodium stimulates the macula densa to produce renin. The various types of diuretics are discussed below and in Chapter 11.

MERCURIAL

The mercurial diuretics, which inhibit reabsorption of sodium and chloride in the ascending limb of the loop of Henle, are infrequently used today. Treatment with mercurials usually produces a metabolic alkalosis because losses of chloride are unaccompanied by equivalent amounts of bicarbonate.

THIAZIDE DIURETICS

Thiazide diuretics accelerate sodium-potassium exchange between the diluting segment in the ascending limb of the loop of Henle and the initial

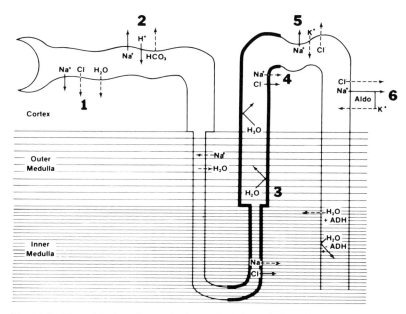

Fig. 14-5. Normal ionic exchanges in the renal tubule are indicated. Numerals indicate the sites of action of the various diuretics where 1—early proximal tubule, 2—late proximal tubule, 3&4—ascending limb, loop of Henle, 5—distal tubule, 6—collecting duct. + indicates a major site of action in the table below. (+) indicates a minor site of action. (From Merin RG, Bastron RD: Diuretics. *In* Smith NT, Corbascio AN (eds): Drug Interactions in Anesthesia. Philadelphia, Lea & Febiger, 1981, p. 148, with permission.)

Diuretic	Site					
	1	2	3	4	5	6
Thiazide		(+)		+	(+)	
Furosemide	(+)	(+)	+	(+)	(+)	
Ethacrynic acid	(+)		+	(+)	(+)	
Spironolactone						+
Triamterene					+	
Metolazone		(+)			+	
Bumetanide			+			

Source: From Merin RG, Bastron RD: Diuretics. *In* Smith NT, Corbascio AN (eds): Drug Interactions in Anesthesia. Philadelphia, Lea & Febiger, 1981, p 148, with permission.

portion of the distal tubule where sodium reabsorption is regulated by aldosterone (Fig. 14-5). Sodium reabsorption is inhibited and potassium secretion enhanced. The carbonic anhydrase activity of thiazides is negligible. Chloride, sodium, and potassium are excreted. Magnesium and, to a small extent, bicarbonate is lost as well.

Like the thiazides, metolazone, a quinethazone derivative, inhibits initial distal and possible proximal tubular reabsorption of sodium. Unlike the thiazides, its effectiveness is maintained even with decreasing renal function.

Thiazides are rapidly absorbed through the gastrointestinal (GI) tract. The onset of action is 1–2 hours with a peak at four hours and duration of action of 6–12 hours. Their action is unaffected by acid-base balance. The dose depends on the particular thiazide compound, but all thiazides have similar pharmacologic effects (Chapter 11). Thiazides are excreted unchanged in the urine by glomerular filtration and proximal tubular secretion.[58] They are also excreted by the liver in the absence of renal function.[59] Once or twice daily administration of 50–100 mg of hydrochlorothiazide, orally, is used for CHF.

The dose of chlorothiazide is 500–1000 mg/day, and its duration of action is 6–12 hours. Chlorthalidone has an onset of action within 2 hours after 25–100 mg/day doses, and its duration of action is 48–72 hours. Metolazone, in doses of 5–10 mg/day, has its onset in one hour and a duration of action of 24–48 hours.

Hypokalemia, hyperuricemia, and glucose intolerance are the most frequent complications of thiazide therapy. Potassium and chloride supplementation may be necessary if dietary intake of these elements is inadequate. Thiazide drugs may exacerbate renal insufficiency and their efficacy is reduced in renal dysfunction.[60] They decrease glomerular filtration rate about 20 percent due either to a direct renal vascular effect or decreased effective filtration pressure from diuretic-induced increased intratubular volume or pressure.[60] Thiazides slightly increase renal vascular resistance, and PRA increases during therapy.

Thiazides are often used for maintenance therapy in ambulatory patients with mild CHF. They are frequently combined with digoxin or vasodilator therapy.

LOOP DIURETICS

Ethacrynic acid, furosemide, and bumetanide are the commonly used loop diuretics. Although their chemical structures are different, their mechanisms of action, inhibition of tubular reabsorption of sodium along the medullary and cortical portions of the loop of Henle, are similar (Fig. 14-5). Bumetanide is a metanilimide derivative, whereas furosemide is a sulfonamide. Because chloride transport in the loop of Henle is inhibited, the gradient permitting water reabsorption in the descending limb and medullary collecting duct is disrupted and free-water clearance is increased. Furosemide also has some carbonic anhydrase activity as well, interfering with reabsorption of bicarbonate and phosphate in the proximal tubule. Inhibition of proximal tubular sodium reabsorption is an unimportant action of furosemide (Fig. 14-5). Ethacrynic acid and furosemide inhibit free-water generation, causing excretion of concentrated urine, which predisposes to hyponatremia. Hyponatremia is also linked to potassium depletion by enhancement of antidiuretic hormone secretion and by movement of sodium intracellularly to replace potassium. Excretion of sodium, potassium, chloride, magnesium, and calcium is increased by these drugs.

Furosemide can increase venous capacitance and decrease left ventricular filling pressure by direct vasodilatation with peripheral venous pooling before

diuresis, even in renal failure.[61,62] Ethacrynic acid, furosemide, and bumetanide increase total renal blood flow by uncertain mechanisms, possibly mediated via the kallikrein system, prostaglandins, or increased proximal tubular pressure.[14] This effect is unrelated to the diuretic effect and results from decreased renal vascular resistance.[14] All three drugs increase plasma renin activity.

The onset of action orally or intravenously is rapid. The following doses of furosemide, 40–120 mg/day, ethacrynic acid 50–100 mg/day, and bumetanide, 0.5–2 mg/day, are used. The onset is within 1 hour and the duration of action about 4–8 hours after oral administration. With intravenous administration, the onset occurs in 5–10 minutes with a duration of 3 hours. The volumes of distribution are the size of the extracellular space.[63] Both furosemide and ethacrynic acid may be effective in patients with renal dysfunction. Furosemide and ethacrynic acid are excreted unchanged in stool and urine.

Furosemide may increase the action of nondepolarizing neuromuscular blocking agents.[64] Adverse effects include hypokalemia, hyponatremia, deafness, leukopenia, hepatic necrosis, hyperuricemia, and contraction alkalosis. The hypokalemic alkalosis occurs with both thiazides and loop diuretics. It results from the loss of sodium, water, potassium and hydrogen ions in the distal tubular fluid. The hydrogen ions generate bicarbonate which is reabsorbed. A reduction of diuretic dose coupled with potassium administration will remedy this condition. Furosemide may also exhibit cross-hypersensitivity reactions with thiazides and their derivatives. In allergic patients, the use of bumetanide eliminates such reactions. Urinary excretion of magnesium is increased by loop and thiazide diuretics, which may increase the possibility of cardiac dysrhythmias secondary to myocardial potassium loss and hypomagnesemia.

POTASSIUM-SPARING DIURETICS

Amiloride, spironolactone, and triamterene are potassium-sparing diuretics. Spironolactone is a competitive inhibitor of aldosterone. It prevents binding of aldosterone to cellular receptors, which prevents aldosterone-induced distal tubule sodium reabsorption. Amiloride and triamterene block a site in the distal convoluted tubule responsible for potassium, sodium and hydrogen exchange independent of aldosterone (Fig. 14-5). Triamterene and amiloride also antagonize the renal tubular effects of aldosterone. Triamterene and amiloride decrease the glomerular filtration rate, whereas spironolactone increases it. Potassium-sparing diuretics are usually given in conjunction with furosemide or ethacrynic acid to reduce the potassium loss associated with thiazides or loop diuretics. Spironolactone is most effective when increased aldosterone is involved in the sodium and water retention.

Spironolactone, 25 mg orally, four times daily, and triamterene, 100 mg orally, once or twice daily, are effective doses. Within 2 hours, triamterene is effective and its action continues for 12–16 hours. Amiloride is given in doses of 5–10 mg daily. Its onset of action may be delayed up to 72 hours. A side effect of all potassium-sparing diuretics is hyperkalemia; thus, they should be given with extreme caution, if at all, to patients with renal dysfunction.

In most patients with moderate CHF either a thiazide or loop diuretic will promote sufficient diuresis to control fluid retention. Combinations of a thiazide and loop diuretic, or triple therapy with the addition of a potassium-sparing agent will be required in resistant cases.

VASODILATORS

The hemodynamic effects of vasodilators are exerted on the arterial, venous, and coronary circulations, or on all three vascular components. Preload is the end-diastolic stress on the ventricle, usually presented as the end-diastolic fiber length. It is not synonymous with, but is related to, end-diastolic volume. Afterload is the wall stress or tension faced by the myocardium during ventricular ejection. Factors determining afterload are the left ventricular radius (determined by chamber volume and preload) and aortic impedance (controlled by arterial compliance and SVR in the case of the left ventricle).[65] Afterload is not synonymous with mean arterial pressure (MAP) or SVR, although both are often used clinically to approximate afterload.

Vasodilators reduce both preload and afterload by decreasing ventricular filling pressure, and systemic and pulmonary resistances. They also decrease the intracavitary radius and increase wall thickness during ventricular ejection. Ventricular emptying improves. In CHF, pure arteriolar dilators increase CO with little or no change in preload. Venous vasodilators principally decrease preload on both sides of the heart with little change in CO. The overall effect of a venodilator will depend upon the initial LVEDP. If it is increased, a decrease in LVEDP may cause a substantial increase in stroke volume. With a low LVEDP, venodilatation and a decreased preload may actually decrease the stroke volume (Fig. 14-4). Dilators affecting both arterioles and veins increase CO and decrease preload in patients with CHF.

Vasodilation can be produced by a number of mechanisms including direct vascular smooth muscle relaxation, reduction of peripheral sympathetic outflow, alpha-adrenergic blockade, ganglionic blockade, calcium entry blockade, beta$_2$-receptor stimulation, competitive antagonism of ANG II, and increased cyclic quanosine monophosphate (cGMP) in vascular smooth muscle. Many vasodilator drugs have multiple mechanisms of vasodilatation (Table 14-4).

Optimal use of vasodilator therapy may require invasive monitoring at least initially until the predominant hemodynamic abnormality (increased LVEDP or SVR) is identified. Invasive monitoring is less essential if neurohumoral antagonists (converting enzyme inhibitors, alpha-adrenergic blockers) are used in patients with valvular regurgitation and marked ventricular dilatation than when direct-acting agents (hydralazine, minoxidil) are given to patients with less ventricular wall stress. If neither clinical nor radiographic evidence of pulmonary congestion

Table 14-4
Vasodilator Therapy in Heart Failure

Drug	Dose	Mechanism	Types of Action
Captopril	6.25–25 mg TID	CEI	A + V
Enalapril	5–10 mg BID	CEI	A + V
Prazosin	2–10 mg QID	α_1-adrenergic blockade	A + V
Minoxidil	10–20 mg BID	Direct	A
Nitroglycerine	Topical 1–4 inches		
	10–60 mg oral QID	Direct	V
Hydralazine	75–200 mg TID or BID	Direct	A
Phentolamine	50–100 mg daily	α-adrenergic blockade	A
Trimazosin	25–100 mg TID	α_1-adrenergic blockade	A + V

A = arteriolar dilator; V = venodilator; CEI = converting enzyme inhibition.

or left ventricular failure are present, hydralazine may be the safest choice for the management of mild-to-moderate CHF. The role of vasodilator therapy in severe CHF is well-documented, while its use in mild or moderate failure is uncertain and requires further evaluation. Vasodilator therapy should generally be avoided in the presence of normal or decreased LVEDP. Indications for vasodilator therapy in addition to heart failure include angina, hypertension, regurgitant mitral or aortic valve disease, and acute myocardial infarction (see Chapters 11, 13 and 26).

ALPHA-ADRENERGIC INHIBITORS

Receptors of the sympathetic nervous system are classified as either alpha or beta. The alpha-receptors include the $alpha_1$ subtype, which is near the neural synaptic cleft, responsive to neuronally released norepinephrine, and causes vasoconstriction. The $alpha_2$ subtype may be either neuronal or vascular receptors. The vascular $alpha_2$-receptor is distant from the synaptic cleft, responsive to circulating or blood-born catecholamines,[66] and also mediates vasoconstriction.

Prazosin. Prazosin, a quinazoline derivative, blocks the vascular alpha-adrenergic receptors. It has marked affinity for the postsynaptic $alpha_1$-receptors, but little affinity for the neuronal $alpha_2$-receptor.[67] Both precapillary resistance and postcapillary venous capacitance vessels are dilated by prazosin, so that it is essentially an "oral nitroprusside" (Table 14-4). The norepinephrine system for negative feedback remains intact since phosphodiesterase inhibition, which interferes with norepinephrine synthesis, is not induced by prazosin in clinical doses.[68]

Cardiac output and stroke volume are increased while SVR and blood pressure decrease. Pulmonary and systemic venous pressures and resistances also decrease[69,70] (Figs. 14-2 and 14-4). Heart rate decreases or is unchanged. In some patients, coronary hemodynamic effects are variable, with increases in coronary blood flow reported despite a decrease in myocardial oxygen demand.[71,72] Hepatic blood flow increases with lower doses and is unchanged at higher doses, while renal vascular resistance and renal blood flow are unaffected.[4] Prazosin may also exert some antiarrhythmic effects.[73]

Prazosin is often used as a long-term afterload reduction agent in doses of 0.5–20 mg daily. It is rapidly absorbed orally with good bioavailability. The mean elimination half-life of 2.5 hours is slightly prolonged in patients with CHF and the pro-

tein binding is reduced.[74] The volume of distribution in humans is 78–118 liters.[75] Hepatic metabolism and excretion in the bile terminate its effects. Adverse effects include postural hypotension, but serious side effects are rare. For unclear reasons, early attenuation of its hemodynamic effects occurs.[76] Clinical tolerance may be managed by: (1) substitution of nitrates and hydralazine temporarily; (2) continuation of the drug and waiting for resumption of response; (3) increasing the dose; or (4) addition of a diuretic. Pretreatment with spironolactone minimizes clinical tolerance.[72]

Trimazosin. This quinazoline derivative increases the CO and stroke volume of patients with CHF.[71] Systemic and pulmonary pressures and resistances decrease, while heart rate and arterial pressure are unchanged.[77] Like prazosin, it exerts a balanced effect on both the venous and arterial circulations (Table 14-4). Even during chronic therapy, the beneficial effects are maintained without development of tolerance or fluid retention.[71] Usual doses are 25 to 100 mg three times daily.

Labetalol. This recently introduced drug blocks both alpha- and beta-receptors. The beta-receptor blockade predominates in a ratio of 7:1.[78] The site of its alpha-blocking effect is the postjunctional vascular alpha-receptors. While a decrease in plasma angiotensin and aldosterone have been demonstrated in some studies,[79] other investigators have been unable to show a substantial change in the renin-angiotensin system.[80] Labetalol also has membrane-stabilizing and antiarrhythmic properties. It is well-absorbed orally, with peak concentrations in 30–60 minutes, and undergoes first-pass hepatic metabolism terminating its effects within 8 to 12 hours.[78] Intravenously, it has a biexponential clearance and an elimination half-life of 4.9 hours.[78]

Hemodynamically, labetalol decreases SVR with a small reduction in CO after intravenous administration. Its alpha-antagonist properties are similar to those of prazosin. However, because it has significant beta-blocking activity, it may be unsuitable for the therapy of CHF and doses for that purpose have not been established.

Phenoxybenzamine. This is a powerful alpha-blocker with a long-lasting effect. Severe hypotension and reflex tachycardia are the major problems with its use, and, therefore, it is employed in the management of CHF very infrequently. Oral doses of 10–60 mg/day are given incrementally.

Phentolamine. Phentolamine has a direct relaxing action on vascular smooth muscle combined with alpha-adrenergic blockade. It blocks both pre-synaptic alpha$_2$- and postsynaptic alpha$_1$-adrenoceptors. The major effect is arteriolar dilatation with less venodilator action than either sodium nitroprusside (SNP) or nitroglycerin (NTG)[81] (Table 14-4). In one of the earliest reports of successful vasodilator therapy, Majid et al found that alpha-adrenergic blockade with phentolamine improved left ventricular function and decreased SVR.[82] Phentolamine increased ejection fraction and CO while decreasing pulmonary venous pressure[82,83] (Figs. 14-2 and 14-4). A positive inotropic effect also occurs when norepinephrine is released from the nerve terminal and is blocked from reuptake at the alpha$_2$-receptor. Phentolamine is most effective for the patient with decreased CO, increased SVR, and normal or near normal ventricular filling pressures.

Phentolamine is usually given in intravenous doses of 1–2 μg/kg/min. Calculation of SVR may be necessary to demonstrate afterload reduction at this low dose.[82,84] Stern et al noted significant reduction of right- and left-sided filling pressures, as well as increased CO and heart rate with doses of 10 μg/kg/min in patients with chronic CHF, and improvement persisted for 53 minutes after discontinuation of the drug.[85]

Oral doses of 50 mg four to six times daily have been used, but experience is limited with an oral preparation.[86] Phentolamine also inhibits the bronchoconstriction associated with CHF.[82] The metabolism of phentolamine is largely unknown, although about 10 percent is excreted in urine.

GANGLIONIC BLOCKERS

Guanethidine. Guanethidine inhibits the depolarization of the postganglionic nerve terminal, blocking norepinephrine release and decreasing peripheral sympathetic outflow.[87] It also partially releases norepinephrine from the intraneuronal storage granules and blocks its reuptake by the nerve terminal.[87] Guanethidine is generally used for hypertension rather than treatment of CHF. The usual antihypertensive oral dose is 35–100 mg, with orthostatic hypotension and diarrhea common adverse effects.[87]

CALCIUM CHANNEL BLOCKERS

Of the numerous calcium channel blockers that are available or being tested, nifedipine is most often used to improve left ventricular function by systemic

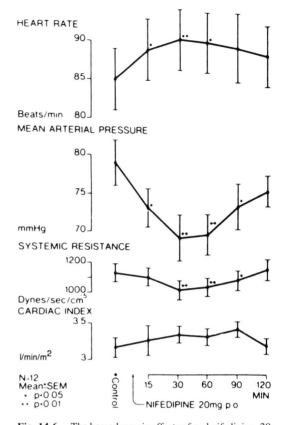

Fig. 14-6. The hemodynamic effects of oral nifedipine, 20 mg, in patients with congestive heart failure. Compared to control values, nifedipine significantly decreases arterial pressure and systemic resistance. Because nifedipine has no direct effect on the sinus node, reflex tachycardia occurs in response to vasodilation. (From Josephson MA, Josephson MA, Singh BN: Use of calcium antagonists in ventricular dysfunction. Am J Cardiol 55:81B–88B, 1985, with permission.)

vasodilation. The adverse effect on ventricular function produced by verapamil does not justify its use as an afterload-reducing agent in patients with ventricular dysfunction. Diltiazem has not been systematically investigated in patients with ventricular dysfunction. Indeed, the ultimate role of calcium channel blockers for afterload reduction is unclear at present because of their associated negative inotropic effect (Chapter 13).

Patients with mildly decreased ejection fractions improved their left ventricular function during rest and exercise in response to vasodilation with nifedipine[88] (Fig. 14-6). Unfortunately, the results are quite different in patients with poor left ventricular function. Sublingual nifedipine may increase CO by afterload reduction, but there is no decrease in filling pressure and the decreased myocardial contractility may precipitate CHF in a poorly functioning heart.[89,90] In recent studies, more than one-third of patients failed to increase CO in response to vasodilation from nifedipine, and 20 percent suffered significant hemodynamic deterioration.[91] These responses were not predicted by baseline left ventricular function, nor were they dose related.[91]

Nifedipine has little effect on automaticity or atrial conduction; but with high doses, AV conduction may be depressed.[92] Because of the lack of a direct depressant effect on the sino-atrial (SA) node and the absence of antisympathetic effects, a reflex increase in heart rate occurs with administration of nifedipine in response to primary vasodilatation. Nifedipine has no direct antiarrhythmic effects.[93,94]

Nifedipine is well absorbed through the gastrointestinal tract. The onset of action is almost as rapid when nifedipine is given orally as intravenously, which is consistent with rapid membrane transport. The peak effect is variable orally, but after intravenous administration, it appears to be about 20 minutes.[95] Extensive protein binding makes nifedipine subject to changes in plasma protein concentration,[95] and competition from other protein-bound drugs that increase the free (active) fraction.[96] Nifedipine is oxidized to a free acid, lactate, and other inactive metabolites in the liver.[96] It is also oxidized by exposure to light. Its pharmacokinetics fit a two-compartment model, with an alpha half-life of 150 to 180 minutes and a beta half-life of 4 to 5 hours.[96] Final elimination of nifedipine and its metabolites is via the urine. Usual oral doses are 10–20 mg three times daily.[96]

The vasodilating effects of calcium channel blockers can be antagonized by increasing the extracellular calcium ion concentration which increases the influx gradient across the remaining unblocked channels.[97] The hemodynamic effects of calcium channel blockers are more easily antagonized than the electrophysiologic effects.[98,99] Catecholamines reverse both the hemodynamic and electrophysiologic effects of calcium channel blockers by increasing the number of calcium channels available for activation.[100]

Renal tubular secretion of digoxin is decreased with concomitant administration of nifedipine, resulting in increased serum concentrations.[48] It is likely that decreased metabolic clearance of digoxin and a decreased volume of distribution occur as well. Thus, digoxin dosage should be decreased.

Cardiodepressant interactions between the calcium channel blockers and potent inhalation anesthetics have been demonstrated,[101,102] and fluid requirements are increased with high-dose fentanyl anesthesia.[103] Potentiation of the effects of succinylcholine,[104] pancuronium,[104,105] d-tubocurarine,[105] atracurium,[105] and vecuronium[105] have been described in vitro.

DIRECT VASODILATORS

Nitrates. Nitrates relax all vascular smooth muscle in a nonspecific fashion irrespective of innervation.[106] The mechanism of action involves a reaction with the cysteine-containing receptor in the vessel wall, which results in the formation of intermediate metabolites activating guanylate cyclase.[107] Guanylate cyclase increases the smooth muscle cyclic guanosine monophosphate (cGMP), which causes sequestration or extrusion of calcium, and thus vascular relaxation.[107] Nitrates may also stimulate prostacyclin production within vessel walls.[106] There may be greater sensitivity of the veins to the vasodilating effects of NTG as an arterial-venous gradient exists during intravenous infusions in humans.[108] Greater vascular uptake of NTG also occurs in the veins.[108] Likewise, the vasodilatory effects are greater in large arteries than in small arteries or arterioles.[4] Therefore, nitrates affect preload to a greater extent than SVR or afterload[109] (Figs. 14-2, 14-4, and 14-7) (see Chapter 13). Pooling of blood in the splanchnic bed also occurs, and renal blood flow tends to parallel the decrease in arterial pressure.[110] Nitrates decrease pulmonary arterial pressure,[37,111] bronchial tone, and PO_2.[112] Nitroglycerin increases dead space-to-tidal volume ratio (V_D/V_T), venous admixture, and the alveolar-arterial oxygen gradient (A-aDO_2).[111] These effects occur in patients with either chronic obstructive lung disease or normal cardiopulmonary function.[113]

The side effects of NTG therapy include headache, dizziness, weakness, and postural hypotension. Dilatation of the meningeal vessels causes the transient pulsating headache, since the slight increase in intracranial pressure is clinically insignificant. Methemoglobinemia can occur, but is rarely seen clinically, although nitrate ion oxidizes hemoglobin to methemoglobin in vivo and in vitro.[114] Prolongation of neuromuscular blockade with pancuronium, but not with other muscle relaxants, has been reported in vitro and is reversible with anticholinesterases.[115]

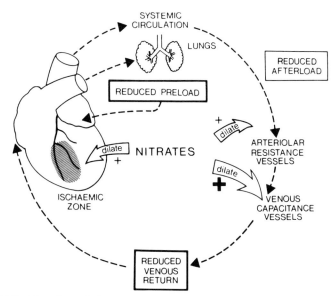

Fig. 14-7. The effects of nitrates on the circulation include prominent venodilation and reduction of preload. Afterload is decreased due to mild arteriolar dilatation. In addition, coronary dilatation occurs to benefit ischemic myocardium. (From Opie LH: Drugs and the heart. II. Nitrates. Lancet 1:750–753, 1980, with permission.)

Nitrates are rapidly denitrated by the glutathione-organic nitrate reductase system during their first pass through the liver. Relatively large oral doses are required to overcome the hepatic degradation,[116] but nitrates administered orally are clinically effective for long periods of time. Although hepatic blood flow is reduced in CHF, there is no alteration of nitrate kinetics. Renal dysfunction likewise fails to influence plasma nitrate concentrations.

A comparison of the various nitrate preparations is presented in Table 14-5.[106,117,118] While NTG is well absorbed through sublingual mucosa, short-acting sublingual preparations are impractical in the treatment of CHF. Nitrates, given orally, sublingually, or in chewable preparations have longer durations of action and are more suitable for vasodilator therapy. Doses of nitrates for vasodilator therapy have not been entirely clarified, but appear to be

Table 14-5

Dosage and Kinetics of Nitroglycerin Preparations

Nitrate	Usual Dosage	Onset of Action	Peak Action	Duration of action
		min	*min*	
Sublingual NTG	0.3–0.8 mg	2–5	4–8	10–30 min
Sublingual ISDN	2.5–10 mg	5–20	15–60	45–120 min
Buccal NTG	1–3 mg	2–5	4–10	30–300 min
Oral ISDN	10–60 mg	15–45	45–120	2–6 hr
Oral NTG	6.5–19.5 mg	20–45	45–120	2–6 hr
Oral PET	40–80 mg	60	60–120	3–6 hr
NTG ointment (2%)	$^1/_2$–2 inch	15–60	30–120	3–8 hr
NTG discs (transdermal)	10–20 mg	30–60	60–180	Up to 24 hr

PET = pentaerythritol tetranitrate; NTG = nitroglycerin; ISDN = isosorbide dinitrate.
Source: From Abrams J: Pharmacology of nitroglycerin and long-acting nitrates. Am J Cardiol 56:12A–18A, 1985, with permission.

between 2.5 and 10 mg of isosorbide dinitrate sublingually, or 20 to 40 mg orally. The minimal venodilating plasma concentration is 1.2 ng/ml.[119] Nitrates are also well absorbed through the skin, and transdermal preparations may be the most effective for the patient with CHF.[37,117,118] Nitrates combined with hydralazine or other arteriolar dilators, without venous capacitance effects, are often efficacious in CHF.

Tolerance may develop to the arterial-dilating effect, but less to the venodilating capacity.[76] Tolerance develops when disulfide bridges form in vascular smooth muscle at the nitrate receptor site, rendering the receptor unresponsive.[120] It does not always result from chronic administration. Discontinuation of nitrates after regular, frequent use may lead to nonatheromatous ischemic heart disease. Both the "withdrawal effect" and tolerance may result from an intrinsic vasoconstrictor mechanism (unrelated to sympathetic nervous or renin-angiotensin systems) activated by nitrate therapy.[121]

In chronic CHF, nitrates decrease pulmonary capillary wedge pressure (PCWP), CVP, pulmonary arterial pressure (PAP), and systemic arterial pressures. Systemic vascular resistance, CO, and stroke volume are variably affected.[122,123] Both vasodilation of resistance vessels and reflex vasoconstriction are impaired in heart failure. Forearm vascular resistance, thus, is unchanged by NTG in patients with CHF.[124] Nitroglycerin increases flow to ischemic myocardium with no effect on subendocardial flow in nonischemic myocardium in experimental preparations.[125] Thus, it does not produce an intracoronary steal as do arteriolar dilators such as nitroprusside, which may divert coronary flow away from ischemic areas.[125]

Hydralazine. Hydralazine directly relaxes arterial smooth muscle, and dilates precapillary resistance vessels.[126] Peripheral resistance decreases with little or no effect on venous smooth muscle. Reflexly, increases in CO and heart rate occur in normal subjects, but heart rate is unchanged in the patient with CHF (Fig. 14-4). In nonfailing hearts, myocardial contractility increases.[127] Arterial pressure is unchanged or decreases slightly, systemic and pulmonary venous pressures are unchanged,[4] but pulmonary vascular resistance usually decreases. There is an increase in renal and limb blood flow without a significant change in hepatic blood flow.[128] Coronary blood flow increases and coronary vascular resistance decreases.[129]

The principal effect of hydralazine in patients with CHF is reduction of left ventricular wall stress,

since little inotropic effect occurs.[130] Patients with the greatest ventricular wall stress (ie, highest LVEDP) are most likely to demonstrate improvement after hydralazine administration.[130] The increase in CO is usually sufficient to minimize or prevent orthostatic hypotension and tachycardia in the patient with CHF.

Usual oral doses are 100 to 150 mg daily, combined with diuretics, but doses up to 1200 mg daily may be required in some patients.[4] It is well absorbed orally with a peak effect in 1–2 hours. Although the plasma half-life is 2–8 hours, its vascular effects are longer lasting due to uptake in the vessel wall. Hydralazine is metabolized in the liver by acetylation and excreted in the urine. Development of a lupus-like syndrome in 15–20 percent of patients results from deficiency of the hepatic enzyme N-acetyl transferase that inactivates hydralazine.[131] The rapidity of acetylation also necessitates an increased dose. Clinically important tolerance unresponsive to increasing dose, intravenous administration, or diuresis occurs in about 30 percent of patients with CHF on long-term hydralazine therapy,[76] which may be due to gradual fluid retention.[132] Other side effects include palpitations, angina, dizziness, gastrointestinal disturbances, polyneuropathy due to pyridoxine deficiency,[133] fluid retention, and headache.

Minoxidil. Minoxidil is a piperidine derivative that acts directly on vascular smooth muscle. Its predominant effect is on arteriolar resistance vessels with little effect on venous capacitance vessels.[134] Since it is a vasodilator, it causes reflex tachycardia in normal individuals, but heart rate is usually unchanged in patients with CHF. Alternatively, beta-blockade may be used to prevent tachycardia. Stroke volume and CO increase, while pulmonary and systemic venous pressures are unchanged. Renin is increased by minoxidil, although the increase can be blocked by propranolol.[14] Although it has beneficial effects in patients with CHF,[135] the side effects of sodium and fluid retention and hirsutism may limit its application.

Minoxidil is completely absorbed orally, with appearance in plasma within 30 minutes, and peaks in 1 hour. The elimination half-life is 4 hours. Usual oral doses for the treatment of CHF are 5 mg once daily, with increases up to 20 mg when required.

ANGIOTENSIN II INHIBITORS

Captopril. Efforts to define the role of renin and angiotensin required the development of the inhibitors of the angiotensin-converting enzyme system. There are many points where the renin cascade can be interrupted. Among these is inhibition of renin release by the juxtaglomerular apparatus with non-specific sympatholytic agents (propranolol, clonidine, and methyldopa) that may also decrease myocardial contractility. The principal area for inhibition is at the level of the converting enzyme (Chapter 11). The oral converting enzyme inhibitor (CEI), captopril, binds specifically to the active site of the converting enzyme (Fig. 14-8). Captopril decreases CVP, PCWP, and MAP while increasing, SV, CO, ejection fraction, and stroke work index (LVSWI) in patients with CHF.[136-138] It also causes prominent peripheral venodilatation[139] (Table 14-4). Due to the blunted baroreceptor reflex response in CHF and withdrawal of sympathetic tone when CHF is treated, heart rate is usually unchanged with captopril therapy. Compared with nitrates, captopril produces less improvement of CO and CVP, although both decrease SVR and LVEDP.[140] Captopril decreases SVR and increases CO less than hydralazine.[140] Myocardial oxygen consumption and coronary blood flow decrease when captopril is given to patients with CHF.[141,142] Cerebral blood flow is increased, but hepatic blood flow is decreased by captopril.[143] Renal blood flow increases due to decreased renal vascular resistance, producing an initial natriuresis, but there is no change or a decrease in glomerular filtration rate. However, later glomerular filtration increases,[142] and further diuresis occurs to decrease body weight.

Decreased SVR is not entirely due to captopril-decreased ANG II levels, since SVR and the initial PRA are only generally correlated.[136,144,145] Both plasma catecholamines and ANG II may be responsible for the decrease in SVR. Plasma catecholamines decrease with captopril administration, which *may* also be responsible for the venodilation seen after captopril.[146] A decrease in catecholamines may also reduce the anxiety associated with sympathetic stimulation and contribute to the feeling of well being experienced by many patients.[4] Recent studies suggest that the renin system modulates vascular tone which is maintained by postsynaptic alpha$_2$-receptors, since captopril blocks the vasopressor effect of norepinephrine only after blockade of vascular alpha$_1$- receptors with prazosin.[147] Another possibility is the inhibition of the destruction of bradykinin, a potent vasodilator[148] (Table 14-6).

Captopril is well absorbed orally, with development of peak blood levels within 1 to 1½ hours, corresponding to peak hemodynamic response.[149]

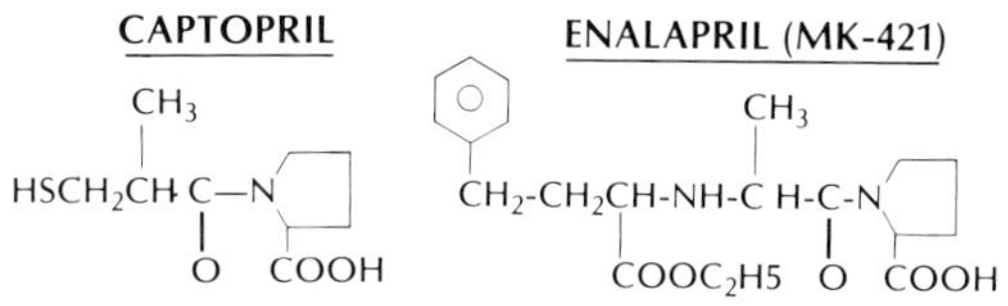

Fig. 14-8. The chemical structures of the converting enzyme inhibitors captopril and enalapril.

The volume of distribution is 0.7 liter/kg. The elimination half-life is 2 hours in patients with either normal renal function or CHF.[150] The usual dose is 6.25–25 mg three times daily, but many patients require daily doses up to 75 or 150 mg.[151] Smaller doses are used in patients with renal dysfunction, due to renal excretion of captopril. The usual duration of action is 3–8 hours, and peak effects are seen within 60–90 minutes of an oral dose. The most important side effect is hypotension. Other side effects include dysgeusia, proteinuria, skin rashes, and neutropenia.[151] Sustained effects are seen even with chronic administration since the renin-angiotensin system is blocked, which is one of the common mechanisms for development of tolerance to vasodilators. This feature makes captopril potentially more useful than direct vasodilators for chronic management of CHF. Withdrawal does not appear to precipitate a rebound phenomenon,[152,153] although sustained withdrawal results in deterioration. Variable responses to captopril therapy such as the triphasic response (initial efficacy, attenuation of response, and spontaneous restoration of benefit), tolerance, or a sustained response have been noted.[154]

Angiotensin II normally inhibits further renin release by completing a negative feedback loop. With CEI, the loop is interrupted and a significant increase in PRA occurs. Hemodynamic response to captopril depends upon the initial PRA, with little response in patients with low plasma renin levels. As circulating ANG II is reduced, aldosterone release from the adrenal glands also decreases. Long-term

Table 14-6

Potential Benefits of CEI in Heart Failure

Decreased formation of ANG II causing arteriolar dilation
Decreased aldosterone release
Decreased norepinephrine synthesis and release
Increased prostaglandin production
Decreased central nervous system adrenergic activity

Source: Modified from Francis GS: Neurohumoral mechanisms involved in congestive heart failure. AJC 55:15A–21A, 1985,

blockade increases systemic and regional blood flow and reduces pulmonary and systemic venous congestion.[155] There is a sustained decrease in SVR that may cause orthostatic hypotension and is responsive to acute volume expansion or sodium repletion.[150]

The magnitude of response of the PVR is considerably less than that of the SVR when captopril is given. In recent work, patients who had substantial decreases in PVR showed greater increases in SVI, CI, and LVSWI than patients who demonstrated predominantly systemic vasodilation.[156] In patents with right ventricular failure, the right ventricular ejection fraction and pulmonary arterial pressure determine the functional status, and correlate better with exercise capacity. Their response to CEI may also result from increased prostaglandins, since ACE also degrades endogenous kinins, which are potent vasodilators through their ability to stimulate renal prostaglandin production. Prostaglandins, particularly E$_1$, affect the pulmonary circulation and cause pulmonary and systemic vasodilation in patients with CHF.[156]

Other effects of ANG II include norepinephrine release, blockade of neuronal uptake of norepinephrine, enhanced norepinephrine synthesis in adrenergic nerve terminals, stimulation of central nervous system norepinephrine activity, and release of epinephrine from the adrenal medulla.[66] All of these actions are blocked by the CEI as well (Table 14-6).

Enalapril (MK-421). Enalapril is an oral synthetic tripeptide CEI with a long duration of action (Fig. 14-8). Its onset of action is slow (about 3–4 hours), because it is a pro-drug which requires hepatic de-esterification for activity. Its hemodynamic effects are similar to those of captopril (Table 14-4). The intravenous preparation, enalaprilat (MK-422), a metabolite of enalaprilic acid, is effective within 15 to 30 minutes. In patients with CHF, oral doses of enalapril, 5–10 mg, increased SV and CO during rest or exercise while decreasing SVR and pulmonary and systemic pressures.[4,157,158] Exercise duration was also increased.[157] Ventricular dysrhythmias decreased during enalapril therapy in patients with CHF, although the mechanism for this benefit is unknown.[159] A possible mechanism is the increased serum potassium occurring after both captopril and enalapril, which may decrease dysrhythmias in diuretic-treated patients. These beneficial effects are maintained with chronic therapy.[4] No untoward effects were attributable to the drugs. A lesser increase in renal blood flow in patients with CHF

occurred after enalapril in doses of 2.5–10 mg IV than with a dopamine infusion of 4 µg/kg/min.[157]

Usual oral doses of enalapril are 5–10 mg twice daily, since the duration of action is 12 hours.[4] A combination of initial intravenous and oral enalapril therapy may be optimum. Intravenous therapy begins at doses of 0.625–1.25 mg.

Inotropic Agents

AMRINONE

Amrinone, a new bipyridine positive inotropic drug, increases the myocardial content of cAMP by stimulation of adenylate cyclase or inhibition of phosphodiesterase activity. Phosphodiesterase inhibition may be limited to phosphodiesterase III.[160] The increased cAMP enhances slow channel calcium inward current, causing greater filling of the sarcoplasmic reticulum with releasable calcium. The increased calcium concentration activates the contractile proteins, increasing myocardial contractility.[161] The higher the external calcium level, the greater the inotropic response to amrinone in isolated papillary muscle[162]; however, at very high external calcium concentrations, the dose-dependent positive inotropic effect of amrinone is attenuated.[163] The force of contraction increases concurrently with the increased myocardial cAMP level in a concentration-dependent manner.[164-166] Improvements in CI, LVSWI, LVEDP, PCWP, PAP, CVP, ejection fraction (EF), and SVR are dose related.[161,164,165,167-180] Heart rate is insignificantly affected, although slight increases occur when there is a marked increase in force of contraction.[181] Venous compliance is increased and forearm vascular resistance reduced.[160] Increases in EF and CI occur, while MAP, LVEDP, and SVR decrease after intravenous administration to humans with CHF.[182] Combined oral therapy with hydralazine and amrinone improved LVSWI and decreased PCWP more than either drug alone[183] (Fig. 14-9). Since all investigators have not found evidence of increased myocardial contractility, some authors have concluded that the major effect of amrinone is direct vasodilation.[171,182]

In addition to the improvement in CO, amrinone increases myocardial blood flow, cortical and medullary renal flow, and hepatic and splenic blood flow in animals with experimentally induced CHF.[160] Vascular responsiveness to amrinone varies in different vascular beds. While hepatic, renal, and splenic flow are increased, central nervous system, pancreatic,

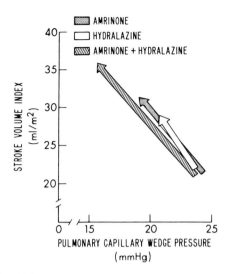

Fig. 14-9. Greater improvement of ventricular function occurs when amrinone is given in combination with hydralazine than when either drug is administered alone to patients with heart failure. (From Siegel LA: Beneficial effects of amrinone-hydralazine combination on resting hemodynamics and exercise capacity in patients with severe congestive heart failure. Circulation 63:838–844, 1981, with permission.)

intestinal, gastric, and cholecystic flow are decreased.[169] Skeletal muscle perfusion is also diminished.[169]

Myocardial ischemia is not worsened since myocardial oxygen demand, coronary blood flow, and arterial lactate levels decrease.[160] However, these effects are species specific, as myocardial oxygen consumption, coronary blood flow, cardiac work, and maximum rate of rise of left ventricular pressure increase in guinea pig hearts, without an increase in heart rate or cardiac efficiency.[162,184] The rate of lactate production was unchanged in these animals, indicating the presence of anaerobic metabolism.[184]

Amrinone does not appear to be dysrhythmogenic. It did not affect resting membrane potential, action potential amplitude, effective refractory period, maximum upstroke or conduction velocities, or depolarization/repolarization phases in canine papillary muscle and Purkinje fibers.[185] The functional refractory period and conduction time through the AV node were shortened.[186] Sinus node recovery time after rapid atrial stimulation was also shortened.[186] Amrinone produced no change in PR, QRS, Qtc, AH, or HV intervals in humans with CHF.[187] Although there was no effect on the ventricular

effective refractory period, amrinone decreases the atrial effective refractory period and atrioventricular nodal functional refractory period, and enhances maximal AV nodal conduction.[187] The improvement in AV nodal conduction is not mediated by adrenergic reflex stimulation. The improvement in AV nodal conduction after amrinone administration may occur by augmented calcium influx via the slow calcium channel. In potassium-depolarized atrial and ventricular guinea pig myocardium, amrinone restores slow channel response.[188] Because of the possibility of a rapid ventricular response secondary to enhanced AV conduction, prophylactic administration of digoxin may be desirable in patients with or likely to develop atrial fibrillation.

Amrinone is well absorbed orally with onset of action within 30 to 120 minutes and peak effect by 4 hours. The elimination half-life in humans is 3.6 hours after oral administration of 0.8–2.2 mg/kg, although it is prolonged after higher oral doses.[177,189] Peak human plasma concentrations of 4 μg/ml occur within 0.5 to 3 hours of 3.5 mg/kg oral doses,[168] and fail to increase further with large doses.[160] Steady-state plasma concentrations appear to be about 1.2–1.7 μg/ml,[168] and the plasma level is linear with cardiac index.[168] The half-life is prolonged in patients with CHF.[168,190,191] Volume of distribution in healthy humans is 1.43 liters/kg and 0.64 to 1.2 liters/kg in patients with CHF.[160] The oral dose of amrinone is 100 mg thrice daily, with increases of 50 mg to a maximum of 450 mg/day. Based on the half-life of the drug, oral administration every eight hours provides adequate plasma levels.[189] Abrupt withdrawal of the drug may produce rapid and significant hemodynamic deterioration, and reinstitution reverses these effects. However, some patients with end-stage disease may be unresponsive to amrinone or may develop tolerance to its effects with prolonged administration.[173]

The primary problem with amrinone is the production of thrombocytopenia to levels of 70,000–90,000/mm^3, which is reversible, dose related, and usually asymptomatic.[192] This occurs in about 20 percent of patients with chronic therapy due to increased peripheral loss of platelets.[193] Amrinone may be a selective thromboxane synthetase inhibitor in platelets, as it decreases production of thromboxane B$_2$ from platelets.[174]

MILRINONE

Although oral amrinone produces significant thrombocytopenia and gastrointestinal side effects, milrinone does not.[193] Milrinone transiently increases CO and reduces afterload by a decrease in SVR and PCWP.[194] Overall ventricular performance is dose related up to a plateau, although the CO of individual patients fails to correlate with plasma milrinone concentration.[194] After intravenous administration, the volume of distribution is 0.35 ± 0.03 liters/kg and elimination half-life is 1.7 hours in patients with CHF.[195] Compared with oral captopril, oral milrinone produced a greater increase in CI, similar decrement in PCWP, a more modest decrease in MAP, and an unchanged heart rate. Captopril caused a greater decrease in SVR than milrinone, and both drugs increased renal blood flow.[195]

GLUCAGON

Glucagon increases intracellular cAMP[196] and inhibits membrane ATPase[197] in the heart. It increases CI, heart rate, systolic blood pressure, PVR, and LV dP/dt,[198] while LVEDP and SVR decrease.[198] The improvement of myocardial contractility occurs in the absence of catecholamines.[199] Glucagon increases heart rate by increasing sinus node and AV node intrinsic pacemaker activity.[196] Atrioventricular conduction time decreases as conduction is enhanced. The drug does not affect Purkinje fiber action potentials, increase ventricular automaticity,[200,201] nor produce dysrhythmias, even in the presence of hypokalemia.[196]

Wilcken and Lvoff used doses of 2.5–7.5 mg/kg to successfully treat CHF after myocardial infarction.[202] Glucagon is potentially useful for cardiac failure, particularly when precipitated by beta-adrenergic blockade because of its different mechanism of action. However, it is used infrequently at the present time.

XANTHINES

Phosphodiesterase inhibitors exert an inotropic effect by causing accumulation of cAMP. Drugs such as caffeine and theophylline have cardiostimulating properties, as well as diuretic effects. They increase urine flow and sodium and chloride excretion. However, their efficacy is limited, tolerance rapidly develops to the diuretic effect, and they are not often used for treatment of CHF. In many ways, these drugs are similar to amrinone.

SYMPATHOMIMETIC AMINES

Sympathomimetic amines increase myocardial contractility by stimulation of beta-receptors on the cardiac cell. These amines stimulate adenyl cyclase, which converts ATP to increase cyclic 3'5'-AMP in cytosol. Cyclic AMP activates a protein kinase enzyme, phosphorylating other proteins, and possibly altering membrane calcium permeability. The administration of sympathomimetic amines shortens the duration of ventricular contraction, increases the velocity and extent of wall shortening, and increases SV. However, stimulation of the beta-receptors also increases sinoatrial node discharge and AV nodal conduction to increase heart rate. In-hospital treatment of severe CHF is based on the use of intravenous beta$_1$-adrenergic drugs such as dobutamine, dopamine, epinephrine, norepinephrine, and isoproterenol (see Chapters 26 and 30). None of these drugs is available for oral use, but ephedrine and L-dopa have been utilized to treat CHF with limited success.

Salbutamol. Salbutamol is a beta$_2$-agonist which promotes arteriolar vasodilation, bronchodilation, and probably a positive inotropic effect. Acute oral administration of 4–8 mg improved CI and reduced SVR.[203] It has been used in patients with left ventricular failure after myocardial infarction[204] or cardiomyopathy.[205] Its cardiac use in the United States is investigational, with the major approved indication being bronchodilation.

Prenalterol. A selective B$_1$-agonist, prenalterol has significant inotropic and slight positive chronotropic effects. It has a half-life of 3 hours. Its beneficial effects have been demonstrated in acute myocardial ischemia, chronic CHF, and septic shock, although ventricular dysrhythmias are increased in acute ischemia.[206] Neither blood pressure, heart rate, nor SVR change in patients with CHF, while CI and SV increase and filling pressure decreases.[207,208] Intravenous doses are 1–5 mg, and oral doses range from 20 to 100 mg. An oral preparation is currently undergoing clinical investigation.

Pirbuterol. Pirbuterol has both beta$_1$ and beta$_2$ properties, so that both an increase in myocardial contractility and peripheral vasodilation occur after its use. The increased dP/dt is either a direct effect or mediated by reflex release of plasma catecholamines. Pulmonary capillary wedge pressure decreases and EF increases. Heart rate and MAP do not increase when pirbuterol is given to patients with CHF in doses of 5–30 mg orally thrice daily.[209-212] Myocardial lactate extraction is unchanged and angina is not exacerbated.[213] An additional benefit is bronchodilation. The beneficial effects may be attenuated with chronic therapy due to a "down regulation" of beta-receptor density in the myocardium.[214] However, investigators have noted sustained improvement with chronic therapy in a majority of patients.[209,210] Pirbuterol has no cardiotoxic interaction with digoxin and substantially increases myocardial contractility in digitalized experimental animals.[215]

COMBINATION THERAPY

Since the hemodynamic abnormalities in patients with CHF are variable, combinations of arteriolar and venodilator drugs, or combinations of vasodilators with positive inotropic drugs may be more beneficial than either alone. Due to the down-regulation of the beta-receptors in chronic CHF, the use of vasodilators rather than sympathomimetic drugs is often preferable. The combination of hydralazine with nitrates increased CO and reduced both systemic and pulmonary venous pressures without changes in heart rate or blood pressure in patients with CHF.[216] Hydralazine by itself increased CO, but failed to reduce systemic and pulmonary venous pressures, while nitrates alone reduced only the CVP and PCWP.[216] Both minoxidil with nitrates and hydralazine with nitrates have been shown to be effective combinations for chronic CHF.[217,218] In some patients vasodilator therapy alone is contraindicated because of further reduction of arterial perfusion. In these patients, combined therapy with inotropic and vasodilator drugs may be effective.

Future Therapeutic Possibilities

MDL 17043

This noncatecholamine, nonglycoside-substituted imidazolone probably acts by either inhibition of phosphodiesterase III or inhibition of sodium-potassium-ATPase.[219] The elimination half-life is 20 hours.[220] Both intravenous doses of 1–3 mg/kg and oral doses of 6 mg/kg increased CO, decreased SVR, and decreased or did not change left ventricular filling pressure. Renin was increased and norepinephrine decreased.[220] Its major side effects were diarrhea

(occurring in 75 percent of patients)[220] and increased ventricular dysrhythmias. Although short-term improvement is good, sustained long-term benefit has been variable with poor results[221] and good results[220] reported by various investigators.

SUMAZOLE (ARL-115-BS)

In animals, this benzimidazole derivative increased myocardial contractility and reduced afterload.[222] Sumazole may increase the affinity of myofibrillar receptors for calcium.[223] It also inhibits phosphodiesterase, an effect similar to the xanthines.

RO 13-6438

This is a new noncatecholamine, nonglycoside imidazoquinazoline derivate that increases CI and LVSWI, and decreases PCWP in humans with CHF after 20-mg oral doses. Heart rate is unchanged and the blood pressure response is variable. Neither myocardial oxygen consumption, coronary sinus flow, nor arterial-coronary lactate difference change after RO 13-6438.[224]

FENOLDOPAM MESYLATE (SKF-82526-J)

This benzazepine derivative, a selective dopamine$_1$-receptor agonist, decreases PCWP and SVR, and increases CI in patients with CHF given oral doses of 200 mg.[225,226] Its duration of action is 3–4 hours and it has renal vasodilating properties six times that of dopamine.[226] It does not activate central dopaminergic receptors and does not readily cross the blood-brain barrier.[226] The only side effect noted was transient nausea in one series.[226]

SUMMARY

In addition to the use of digitalis, diuretics, positive inotropic, and vasodilator drugs, certain patients with chronic CHF may have to be considered for cardiac transplantation or insertion of a mechanical heart. Management of these patients with severe end-stage CHF or acute cardiac decompensation is discussed in Chapters 23, 26, 27, 28, and 30.

REFERENCES

1. Little RC, Ginsburg JM: The physiologic basis for clinical edema. Arch Intern Med 144:1661–1664, 1984
2. Weber KT, Janicki JS: Cardiopulmonary exercise testing for evaluation of chronic cardiac failure. Am J Cardiol 55:22A–31A, 1985
3. Cohn JN, Hamosh P: Experimental observations on pulsus paradoxus and hepatojugular reflux. In Reddy PS, Leon DF, Shaver JA (eds): Pericardial Disease. New York, Raven Press, 1982, pp 249–258
4. Cohn JN (ed): Drug Treatment of Heart Failure. New York, Yorke Medical Books, 1983

5. Parmley WW: Pathophysiology of congestive heart failure. Am J Cardiol 55:9A–14A, 1985

6. Mason DT, Awan NA, Joyce JA, et al: Treatment of acute and chronic congestive heart failure by vasodilator-afterload reduction. Arch Intern Med 140:1577–1581, 1980

7. Pepine CJ, Nichols WW, Conti CR: Aortic input impedance in heart failure. Circulation 58:460–465, 1978

8. Levine TB, Francis GS, Goldsmith SR, et al: Activity of the sympathetic nervous system and renin-angiotensin system assessed by plasma hormone levels and their relationship to hemodynamic abnormalities in congestive heart failure. Am J Cardiol 49:1659–1666, 1982

9. Swedberg K, Viquerat C, Rouleau J–L, et al: Comparison of myocardial catecholamine balance in chronic congestive heart failure and in angina pectoris without failure. Am J Cardiol 54:783–786, 1984

10. Chidsey CA, Braunwald E, Morrow AG: Catecholamine excretion and stores of norepinephrine in congestive heart failure. Am J Med 39:442–451, 1965

11. Spann JF Jr, Sonnenblick EH, Cooper T, et al: Cardiac norepinephrine stores and the contractile state of heart muscle. Circ Res 19:317–325, 1966

12. Goldsmith SR, Francis GS, Cohn JN: Norepinephrine infusions in congestive heart failure. Am J Cardiol 56:802–804, 1985

13. Peach MJ: Renin-angiotensin system. Biochemistry and mechanisms of action. Physiol Rev 57:313–370, 1977

14. Keeton TK, Campbell WB: Control of renin release and its alteration by drugs. In Antonaccio M (ed): Cardiovascular Pharmacology. New York: Raven Press, 1984, pp 65–118

15. Reid IA: The renin-angiotensin system and body function. Arch Intern Med 145:1475–1479, 1985

16. Curtiss C, Cohn JN, Vrobel T, et al: Role of the renin-angiotensin system in the systemic vasoconstriction of chronic congestive heart failure. Circulation 58:763–770, 1978

17. Laragh JH, Seeley JE: The renin-angiotensin-aldosterone hormonal system and regulation of sodium, potassium and blood pressure homeostasis. In Orlaff J, RW Berliner (eds): Handbook of Physiology Section 8, Renal Physiology, Baltimore, Williams and Wilkins Co., 1973, pp 831–908

18. Levine TB, Franciosa JA, Vrobel T, et al: Hyponatremia as a marker for high-renin heart failure. Br Heart J 47:161–166, 1982

19. Schaer GL, Covit AB, Laragh JH, et al: Association of hyponatremia with increased renin activity in chronic congestive heart failure: Impact of diuretic therapy. Am J Cardiol 51:1635–1638, 1983

20. Cody RJ, Franklin KW, Kluger J, et al: Mechanisms governing the postural response and baroreceptor abnormalities in chronic congestive heart failure: Effects of acute and long-term converting enzyme inhibition. Circulation 66:135–142, 1982

21. Cannon PJ: The kidney in heart failure. N Engl J Med 296:26–32, 1977

22. Goldsmith SR, Francis GS, Cowley AW, et al: Increased plasma arginine vasopressin in patients with congestive heart failure. J Am Coll Cardiol 1:1385–1390, 1983

23. Zucker IH, Share L, Gilmore JP: Renal effects of left atrial distention in dogs with chronic congestive heart failure. Am J Physiol 236:H554–H560, 1979

24. Zelis R, Flaim SF: Alterations in vasomotor tone in congestive heart failure. Prog Cardiovasc Dis 24:437–459, 1982

25. Sordahl LW, Wood WG, Schwartz A: Production of cardiac hypertrophy and failure in rabbits with ameroid clips. J Mol Cell Cardiol 1:341–344, 1970

26. Morkin E, LaRaia PJ: Biochemical studies on the regulation of myocardial contractility. N Engl J Med 290:445–451, 1974

27. Chidsey CA, Weinbach EC, Pool PE, et al: Biochemical studies of energy production in the failing human heart. J Clin Invest 45:40–50, 1966

28. Suko J, Vogel JHK, Chidsey CA: Reduced calcium uptake and ATPase of the sarcoplasmic reticular fraction prepared from chronically failing calf hearts. Circ Res 27:235–247, 1970

29. Merrill AJ: Edema and decreased renal blood flow in patients with chronic congestive heart failure. Evidence of "forward failure" as the primary cause of edema. J Clin Invest 25:389–400, 1946

30. Vander AJ, Malvin RL, Wilde WS, et al: Re-examination of salt and water retention in congestive heart failure. Am J Med 25:497–502, 1958

31. Woodson RD, Torrance JD, Shappell SD, et al: The effect of cardiac disease on hemoglobin-oxygen binding. J Clin Invest 49:1349–1356, 1970

32. Higgins CB, Vatner SF, Millard RW, et al: Alterations in regional hemodynamics in experimental heart failure in conscious dogs. Trans Assoc Am Physicians 85:267–278, 1972

33. Smith TW: Digitalis glycosides. N Engl J Med 288:719–722, 1973; 288:942–946, 1973

34. Smith TW, Haber E: Digitalis. N Engl J Med 289:945–952; 1011–1015; 1063–1072; 1125–1129, 1973

35. Sonnenblick EH, Williams JF, Glick G, et al: Studies on digitalis. XV. Effects of cardiac glycoside on myocardial force-velocity relations in the nonfailing human heart. Circulation 34:532–539, 1966

36. Rosen MR, Wit AL, Hoffman BF: Electrophysiology and pharmacology of cardiac arrhythmias. IV. Cardiac antiarrhythmic and toxic effects of digitalis. Am Heart J 89:391–399, 1975

37. Goodman LS, Gilman A: The pharmacological basis of therapeutics. New York, Macmillan, 1975

38. Mason DT, Braunwald E: Studies on digitalis. X. Effects of ouabain on forearm vascular resistance

and venous tone in normal subjects and in patients with heart failure. J Clin Invest 43:532–543, 1964

39. Sodums MT, Walsh RA, O'Rourke RA: Digitalis in heart failure. JAMA 246:158–160, 1981

40. Lindenbaum J: Greater bioavailability of digoxin solutions in capsules. Clin Pharmacol Ther 21:278–282, 1977

41. Doherty JE, Hall WH, Murphy ML, et al: New information regarding digitalis metabolism. Chest 59:433–437, 1971

42. Doherty JE, Perkins WH, Wilson MC: Studies with tritiated digoxin in renal failure. Am J Med 37:536–544, 1964

43. Doherty JE, Perkins WH: Studies following intramuscular tritiated digoxin in human subjects. Am J Cardiol 15:170–174, 1965

44. Ewy GA, Kapadia GG, Yao L, et al: Digoxin metabolism in the elderly. Circulation 39:449–453, 1969

45. Morrow DH, Gaffney TE, Braunwald E: Studies on digitalis. VII. Influence of hyper- and hypothyroidism on the myocardial response to ouabain. J Pharmacol Exp Ther 140:324–328, 1963

46. Rakita L, Sobol SM: Amiodarone in the treatment of refractory ventricular arrhythmias. JAMA 250:1293–1295, 1983

47. Zipes DP, Prystowsky EN, Heger JJ: Amiodarone: Electrophysiologic actions and clinical effects. J Am Coll Cardiol 3:1059–1071, 1984

48. Kapur PA: Cardiovascular pharmacology. Beta-receptor blockers and slow calcium channel inhibitors. Semin Anesthesia 1:196–206, 1982

49. Pederson KE, Dorph-Pederson A, Hvidt S, et al: Digoxin-verapamil interaction. Clin Pharmacol Ther 30:311-316, 1981

50. Doering W: Digoxin-quinidine interaction. N Engl J Med 301:400–404, 1979

51. Burchell HB: Digitalis poisoning: Historical and forensic aspects. J Am Coll Cardiol 1:506–516, 1983

52. Moorman JR, Pritchett ELC: The arrhythmias of digitalis intoxication. Arch Intern Med 145:1289–1292, 1985

53. Beller GA, Smith TW, Abelmann WH, et al: Digitalis intoxication—a prospective clinical study with serum level correlations. N Engl J Med 284:989–997, 1971

54. Smith TW, Braunwald E: The management of heart failure. In Braunwald E (ed): Heart Disease A Textbook of Cardiovascular Medicine. Philadelphia, WB Saunders, 1980, pp 509–570

55. Cook LS, Doherty JE, Straub KD, et al: Digoxin uptake into peripheral cardiac nerves. A possible mechanism for antiarrhythmic and toxic cardiac actions. Am Heart J 102:58–62, 1981

56. Lown B, Kleiger R, Williams J: Cardioversion and digitalis drugs: Changed threshold to electric shock in digitalized animals. Circ Res 17:519–531, 1966

57. Ivankovich AD, Miletich DJ, Grossman RK, et al: The effect of enflurane, isoflurane, fluoroxene, methoxyflurane, and diethyl ether anesthesia on ouabain tolerance in the dog. Anesth Analg 55:360–365, 1976

58. Kessler RH, Hierholzer K, Gurd RS, et al: Localization of the action of chlorothiazide in the nephron of the dog. Am J Physiol 196:1346–1351, 1959

59. Beyer KH: The mechanism of action of chlorothiazide. Ann NY Acad Sci 71:363–379, 1958

60. Villareal H, Revollo A, Exaire JE, et al: Effects of chlorothiazide on renal hemodynamics. Circulation 26:409–412, 1962

61. Bourland WA, Day DK, Williamson HE: The role of the kidney in the early nondiuretic action of furosemide to reduce elevated left atrial pressure in the hypervolemic dog. J Pharmacol Exp Ther 202:221–229, 1977

62. Dikshit K, Vyden JK, Forrester JS, et al: Renal and extrarenal effects of furosemide in congestive heart failure after myocardial infarction. N Engl J Med 188:1087–1090, 1973

63. Beyer KH, Baer JE, Michaelson JR, et al: Renotropic characteristics of ethacrynic acid. A phenoxyacetic saluretic diuretic agent. J Pharmacol Exp Ther 147:1–22, 1965

64. Miller RD, Sohn YJ, Matteo RS: Enhancement of d-tubocurarine neuromuscular blockade by diuretics in man. Anesthesiology 45:442–445, 1976

65. Little RC, Little WC: Cardiac preload, afterload, and heart failure. Arch Intern Med 142:819–922, 1982

66. Francis GS: Neurohumoral mechanisms involved in congestive heart failure. Am J Cardiol 55:15A–21A, 1985

67. Graham RM, Pettinger WA: Prazosin. N Engl J Med 300:232–236, 1979

68. Stanaszek WP, Kellerman D, Brogden RN, et al: Prazosin update. Drugs 25:339–384, 1983

69. Mehta J, Iacona M, Pepine C, et al: Comparison of hemodynamic effects of oral prazosin, oral hydralazine and intravenous nitroprusside in the same patients with chronic heart failure. Br Heart J 42:664–670, 1979

70. Miller RR, Awan NA, Maxwell KS, et al: Sustained reduction of cardiac impedance and preload in congestive heart failure with the antihypertensive vasodilator prazosin. N Engl J Med 297:303–307, 1977

71. Chatterjee K, Parmley WW: Vasodilator therapy in chronic heart failure. Annu Rev Pharmacol Toxicol 20:475–512, 1980

72. Rouleau JL, Warnica JW, Burgess JH: Prazosin and congestive heart failure. Short- and long-term therapy. Am J Med 71:147–152, 1981

73. Kumpuris AG, Miller RR, Quinones MA, et al: Salutary effects of cardiac unloading on ventricular ectopy in congestive cardiomyopathy. Am J Cardiol 43:360, 1979

74. Jaillon P: Clinical pharmacokinetics of prazosin. Clin Pharmacokinetics 5:365–376, 1980

75. Wood AJ, Bolli P, Simpson FO: Prazosin in normal subjects. Plasma levels, blood pressure and heart rate. Br J Clin Pharmacol 3:199–201, 1976

76. Packer M: Vasodilator and inotropic therapy for severe chronic heart failure. J Am Coll Cardiol 2:841–852, 1983

77. Chatterjee K, Rouleau J-L: Hemodynamic and metabolic effects of vasodilators, nitrates, hydralazine, prazosin, and captopril in chronic ischemic heart failure. Acta Medica Scand 210(Suppl 651):295–303, 1981

78. Wallin JD, O'Neill WM: Labetalol, current research and therapeutic status. Arch Intern Med 143:485–490, 1983

79. Trust PM, Rosei EA, Brown JJ, et al: Effects of blood pressure, angiotensin II and aldosterone concentrations during treatment of severe hypertension with intravenous labetalol: Comparison with propranolol. Br J Clin Pharmacol 3(4 Suppl 3):799–803, 1976

80. Lijnen PJ, Amery AK, Fagard RH, et al: Effects of labetalol on plasma renin, aldosterone, and catecholamines in hypertensive patients. J Cardiovasc Pharmacol 1:625–632, 1979

81. Miller RR, Vismara LA, Williams DO, et al: Pharmacological mechanisms for left ventricular unloading in clinical congestive heart failure. Differential effects of nitroprusside, phentolamine, and nitroglycerin on cardiac function and peripheral circulation. Circ Res 39:127–133, 1976

82. Majid PA, Sharma B, Taylor SH: Phentolamine for vasodilator treatment of severe heart failure. Lancet 2:719–723, 1971

83. Walinsky P, Chatterjee K, Forrester J, et al: Enhanced left ventricular performance with phentolamine in acute myocardial infarction. Am J Cardiol 33:37–41, 1974

84. Nagasawa K, Vyden JK, Forrester JS, et al: Effect of phentolamine on cardiac performance and energetics in acute myocardial infarction. Circulatory Shock 2:5–11, 1975

85. Stern MA, Gohlke HK, Loeb HS, et al: Hemodynamic effects of intravenous phentolamine in low output cardiac failure. Circulation 58:157–163, 1978

86. Opie LH, Harrison DC: Vasodilating drugs. In Opie LH (ed): Drugs for the heart. Orlando, FL, Grune & Stratton, 1985, pp 129–151

87. Frohlich ED: Inhibition of adrenergic function in the treatment of hypertension. Arch Intern Med 133:1033–1048, 1974

88. Zacca NM, Verani MS, Chahine RA, et al: Effect of nifedipine on exercise-induced left ventricular dysfunction and myocardial hypoperfusion in stable angina. Am J Cardiol 50:689–695, 1982

89. Ludbrook PA, Tiefenbrunn AJ, Reed FR, et al: Acute hemodynamic responses to sublingual nifedipine: Dependence on left ventricular function. Circulation 65:489–498, 1982

90. Matsumoto S, Ito T, Sada T, et al: Hemodynamic effects of nifedipine in congestive heart failure. Am J Cardiol 46:476–480, 1980

91. Elkayam U, Weber L, McKay C, et al: Spectrum of acute hemodynamic effects of nifedipine in severe congestive heart failure. Am J Cardiol 56:560–566, 1985

92. Henry PD: Comparative pharmacology of calcium antagonists; nifedipine, verapamil, and diltiazem. Am J Cardiol 46:1047–1058, 1980

93. Ellrodt GG, Chew CYC, Singh BN: Therapeutic implications of slow-channel blockade in cardiocirculatory disorders. Circulation 62:669–679, 1980

94. Henry PD: Calcium ion (Ca^{++}) antagonists. Mechanisms of action and clinical applications. Prac Cardiol 5:145–146, 1979

95. Horster FA, Duhm B, Maul W, et al: Klinische untersuchungen zur Pharmakokinetik von radioaktiv markiertem 4-(2'-nitrophenyl)-2, 6-dimethyl-1, 4-dihydropyridin-3, 5-dicarbonsauredim-ethylester. Arzneim Forsch 22:330–334, 1972

96. Reves JG, Kissin I, Lell WA, et al: Calcium entry blockers: Uses and implications for anesthesiologists. Anesthesiology 57:504–518, 1982

97. Morris DL, Goldschlager N: Calcium infusion for reversal of adverse effects of intravenous verapamil. JAMA 249:3212–3213, 1983

98. Nugent M, Tinker JH: Verapamil worsens rate of development and hemodynamic effects of acute hyperkalemia in halothane-anesthetized dogs. Effects of calcium therapy. Anesthesiology 60:435–439, 1984

99. Hariman RJ, Mangiardi LM, McAllister RG, et al: Reversal of the cardiovascular effects of verapamil by calcium and sodium: Differences between electrophysiologic and hemodynamic responses. Circulation 59:797–804, 1979

100. Reuter H, Scholz H: The regulation of the calcium conductance of cardiac muscle by adrenaline. J Physiol 264:49–62, 1977

101. Kates RE, Kaplan JA: Cardiovascular responses to verapamil during coronary artery bypass graft surgery. Anesth Analg 62:821–826, 1983

102. Tosone S, Reves JG, Kissin I, et al: Hemodynamic responses to nifedipine in dogs anesthetized with halothane. Anesth Analg 62:903–908, 1983

103. Freis ES, Lappas DG: Chronic administration of calcium entry blockers and the cardiovascular responses to high doses of fentanyl in man. Anesthesiology 57:A295, 1982

104. Durant NN, Nguyen N, Katz RL: Potentiation of neuromuscular blockade by verapamil. Anesthesiology 60:298–303, 1984

105. Bikhazi GB, Leung I, Foldes FF: Interaction of neuromuscular blocking agents with calcium channel blockers. Anesthesiology 57:A268, 1982

106. Abrams J: Pharmacology of nitroglycerin and long-acting nitrates. Am J Cardiol 56:12A–18A, 1985

107. Gazes PC, Assey ME: The management of congestive heart failure. Curr Prob Cardiol 8(11):8–70, 1984

108. Armstrong PW, Moffat JA, Marks GS: Arterial-venous nitroglycerin gradient during intravenous infusion in man. Circulation 66:1273–1276, 1982

109. Flaherty JT, Reid PR, Kelly DT, et al: Intravenous nitroglycerin in acute myocardial infarction. Circulation 51:132–139, 1975

110. Winbury MM: Redistribution of left ventricular blood flow produced by nitroglycerin. Circ Res (Suppl 1):140–147, 1971

111. Mookherjee JEE, Fuleihan D, Warner RA, et al: Effects of sublingual nitroglycerin on resting pulmonary gas exchange and hemodynamics in man. Circulation 57:106–110, 1978

112. Kopman EA, Weygandt GR, Bauer S, et al: Arterial hypoxemia following the administration of sublingual nitroglycerin. Am Heart J 96:444–447, 1978

113. Chick TW, Kochukosky KN, Matsumoto S, et al: The effect of nitroglycerin on gas exchange, hemodynamics, and oxygen transport in patients with chronic obstructive lung disease. Am J Med Sci 276:105–111, 1978

114. Zurick AM, Wagner RH, Starr NJ, et al: Intravenous nitroglycerin, methemoglobinemia, and respiratory status in a postoperative cardiac surgical patient. Anesthesiology 61:464–466, 1984

115. Glisson SN, Sanchez MM, El Etr AA, et al: Nitroglycerin and the neuromuscular blockade produced by gallamine, succinylcholine, tubocurarine and pancuronium. Anesth Analg 59:117–122, 1980

116. Opie LH: Nitrates. Lancet 1:750–753, 1980

117. Armstrong PW, Mathew MT, Boroomand K, et al: Nitroglycerin ointment in acute myocardial infarction. Am J Cardiol 38:474–478, 1976

118. Taylor WR, Forrester JS, Magnusson P, et al: Hemodynamic effects of nitroglycerin ointment in congestive heart failure. Am J Cardiol 38:469–473, 1976

119. Armstrong PW, Armstrong JA, Marks GS: Pharmacokinetic-hemodynamic studies of intravenous nitroglycerin in congestive cardiac failure. Circulation 62:160–166, 1980

120. Zelis R, Flaim SF, Moskowitz RM, et al: How much can we expect from vasodilator therapy in congestive heart failure? Circulation 59:1092–1097, 1979

121. Olivari MT, Carlyle PF, Levine TB, et al: Hemodynamic and hormonal response to transdermal nitroglycerin in normal subjects and in patients with congestive heart failure. J Am Coll Cardiol 2:872–878, 1983

122. Franciosa JA, Cohn JH: Sustained hemodynamic effects of nitrates without tolerance in heart failure. Circulation 58 (Suppl II):II-28, 1978

123. Cohn JN: Nitrates for congestive heart failure. Am J Cardiol 56:19A–23A, 1985

124. Imaizumi T, Takeshita, A, Ashihara T, et al: The effects of sublingually administered nitroglycerin on forearm vascular resistance in patients with heart failure and in normal subjects. Circulation 72:747–752, 1985

125. Chiariello M, Gold HK, Leinbach RC, et al: Comparison between the effects of nitroprusside and nitroglycerin on ischemic injury during acute myocardial infarction. Circulation 54:766–773, 1976

126. Albrecht RF, Toyooka ET, Polk SLH, et al: Hydralazine therapy for hypertension during anesthetic and postanesthetic periods. Int Anesth Clin 16:299–312, 1978

127. Khatri I, Uemura N, Notargiacomo A, et al: Direct and reflex cardiostimulating effects of hydralazine. Am J Cardiol 40:38–42, 1977

128. Leier CV, Magorien RD, Desch CE, et al: Hydralazine and isosorbide dinitrate: Comparative central and regional hemodynamic effects when administered alone or in combination. Circulation 63:102–109, 1981

129. Magorien RD, Brown GP, Unverferth DV, et al: Effects of hydralazine on coronary blood flow and myocardial energetics in congestive heart failure. Circulation 65:528–533, 1982

130. Smucker ML, Sanford CF, Lipscomb KM: Effects of hydralazine on pressure-volume and stress-volume relations in congestive heart failure secondary to idiopathic dilated cardiomyopathy. Am J Cardiol 56:690–695, 1985

131. Talseth T: Serum concentrations of hydralazine in man after a single dose and at steady state. Eur J Clin Pharm 10:183–187, 1976

132. Packer M, Meller J, Medina N et al: Hemodynamic characterization of tolerance to long-term hydralazine therapy in severe chronic heart failure. N Engl J Med 306:57–62, 1982

133. Kirkendall WM, Page EB: Polyneuritis occurring during hydralazine therapy. JAMA 167:427–432, 1958

134. Kosman ME: Evaluation of a new antihypertensive agent. JAMA 244:73–75, 1980

135. Franciosa JA, Cohn JN: Effects of minoxidil on hemodynamics in patients with congestive heart failure. Circulation 63:652–657, 1981

136. Ader R, Chatterjee K, Ports T, et al: Immediate and sustained hemodynamic and clinical improvement in chronic heart failure by an oral angiotensin-converting enzyme inhibitor. Circulation 61:931–937, 1980

137. Cannon PT, Powers ER, Reison DS, and the Captopril Multicenter Research Group: A placebo-controlled trial of captopril in refractory chronic congestive heart failure. J Am Coll Cardiol 2:755–763, 1983

138. Levine TB, Franciosa JA, Cohn JN: Acute and longterm response to an oral converting enzyme

inhibitor, captopril, in congestive heart failure. Circulation 62:35–41, 1980

139. Awan NA, Mason DT: Vasodilator therapy of severe congestive heart failure. The special importance of angiotensin-converting enzyme inhibition with captopril. Am Heart J 104:1127–1136, 1982

140. Packer M, Medina N, Yushak M: Contrasting hemodynamic responses in severe heart failure: Comparison of captopril and other vasodilator drugs. Am Heart J 104:1215–1223, 1982

141. Chatterjee K, Rouleau J-L, Parmley WW: Captopril in congestive heart failure: Improved left ventricular function with decreased metabolic cost. Am Heart J 104:1137–1146, 1982

142. Dzau VJ, Colucci WS, Williams GH, et al: Sustained effectiveness of converting enzyme inhibition in patients with severe congestive heart failure. N Engl J Med 302:1373–1379, 1980

143. Levine TM, Olivari MT, Cohn JN: Hemodynamic and regional blood flow response to captopril in congestive heart failure. Am J Med 76:38–42, 1984

144. Faxon DP, Halperin JL, Creager MA, et al: Angiotensin inhibition in severe heart failure. Acute central and limb hemodynamic effects of captopril with observations on sustained oral therapy. Am Heart J 101:548–556, 1981

145. Davis R, Ribner HS, Keung E, et al: Treatment of chronic congestive heart failure with captopril. An oral inhibitor of angiotensin converting enzyme. N Engl J Med 301:117–121, 1979

146. Kubo S, Nishioka A, Nishimura H, et al: The renin-angiotensin-aldosterone system and catecholamines in chronic congestive heart failure. Effect of angiotensin I-converting enzyme inhibitor, SQ-14225 (Captopril). Jpn Circ J 44:427–437, 1980

147. DeJonge A, Wiffert B, Kalkman HO, et al: Captopril impairs the vascular smooth muscle contraction mediated by post-synaptic alpha$_2$-adrenoceptor in the pithed rat. Eur J Pharmacol 74:385–386, 1981

148. Sweet CS, Blaine EH: Angiotensin-converting enzyme and renin inhibitors. In Antonacci M (ed): Cardiovascular Pharmacology. New York, Raven Press, 1984, pp 119–154

149. Duchin KL, Singhvi SM, Willard DA, et al: Captopril kinetics. Clin Pharmacol Ther 31:452–458, 1984

150. Cody RJ, Franklin KW, Laragh JH: Postural hypotension during tilt with chronic captopril and diuretic therapy of severe congestive heart failure. Am Heart J 103:480–484, 1982

151. Ram CVS: Captopril. Arch Intern Med 142:914–916, 1982

152. Fouad FM, Tarazi RC, Bravo EL, et al: Long-term control of congestive heart failure with captopril. Am J Cardiol 49:1489–1496, 1982

153. Maslowski AH, Nicholls MG, Ikram H, et al: Haemodynamic, hormonal and electrolyte responses to withdrawal of long-term captopril treatment for heart failure. Lancet 2:959–961, 1981

154. Packer M, Medina N, Yushak M, et al: Hemody-

namic patterns of response during long-term captopril therapy for severe chronic heart failure. Circulation 68:803–812, 1983

155. Powers ER, Bannerman KS, Stone J, et al: The effect of captopril on renal, coronary, and systemic hemodynamics in patients with severe congestive heart failure. Am Heart J 104:1203–1210, 1982

156. Packer M, Lee WH, Medina N, et al: Hemodynamic and clinical significance of the pulmonary vascular response to long-term captopril therapy in patients with severe congestive heart failure. J Am Coll Cardiol 6:635–645, 1985

157. Maskin CS, Ocken S, Chadwick B, et al: Comparative systemic and renal effects of dopamine and angiotensin-converting enzyme inhibition with enalaprilat in patients with heart failure. Circulation 72:846–852, 1985

158. Creager MA, Massie BM, Faxon DP, et al: Acute and long-term effects of enalapril on the cardiovascular response to exercise and exercise tolerance in patients with congestive heart failure. J Am Coll Cardiol 6:163–170, 1985

159. Webster MWI, Fitzpatrick A, Nicholls G, et al: Effect of enalapril on ventricular arrhythmias in congestive heart failure. Am J Cardiol 56:566–569, 1985

160. Ward A, Brogden RN, Heel RC, et al: Amrinone. A preliminary review of its pharmacological properties and therapeutic use. Drugs 26:468–502, 1983

161. Kondo N, Shibata S, Kodama I, et al: Electrical and mechanical effects of amrinone on isolated guinea pig ventricular muscle. J Cardiovasc Pharmacol 5:903–912, 1983

162. Onuaguluchi G, Tanz RD: Cardiac effects of amrinone on rabbit papillary muscle and guinea pig Langendorff heart preparations. J Cardiovasc Pharmacol 3:1342–1355, 1981

163. Rendig SV, Amsterdam EA: Positive inotropic action of amrinone: Effect of elevated external Ca^{++} J Cardiovasc Pharmacol 6:293–299, 1984

164. Endoh M, Yamashita S, Taira N: Positive inotropic effect of amrinone in relation to cyclic nucleotide metabolism in the canine ventricular muscle. J Pharmacol Exp Ther 221:775–783, 1982

165. Honerjager P, Shafer-Korting M, Reiter M: Involvement of cyclic AMP in the direct inotropic action of amrinone. Naunyn-Schmiedeberg's Arch Pharmacol 318:112–120, 1981

166. Shibata S, Kondo N, Kodama I, et al: Electrical and mechanical effects of amrinone on isolated guinea-pig papillary muscle. Fed Proc 40:711, 1981

167. Likoff MJ, Weber KT, Andrews V, et al: Amrinone in the treatment of chronic cardiac failure. J Am Coll Cardiol 3:1282–1290, 1984

168. Edelson J, LeJemtel TH, Alousi T, et al: Relationship between amrinone, plasma concentration and cardiac index. Clin Pharmacol Ther 29:723–728, 1981

169. Einzig S, Rao GHR, Pierpoint ME, White JG: Acute

effects of amrinone on regional myocardial and systemic blood flow distribution in the dog. Can J Physiol Pharmacol 60:811–818, 1982

170. Grupp I, Grupp G, Fowler NO, et al: Hemodynamic and inotropic responses of normal and depressed dog hearts to amrinone. Fed Proc 39:976, 1980

171. Hermiller JB, Leithe ME, Magorien RD, et al: Amrinone in congestive heart failure; Another look at an intriguing new cardioactive drug. J Pharmacol Exp Ther 228:319–326, 1984

172. Jentzer JH, LeJemtel TH, Sonnenblick EH, et al: Beneficial effect of amrinone on myocardial oxygen consumption during acute left ventricular failure in dogs. Am J Cardiol 48:75–83, 1981

173. Kinney EL, Carlin B, Ballard JO, et al: Clinical experience with amrinone in patients with advanced congestive heart failure. J Clin Pharmacol 22:433–440, 1982

174. Kinney EL, Draganis T, Luderer JR, et al: Mechanisms of action of amrinone: Role of thromboxane synthetase. Prostaglandins, Leukotrienes, Medicine 11:213–224, 1983

175. Klein NA, Siskind SJ, Frishman WH, et al: Hemodynamic comparison of intravenous amrinone and dobutamine in patients with chronic congestive heart failure. Am J Cardiol 48:170–175, 1981

176. Kullberg MP, Dorrbecker B, Lennon J, et al: High-performance liquid chromatographic analysis of amrinone and its N-acetyl derivative in plasma. Pharmacokinetics of amrinone in the dog. J Chromatog 187:264–270, 1980

177. Kullberg MP, Freeman GB, Biddlecombe C, et al: Amrinone metabolism. Clin Pharmacol Ther 29:394–401, 1981

178. Leier CV, Dalpaz K, Huss P, et al: Amrinone therapy for congestive heart failure in outpatients with idiopathic dilated cardiomyopathy. Am J Cardiol 52:304–308, 1983

179. LeJemtel TH, Keung E, Robner HS, et al: Sustained beneficial effect of oral amrinone on cardiac and renal function in patients with severe congestive heart failure. Am J Cardiol 45:123–129, 1980

180. LeJemtel TH, Keung EC, Schwartz WJ, et al: Hemodynamic effects of intravenous and oral amrinone in patients with severe heart failure: Relationship between intravenous and oral administration. Trans Assoc Am Physicians 92:325–333, 1979

181. Satoh K, Maruyama M, Taira N: The improvement of cardiac performance by amrinone, a new cardiotonic drug, in an experimental failing heart preparation of the dog. Jpn Heart J 23:975–980, 1982

182. Wilmshurst PT, Thompson DS, Jenkins BS, et al: Haemodynamic effects of intravenous amrinone in patients with impaired left ventricular function. Br Heart J 49:77–82, 1983

183. Siegel LA, Keung E, Siskind SJ, et al: Beneficial effects of amrinone-hydralazine combination on resting hemodynamics and exercise capacity in patients with severe congestive heart failure. Circulation 63:838–844, 1981

184. Zannand F, Juillere Y, Royer RJ: The effects of amrinone on cardiac function, oxygen consumption, and lactate production of an isolated, perfused, working guinea-pig heart. Arch Int Pharmacodyn 263:264–271, 1983

185. Alousi A, Farah AE, Lesher GY, Opalka CJ: Cardiotonic activity of amrinone-Win 40680 (5-amino-3, 4'-bipyridin-6-(1H)-one). Circ Res 45:666–677, 1979

186. Nusrat A, Tepper D, Hertzberg J, et al: Effects of amrinone on atrioventricular conduction in the intact canine heart. J Clin Pharmacol 23:257–265, 1983

187. Naccarelli GV, Gray EL, Dougherty AH, et al: Amrinone: Acute electrophysiologic and hemodynamic effects in patients with congestive heart failure. Am J Cardiol 54:600–604, 1984

188. Adams HR, Rhody J, Sutko JL: Amrinone activates K^+-depolarized atrial and ventricular myocardium of guinea pigs. Circ Res 51:662–665, 1982

189. Park GB, Kershner RP, Angellotti J, et al: Oral bioavailability and intravenous pharmacokinetics of amrinone in humans. J Pharm Sci 72:817–819, 1983

190. Bennotti JR, Grossman W, Braunwald E, et al: Effects of amrinone on myocardial energy metabolism and hemodynamics in patients with severe congestive heart failure due to coronary artery disease. Circulation 62:28–34, 1980

191. Benotti JR, Lesko LJ, McCue JE: Acute pharmacodynamics and pharmcokinetics of oral amrinone. J Clin Pharmacol 22:425–432, 1982

192. Wilmshurst PT, Al-Hasani SFA, Semple MJ, et al: The effects of amrinone on platelet count, survival and function in patients with congestive cardiac failure. Br J Clin Pharmacol 17:317–324, 1984

193. Ansell J, Tiarks C, McCue J, et al: Amrinone-induced thrombocytopenia. Arch Intern Med 144:949–952, 1984

194. Benotti JR, Lesko LJ, McCue J, et al: Pharmacokinetics and pharmacodynamics of milrinone in chronic congestive heart failure. Am J Cardiol 56:685–689, 1985

195. Le Jemtel TH, Maskin CS, Mancini D, et al: Systemic and regional hemodynamic effects of captopril and milrinone administered alone and comcomitantly in patients with heart failure. Circulation 72:364–369, 1985

196. Ivankovich AD: Anesthetic management problems posed by therapeutic advances. II. Digitalis and glucagon. Anesth Analg 51:607–616, 1972

197. Scallan MJH, Gothard JWW, Branthwaite MA: Inotropic agents. Br J Anaesth 51:649–658, 1979

198. Diamond G, Forrester J, Danzig R, et al: Hemodynamic effects of glucagon during acute myocardial infarction with left ventricular failure in man. Br Heart J 33:290–295, 1971

199. Kosinski EJ, Malindzak GS: Glucagon and isopro-

terenol in reversing propranolol toxicity. Arch Intern Med 132:840–843, 1973

200. Lucchesi BR, Stutz DR, Winfield RA: Glucagon: Its enhancement of atrioventricular nodal pacemaker activity and failure to increase ventricular automaticity in dogs. Circ Res 25:183–190, 1969

201. Prasad K: Electrophysiologic effects of glucagon on human cardiac muscle. Clin Pharmacol Ther 18:22–30, 1975

202. Wilcken DEL, Lvoff R: Glucagon in resistant heart failure and cardiogenic shock. Lancet 1:1315–1318, 1970

203. Mifune J, Kuramoto K, Ueda K, et al: Hemodynamic effects of salbutamol, an oral long-acting beta stimulant in patients with congestive heart failure. Am Heart J 104:1011–1015, 1982

204. Timmis AD, Stark SK, Chamberlin DA: Hemodynamic effects of salbutamol in patients with acute myocardial infarction and severe left ventricular dysfunction. Br Med J 2:11:1–1103, 1979

205. Sharma B, Goodwin JF: Beneficial effect of salbutamol on cardiac function in severe congestive cardiomyopathy: Effect of systolic and diastolic function of the left ventricle. Circulation 58:449–460, 1978

206. Kirlin PC, Pitt B, Lucchesi BR: Comparative effects of prenalterol and dobutamine in a canine model of acute ischemic heart failure. J Cardiovasc Pharmacol 3:896–905, 1981

207. Petch MC, Wisbey C, Ormerod O, et al: Acute hemodynamic effects of oral prenalterol in severe heart failure. Br Heart J 52:49–52, 1984

208. Erbel R, Meyer J, Lambertz H, et al: Hemodynamic effects of prenalterol in patients with ischemic heart disease and congestive cardiomyopathy. Circulation 66:361–369, 1982

209. Awan NA, Needham K, Evenson MK, et al: Therapeutic efficacy of oral pirbuterol in severe chronic congestive heart failure. Acute hemodynamic and long-term ambulatory evaluation. Am Heart J 102:555–563, 1981

210. Pamelia FX, Georghiade M, Beller GA, et al: Acute and long-term hemodynamic effects of oral pirbuterol in patients with chronic severe congestive heart failure: Randomized double-blind trial. Am Heart J 106:1369–1376, 1983

211. Colucci WS, Alexander RW, Mudge GH, et al: Acute and chronic effects of pirbuterol on left ventricular ejection fraction and clinical status in severe congestive heart failure. Am Heart J 102:564–568, 1981

212. Sharma B, Hoback J, Francis GS, et al: Pirbuterol: A new oral sympathomimetic amine for the treatment of congestive heart failure. Am Heart J 102:533–541, 1981

213. Rude RE, Turi Z, Brown EJ, et al: Acute effects of oral pirbuterol on myocardial oxygen metabolism and systemic hemodynamics in chronic congestive heart failure. Circulation 64:139–145, 1981

214. Colucci WS, Alexander RW, Williams GH, et al: Decreased lymphocyte beta-adrenergic-receptor density in patients with heart failure and tolerance to the beta-adrenergic agonist pirbuterol. N Engl J Med 305:185–190, 1981

215. Taylor CR, Baird JRC, Blackburg KJ et al: Comparative pharmacology and clinical efficacy of newer agents in treatment of heart failure. Am Heart J 102:515–532, 1981

216. Massie B, Chatterjee K, Werner J, et al: Hemodynamic advantage of combined administration of hydralazine orally and nitrates nonparenterally in the vasodilator therapy of chronic heart failure. Am J Cardiol 40:794–801, 1977

217. Chatterjee K, Drew D, Parmley WW, et al: Combination vasodilator therapy for severe chronic congestive heart failure. Ann Inter Med 85:467–470, 1976

218. Massie B, Ports T, Chatterjee K, et al: Longterm vasodilator therapy for congestive heart failure. Clinical response and its related hemodynamic measurements. Circulation 63:269–278, 1981

219. Kariya T, Wille LJ, Dage RC: Biochemical studies on the mechanism of cardiotonic activity of MDL 17043. J Cardiovasc Pharmacol 4:509–514, 1982

220. Uretsky BF, Generalovich T, Verbalis JG, et al: MDL 17043 therapy in severe congestive heart failure: Characterization of the early and late hemodynamic, pharmacokinetic, hormonal, and clinical response. J Am Coll Cardiol 5:1414–1421, 1985

221. Rubin SA, Tabak L: MDL 17043: Short- and long-term cardiopulmonary and clinical effects in patients with heart failure. J Am Coll Cardiol 5:1422–1427, 1985

222. Diederen W, Kadatz R: Effects of AR-L 115 BS, a new cardiotonic compound, on cardiac contractility, heart rate, and blood pressure in anesthetized and conscious animals. Arzneim Forsch 31:146–150, 1981

223. Herzig JW, Feile K, Ruegg JC: Activating effects of AR-L 115 BS on the Ca^{++} sensitive force, stiffness, and unloaded shortening velocity (V_{max}) in isolated contractile structures from mammalian cardiac muscle. Arzneim Forsch 31:188–191, 1981

224. Daly RA, Chatterjee K, Viquerat CE, et al: R013-6438, a new inotropic-vasodilator. Systemic and coronary hemodynamic effects in congestive heart failure. Am J Cardiol 55:1539–1544, 1985

225. Leon CA, Suarez JM, Aranoff RD, et al: Fenoldopam: Efficacy of a new orally active dopamine analog in heart failure. Circulation 70:(Suppl II) II-307, 1984

226. Young JB, Leon CA, Pratt CM, et al: Hemodynamic effects of an oral dopamine receptor agonist (Fenoldopam) in patients with congestive heart failure. J Am Coll Cardiol 6:792–796, 1985

Index

Page numbers in *italics* indicate illustrations.
Page numbers followed by t indicate tables.